Essentials of
Neuroimaging

Essentials of Neuroimaging

J. Robert Kirkwood, M.D.

Associate Clinical Professor
Department of Radiology
Tufts University School of Medicine
Tufts-New England Medical Center
Boston, Massachusetts
Vice Chairman and Chief
Division of Neuroradiology
Department of Radiology
Baystate Medical Center
Consultant in Radiology
Shriners Hospital
Springfield, Massachusetts

Churchill Livingstone
New York, Edinburgh, London, Melbourne, Tokyo

Library of Congress Cataloging-in-Publication Data

Kirkwood, J. Robert.
   Essentials of neuroimaging / J. Robert Kirkwood.
     p. cm.
   Includes bibliographical references.
   Includes index.
   ISBN 0-443-08479-3
   1. Brain—Imaging. 2. Skull—Imaging. 3. Spinal cord—Imaging.
I. Title.
   [DNLM: 1. Diagnostic Imaging. 2. Nervous System Diseases–diagnosis.   WL 141 K59e]
RC386.6.D52K57 1990
616.8 ′04754—dc20
DNLM/DLC
for Library of Congress   90-1983
                                                CIP

© Churchill Livingstone Inc. 1990

Distributed in the United Kingdom by Churchill Livingstone, Robert Stevenson House, 1–3 Baxter's Place, Leith Walk, Edinburgh EH1 3AF, and by associated companies, branches, and representatives throughout the world.

Accurate indications, adverse reactions, and dosage schedules for drugs are provided in this book, but it is possible that they may change. The reader is urged to review the package information data of the manufacturers of the medications mentioned.

The Publishers have made every effort to trace the copyright holders for borrowed material. If they have inadvertently overlooked any, they will be pleased to make the necessary arrangements at the first opportunity.

Acquisitions Editor: *Robert A. Hurley*
Copy Editor: *Ann Ruzycka*
Production Designer: *Jill Little*
Production Supervisor: *Sharon Tuder*
Production Services provided by Bermedica Production

Printed in the United States of America

First published in 1990   7 6 5 4 3 2

*With my love
for Gale
and our children
Rusty, Tim, Allison, and Chris*

Preface

In the process of teaching neuroimaging to radiology residents, I find it difficult to direct them to one manageable source that can serve as a basic text. To be sure, there are excellent texts on CT scanning, MRI, and angiography; but to study the entire topic from these sources requires considerable expense and effort. The information is frequently too exhaustive and the multiplicity of texts often results in considerable repetition.

This book is intended to provide a good understanding of neuroimaging from a single readable source. It is more than an introduction, as it provides in-depth discussions of the basic principles of neurodiagnosis and gives the information necessary to diagnose accurately almost all processes that involve the nervous system and the spine without being overly lengthy. The book is primarily designed for use by residents in radiology as both a learning and board review text. Fellows in neuroradiology, radiologists in general practice, neurologists, and neurosurgeons may also find the book helpful.

The book is heavily illustrated. The cases are carefully selected to demonstrate specific points necessary for diagnosis and clinical management of the patient. MRI, CT scanning, and angiography are given the most emphasis. Commonly, an entity is compared as it appears on multiple modalities, mostly using images from the same patient. The most common diseases are given a larger number of illustrations so that the full spectrum of the process can be seen. A plain-film example is used only when it is essential to the disease process. The images are labeled to make important points and the captions are relatively detailed. However, the diagnosis of each illustration is given in bold print at the beginning of the caption to make identification easy.

The text is weighted according to the importance of the disease process; thus, stroke, glioma, and trauma receive much more detailed discussion than more obscure entities. Many tables and boxes are used to set off important lists of differential diagnoses or components of a disease process. In the text specific diseases are indicated in bold type. These features will allow one to thumb through the pages for board review.

A single-author book has the advantage of consistency of style. However, it also presents certain potential hazards. To lessen these pitfalls, I have had the entire text reviewed for accuracy and completeness by other neuroradiologists and neurologists, and for clarity and length by general radiologists and radiology residents. I hope that the reader will find the result satisfactory.

J. Robert Kirkwood, M.D.

Acknowledgments

This book could not have been conceived and written without the help of a number of people. Dr. Robert A. Grugan, the former Chairman of the Department of Radiology of Baystate Medical Center, gave me continuous encouragement and facilitated the progression of the project. Radiology and Imaging, Inc., allowed me time away from a busy practice. Larry Flaccus and Neil Markowitz of Media Services of Baystate Medical Center carefully organized the process of image reproduction. Harry Maskell, Bob Sheehan, and Martha Leaver of the Educational Media Center at Tufts -New England Medical Center made the reproductions from hard copy films. Kathy Cosgrove and Louise Williams retrieved journal articles and transcribed the text and the editorial comments of multiple readers. The excellent and experienced staff of technologists of the Radiology Department were responsible for almost all of the images used in the book.

Many colleagues helped with the content of the book. Special thanks go to Drs. Said Zu'bi (Nuclear Medicine), Howard Raymond (Ultrasound), and Richard Hicks (Neuroradiology). Others who made significant contributions are Drs. Sam Mayerfield, of the Medical College of New Jersey; Frank White and Robert Chiulli, from Worcester, Massachusetts; Ronald Eisenberg, from Shreveport, Louisiana; and Drs. Edward Sweet, Lawrence Goodman, James Polga, Bruce Haskin, David Marinelli, Stanley Polansky, Jehangir Patel, Robert Austin, Fred Hampf, Alan Brown, Thomas Parker, Lawrence Metz, Bernard Pleet, and Joseph Sklar, all from Springfield, Massachusetts. I am also indebted to the Radiology Residents who carefully read the numerous drafts of the manuscript and honestly offered help with the clarity of style and level of content.

Contents

1
Techniques and Anatomy

CEREBRAL ANGIOGRAPHY

Cerebral angiography is serial radiography of the skull during opacification of the blood vessels with an aqueous contrast agent. Diagnosis of intracranial pathology is then made by (1) observation of abnormalities involving the blood vessels themselves (aneurysm, vascular malformation, occlusion, arteritis, tumor neovascularity) or (2) inferring the presence of pathology by the observation of vascular displacements (tumor, hematoma, edema, abscess, hydrocephalus). Because the technique cannot directly image the brain parenchyma and it is difficult, dangerous, and expensive, angiography has largely been displaced by computed tomography (CT) and magnetic resonance imaging (MRI). Nevertheless, cerebral angiography remains as the main technique for a number of CNS problems.

The contrast is most effectively delivered by a catheter selectively placed in the carotid and vertebral arteries via the femoral approach. Rarely, catheterization through the axillary artery or direct brachial or common carotid needle placement may be used if the femoral route is not available. Magnification filming is employed when possible, but it is not essential for most diagnostic work. Subtraction films can better demonstrate the vascular anatomy, particularly at the base of the skull. The smallest-diameter catheter possible is used as it decreases the incidence of thrombus formation on the surface of the catheter. Heparin and Teflon-coated wire guides are generally preferred. Once within the arterial system, the catheter is "double flushed" with a heparinized saline solution every 1 minute to keep it clear of blood. A continuous high pressure infusion may also be used. The non-ionic contrast agents do not prevent blood clotting, and so they cannot be used as a flush solution or catheter filling agent. The ionic contrast agents prevent clotting. Meglumine iothalamate or any one of the low-osmolar contrast agents are recommended for contrast. Air must never enter a cerebral catheter.

Significant complications may occur from angiography. The most common severe complication is a stroke

---

INDICATIONS FOR CEREBRAL ANGIOGRAPHY

Diagnosis of cerebrovascular disease
> Extracranial and intracranial atherosclerosis, stenosis, and occlusion
>
> Aneurysms: "berry," mycotic, dissecting
>
> Vasculitis
>
> Embolization
>
> Venous thrombosis
>
> Vascular malformations

Definition of tumor type: Glioma, metastasis, meningioma, hemangioblastoma

Definition of vascular supply of a tumor

Topographic localization of cerebral lesions

Detection of vascular tumors (hemangioblastoma)

Trauma to vessels, particularly extracranial

Determination of cerebral death

---

from embolization of clot or air into a cerebral vessel. This problem may occur despite seemingly impeccable technique (Fig. 1-1). Once an embolism has occurred, there is little that can be done to alter the condition except to apply steroid therapy and routine support of blood pressure and oxygenation. This complication occurs with about a 1 : 1,000 frequency when the procedure is performed by an experienced angiographer. Death may occur from stroke, cardiac arrest, severe contrast anaphylaxis, undetected femoral hemorrhage, or diffuse atheromatous embolization from a severely diseased aorta into visceral organs. The complications of angiography and preventive measures are given in Tables 1-1 and 1-2 (Fig. 1-2).

Aortic Arch

The most proximal branch of the aortic arch is the innominate artery (Fig. 1-3). It arises as a wide trunk from the superior margin of the anterior aortic arch

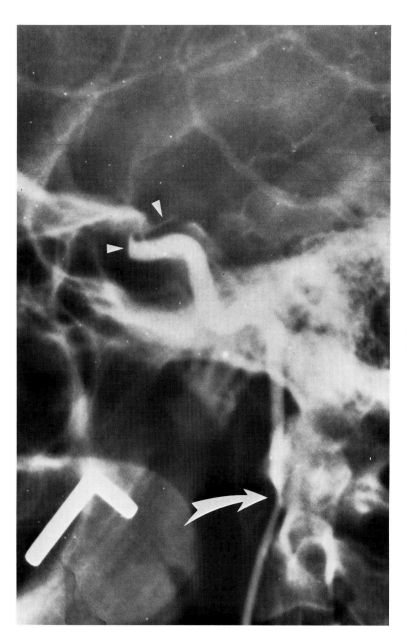

Fig. 1-1 Catheter-induced spasm in ICA. The distal ICA has contracted about the catheter tip (arrow) causing complete cessation of flow. A stagnant column of contrast is seen distal to the catheter. Gravity forms a fluid level at the termination of the contrast column and causes a small trickle of contrast to flow into the supraclinoid segment (arrowheads). This problem tends to occur in young women and children.

Table 1-1 Complications of Cerebral Angiography

Complication	Approximate Rate
Death	1 : 5,000+
Stroke	1 : 1,000
Transient cortical blindness	1 : 1,000
TIA	1 : 500
Contrast reaction	1 : 100
Femoral hematoma, pseudoaneurysm, fistula (Fig. 1-2)	1 : 50

and, after about 1.5 cm, divides into the right common carotid artery (CCA) and the right subclavian artery. Normally, the right CCA is the anterior branch. The left common carotid artery normally originates as a separate vessel from the superior margin of the aortic arch just distal to the innominate artery. The left common carotid artery frequently has a partial or complete common origin from the brachiocephalic artery. The left subclavian artery arises constantly just distal to the

Table 1-2 Prevention of Complications of Angiography

Preventive Measure	Rationale
Pretreatment with aspirin	Prevent platelet thrombus on wire guide and catheter
Heparin and Teflon-coated wire guides	Prevent thrombus on guide
Pretreatment with steroid	Stabilize endothelium; prevent transient cortical blindness and seizures
Systolic blood pressure < 180 mmHg	Decrease incidence of stroke and hematoma
Preangiography hydration and mannitol	Prevent contrast-induced renal failure in those with renal compromise, diabetes, or myeloma
Low-osmolar contrast	Prevent cardiac decompensation in those with heart disease; decrease chance for adverse reaction in those with prior contrast reaction
Monitor ECG	Detect and control cardiac arrhythmia
Keep procedure less than 2 hours in duration	Incidence of complications increases after 2 hours
Keep catheter low in ICA and vertebral arteries	Prevent catheter-induced spasm around catheter (Fig. 1-1)
Avoid injecting costocervical trunk	Prevent quadriplegia from contrast toxicity to cervical spinal cord

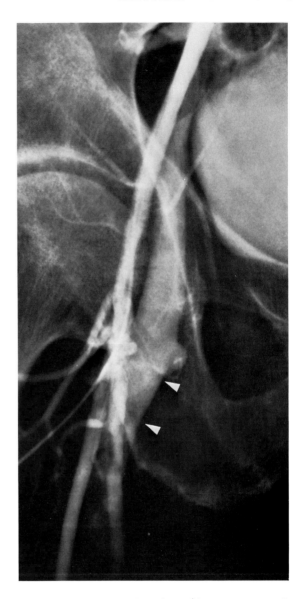

Fig. 1-2 Postangiographic femoral artery–vein fistula. An arteriovenous fistula may form at a puncture site. Here the femoral vein fills rapidly (arrowheads) during right femoral arteriography. Usually both artery and vein must be punctured for a fistula to form.

left common carotid artery. An aberrant right subclavian artery may rarely arise from the posterior aorta distal to the origin of the left subclavian artery.

The right and left vertebral arteries (VAs) originate from the corresponding subclavian arteries, posteromedially about 2 cm distal to the aortic arch. The exact site of origin is variable. Occasionally, the left vertebral

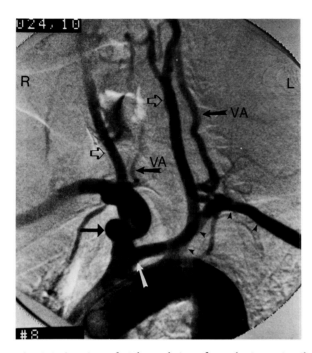

Fig. 1-3 Aortic arch. The study is performed using a pigtail catheter placed as far anterior in the aortic arch as possible. The left common carotid artery has an anomalous origin from the base of the innominate artery (white arrow). The right subclavian artery arises from the posterior wall of the innominate artery (black arrow). The vertebral arteries can be seen (VA, arrow) and the left vertebral artery is dominant. Both common carotid arteries (open arrows) and the left subclavian arteries are seen (arrowheads).

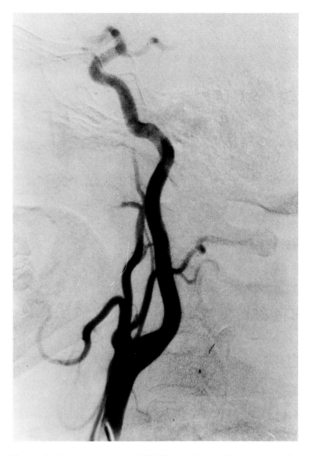

Fig. 1-4 Common carotid bifurcation. The CCA divides into the external carotid artery (smaller anterior branch) and the ICA (larger posterior branch). The origin of the ICA is usually dilated and is called the "bulb." Normally, the vessel margins are perfectly smooth. (From Heinz, 1984, with permission.)

artery arises directly from the aorta from a position between the left common carotid and left subclavian arteries. The left vertebral artery is usually dominant. It is preferable to catheterize the dominant vertebral artery for posterior fossa angiography.

Common Carotid Artery

The common carotid artery (CCA) is that portion of the vessel from the origin at the aorta to the common carotid bifurcation (Fig. 1-3). The bifurcation divides the vessel into the internal and external carotid arteries (Fig. 1-4). The internal carotid artery (ICA) is larger and is almost always posterior. The bifurcation is most commonly at the C4 vertebral level but may be low in the neck.

External Carotid Artery

The external carotid artery (ECA) is the smaller of the two branches arising from the carotid bifurcation. It normally courses anteromedially to the internal carotid artery. It gives rise to numerous important branches (Fig. 1-5).

1. Internal maxillary artery. The internal maxillary artery is the main trunk of the ECA and begins by coursing superiorly parallel to the ICA. It gives rise to the external occipital, superficial temporal, and middle meningeal arteries. It then goes deep into the pterygoid fossa to supply the maxillary sinuses. The distal branches of the internal maxillary artery anastomose

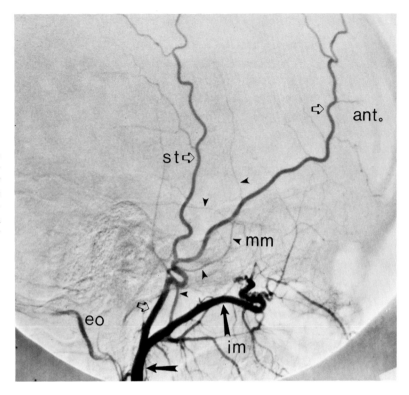

Fig. 1-5 External carotid artery. The major branch of the external carotid artery is the internal maxillary artery (im, black arrows). It gives rise to the external occipital artery (eo), superficial temporal artery (st, open arrows), and middle meningeal artery (mm, arrowheads).

with the distal branches of the ophthalmic artery, providing an important collateral arterial pathway to the intracranial ICA.

2. Middle meningeal artery. The middle meningeal artery arises from the internal maxillary artery and goes superiorly through the foramen spinosum to enter the skull. From there it courses between the dura and the inner table of the skull along the floor of the temporal fossa and the greater sphenoid wing to reach the region of the pterion. Here it normally divides into the anterior and posterior meningeal branches, supplying the dura of the frontal and parietal convexities. The branches are normally accompanied by one or two parallel extradural veins. Together these vessels produce the meningeal vascular channels seen on lateral skull radiography.

The middle meningeal artery is important for the diagnosis of intracranial pathology. This vessel and its branches enlarge with dural pathology, including meningioma and vascular malformation. Rarely, meningeal vessels contribute collateral circulation to the middle cerebral artery after stroke or to the blood supply of peripheral invasive intracerebral tumors (glio-

blastoma, gliosarcoma) that reach the cortical surface of the brain. Laceration and hemorrhage from a middle meningeal artery is the most common cause of a posttraumatic epidural hematoma.

3. External occipital artery. This artery is a posterior branch of the internal maxillary artery, which supplies the deep posterior muscles of the upper neck and the posterior scalp. It has important anastomoses with the deep muscular branches of the ipsilateral vertebral artery that may provide collateral pathways from the vertebral artery. The occipital artery may also supply a meningioma that has invaded the posterior calvarium.

4. Superficial temporal artery. This artery is the largest branch of the internal maxillary artery. It courses superiorly over the temporalis muscle to supply the anterior scalp. Its importance lies mainly in the diagnosis of temporal arteritis. It may also supply a meningioma that has invaded the calvarium.

5. Ascending pharyngeal artery. This small artery arises from the proximal internal maxillary artery and courses superiorly to the base of the skull. It sometimes hypertrophies to supply meningeal or acoustic tumors adjacent to the petrous pyramid.

Selective external carotid arteriography is performed to evaluate meningioma, vasculitis, glomus tumors, juvenile angiofibroma, and abnormalities of the calvarium or scalp. The catheter is rotated away from the internal carotid artery and advanced a small way into the proximal internal maxillary artery just distal to the lingual artery. Placing the catheter too far up the internal maxillary artery will likely result in localized spasm. The usual contrast injection is 2 ml of 60 percent contrast for a total of 6 to 8 ml, followed by filming for 12 seconds at a 1/sec rate. With the standard ionic contrast agents the selective external carotid injection is intensely painful, likened to a hot iron placed on the face. The use of low-osmolar contrast agents significantly reduces the pain of ECA angiography and improves film quality from reduced patient motion.

Internal Carotid Artery

The internal carotid artery courses posterolaterally from the bifurcation within the carotid sheath. It lies medial to the internal jugular vein. The vessel is divided anatomically into segments.

CERVICAL SEGMENT

The cervical segment extends from the bifurcation to the entrance into the carotid canal of the petrous bone. Cervical sympathetic nerves course along this segment. Normally, there are no angiographically visible branches along this portion. Insignificant loops may occur (Fig. 1-6).

Atherosclerosis occurs at the proximal portion at the bifurcation, whereas fibromuscular disease, dissection, and traumatic lesions occur in the middle cervical segment. The highly vascular carotid body tumor occurs in the crotch of the bifurcation. The primitive hypoglossal artery may rarely be seen coursing through the hypoglossal canal, connecting the cervical portion of the internal carotid artery with the basilar artery.

PETROUS SEGMENT

The petrous segment extends from the entrance to the carotid canal at the base of the petrous bone to the entrance to the cavernous sinus. The vessel first courses horizontally and anteromedially through the bony canal, lies just intracranially adjacent to the foramen lacerum, and then courses superiorly along the lateral

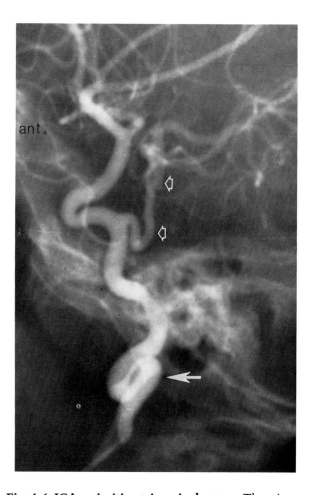

Fig. 1-6 ICA, primitive trigeminal artery. There is an insignificant loop in the cervical portion of the ICA (arrow). There is also a primitive trigeminal artery arising from the proximal cavernous portion to connect with the basilar artery (open arrows).

clivus to the entrance to the cavernous sinus. This segment gives rise to two small branches: (1) The caroticotympanic branch, which supplies the tympanic cavity, is not seen unless it is enlarged to supply a glomus tympanicum tumor. (2) The pterygoid branch (vidian artery) arises from the horizontal canalicular portion to anastomose with pterygoid branches of the internal maxillary artery. It is sometimes seen angiographically as a collateral vessel faintly filling the petrous portion of the ICA when the proximal portion is occluded (see Fig. 2-27B).

The petrous segment is rarely involved with disease. Spontaneous dissection occurs usually as an extension from dissection in the cervical portion. The upper clival portion is in close relation with the inferior border of the gasserian ganglion, and a neuroma in this region may anteriorly displace this segment (see Fig. 5-47). A primitive acoustic artery may rarely be seen connecting the petrous portion of the ICA with the basilar artery.

CAVERNOUS SEGMENT

The cavernous segment lies within the cavernous sinus, lateral to the sella and medial to cranial nerve (CN) III, CN IV, branches of CN V, and CN VI. The carotid artery turns sharply anterior as it enters the posterior cavernous sinus and then turns sharply superior to enter the dura just above and medial to the anterior clinoid process. This segment is also referred to as the *carotid siphon*. A primitive trigeminal artery may arise at the posterior siphon and connect with the basilar artery (Fig. 1-6).

The cavernous segment gives rise to two important vessel groups.

1. The meningohypophyseal vessels arise from the proximal curve of the cavernous portion of the ICA. There are usually three branches: (1) the tentorial branch, coursing posteriorly near the free edge of the tentorial hiatus; (2) the dorsal (clival) branch, coursing along the dura of the posterior clinoid process and the clivus; and (3) the inferior hypophyseal branch, which supplies the pituitary gland. There is anastomosis with the opposite side. These vessels, seen normally as small twigs, can hypertrophy to supply meningiomas or dural arteriovenous malformations of the tentorium, cerebellopontine angle, or clivus, providing important angiographic information (Fig. 1-7; see also Fig. 5-35).

2. The cavernous branches are numerous, small, short vessels arising from the cavernous portion of the ICA, supplying the dura of the cavernous sinus and

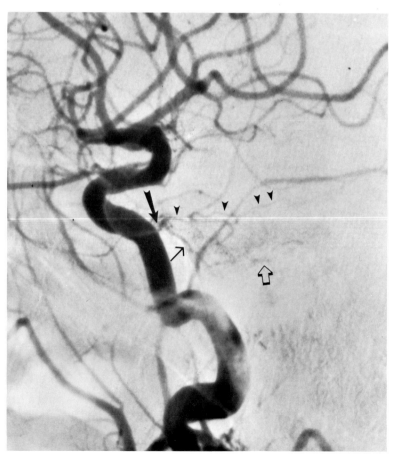

Fig. 1-7 Meningohypophyseal vessels, cerebellopontine angle meningioma. The meningohypophyseal vessels are hypertrophied to supply a meningioma, which is seen as a blush (open arrow). The trunk (thick black arrow) arises from the proximal cavernous portion of the ICA. A tentorial branch courses straight posteriorly (arrowheads). The dorsal branch courses inferiorly (thin arrow).

gasserian ganglion. As with any dural branches, they hypertrophy to supply meningiomas or neurinomas of the paracavernous region. They may also enlarge as part of external carotid collateral circulation to the ICA when the proximal ICA is occluded (see Fig. 2-27A) or as a dural arteriovenous malformation, emptying directly into the cavernous sinus.

SUPRACLINOID SEGMENT

The supraclinoid (intradural) segment extends from the anterior clinoid to the terminal bifurcation into the middle and anterior cerebral arteries. This segment gives rise to three important vessels (Fig. 1-8).

1. The ophthalmic artery arises first from the anteromedial aspect of the ICA, usually within the subdural space just as the ICA enters the intradural intracranial space. It courses anteriorly underneath the anterior clinoid process, through the optic canal, and into the orbit. From a lateral inferior position, it curves superiorly over the optic nerve to the anterosuperior and medial portion of the orbit. It exits the orbit anteriorly near the trochlea. It gives off anterior and posterior ethmoidal branches, which supply the ethmoid sinuses and the dura of the anterior falx (anterior falx artery), the cribriform plate, and the planum sphenoidale. These branches hypertrophy to supply meningiomas, which commonly occur in these regions. The recurrent

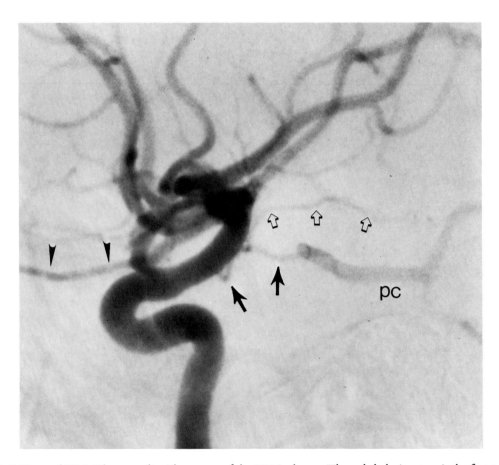

Fig. 1-8 Normal ICA. The supraclinoid segment of the ICA is shown. The ophthalmic artery is the first to arise from this segment, coursing anteriorly into the orbit. The second vessel to arise is the posterior communicating artery (arrows), coursing posteriorly to the ipsilateral posterior cerebral artery (pc). The third vessel to arise is the anterior choroidal artery (open arrows).

meningeal artery arising from the proximal ophthalmic artery may give rise to the entire middle meningeal artery. The ocular complex, including the central retinal artery, supplies the globe. It produces the "choroidal blush" outlining the posterior globe. Berry-type aneurysms occasionally arise from the ICA at the origin of the ophthalmic artery or just beyond. The artery may be involved with temporal arteritis.

2. The posterior communicating artery (PCA) is the next branch to arise from the supraclinoid ICA. It undulates backward to join the proximal portion of the posterior cerebral artery. This artery forms the lateral segment of the anastomotic circle of Willis. The PCA may be large, hypoplastic, or atretic. It is an important vessel for potential collateral blood flow to maintain ICA flow when there is proximal ICA stenosis or occlusion. When it is large, it continues without caliber change into the posterior cerebral artery, forming the "fetal type" origin of the posterior cerebral artery from the ICA. In this instance, the connection of the posterior cerebral artery to the basilar artery is lost. This anatomic variation occurs about 30 percent of the time. When present, this connection allows occipital infarction due to carotid vascular disease (Fig. 1-15B).

A "funnel-shaped" origin of the PCA is common. It is termed an *infundibulum* (see Fig. 2-21). It should not be considered an aneurysm unless the enlargement is more than 3 mm on nonmagnified films and if the margins are more rounded than triangular. ICA berry aneurysms are common at the origin of the PCA. The PCA is stretched downward by transtentorial herniation of brain tissue and severe hydrocephalus.

3. The anterior choroidal artery arises a few millimeters distal to the PCA (Figs. 1-8 and 1-9). It is a small vessel that undulates posteriorly adjacent to the optic tract within the suprasellar cistern. After giving off tiny branches to the optic tracts and geniculate bodies, it dives into the choroidal fissure of the medial temporal lobe. Here it forms a characteristic kink, seen on the lateral angiographic projection. It supplies the choroid plexus, primarily within the temporal horn, as well as portions of the glomus within the atrium. Its posterior curve outlines the inferior portion of the pulvinar of the thalamus.

The anterior choroidal artery enlarges to supply intraventricular tumors, particularly meningioma or choroid plexus papilloma, and it occasionally contributes to vascular malformations of the temporal lobe or thalamus. It becomes stretched and displaced downward

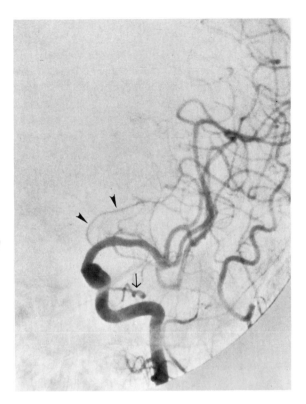

Fig. 1-9 Anterior choroidal artery, AP projection. The anterior choroidal artery is well seen with its characteristic course (arrowheads). Note the ophthalmic artery running anteriorly into the orbit (arrow). The anterior cerebral artery is atretic.

and medially with uncal herniation of the temporal lobe (see Fig. 1-12B).

Anterior Cerebral Artery Complex

The anterior cerebral artery complex is composed of the short anterior cerebral artery (A-1 segment), the very short anterior communicating artery, and the pericallosal artery and its branches. The anterior cerebral artery is the medial of the two terminal branches of the ICA. It arcs anteromedially from the distal ICA to the midline underneath the inferior portion of the genu of the corpus callosum just anterior to the thin lamina terminalis. At this point, the very short (2 mm) anterior communicating artery connects it with the opposite anterior cerebral artery. The anterior cerebral artery may be hypoplastic or atretic (Fig. 1-9). When it is, both pericallosal arteries fill from an angiographic injection of the contralateral ICA. Portions of the pericallosal group may arise from contralateral pericallosal arteries.

The anterior cerebral artery gives rise to small lenticulostriate branches and the larger recurrent artery of Heubner, which supply the medial and anterior portion of corpus striatum (caudate nucleus, globus pallidus, and putamen), the anterior inferior internal capsule, and the septum pellucidum.

The pericallosal artery is the principal continuation of the anterior cerebral artery (Fig. 1-10). It undulates within the interhemispheric fissure, curving close to the perimeter of the corpus callosum. Posteriorly, it

breaks up into a plexus of small vessels that extend slightly laterally above the corpus callosum in the pericallosal sulcus inferior to the cingulate gyrus. This plexus is seen on the frontal angiographic projection as laterally directed horizontal vessels resembling a mustache (Fig. 1-10). The "mustache" is tilted downward by masses that occur medially within the parietal lobe. This trait may be the only angiographic sign of such a mass.

Other branches of the pericallosal artery are the orbital-frontal branch, supplying the inferior medial frontal lobe, and the variable callosal marginal artery, which generally runs in the sulcus just peripheral to the

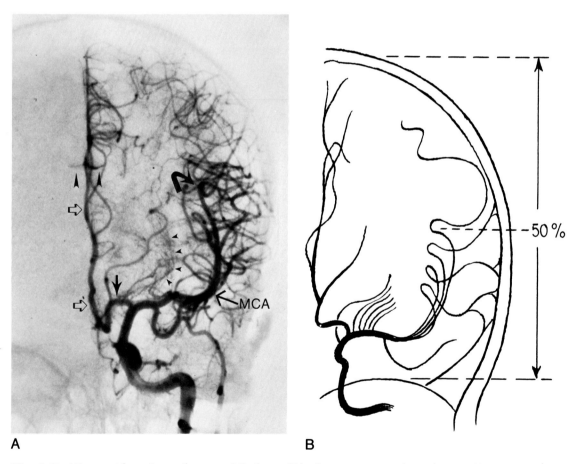

A   B

Fig. 1-10 AP carotid angiography, arterial phase. (A) The A-1 segment (arrow), pericallosal artery (open arrows), and callosal cistern blush called the "mustache" (arrowheads) are shown. The curved arrow points to the sylvian point, which is in the posterior portion of the sylvian fissure. The angiographic sylvian point is usually halfway between the vertex and the ipsilateral roof of the orbit. Note the lenticulostriate arteries (small arrowheads). **(B)** Diagram of AP projection. (Fig. B from Heinz, 1984, with permission.)

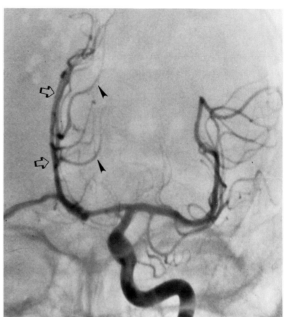

Fig. 1-11 "Round" shift, frontal lobe mass. (A) AP arterial angiography shows a rounded contralateral shift of the pericallosal group of vessels (arrows). Note the "frontal polar sign" as the more peripheral vessels return to the midline before the pericallosal artery because of the falx (arrowheads). **(B)** The pericallosal artery is stretched as it is displaced across the midline (arrows). The sylvian vessels are displaced posteriorly and inferiorly (arrowheads). There is wide separation and stretching of all the frontal vessels.

A

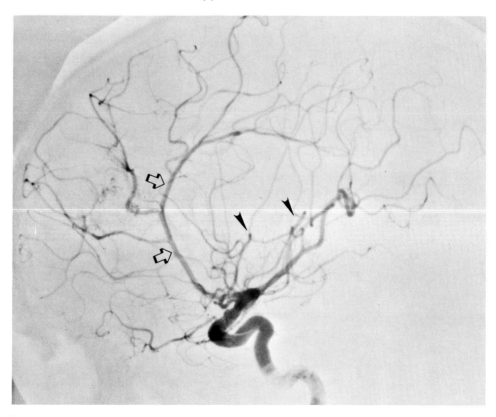

B

cingulate gyrus. These vessels continue over the medial convexity of the frontal and parietal lobes to supply the parasagittal convexity for 2 cm lateral to the midline.

The pericallosal arterial complex is the major arterial midline marker. It shifts to correspond with herniation of the brain across the midline through the large opening in the more anterior portion of the relatively rigid midline falx. This shift is termed *subfalcial herniation* and occurs secondary to unilateral mass lesions within the calvarium. The shape of the shifted pericallosal artery varies with the location of the unilateral mass. There are three basic patterns encountered.

1. "Round" shift (frontal masses) (Fig. 1-11). The round shift is recognized as a curve of the pericallosal artery across the midline with the greatest amount of shift in the anterior segment of the complex. It occurs secondary to a mass in the frontal region usually anterior to the coronal suture. The curve is reflecting the mass itself (tumor plus surrounding edema).

2. "Square" shift (temporal, large posterior parietal masses) (Fig. 1-12). The square shift results from a mass within the temporal fossa or a large mass in the posterior parietal or occipital region. The square appearance is caused by the forward portion of the brain herniating as a whole.

3. Posterior shift (all posterior locations) (Fig. 1-13). With the posterior (distal) shift, only the more posterior portion of the brain is displaced across the midline. The anterior portion may remain in the midline. The shift results from a mass in the parietal or occipital region.

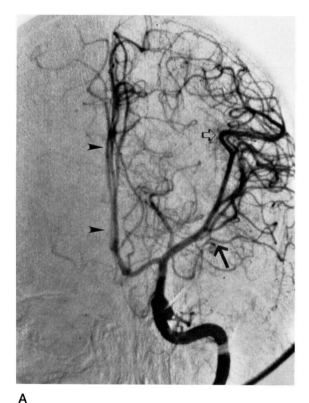

A

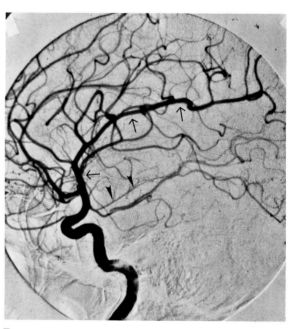

B

Fig. 1-12 "Square" shift, temporal lobe mass. (A) AP arteriography shows a slight "square" shift of the pericallosal group of vessels across the midline (arrowheads). Little shift compared with the size of the mass is typical for temporal lobe lesions. The middle cerebral artery is elevated, and the sylvian vessels are displaced medially (black arrow). The sylvian point is elevated (open arrow). **(B)** Lateral arteriography shows marked elevation of the middle cerebral artery and sylvian vessels (arrows). Note the stretching and downward displacement of the anterior choroidal artery, indicating uncal herniation.

Fig. 1-13 Posterior shift, posterior parietal mass. (A)
AP angiography shows the posterior portion of the pericallosal artery shifted more than the anterior portion (arrowheads). Note the downward displacement of the sylvian point (arrow). **(B)** A large mass is present posteriorly, causing anterior and downward displacement of the sylvian vessels (arrow) and stretching of the posterior parietal convexity vessels (arrowheads).

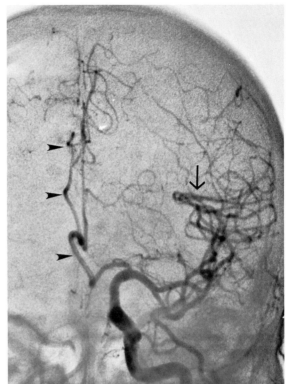

A

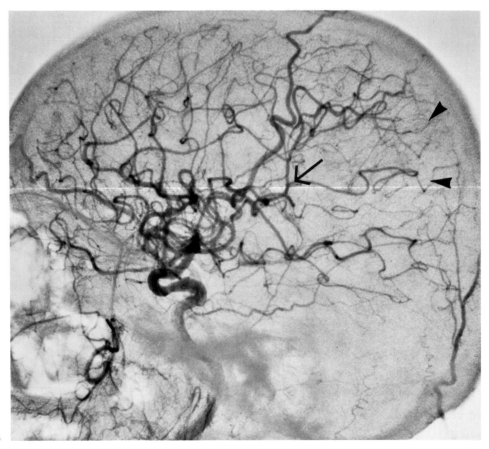

B

The anterior cerebral artery complex may be affected by hydrocephalus, arterial occlusive disease, and masses in the suprasellar, subfrontal, or deep midline regions.

Circle of Willis

The circle of Willis is the anastomotic pentagon of vessels at the base of the brain lying within the suprasellar cistern. It is composed of the anterior communicating artery, both anterior cerebral arteries, both posterior communicating arteries, and the proximal segment of both posterior cerebral arteries. The anastomotic arch is complete and equal about 20 percent of the time. Commonly, one or more of the anastomotic segments is absent or hypoplastic (Fig. 1-14).

Middle Cerebral Artery

The middle cerebral artery (MCA) is the more lateral of the two terminal branches of the internal carotid artery (Figs. 1-10 and 1-15). It curves laterally immediately underneath the anterior perforated substance of the

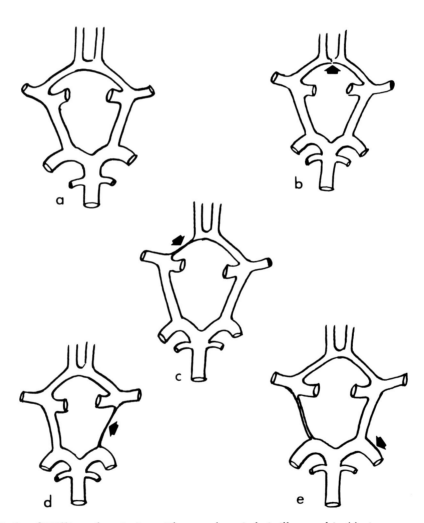

Fig. 1-14 Circle of Willis and variations. The complete circle is illustrated in (a). A common variation not illustrated is atresia of the proximal segment of the posterior cerebral artery so that the posterior communicating artery becomes the sole supply of its distal segment. This variation is the "fetal type" of communication (see Fig. 1-15B). (From Heinz, 1984, with permission.)

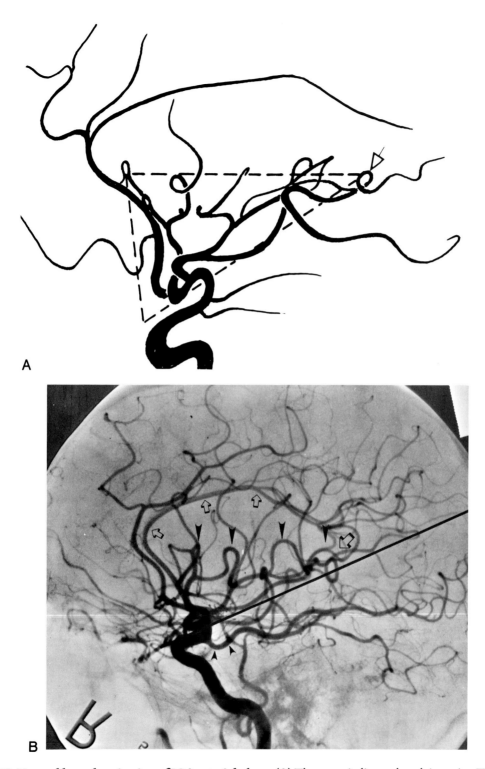

Fig. 1-15 Normal lateral projection of ICA arterial phase. (A) The arrow indicates the sylvian point. The two vessels arising from the supraclinoid ICA are the proximal posterior communicating artery and the more distal anterior choroidal artery. **(B)** Lateral angiography outlines the normal sylvian vessels. The posteroinferior border of the sylvian triangle is defined by the clinoparietal line paralleling the posterior branch of the MCA within the sylvian fissure. The superior border of the triangle is outlined by the opercular branches (large arrowheads). The sylvian point is indicated (large open arrow). Note the normal sweep of the pericallosal artery (small open arrows). There is a "fetal type" posterior cerebral artery (small arrowheads). Note the normal undulating course of all the cortical arteries. Mass lesions cause straightening as well as displacement of cortical vessels. (Fig. A from Heinz, 1984, with permission.)

brain (inferior surface of the basal ganglia) and above the temporal lobe. Numerous perforating small end-arteries arise from the horizontal segment of the MCA and are called the lenticulostriate arteries. These supply the basal ganglia. Laterally, it curves around the insula to enter the sylvian fissure. It normally bifurcates into anterior and posterior branches. These branches then undulate posterosuperiorly within the sylvian fissure lying on the surface of the insula. They give off additional branches which turn sharply laterally to exit the sylvian fissure between the parietal and temporal opercula (overhanging covering) to distribute over the cortical surface of the hemisphere. The anterior branch gives origin to the orbital frontal, precentral, central, and anterior parietal arteries, which supply the lateral frontal and anterior parietal hemisphere. They anastomose with distal branches of the anterior cerebral complex over the medial hemispheric convexity. The posterior branch gives origin to the posterior parietal, parieto-occipital, and posterior temporal branches, which supply the lateral posterior parietal, occipital, and temporal lobes. They anastomose with distal branches of the posterior cerebral artery over the posterior occipital convexity and the lateral and inferior surface of the temporal lobe.

The *sylvian point* refers to the point at which the most posterosuperior of the arteries on the insula makes its initial turn laterally to exit the sylvian fissure. On the frontal view it is most easily recognized as the most posterior and medial loop of the middle cerebral group within the sylvian fissure (Fig. 1-10). It normally lies at a point halfway between horizontal lines drawn from the external table at the vertex and the orbital roof and is about one-third of the distance from the inner table to the midline. The sylvian point is elevated by masses within or underneath the temporal lobe (Fig. 1-12). It is depressed by masses within or adjacent to the parietal lobe (Fig. 1-13A). It is pushed forward by masses in the posterior parietal or occipital lobes (Fig. 1-13B).

The *sylvian triangle* is an upside-down triangle defined angiographically on the lateral projection (Fig. 1-15). The superior border of the triangle is formed by a line drawn connecting the points at which each of the middle cerebral arteries makes its turn deep within the sylvian fissure to course laterally around the parietal operculum. This line roughly parallels the planum sphenoidale and bifurcates the sweep of the pericallosal artery. The apex of the triangle is at the anterior clinoid process. The posterior side of the triangle is defined by the *clinoparietal line* (a line drawn from a point 2 cm

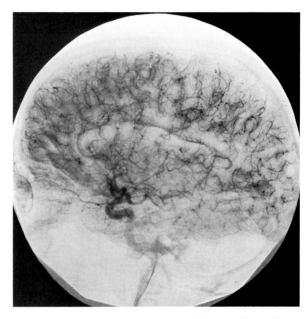

Fig. 1-16 Normal ICA arteriography, capillary phase. The capillary, or "brain stain," phase is intermediate between the arterial and venous phases. It shows a cortical blush for all normally perfused regions of the brain. The perfusion pattern should be homogeneous. Because mass lesions decrease regional blood flow, they can be identified by voids in the brain stain phase. (From Heinz, 1984, with permission.)

anterior to the lambda to the anterior clinoid process on nonmagnified angiography). The sylvian triangle is deformed by masses in the frontal (Fig. 1-11), parietal (Fig. 1-13), occipital, and temporal lobes (Fig. 1-12). The horizontal segment of the MCA is also elevated by masses within the temporal lobe (Fig. 1-12A).

The capillary or intermediate phase of the angiogram represents the flooding of the capillaries with contrast, which occurs at 3 to 6 seconds on normal angiography, best seen with the subtraction technique. It produces a *brain stain,* which is useful for defining small mass effects or ischemic regions. The normal "brain stain" is uniform in density throughout the hemisphere (Fig. 1-16). Masses, edema or infarctions are seen as regions of void within the "stain."

Cerebral Veins

The cerebral veins are important for angiographic diagnosis. They are altered by cerebral masses, vascular malformations, extracerebral fluid accumulations, and thrombosis. They can be anatomically classified into superficial and deep veins.

SUPERFICIAL CEREBRAL VEINS

The superficial veins course over the surface of the gyri of the cerebral hemisphere (Fig. 1-17) and drain to the dural sinuses. The veins fill with contrast sequentially in an order determined by their distance from the terminal carotid artery. Thus the frontal and temporal veins fill first followed by the parietal veins and finally the occipital veins. Frequently, there is a large vein of Trolard, which drains the parietal lobe superiorly to the sagittal sinus; a vein of Labbe, which drains the posterior temporal lobe into the lateral sinus; and a sylvian vein, which drains the insula and opercular regions into the cavernous sinus. The sylvian veins fill relatively early. Numerous unnamed smaller cortical veins drain the lateral and interhemispheric cortical surfaces to the nearest dural sinus.

The presence of an early-filling vein is a basic angiographic sign and is always an abnormal finding. For a vein to be classified as early-filling, it must fill at least 1 second earlier than the veins in its immediate vicinity. It is most commonly seen with a malignant primary or metastatic brain tumor (see Fig. 5-25B) or arteriovenous malformation (see Fig. 4-4). It may also be seen whenever there is an increase in the regional blood flow that occurs with the "luxury perfusion" surrounding an infarction (see Fig. 2-19B), an abscess, or recent seizure. In some cases, it may be the only angiographic abnormality demonstrated. When seen alone it is nonspecific, and the nature of the abnormality then cannot be diagnosed.

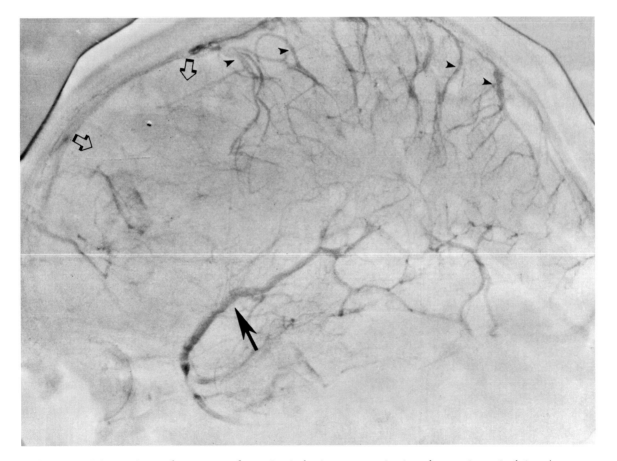

Fig. 1-17 ICA arteriography, venous phase. Cortical veins are emptying into the superior sagittal sinus (arrowheads). A large sylvian vein is seen (black arrow). There is decreased venous filling in the frontal lobe because of a tumor mass (open arrows).

The cortical veins are the best markers of the brain surface on angiography. Whereas the cortical arteries course within the depths of the cerebral sulci and so may be at some distance from the inner table of the skull, the veins run on the cortical surface and are normally close to the inner table of the calvarium. They are displaced inwardly from the inner table by extracerebral fluid collections (subdural and epidural hematoma), meningioma, or epidural extension of a calvarial metastasis.

Although a relatively infrequent occurrence, sagittal sinus thrombosis may cause cerebral infarction. The dural sinuses, especially the sagittal and lateral sinuses, must be specifically observed to determine normal contrast filling. Normally, there is greater filling of the posterior portion of the sagittal sinus. However, there are always some contrast "defects" in the opacified sinus because of the entry of unopacified blood from the contralateral side or the posterior fossa. There is also considerable asymmetry of the lateral sinuses, and one side is usually dominant. Reversal of flow in the cortical veins and collateral deep venous drainage must be seen to reliably diagnose sinus thrombosis (see Chapter 2).

DEEP CEREBRAL VEINS

The deep venous system refers to the paired midline internal cerebral veins, the subependymal veins of the lateral ventricles, and the deep medullary veins of the cerebral white matter. They have importance in the diagnosis of midline brain shifts, hydrocephalus, and white matter cerebral pathology.

The paired internal cerebral veins course within the cavum velum interpositum immediately above the roof of the third ventricle. They comprise the most important angiographic midline marker and are generally more sensitive to the detection of midline shifts than the pericallosal arteries. The posterior portion of the internal cerebral veins are held close to the midline by their entry into the vein of Galen, but the anterior portion is free to pivot with midline herniations of the brain. Therefore, with hemispheric shifting, the anterior portion pivots away from the side of the mass lesion. This situation can be recognized on the frontal projection of the angiogram (Fig. 1-18). The internal cerebral vein is normally seen as a thick, short band of contrast superimposed on the vein of Galen and the straight sinus. With shift, the internal cerebral vein can be seen as a humped, foreshortened channel displaced across the midline away from the mass.

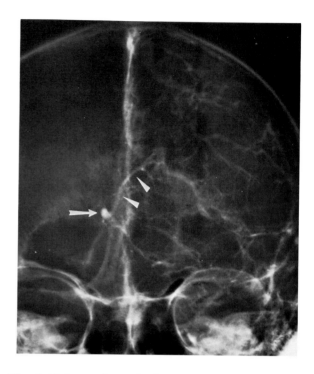

Fig. 1-18 Internal cerebral vein, contralateral shift. The anterior portion of the internal cerebral vein is shifted across the midline (arrow). There also is contralateral displacement of the thalamostriate vein (arrowheads).

The subependymal veins are numerous, relatively constant veins that run just underneath the ependyma of the lateral ventricles. The most important, the thalamostriate vein (Fig. 1-19A), drains from the lateral superior angle of the body of the lateral ventricle and courses anteromedially and inferiorly in the groove between the tail of the caudate nucleus and the thalamus to meet the internal cerebral vein at the foramen of Monro. Usually the anterior septal midline vein also enters at this point, which is called the *deep venous angle* (Fig. 1-19B). Frequently, the thalamostriate vein is not present, and its draining function is replaced by a direct lateral ventricular vein. This vein also drains from the lateral superior angle but then courses directly medially along the lateral wall and then the floor of the body of the lateral ventricle to enter the internal cerebral vein at some point posterior to the foramen of Monro. Its point of entry is called the *false venous angle* (Fig. 1-19C). It is important to recognize this variant so that displacement of the venous angle is not mistakenly diagnosed.

Because they course along the walls of the lateral ventricles, the subependymal veins are excellent

Fig. 1-19 Normal deep veins. (A) AP view obliqued slightly to the right shows the midline septal vein (black arrowheads), internal cerebral vein (open arrow), and vein of Galen (thin black arrow). The tiny deep medullary veins (white arrowheads) are seen draining into the thalamostriate vein (white arrows), which outlines the lateral margin of the posterior frontal horn. **(B)** Lateral projection. The deep medullary veins (white arrowheads) drain into the thalamostriate vein (white arrow), which courses anteroinferiorly to meet the internal cerebral vein (black open arrow) at the venous angle (white open arrow). The septal vein courses along the septum pellucidum (arrowheads). In this patient the septal vein enters the internal cerebral vein posterior to the venous angle. The vein of Galen (thin black arrows) is a short, large vein in the midline draining into the straight sinus (black arrow). **(C)** False venous angle. Here the thalamostriate vein is atretic, and there is a direct lateral vein (white arrow) emptying into the internal cerebral vein at the false venous angle (white open arrow). Note the anterior caudate vein (thin black arrow) and the septal vein (arrowheads).

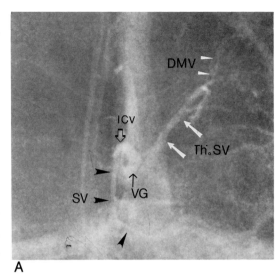

A

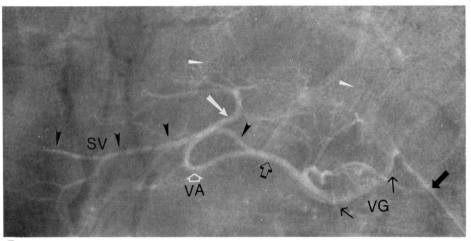

B

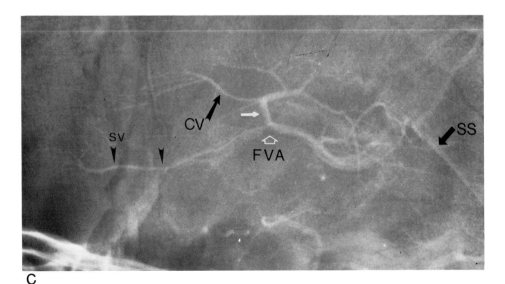

C

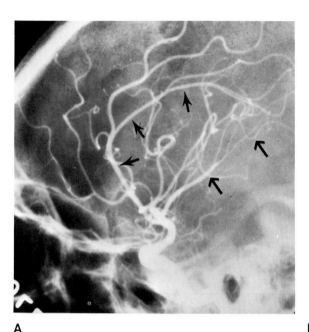
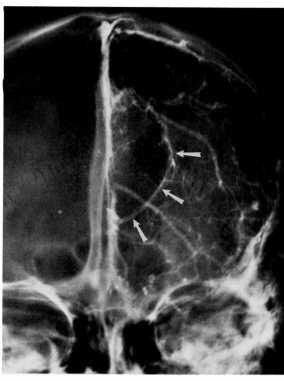

A
B

Fig. 1-20 Hydrocephalus. (A) Lateral arterial phase carotid angiography shows stretching of the pericallosal vessels (sharp arrows) and elevation of the sylvian vessels from temporal horn enlargement (blunt arrows). **(B)** AP venous phase shows lateral displacement and stretching of the thalamostriate vein (arrows), representing frontal horn enlargement.

markers of ventricular size. The deep veins form what is referred to as the *cast of the ventricular cavities.* As seen on the frontal projection, the thalamostriate vein outlines the lateral margin of the frontal horn. With ventricular enlargement, the thalamostriate vein is stretched and bowed laterally (Fig. 1-20). The width across the top of a lateral ventricle is normally less than 20 mm when measured on the nonmagnified frontal view. The outline of the ventricle can also be seen on the lateral projection.

The deep medullary veins of the white matter course along the parallel fibers of the corona radiata and drain deep into the subependymal veins at the lateral superior angle of the ventricular system. On high quality films they may be seen normally as a series of short, faint, brush-like veins perpendicular to the ventricle fading off into the paraventricular white matter (Fig. 1-19). They enlarge and become much more visible in the presence of any process that results in an increase in the

blood flow through the white matter. Prominent deep medullary veins most commonly indicate a glioblastoma. They may be less commonly seen with deep arteriovenous malformations, cortical venous or venous sinus thrombosis (collateral flow), venous occlusive abnormalities, lymphoma, progressive multifocal leukoencephalopathy, deep infection, and fulminant multiple sclerosis.

Cerebral angiography is now used primarily to define the etiology of an abnormality that has been defined clinically or by another imaging modality. A checklist for reviewing an angiogram follows (see box).

VERTEBRAL ANGIOGRAPHY

Vertebral angiography defines the vessels that supply all of the posterior fossa, the posterior thalamic nuclei, the choroid plexus of the atria of the lateral ventricles,

CHECKLIST FOR REVIEWING A
CAROTID ANGIOGRAM

1. Venous and arterial midline markers for shift
2. Sylvian point and triangle for position
3. Position of horizontal portion of the middle cerebral artery
4. Position of venous angle
5. Capillary "brain stain" phase for subtle masses
6. Relation of the cortical veins to the inner table
7. Late arteries and collateral flow
8. Early veins
9. Aneurysm, characteristic locations
10. Extracranial carotid and vertebral arteries
11. DMV, size
12. Vascular lumen (atherosclerosis, vasculitis)
13. Neovascularity

and the occipital and posterior inferior temporal lobes unless the posterior cerebral artery arises directly from the carotid artery.

ANGIOGRAPHIC CHARACTERIZATION
OF A MASS LESION

1. Locate the mass using angiographic principles.
2. Define the etiology of the mass by identifying the following:
   a. Neovascularity (characterize)
   b. Deep medullary veins present?
   c. Tumor stain (meningioma, metastasis)
   d. Occluded vessel or thrombus within the vessel
   e. Intracerebral or extracerebral location
   f. Dural vascular supply

Vertebral Artery

Throughout its course along the cervical spine, the vertebral artery passes through the transverse foramina of the upper six vertebral segments. It gives off numerous segmental muscular branches. These branches anastomose with the cervical muscular branches of the ipsilateral external carotid artery and so provide a potential for collateral circulation. If the proximal vertebral artery is occluded, blood flows from the external carotid system through the muscular branches to fill the distal vertebral artery (see Fig. 2-31). If the common carotid artery is occluded, blood flows from the vertebral into the external carotid artery and then to the internal carotid artery via the bifurcation (see Fig. 2-29B).

After making its characteristic zigzag to pass through the transverse process of the atlas, it curves posteriorly to the atlanto-occipital joint to pierce the dura and pass superiorly through the foramen magnum. The vertebral artery often becomes smaller as it enters the intradural space. The vertebral arteries give off anterior and posterior meningeal branches, which supply the dura of the foramen magnum, the falx cerebelli, and the occipital dura.

Basilar Artery

The large basilar artery is formed from the junction of the two vertebral arteries. It continues superiorly more or less in the midline posterior to the clivus and close to the anterior surface of the pons. It tends to curve away from the side of the dominant vertebral artery; but it may meander, especially if it becomes ectatic from atherosclerosis. At a point slightly above the dorsum sellae it divides into the bilateral posterior cerebral arteries. Along its course the basilar artery gives off numerous small pontine perforating arteries, analogous to the perforating arteries from the MCA to the basal ganglia.

The basilar artery may be significantly diseased with atherosclerosis, resulting in the numerous symptoms of vertebrobasilar insufficiency. Severe atherosclerosis may result in a giant aneurysm of the entire basilar artery (see Fig. 3-17). Berry aneurysms occur at the distal tip of the basilar artery (see Fig. 3-11) and at the origins of the posterior inferior cerebellar arteries (PICA) and the anterior (AICA) inferior cerebellar arteries. The basilar artery is displaced forward against the clivus by masses in the pons or cerebellum (see Fig.

1-23) and backward by extra-axial masses near the clivus (see Fig. 5-58).

Posteroinferior Cerebellar Arteries

The important bilateral posteroinferior cerebellar arteries (PICAs) arise from each distal vertebral artery as it lies anterolateral to the upper medulla (Fig. 1-21). The level of origin and the course of the PICA is variable, but certain generalities obtain. The PICA begins by making a short superior curve to reach the lateral surface of the medulla and then courses downward along the lateral surface of the medulla ending in an upward curve. These portions are called the anterior and the lateral medullary segments. The inferior curve is usually referred to as the *caudal loop*. At the caudal loop the artery normally divides into medial and lateral branches.

The medial branch continues superiorly and me-dially to run along the anterior surface of the cerebellar tonsil and then on the inferior surface of the posterior medullary velum (inferior roof) of the fourth ventricle to reach the apex of the triangle of the roof of the fourth ventricle (the *fastigium*). It then loops backward and downward over the posterior surface of the tonsil and continues posteriorly near the midline along the undersurface of the vermis. The relatively broad superior curve of the medial branch is called the *choroidal loop*. Usually at its apex it gives off small variable branches to the choroid plexus of the fourth ventricle. This area is called the *choroidal point* and is an important marker of the position and size of the fourth ventricle.

The choroidal point is generally considered to lie at the apex of the curve of the choroidal loop. There are numerous systems to measure its position. The one that is preferred because it is proportional and not subject to the vagaries of different magnification, is the *F–T line* (Fig. 1-22). This line is drawn from the anterior margin of the foramen magnum to the torcula. The choroidal

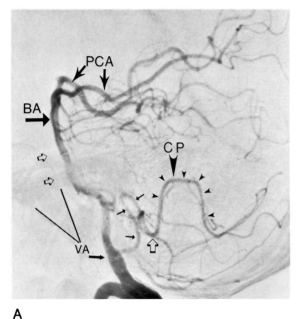

A

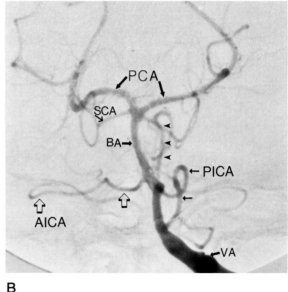

B

Fig. 1-21 Normal vertebral arteriography, arterial phase. (A) Lateral arterial projection shows the basilar artery (BA) separated from the posterior margin of the clivus (small open arrows). The lateral medullary segment of the PICA (small arrows) arises from the distal vertebral artery (VA). The caudal loop of the posterior medullary segment is indicated (large open arrow). The choroidal loop is well formed in this patient (arrowheads), and the choroidal point is indicated (CP). **(B)** Towne projection, showing the lateral medullary segment (small arrows) and the choroidal loop (arrowheads) of the PICA. The choroidal loop is in its normal position just lateral to the midline. The AICA is well seen on the opposite side (open arrows).

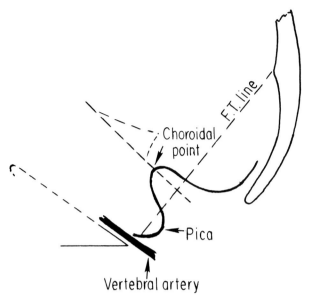

Fig. 1-22 Lateral vertebral arteriogram and choroidal point. The lateral vertebral angiogram illustrates the (PICA) and the relation of the choroidal point to the fourth ventricle. The choroidal point should fall at the juncture of the anterior and middle thirds of a line (F.T. line) drawn between the anterior lip of the foramen magnum (F) and the torcular herophili (T). (From Heinz, 1984, with permission.)

point should lie close to the junction of the anterior and middle thirds of the line. There are numerous variations to the appearance of the choroidal loop, and at times the position of the choroidal point is an estimate.

The PICA is the arterial marker for the position and size of the fourth ventricle. Masses within the posterior compartment of the posterior fossa (cerebellar hemispheres and vermis) displace the fourth ventricle and thus the choroidal loop anteriorly and inferiorly (Fig. 1-23; see also Fig. 6-5). Masses in the anterior compartment (pons, clivus) displace the choroidal loop posteriorly. Masses within the fourth ventricle separate and broaden the two PICA loops (see Fig. 1-28, 6-2, and 6-7).

The PICA is the most important midline marker within the posterior fossa. On the AP projection, the choroidal loop and the inferior vermian branch are displaced contralaterally by cerebellar hemispheric masses (Fig. 1-24).

Anteroinferior Cerebellar Arteries

The paired anteroinferior cerebellar arteries (AICAs) arise from the lower portion of the basilar artery. They course laterally around the pons to meet the exiting CN

Fig. 1-23 Posterior compartment hemispheric mass. The lateral vertebral study shows anterior and inferior displacement of the choroidal loop of the PICA (arrow). The overall mass causes stretching of hemispheric branches throughout and anterior displacement of the basilar artery against the clivus (open arrows). Scattered vasospasm is also seen (arrowheads), the etiology of which was never determined.

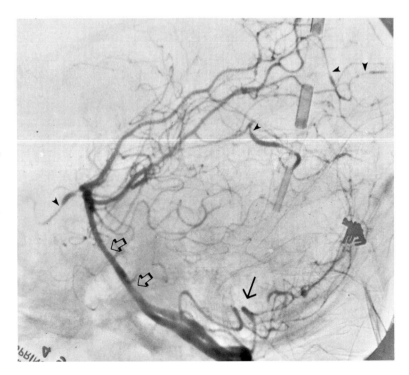

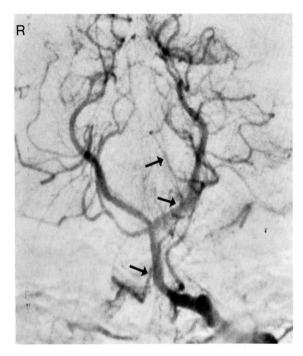

Fig. 1-24 Right hemispheric cerebellar mass. A large right hemispheric mass is causing contralateral displacement of both PICAs (arrows).

VII and CN VIII. The artery follows the nerves into the internal auditory canal, makes a loop, and continues laterally over the anterior cerebellar hemisphere (Fig. 1-21B; see also Fig. 1-27B). The size of the AICA is usually reciprocal with the size of the ipsilateral PICA. At times the PICA may be absent on one side, and the AICA supplies the distribution of both the AICA and PICA (Fig. 1-25).

The AICA lies within the cerebellopontine angle cistern and is displaced by large tumors in this region, e.g., acoustic neurinoma (see Fig. 5-58) and meningioma. Berry aneurysms may rarely occur at its origin.

Superior Cerebellar Arteries

The paired superior cerebellar arteries arise from the distal basilar artery. They pass around the upper pons or mesencephalon within the ambient cisterns just below the tentorium and then divide into medial and lateral branches. The medial branches reach the midline in the quadrigeminal plate cistern and then continue over the superior surface of the vermis. These arteries outline the superior margin of the vermis and cerebellar hemi-

spheres (Fig. 1-26). They are most useful in the diagnosis of herniation, either upward of the vermis due to a cerebellar mass or downward due to transtentorial herniation of the cerebrum. The lateral branches spreading out over the top of the cerebellar hemispheres are stretched by intracerebellar masses.

Posterior Cerebral Arteries

The large paired posterior cerebral arteries (PCAs) arise from the terminal bifurcation of the basilar artery (Fig. 1-21). Each circles the mesencephalon just above the level of CN III and the tentorium. Early in its course it is joined by the posterior communicating artery. About 30 percent of the time, the posterior communicating artery is the dominant supplier of the PCA. Sometimes the PCA maintains its origin from the internal carotid artery and the proximal PCA is atretic. This is referred to as a "fetal" type PCA (Fig. 1-15B). On vertebral studies unopacified blood may enter the PCA from the posterior communicating artery. The "washout" effect causes an apparent "filling defect" and should not be misinterpreted as an intraluminal clot.

The PCA continues to supply the medial portion and posterior tip of the occipital lobe. The two major branches to the occipital lobe are the more superior parieto-occipital branch and the inferior calcarine branch (Fig. 1-25). The PCA also gives off many branches to the medial and inferior surfaces of the temporal lobe, supplying the region of the hippocampus.

Displacement of these vessels is difficult to recognize, but they may be seen to be stretched in response to a mass in the occipital or posterior temporal lobe. Occlusive disease is common in this group, and one should look carefully for the absence of major branches.

Other important branches arise from the proximal PCA. The medial posterior choroidal artery arises from the proximal PCA, courses around the brain stem, and passes along the colliculi to reach the pineal. It then continues anteriorly over the roof of the third ventricle along with the internal cerebral veins (Fig. 1-27). This vessel is elevated by thalamic or pineal masses. The lateral posterior choroidal arteries arise from the proximal PCA and curve superiorly behind the pulvinar of the thalamus, supplying the choroid plexus of the atrium of the lateral ventricle and the posterior superior thalamus. These vessels are displaced and stretched posteriorly by thalamic masses and contribute to intraventricular tumor or vascular malformations in the region.

Fig. 1-25 Normal vertebral angiography, AICA. (A) Towne arterial phase shows the AICA on the right continuing inferiorly to supply the region of the PICA (arrowheads). The left superior cerebellar artery (SCA) is well seen because the proximal segment of the left PCA is atretic and does not fill from the vertebral injection. Hemispheric branches of the left PICA are seen (small arrows). **(B)** Lateral projection shows the inferior continuation of the AICA to supply the region of the PICA on its side (arrowheads). The choroidal point of the PICA is well seen (open arrow), although the choroidal loop is poorly formed. Hemispheric branches (small arrows) and the inferior vermian branches (large arrows) are well seen. PO = parietal occipital branch of the PCA; CAL = calcarine branch of the PCA; Th.P = thalamoperforate branches.

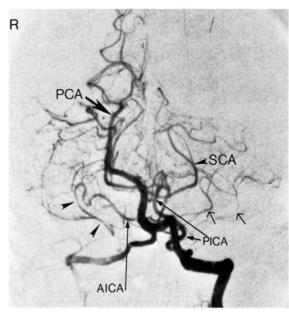

A

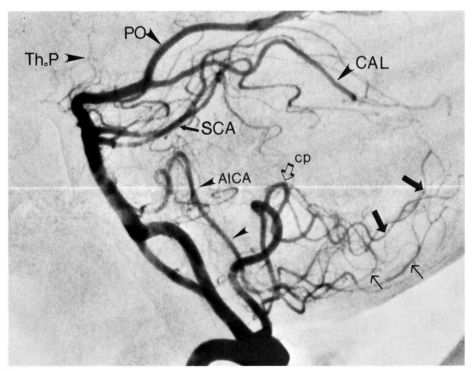

B

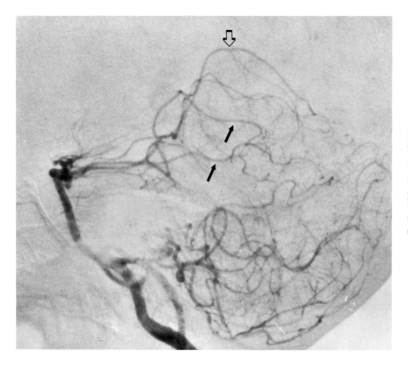

Fig. 1-26 Normal superior cerebellar arteries. Neither PCA fills from the vertebral injection. This view shows the SCA distribution to good advantage. The superior vermian branch (open arrow) and the hemispheric branches (arrows) are indicated.

The posterior pericallosal arteries arise from the PCA and then course in the midline posterior to the splenium of the corpus callosum. They mark the posterior margin of the splenium and are displaced posteriorly by tumors extending into the splenium and by hydrocephalus (Fig. 1-28). The thalamoperforate arteries arise from the medial part of the PCA and fan out superiorly to supply the inferior thalamus, subthalamus, hypothalamus, and red nucleus. They are displaced by tumors in this region. They may also contribute vascular supply to tumors and vascular malformations.

Veins of the Posterior Fossa

There are only a few important veins of the posterior fossa (Fig. 1-29). The anterior pontomesencephalic vein is important as a marker of the position of the anterior margin of the pons. Because it is more closely applied to the pons than to the basilar artery, it more accurately defines displacement of the pons. Superiorly the vein begins in the subthalamic region in the upper suprasellar cistern. It then courses posteroinferiorly in the mid-line within the interpeduncular sulcus on the anterior surface of the mesencephalon. At the superior belly of the pons, it abruptly curves anteriorly to round

the pons and continue inferiorly on its anterior surface. The vein is displaced forward by masses within the pons or cerebellum and backward by prepontine masses.

The precentral cerebellar vein courses superiorly, convex anteriorly, in the space immediately anterior to the superior vermis (Fig. 1-29A&B). It marks this structure and the posterior margin of the superior medullary velum of the fourth ventricle (the superior roof). The vein is "hooked" upward in a characteristic fashion by masses within the fourth ventricle (Fig. 1-30). It is displaced superiorly by upward transtentorial herniation, stretched anteriorly by masses within the vermis or cerebellar hemispheres, and stretched backward by masses within or in front of the pons.

The large, paired inferior vermian veins run in the midline underneath the inferior margin of the vermis. Anteriorly, the superior and inferior tonsillar veins enter the vermian veins. The veins are displaced downward by inferior herniation of the cerebellum or vermis, pushed backward close to the inner table of the occipital bone by masses within the vermis, and shifted to one side by contralateral masses within the cerebellar hemisphere.

The petrosal vein is a short trunk that receives multi-

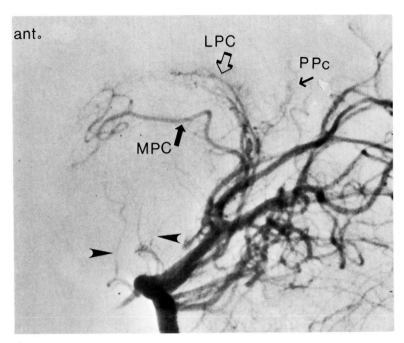

A

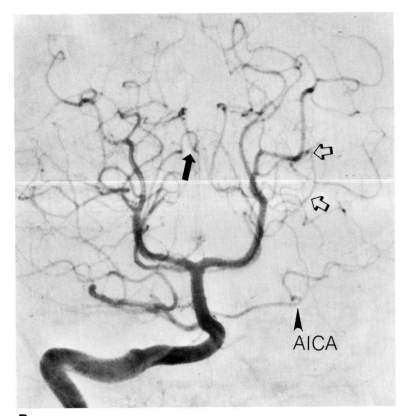

B

Fig. 1-27 Posterior choroidal vessels. **(A)** Lateral vertebral arteriogram shows the characteristic course of the medial posterior choroidal artery (MPC). The sharp curves posteriorly are near the colliculi and pineal gland. The lateral posterior choroidal arteries (LPC) curve broadly behind the pulvinar of the thalamic nuclei. The posterior pericallosal arteries (PPc) course posterior to the splenium of the corpus callosum. The thalamoperforate arteries are seen (arrowheads). **(B)** Towne view shows the medial posterior choroidal artery on the right (arrow) and the lateral posterior choroidal artery on the left (open arrows). The characteristic loop of the AICA is seen as it enters the internal auditory canal (arrowhead).

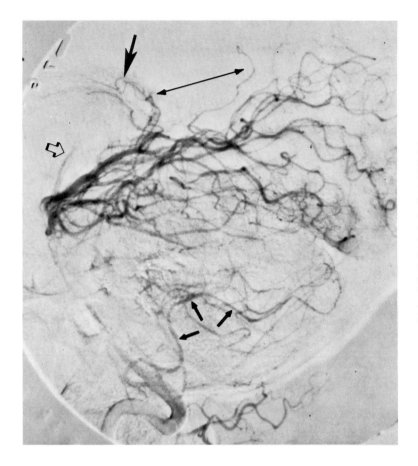

Fig. 1-28 Fourth ventricular mass and hydrocephalus. Lateral vertebral arteriogram shows widening of the choroidal loop by the intraventricular mass (small arrows). Hydrocephalus with lateral ventricular enlargement produces downward displacement of the choroidal vessels (arrow) and increased distance between the choroidal and posterior pericallosal arteries (opposed arrows). The thalamoperforate arteries are displaced and stretched by enlargement of the third ventricle (open arrow).

ple veins from the anteroinferior cerebellum. It lies within the cerebellopontine angle cistern immediately above the porus acusticus and drains into the superior petrosal sinus. Its major importance is in the diagnosis of cerebellar pontine angle masses, particularly acoustic neurinoma. The vein either is displaced and stretched upward in an arc or is occluded by the tumor.

Fortunately, it is no longer essential to be able to diagnose small masses within the posterior fossa with the vertebral angiogram. It can be done much better with MRI or CT scanning. The vertebral angiogram is now used for the reasons given in the box.

MRI

Overall, MRI is the most sensitive imaging technique for the detection of central nervous system pathology. Whenever possible, it is the preferred initial image examination, except for the detection of sub-

arachnoid hemorrhage or bone lesions. The routine MRI examination is performed using spin echo technique (SE) including a T_1-weighted study (SE300–600/20 or IR 500), a T_2-weighted study (SE2000–

USES OF VERTEBRAL ANGIOGRAPHY

Aneurysm

Vascular malformation

Hemangioblastoma, particularly after prior surgery

Atherosclerosis

Arteritis

Preoperative mapping of vessels

Differentiate meningioma from acoustic neurinoma

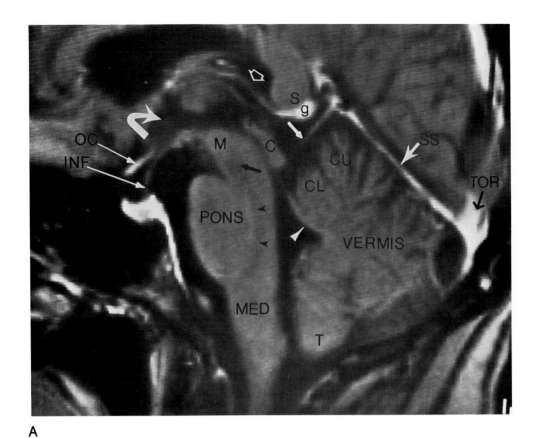

A

Fig. 1-29 Veins of the posterior fossa. (A) Sagittal T_1-
weighted Gd-DTPA contrast-enhanced MRI shows the important anatomy of the posterior fossa. The precentral vein
(white arrow) courses anterior to the superior vermis. It
begins at the level of the superior medullary velum of the
fourth ventricle (white arrowhead). The internal cerebral
vein is demonstrated (open arrow), as is the medial lemniscus
(small black arrowheads) and decussation of the superior cerebellar peduncles (black arrow). S = splenium; M =
mesencephalon; C = collicular plate; MED = medulla; T =
cerebellar tonsil; CL = central lobule; CU = culmen;
SS = straight sinus; TOR = torcula; OC = optic chiasm;
INF = infundibulum; curved arrow = third ventricle. **(B)**
Lateral venous phase shows the normal course of the anterior
pontomesencephalic vein (APM). The precentral vein (PC) is
seen coursing anterior to the vermis. The inferior vermian
vein (IV) runs behind the vermis inferiorly (arrow). The vein
of Galen (curved arrow) is large and drains into the straight
sinus (SS). Th = retrothalamic veins; SV = superior vermian
veins; PV = petrosal vein. *(Figure continues.)*

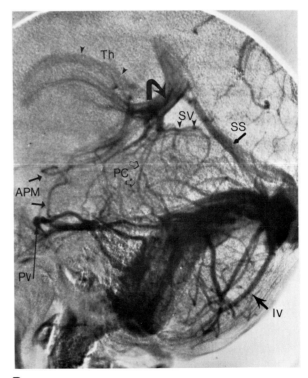

B

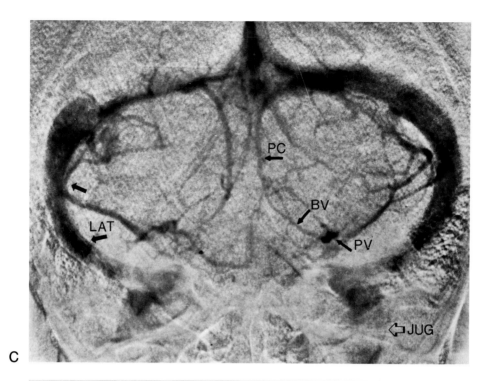

C

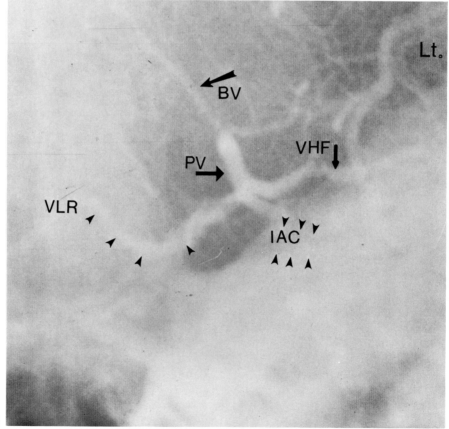

D

Fig. 1-29 *(Continued)* **(C)** Towne projection. PC = precentral vein; BV = brachial vein; PV = petrosal vein; LAT = lateral sinus; JUG = jugular vein. Inferior vermian veins are not present in this patient. **(D)** Magnification of the Towne projection of the left petrosal vein. The petrosal vein (PV) is short. The major tributaries are the vein of the lateral recess of the fourth ventricle (VLR, arrowheads), the brachial vein (BV), and the vein of the horizontal fissure (VHF). IAC = internal auditory canal.

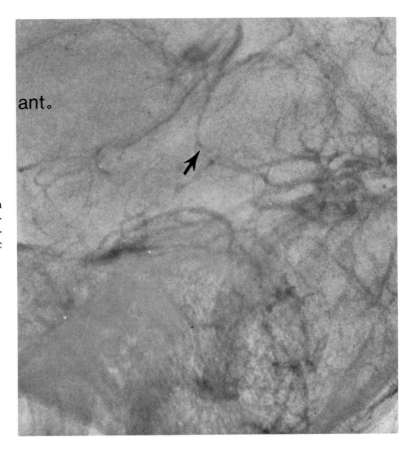

Fig. 1-30 Mass within the fourth ventricle. The precentral vein is displaced superiorly by the intraventricular mass (arrow), with a characteristic "hook."

3000/60–100), and a proton density study SE (TR 2000–3000/25–50) (Table 1-3). Relatively thin (6 to 8 mm) slice thickness is used with as little interslice gap as possible while still allowing for complete coverage of the brain within a reasonable period of time. Transaxial sections are usually routine. Coronal sections have an advantage when imaging the convexities, the temporal lobes, and the sella region. Sagittal sections are best for the subfrontal region, the colliculi, and the foramen magnum.

The T_1-weighted sequence produces a strong MRI signal that results in a clear anatomic image. This sequence is therefore best for evaluating the anatomic structure of the brain. Ventricular size and anatomic distortions are optimally displayed. The relatively short TR that is used also means that the total scanning time for the image is also relatively short. Fat is intensely bright on T_1 images, which is an advantage when outlining the epidural space or marrow in the spinal column. Subacute and chronic hematomas are seen as high density (see Ch. 2). However, the T_1-weighted images are relatively insensitive to small changes in the water content of tissue. Therefore small or early lesions of the brain that do not cause anatomic distortion are often invisible on T_1 images.

The T_2-weighted sequences produce images that are much more sensitive in the detection changes in the water content of the tissue imaged. Because water has a

Table 1-3 T_1 and T_2 Weighting, SE Sequences

T_1 Weighted	
TR short	< 600 msec
TE short	< 25 msec
T_2 Weighted	
TR long	> 2,000 msec
TE long[a]	> 60 msec
Proton Density	
TR long	> 1,000 msec
TE short	< 30 msec

[a] The longer the TE, the greater the T_2 based contrast.

long T_2 relaxation time, the T_2 signal of water lasts into the late echo times after the signal of the background tissue has died away. Regions of increased water content (edema) are imaged as regions of high signal superimposed on a dark background. However, because the signal of the background tissue is not strong, the T_2-weighted sequence is not as useful for displaying anatomy. The high sensitivity of T_2-weighted MRI for the detection of changes in tissue water content is the primary reason for the increased sensitivity of MRI over CT scanning for the detection of brain and spinal cord pathology. The signal characteristics of various tissues is given in Table 1-4.

Gradient refocused echo (GRE) imaging may be used to save imaging time. With this technique the MRI signal is produced by the application of sequential but opposite dephasing gradients. Variable "flip" angles and short TR and TE are used. T_1 or T_2 weighting can be produced depending on the relation of the "flip" angle to the TR. Small "flip" angles (10 to 30 degrees) and short TR (100 to 300 msec) with TE of 10 to 15 msec create T_2-weighted images. Large "flip" angles and short TR produce T_1-weighted images. GRE sequences are useful for producing three-dimensional images in a reasonable period of time. GRE and the three-dimensional technique may prove useful in MRI "angiography."

Intravenous contrast enhancement may be used with MRI of the central nervous system. Gadolinium, a paramagnetic agent, chelated to DTPA (Gd-DTPA) is the agent employed at this time. The paramagnetic agent, when deposited within tissue, greatly decreases the T_1

relaxation time of that tissue, resulting in a strong T_1 signal wherever the contrast has accumulated. Gd-DTPA has been shown to be safe, having produced few adverse reactions. T_1-weighted imaging is used after contrast infusion.

The aim is to deliver the paramagnetic agent to regions of abnormality within the brain and spinal cord. In general, the contrast accumulates within regions of

Table 1-4 MRI Signal Intensity of Cerebral Contents

Tissue	T_1	T_2
CSF	Low	High
White matter	Mod. high	Mod. low
Gray matter	Mod. low	Mod. high
Edema fluid	Mod. low	Very high
Fat	High	Mod. high
Tumors	Low	Mod. high
Fast-flowing blood	Very low	Very low
Slow-flowing blood	High	Variable
Bone	Very low	Very low
Bone marrow	High	Mod. low
Air	Very low	Very low
Cyst fluid, clear	Low	High
Cyst Fluid, protein	Sl. low	Very high
Clotted blood	Complex (see text and Ch. 2)	

INDICATIONS FOR CONTRAST ENHANCEMENT WITH MRI OR CT SCANNING

Signs/symptoms
    Focal neurologic signs or symptoms
        Hemiparesis
        Aphasia
    Focal sensory deficit
        Visual deficit
        Anosmia
        Hemisensory deficit
        Tic douloureux
        Hemifacial spasm
    Cranial nerve dysfunction
        Unilateral hearing loss
        Ophthalmoplegia
    New onset seizures, age > 20 years
    Ataxia
    Vertigo
    Behavior change, age < 50 years
Suspected pathology
    Primary brain tumor
    Metastatic brain tumor
    Meningeal carcinomatosis
    Pituitary adenoma
    Acoustic neurinoma
    Brain abscess or granuloma
    Epidural abscess
    Arteriovenous malformation
    Aneurysm
    Multiple sclerosis
    Infarction, not seen on nonenhanced examination
    Recurrent brain tumor
    To define mass lesions seen on the nonenhanced examination

INDICATIONS FOR NONENHANCED MRI OR CT SCANNING

Symptoms/Clinical Setting
    Headache, nonspecific
    Chronic seizures
    Seizures, age < 20 years
    Immediate postoperative period
    Acute head trauma
    Dementia
Suspected pathology
    Hydrocephalus
    Shunt malfunction
    Intracranial hemorrhage
    Congenital malformation

breakdown of the blood-brain barrier. It is a nonspecific alteration with pathology within the brain and occurs with tumors, infection, and infarction. However, the use of contrast increases the sensitivity of MRI for detecting specific disease processes, particularly small tumors. The indications for contrast and the interpretation of the findings is essentially the same as for contrast enhancement with CT, as outlined above. Specific information is given about the use of enhancement under specific disease headings. The pattern of contrast enhancement with MRI may permit better tissue characterization, similar to the use of contrast with CT. Slowly flowing blood (veins, cavernous sinus) shows greatly enhanced T_1 signal after Gd-DTPA infusion (Fig. 1-29A). Dural membranes do not show enhancement.

Hemorrhage

The MRI technique is generally sensitive for the detection of intracerebral hemorrhage, except subarachnoid hemorrhage and possibly hyperacute hematoma. The MRI image varies with the age and cause of the hemorrhage. Its appearance changes with different pulse sequences. Higher field strength produces better images, but this statement is more theoretical than empiric. Subacute hematomas can be adequately imaged at low field strength. Gradient echo techniques may also be used and have increased sensitivity to the magnetic sus-

ceptibility effect of hemosiderin. The theory of evolution of hematomas is complex (see Ch. 2).

Flowing Blood

The appearance of flowing blood depends on a number of factors, including the pulse sequences used, the order of slice acquisition, the velocity, and the direction of the flow relative to the plane of the imaging. The underlying principles are (1) the "washout" of spins from selectively excited regions during the interval between the initial and the echo-producing pulses, and (2) phase shifting of spins as they transverse magnetic field gradients.

In general, rapidly flowing blood appears dark (flow void) on SE sequences, a phenomenon that has been termed *high velocity signal loss.* Turbulence, also associated with high velocity flow, contributes to the loss in signal. For most instances, when signal void is present within a vessel, it can be determined to be patent. Rarely, hemosiderin within a chronically clotted vessel may produce signal void.

A number of factors, however, may result in increased signal within a vessel that is patent. "Flow-related enhancement" occurs when unsaturated, fully magnetized blood enters the first few slices in a multislice series so that, with reexcitation in the next pulse, maximum signal is obtained on the echo. Another po-

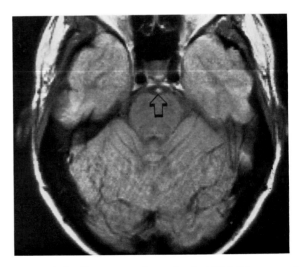

Fig. 1-31 Basilar artery thrombosis, MRI. The normal "flow void" is not present. High signal (arrow) is present within the lumen, indicating thrombosis.

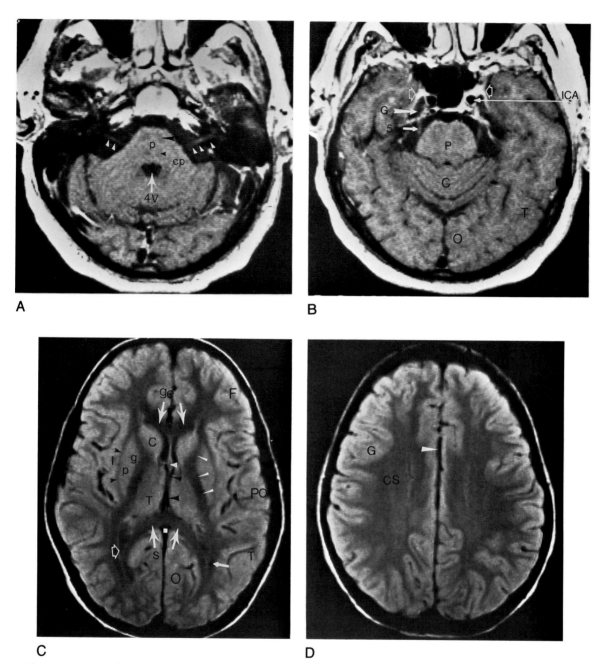

Fig. 1-32 Normal MRI anatomy. (A) Posterior fossa. Transaxial view through the mid-pons level shows the fourth ventricle (white arrow) behind the pons (p). Cortical spinal tracts (large black arrowhead) and the medial lemniscus (small black arrowhead) can be seen as regions of slight hypointensity. The cerebellar peduncles (cp) are large bilateral structures. The branches of the eighth nerve (CN VIII) can be seen in the cerebellar pontine angle cistern entering the internal auditory canals (white arrowheads). **(B)** Transaxial view of a slightly higher level, Gd-DTPA-enhanced. This view shows the level of the upper pons (P). The fifth cranial nerves are seen extending anteriorly (small arrow) to enter Meckel's cave and the gasserian ganglion (large arrow, G). There is normal enhancement (high signal) within the cavernous sinus (open arrow). The internal carotid artery is seen as the round region of flow-void (ICA, long arrow). C = cerebellum; O = occipital lobe; T = temporal lobe. **(C)** MRI. SE2500/ 25 at the level of the foramina of Monro. The corpus callosum (large white arrows) is well seen. (*Figure continues.*)

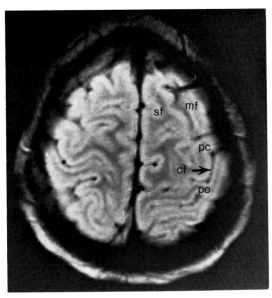

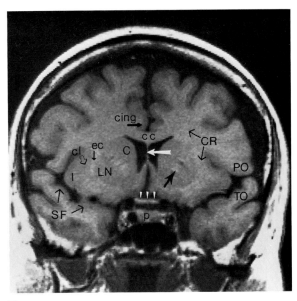

E   F

Fig. 1-32 *(Continued)* The anterior portion is the genu (ge) and the posterior portion is the splenium (s). The frontal horns of the lateral ventricles lie just behind the genu and are separated by the septum pellucidum. At the posterior point of the septum pellucidum there is an enlargement, the fornix (small white arrowhead). The paired internal cerebral veins run in the roof of the third ventricle (black arrowheads) and eventually empty into the vein of Galen (white square). The basal ganglia consist of the caudate nucleus (C), putamen (p), and globus pallidus (g). The internal capsule (thin white arrowheads) is divided into the anterior limb, the genu, and the posterior limb. The external capsule (small black arrowheads), which is lateral to the lenticular nuclei (globus pallidus and putamen), lies just deep to the insula (I). The atrium and occipital horn of the right lateral ventricle are seen (open arrow). The optic radiation is just lateral to this area (small white arrow). F = frontal lobe; PO = parietal operculum; T = temporal lobe; O = occipital lobe. **(D)** MR SE/2500/25 through the centrum semiovale (CS), the large central portion of the hemispheric white matter. The cortical gray matter is seen as slightly higher intensity (G). The pericallosal vessels run in the interhemispheric fissure (white arrowhead.) **(E)** MRI through the vertex shows the sulcal anatomy. The superior frontal gyrus (sf) and the middle frontal gyrus (mf) are separated by a fissure. The precentral gyrus (pc) and the postcentral gyrus (po) are separated by the central fissure (cf, arrow). **(F)** Coronal T_1-weighted MRI through the basal ganglia, showing the pituitary gland (p) and the optic chiasm (white arrowheads). The frontal horns of the lateral ventricle are seen separated by the septum pellucidum (white arrow). The internal capsule (black arrow) receives the fibers from the corona radiata (CR). The insula (I) lies just deep to the sylvian fissure (SF). The claustrum (cl) is a small region of deep gray matter just lateral to the external capsule (ec). LN = lenticular nuclei; C = caudate nucleus; PO = parietal operculum; TO = temporal operculum; cc = corpus callosum; cing = cingulate gyrus.

tential cause of high signal within patent vessels is "even-echo rephasing," where the vessel lumen becomes bright on the second of two evenly spaced echoes. "Diastolic pseudogating" may also occur if, by chance, the repetition time of the sequence chosen approximates the cardiac rate of the patient. In this situation, slices that are consistently produced during the diastolic (slow flow) phase of the cardiac cycle show high signal within arteries that normally would show high flow signal loss. Care must always be taken to exclude these physical factors as the cause of a high intraluminal vascular signal before vessel thrombosis or slow flow is diagnosed.

Flow-related enhancement (FRE) can also be intentionally produced by using GRE imaging sequences with single slice acquisition. FRE occurs because the gradient reversal echo technique utilizes a nonselective gradient so that the time-of-flight effects of washout do not occur. Vessels with flowing blood become bright. If this effect is found, it proves the patency of the vessel.

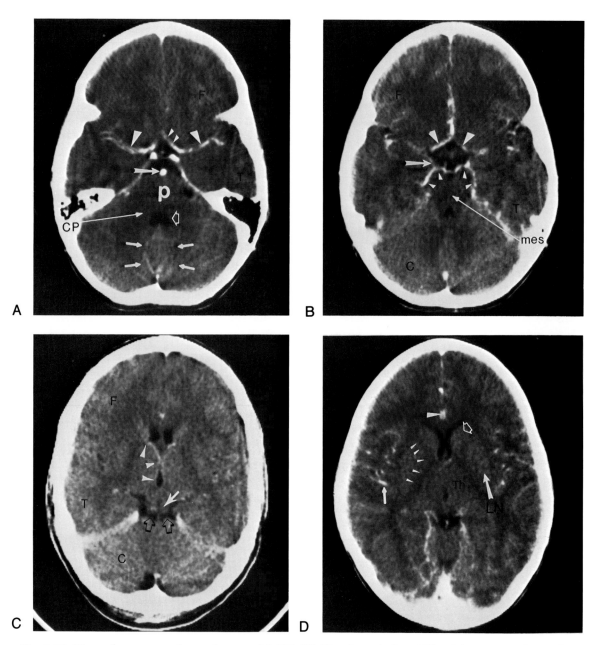

Fig. 1-33 Normal contrast-enhanced transaxial CT. (A) Slice through the middle of the posterior fossa. The vermis shows increased density both before and after contrast enhancement (small white arrows). The fourth ventricle is a small trapezoidal cavity in the midline (open arrow). It lies behind the pons (p). Contrast is seen in the basilar artery (large white arrow). The horizontal portion of the MCA is seen bilaterally (large arrowheads) as is the ACA (small arrowheads). The cerebellar peduncle (CP) connects the pons with the cerebellar white matter. **(B)** Scan through the suprasellar cistern, which is seen as a pentagon at the center of the scan containing fluid of CSF density. It is surrounded by the ACA (large arrowheads), posterior communicating artery (large arrow), and posterior cerebral arteries (small arrowheads). The more distal portions of the PCA surround the mesencephalon (mes). **(C)** Scan slightly higher shows the thalamostriate vein draining into the internal cerebral vein (arrowheads). The vein skirts the top of the third ventricle. The colliculi (large arrow) are seen protruding into the quadrigeminal plate cistern (open arrows). C = cerebellum. **(D)** Scan slightly higher shows the basal ganglia. The caudate nucleus (open arrow) shows slight hyperdensity and forms the lateral border of the frontal horn of the lateral ventricle. The lenticular nuclei (white arrow, LN) are seen slightly posteriorly and laterally. The thalamus is a paired structure on either side of the third ventricle posteriorly (Th). The internal capsule (small arrowheads) separates the lenticular nuclei from the caudate nucleus anteriorly and the thalamus posteriorly. The pericallosal arteries (large arrowhead) and the middle cerebral arteries in the sylvian fissure (small arrow) are seen. *(Figure continues.)*

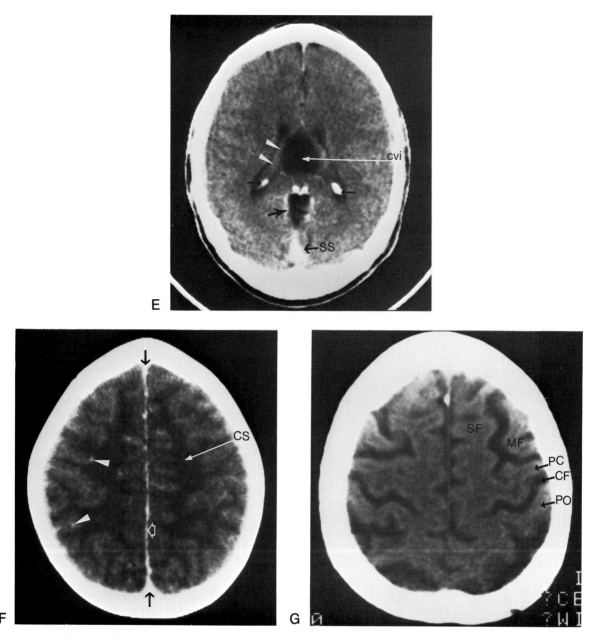

Fig. 1-33 *(Continued)* **(E)** Scan through the level of the bodies of the lateral ventricles show the anterior extension of the choroid plexus (arrowheads) and calcification within the glomus (small black arrows). The ventricular cavities are separated by an enlarged cavum velum interpositum (cvi), which is an extension of the subarachnoid space over the roof of the third ventricle. The supracerebellar cistern extends superiorly through a fenestration in the anterior tentorium (black arrow). The vein of Galen is divided into paired structures. The straight sinus (SS) runs posteriorly toward the torcula. **(F)** Scan through the centrum semiovale. The crotical gyral pattern is prominent. Cortical arteries are seen at the base of the sulci (arrowheads). The falx shows enhancement (open arrow). The sagittal sinus is seen as a triangular, contrast-filled structure (black arrows). CS = centrum semiovale. **(G)** Scan through the vertex shows the major posterior frontal and anterior parietal sulci. SF = superior frontal gyrus; MF = middle frontal gyrus; PC = precentral gyrus; CF = central fissure; PO = postcentral gyrus.

This technique is used to define vessels within an arteriovenous malformation where vascular channels may be difficult to distinguish from the signal void of calcium deposition or within vessels where other sequences suggest thrombosis or slow flow but the diagnosis is not clear.

Presently, only major vessel thrombosis or slow flow can be diagnosed by the absence of high velocity signal loss (Fig. 1-31). Calculation of blood velocity and flow volume is theoretically possible but difficult and time-consuming. Even more difficult is the measurement of actual tissue perfusion because of the slower velocity and multidirectional nature of the capillary flow. At present, it is not possible. MRI angiographic techniques are under development and may prove to be useful for screening patients for large-vessel disease.

Blood flow and CSF pulsation can be troublesome during MRI as artifacts are produced. It is especially a problem on T_2-weighted imaging with longer echo times and complex fluid motion such as the to-and-fro pulsating motion of the CSF. Cardiac gating (to make the effect of flow consistent for each slice), gradient motion refocusing (to rephase spins perturbed by motion) and presaturation techniques are used to reduce the artifacts and are useful especially for spine imaging. MRI is relatively insensitive for the detection of calcium.

A simplified review of brain anatomy as imaged with MRI is presented in Figure 1-32.

CT SCANNING

Computed tomography has been the main neuro-diagnostic imaging technique since its introduction in 1972. Because it is more readily available and less expensive than MRI, it will likely remain the most widely used modality for some time. It is accurate, fast, and versatile. It retains its advantage over MRI for detecting subarachnoid hemorrhage and bone destruction. It is much easier to use on patients who have difficulty remaining motionless or who require life support sys-

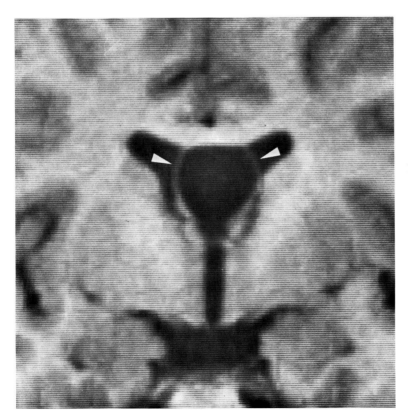

Fig. 1-34 Cyst of septum pellucidum, MRI. Fluid may separate the leaves of the septum pellucidum. If it communicates with the ventricular system, it is a cavum septum pellucidum. If no communication is present a cyst may form (arrowheads) that may obstruct the foramina of Monro.

Table 1-5 Density of Cranial Tissue on CT Scans

Tissue	Appearance Relative to Water	HU
Bone	Very dense	>500
Gray matter	Intermediate density	35–40
White matter	Intermediate density	28–35
CSF	Isodense	0–10
Fat	Hypodense	<−90
Air	Very hypodense	<−500
Tumors	Intermediate density	20–50
Cysts	Isodense	5–15
Calcification	Hyperdense	>80
Clotted blood	Moderately hyperdense	50–100
Blood	Intermediate density	38–48

tems. Overall, CT is slightly less sensitive than MRI for detection of intracranial and spinal pathology, although it is sometimes capable of giving more specific tissue information.

The CT image is based on the same principles as all radiography. Tissue that has greater electron density and therefore greater radioabsorption is normally displayed as a high density area on the CT image. Those tissues with little radioabsorption are displayed as a low density area (Table 1-5). Relatively narrow windows are used for viewing brain tissue, and wide windows are used for viewing bone.

Transaxial 10-mm slices through the entire brain are performed for the routine scan (Figs. 1-33 and 1-34). Thin sections and coronal planes are used for detailed imaging, particularly of the posterior fossa and sella turcica. Intravenous contrast enhancement, using iodinated contrast agents, is frequently used for specific indications (see previous box). It not only increases the sensitivity for the detection of pathology but often gives specific information for histologic diagnosis. The use of contrast enhancement is discussed in more detail under specific diseases.

SUGGESTED READING

General Texts

Brant-Zawadzki M, Norman D: Magnetic Resonance Imaging of the Central Nervous System. Raven Press, New York, 1987

Burrows EH, Leeds NE: Neuroradiology; The Skull. Churchill Livingstone, New York, 1981.

Heinz ER: The Clinical Neurosciences: Neuroradiology. Churchill Livingstone, New York, 1984

Lee SH, Rao KCVG: Cranial Computed Tomography and MRI. 2nd Ed. McGraw-Hill, New York, 1987

Osborn AG: Introduction to Cerebral Angiography. Harper & Row, Hagerstown, MD, 1980

Ramsey RG: Neuroradiology. WB Saunders, Philadelphia, 1987

Stark DD, Bradley WG Jr: Magnetic Resonance Imaging. CV Mosby, St. Louis, 1988

Williams AL, Haughton VM: Cranial Computed Tomography. CV Mosby, St. Louis, 1985

Wong WS, Tsruda JS, Kortman KE, Bradley WG Jr: Practical MRI. Aspen Publishers, Rockville, MD, 1987

Additional Reading

Axel L: Blood flow effects in magnetic resonance imaging. In Kressel HY (ed): Magnetic Resonance Annual 1986. Raven Press, New York, 1986

Bradley WG Jr: Magnetic resonance imaging in the central nervous system: comparison with computed tomography. In Kressel HY (ed): Magnetic Resonance Annual. Raven Press, New York, 1986

Brooks RA, Di Chiro G, Patronas N: MR imaging of cerebral hematomas at different field strengths: theory and applications. J Comput Assist Tomogr 13:194, 1989

Burman S, Rosenbaum AE: Rationale and techniques for intravenous enhancement in computed tomography. Radiol Clin North Am 20:15, 1982

Bydder GM: Clinical application of gadolinium-DTPA. p. 182. In Stark DD, Bradley WG Jr (eds): Magnetic Resonance Imaging. CV Mosby, St. Louis, 1988

Clark JA II, Kelly WM: Common artifacts encountered in magnetic resonance imaging. Radiol Clin North Am 26:393, 1988

Council on Scientific Affairs: Magnetic resonance imaging of the central nervous system. JAMA 259:1211, 1988

Daniels DL: Normal cerebral anatomy. In Williams AL, Haughton VM (eds): Cranial Computed Tomography. CV Mosby, St. Louis, 1985

Daniels DL, Haughton VM, Naidich TP: Cranial and Spinal Magnetic Resonance Imaging: An Atlas and Guide. Raven Press, New York, 1987

Debrun GM (ed): Interventional neuroradiology. Semin Intervent Radiol 4:219, 1987

Erba M, Jungreis CA, Horton JA: Nitropaste for prevention and relief of vasospasm [during angiography]. AJNR 10:155, 1989

Gado MH: Supratentorial anatomy. p. 269. In Stark DD, Bradley WG Jr (eds): Magnetic Resonance Imaging. CV Mosby, St. Louis, 1988

George AE: A systematic approach to the interpretation of

posterior fossa angiography. Radiol Clin North Am 12:371, 1974

Grossman RI, Gomori JM, Goldberg HI, et al: MR imaging of hemorrhagic conditions of the head and neck. Radiographics 8:441, 1988

Hyman RA, Gorey MY: Imaging strategies for MRI of the brain. Radiol Clin North Am 26:471, 1988

Jones JP, Partain CL, Mitchell MR: Principles of magnetic resonance. In Kressel HY (ed): Magnetic Resonance Annual. Raven Press, New York, 1985

Lane B: Erosions of the skull. Radiol Clin North Am 12:257, 1974

Makow LS: Magnetic resonance imaging: a brief review of image contrast. Radiol Clin North Am 27:195, 1989

Oot RF, New PFJ, Pile-Spellman J, et al: The detection of intracranial calcifications by MR. AJNR 7:801, 1986

Rubenfeld M, Wirtshafter JD: The role of medical imaging in the practice of neuroophthalmology. Radiol Clin North Am 25:863, 1987

Runge VM, Wood ML, Kaufman DM, et al: The straight and narrow path to good head and spine MRI. Radiographics 8:507, 1988

Russell EJ, Schaible TF, Dillon W, et al: Multicenter double-blind placebo-controlled study of gadopentate dimeglumine as an MR contrast agent: evaluation in patients with cerebral lesions. AJNR 10:53, 1989

Sage MR: Review: blood-brain barrier: phenomenon of increasing importance to the imaging clinician. AJNR 3:127, 1982

Schnitzlein HN, Murtaugh FR: Imaging Anatomy of the Head and Spine. Urban & Schwarzenberg, Baltimore, 1985

Taveras JM: Interventional neuroradiology symposium on preoperative embolization. AJNR 7:926, 1986

Unsold R, Ostertag CB, de Groot J, Newton TH: Computer Reconstructions of the Brain and Skull Base. Springer-Verlag, Berlin, 1982

Villafana T: Fundamental principles of magnetic resonance imaging. Radiol Clin North Am 26:701, 1988

Wolf GL, Burnett KR, Goldstein EJ, Joseph PM: Contrast agents for magnetic resonance imaging. In Kressel HY (ed): Magnetic Resonance Annual. Raven Press, New York, 1985

Wong WS, Tsuruda JS, Kortman KE, Bradley WG Jr: Fundamentals of MR image interpretation. In: Practical MRI: A Case Study Approach. Aspen Publishers, Rockville, MD, 1987

Yock DH: The skull. In Heinz ED (ed): The Clinical Neurosciences: Neuroradiology. Churchill Livingstone, New York, 1984

2
Cerebrovascular Disease

The term cerebrovascular disease refers to any process that results in abnormality of the cerebral blood vessels or cerebral blood flow. It includes both intracranial and extracranial vessels, as well as embolization, effects of hypertension, hyperviscosity, changes in global blood flow, and hypoxemia. Cerebrovascular disease is by far the most common of all neurologic problems, accounting for up to 70 percent of admissions to the neurologic service. Stroke is the most devastating consequence of cerebrovascular disease and is the third most common cause of death in the United States.

Stroke denotes the sudden development of a neurologic deficit, usually focal in nature. The neurologic manifestation of stroke depends on the volume and location of the tissue involved. About 80 percent of strokes are the result of ischemia and infarction caused by vascular occlusion. The remainder are mostly the result of hemorrhage or a decrease in global blood flow. Thrombosis is thought to be the most common cause of vascular occlusion and is three times as common as embolization. *Ischemia* refers to a metabolically significant decrease in blood flow. *Infarction* refers to the death of tissue as a result of ischemia.

Because the brain cannot repair itself, medical and surgical intervention is directed primarily toward prevention. The aims are to remove an underlying pathologic process, limit brain damage by improving perfusion to marginal regions, and reduce risk factors. The radiologist is responsible for defining the cause and location of the infarction, demonstrating focal extracranial and intracranial vascular pathology, excluding other pathology that might mimic infarction, and evaluating the response to treatment.

CEREBRAL INFARCTION

Classification

A useful clinical categorization of cerebral ischemic events is outlined in the following sections.

TRANSIENT ISCHEMIC ATTACK

Transient ischemic attack (TIA) refers to a transient focal neurologic deficit of sudden onset lasting a few seconds or minutes and always clearing within 24 hours. Symptoms related to the internal carotid artery (ICA) distribution are hemiparesis, aphasia, and amaurosis fugax. Those relating to the vertebral basilar (VB) distribution are bilateral or alternating motor or sensory deficits, transient global amnesia, vertigo, diplopia, dysphagia, and ataxia. Hemianopsia and dysarthria may result from disease in either the ICA or VB circuits. TIA is generally thought to be a result of transient ischemia and reversible damage in the brain, but small infarctions can also cause TIAs and may be detected with MRI. Rarely, what appears to be a TIA is caused by a tumor or chronic subdural hematoma.

A TIA may be thought of as the first manifestation of underlying cerebrovascular disease. It has significant prognostic implications. Persons who have had a TIA have about a 5 percent per year incidence of a completed stroke. Additionally, there is also a 5 percent per year incidence of myocardial infarction. Coronary heart disease is the most common cause of death in this group.

About 50 percent of those with an ICA type of TIA

have a demonstrable lesion in the ipsilateral ICA. Most lesions are atherosclerotic plaques at the origin of the ICA in the neck. However, only about one-half of these lesions are candidates for surgical intervention under the present guidelines. Overall, only about 15 percent of strokes are preceded by a TIA. It is presently recommended that persons with TIAs undergo duplex ultrasonography or angiography of the extracranial circulation. Endarterectomy of appropriate lesions of the ICA will significantly decrease the incidence of TIAs and subsequent stroke.

REVERSIBLE ISCHEMIC NEUROLOGIC DEFICIT

Reversible ischemic neurologic deficit (RIND) refers to a focal neurologic deficit that is similar to a TIA but lasts longer than 24 hours and subsequently clears. It has the same implications as a TIA.

STROKE IN EVOLUTION

Stroke in evolution (SIE) refers to a stepwise worsening of a sudden neurologic deficit occurring over 24 hours. It is thought to be a result of embolization. Many neurologists recommend anticoagulation for this group of patients.

COMPLETED STROKE

A completed stroke is the sudden onset of a focal neurologic deficit that persists and is stable. It is the most common end result of cerebrovascular disease.

LACUNAR INFARCTION

Lacunar infarctions are relatively small (0.5 to 2.0 cm) and result from occlusion of the small penetrating end vessels that supply the deep gray and white matter of the brain and brain stem. The infarcts progress to cysts — hence the name lacune or cyst. The major groups of perforating vessels are (1) lenticulostriate vessels, supplying the basal ganglia and internal capsule; (2) thalamoperforate vessels, supplying the thalamus; and (3) pontine perforate vessels, supplying the pons and mesencephalon.

Lacunar infarction is mainly the result of the effects of hypertension. Prolonged hypertension causes lipohyalinosis of the small perforating arteries. These changes result in narrowing of the vessels and their subsequent occlusions. Small microaneurysms form but are only rarely seen with angiography.

Lacunar infarctions cause specific clinical syndromes. A pure motor deficit is the most common, resulting from infarction in the internal capsule or pons. Pure sensory deficit indicates infarction within the thalamus. Other syndromes include dysarthria with hand clumsiness (genu and anterior limb of internal capsule), ataxic hemiparesis (pons), hemiballismus (subthalamic), and mutism (bilateral nonsimultaneous lacunes). Most lacunar infarctions can be identified with MRI.

NONLACUNAR INFARCTION

The nonlacunar infarction is one that occurs in the cerebral hemispheres or cerebellum.

Pathophysiology

The brain has constant demand for oxygen; but it has little oxygen reserve, so oxygen must be continually supplied in sufficient quantity. Total anoxia for 10 minutes results in total tissue death. Shorter periods may cause incomplete or reversible change. Neurons are more sensitive to anoxia than the supporting astrocytes.

Normally the cerebral blood flow (CBF) is maintained at an average of 50 ml/100 g/min. The gray matter receives 80 ml/100 g/min, whereas the white matter receives only 20 ml/100 g/min. Ischemia begins when the blood flow becomes less than 18 ml/100 g/min. Flow in the white matter is normally dangerously close to this level, and a slight decrease in flow results in white matter damage. This situation explains the greater damage done to the white matter in "watershed" regions after transient global ischemia. Conversely, gray matter is more sensitive to the effects of ischemia once the critical level has been reached. However, the outer cortex is more resistant to ischemia and may be preserved even though the underlying tissue is severely damaged.

Autoregulation occurs so that CBF is nearly constant between the arterial mean pressures of 60 and 180 mmHg. Above and below these levels the regulation breaks down and flow increases or decreases. With chronic hypertension the window of autoregulation is set at a higher level. CBF is also proportional to the

CO_2 content of the blood. Local increase in CO_2 and lactate cause an increase in regional CBF, resulting in "luxury perfusion."

Glucose is the major metabolic substrate of the brain. Up to a point, with decreasing CBF, metabolism is maintained by increased extraction of glucose from the blood. Beyond this point, anaerobic metabolism of glucose occurs, leading to regional lactic acid buildup.

When critical ischemia occurs, a cascade of events is initiated. This cascade runs to completion regardless of reestablishment of flow. The shift to anaerobic metabolism causes an increase in the regional lactic acid and a decrease in the production of adenosine triphosphate (ATP). The integrity of the cell membrane and the function of the sodium pump is impaired, which results in cytotoxic edema. Local endothelial damage is also produced by the abnormal regional metabolites, resulting in the loss of the blood-brain barrier and the production of vasogenic edema. Loss of the blood-brain barrier allows leakage of intravenous contrast into the infarcted tissue, provided there is sufficient blood flow.

The postischemic edema begins within the gray matter during the first 3 hours after the ischemia. Later,

it occurs within the white matter. The edema gets progressively worse until reaching a maximum at about 4 days. If the infarction is large, there may be sufficient edema to cause craniocaudal herniation and death. Steroid treatment has little effect on the edema once the process has begun. A steroid given prior to an ischemic event decreases the amount of edema that may result from infarction.

After about 5 days the edema begins to subside. Proliferation of microglia begins around the periphery and extends centrally into the infarcted tissue. These cells become lipid-laden macrophages. Within 6 weeks the cellular debris is cleared. The region of the infarction becomes soft from a loss of cells (*encephalomalacia*). Complete loss of cells results in a fluid-filled cystic cavity, which is seen most commonly after lacunar infarction. Rarely, calcium is deposited within infarcted tissue.

Small hemorrhages are common within infarctions, particularly those caused by embolization. They usually occur sometime after the stroke, when blood flow to infarcted tissue is reestablished. The hemorrhage is usually petechial but may become confluent. Hemor-

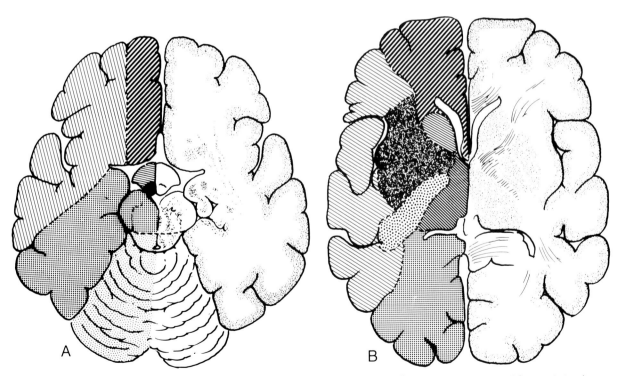

Fig. 2-1 Brain regions supplied by the major intracranial arteries. (From Drayer, 1984, with permission.) (*Figure continues.*)

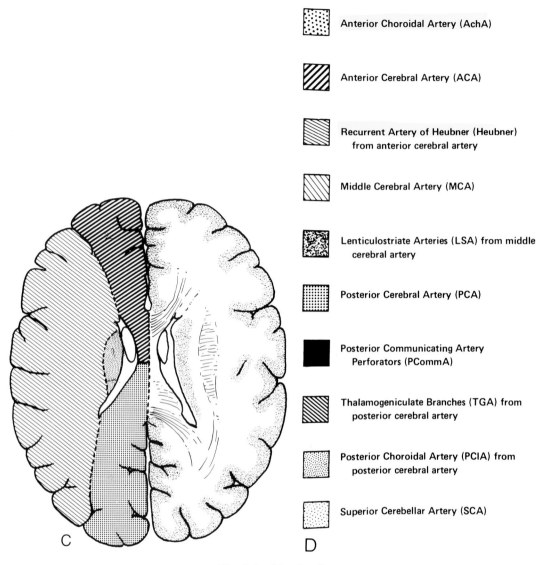

Fig. 2-1 (*Continued*).

rhage is most commonly seen in the cortical gyri. Large hematomas are unusual.

New capillaries are formed about the periphery and extend inward to a slight degree as well. Initially, these vessels do not have a blood-brain barrier, which allows leakage of injected contrast so there is often peripheral enhancement about infarctions beginning at the end of the first week and continuing for a month or more.

In the final stage, the infarction is sharply demarcated from the surrounding brain. Loss of brain tissue results in focal atrophy with dilatation of both the cortical sulci and the subjacent ventricle.

Sodium accumulates in the extracellular and the intracellular fluid so that the concentration of sodium within a volume of infarcted brain tissue is increased 300 percent over normal. This increase in sodium concentration can be imaged with sodium (^{23}Na) MRI, but presently this method has little advantage over proton MRI.

It is important to recognize the common vascular

territories of the brain, as a cerebral infarction most often corresponds with one of these territories. With imaging, territorial patterns help to define the abnormality as infarction rather than some other pathology. The territories are shown in Figure 2-1.

MRI

The most sensitive imaging test for the detection of cerebral infarction is MRI because of its high sensitivity to edema. The edema associated with infarction causes prolongation of both T_1 and T_2 relaxation times. It can be seen as early as 1 hour after the infarction but more consistently at 6 hours. About 80 percent of clinical strokes can be defined with MRI within the first 24 hours.

The infarction is best seen on T_2-weighted images as a region of high signal intensity (Fig. 2-2). The region of edema corresponds with the region of infarcted tissue. T_1-weighted images show infarction as a region of low intensity. Swelling is recognized by compression and a shift of the ventricles and sulci.

Hemorrhage within the infarction is best recognized during the acute phase with high field strength T_2-weighted SE or GRE images (see Ch. 1). Focal low signal intensity is seen within the high signal intensity of the edema because of the magnetic susceptibility of deoxyhemoglobin still within red blood cells (see Fig. 7-3). Low field strength SE images and T_1-weighted images do not consistently show these acute hemorrhages. Subacute hemorrhage is well demonstrated on the T_1-weighted images as high signal within the low

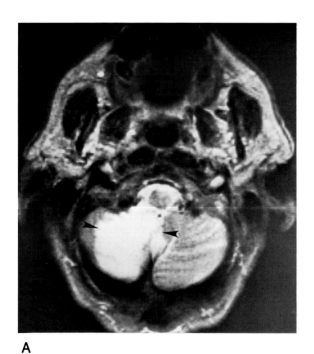

A

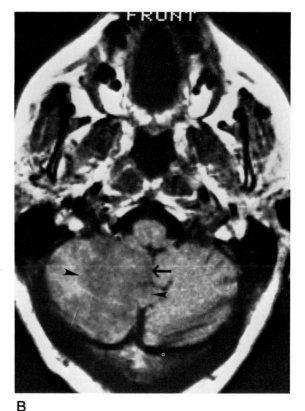

B

Fig. 2-2 Acute ischemic cerebellar infarction, MRI. (A) Transaxial T_2-weighted MRI shows the infarction as a sharply demarcated region of hyperintensity in the distribution of the right PICA. The hyperintensity represents cytotoxic and vasogenic edema that corresponds with the region of infarcted tissue (arrowheads). **(B)** T_1-weighted image shows the infarction as a region of hypointensity (arrowheads). Slight swelling is present with compression of the vallecula (arrow). There are no signal changes of hemorrhage.

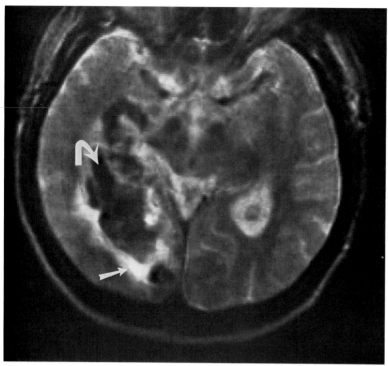

A

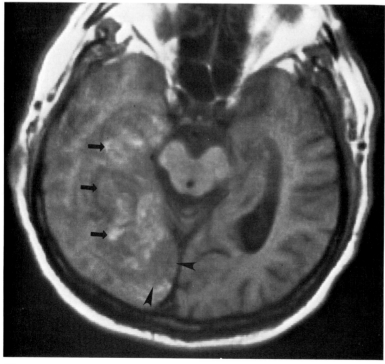

B

Fig. 2-3 Hemorrhagic infarction, MRI and CT scanning. (A) T₂-weighted MRI shows edema in the distribution of the right PCA within the occipital and medial temporal lobes (arrow). The hemorrhage within the infarcted inferior gyri is demonstrated by central low signal intensity (curved arrow). **(B)** T₁-weighted image shows the early subacute hemorrhage as regions of isointense and hyperintense signals (arrows). The edema of the infarction is seen as slight signal hypointensity, which is extending to the cortical surface (arrowhead). The MRI scan was obtained 4 days after the stroke. (*Figure continues.*)

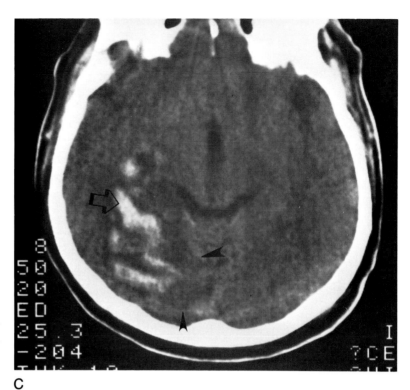

C

Fig. 2-3 (*Continued*) **(C)** CT scan performed on the day of the stroke shows acute serpiginous hemorrhagic high density in the right posterior inferior temporal and occipital lobe gyri (open arrow). The edema of the infarction is imaged as low density (arrowheads). **(D)** T$_2$-weighted MRI scan performed at a higher level demonstrates the edema of infarction of the right thalamus (arrowheads). The central lower intensity may represent slight hemorrhage. Faint high signal intensity is seen in the upper right occipital lobe representing the edge of the infarction. Combination of an infarction involving the ipsilateral medial temporal lobe, occipital lobe, and thalamus indicates occlusion of the right PCA.

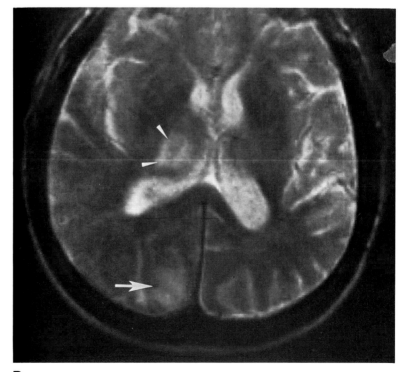

D

intensity signal of the edema. Low signal in the hemorrhage persists on the T$_2$-weighted images into the subacute phase (Fig. 2-3). (For details of brain hemorrhage, see later section.)

Regions of break in the blood-brain barrier can be demonstrated with Gd-DTPA contrast enhancement. The paramagnetic contrast agent leaks through the vessels and is seen on the T$_1$-weighted images as an intense signal within the low signal edema of infarction. The enhancement may be blotchy or show a char-

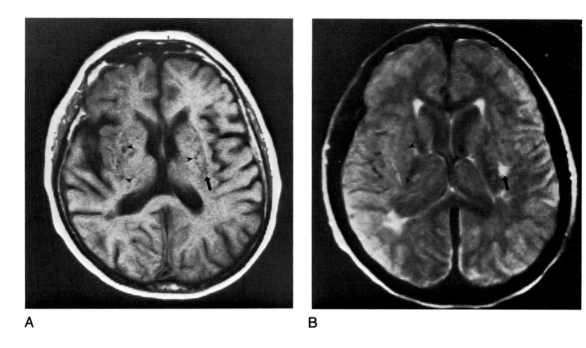

A

B

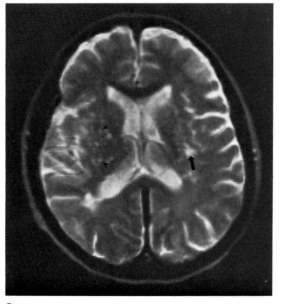

C

Fig. 2-4 Acute lacunar infarction and Virchow-Robin spaces, MRI. (A) T$_1$-weighted MRI through the basal ganglia shows multiple round hypointensities representing the dilated perivascular Virchow-Robin spaces around the perforating arteries (arrowheads). The lacunar infarction in the posterior left lentiform nucleus is virtually impossible to diagnose on this sequence (arrow). **(B)** Proton density image (SE 2500/30) demonstrates the Virchow-Robin spaces as being slightly hypointense and equivalent with CSF (arrowheads). The lacunar infarction is well demonstrated as a region of hyperintensity (arrow). **(C)** T$_2$-weighted study (SE 2500/90) shows the Virchow-Robin spaces as rounded regions of high signal intensity equivalent with CSF. The lacunar infarction is also of high signal intensity but is larger and less rounded than the pervascular spaces (arrow).

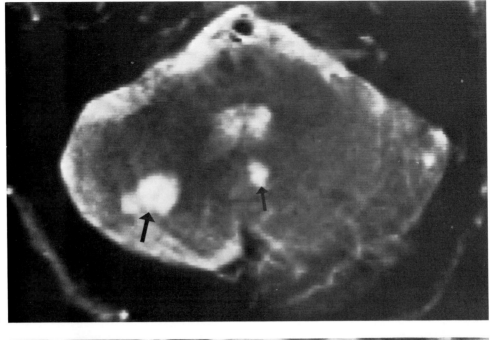

A

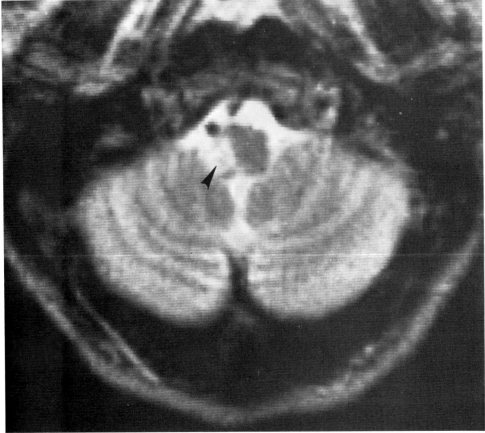

B

Fig. 2-5 Multiple acute cerebellar infarctions, lateral medullary infarction, MRI. (A) T$_2$-weighted MRI demonstrates two rounded regions of high signal intensity in the cerebellum (arrows). Small infarctions in the cerebellum are frequently rounded in configuration and must be differentiated from metastases. **(B)** Lateral medullary infarction. T$_2$-weighted MRI shows high signal intensity in the right side of the medulla. This lesion is a relatively common infarction from a branch occlusion of the PICA (arrowhead).

acteristic ribbon-like pattern of gyral enhancement similar to that seen on contrast-enhanced CT scans (see Fig. 2-15). Gd-DTPA enhancement may be seen within the first 24 hours and helps make a specific diagnosis of infarction. The enhancement may persist for 2 months.

For the detection of lacunar infarctions, MRI is considerably more sensitive than CT. The acute lacune is seen best as high signal intensity on T_2-weighted images (Fig. 2-4). After 1 week lacunes are seen on T_1-weighted images as focal regions of hypointensity. During the chronic stage the lacune has signal intensity equivalent to that of CSF (See also Figs. 10-5, 10-6).

Lacunes must be differentiated from enlarged Virchow-Robin spaces (Fig. 2-4). These spaces, present normally, may enlarge in older persons with chronic hypertension. The mechanism and significance are unknown. The spaces appear as multiple small (less than 5 mm), round structures of CSF-equivalent intensity on all MRI pulse sequences, most prominently in the lateral portion of the putamen. Lacunar infarcts tend to be larger and more oval in shape, and during the acute phase they show high signal on the proton density images (long TR/short TE).

The MRI technique is especially sensitive, compared with other modalities, for the detection of infarction within the cerebellum (Fig. 2-5), pons, and medulla. The infarctions correspond with specific vascular territories. Pontine infarctions are almost always unilateral and paramedian, corresponding with the distribution of the paramedian perforating vessels from the basilar artery (see Fig. 2-11B). Bilateral abnormality is more likely to represent myelinolysis or the high T_2 signal frequently found with aging (Fig. 2-6).

It is difficult to determine the precise age of an infarction using MRI. With time, infarctions become soft and relatively acellular. Cystic cavities may form and, when seen, indicate chronicity (Figs. 2-7 and 2-8). Cystic cavities have signal intensity similar to that of CSF.

Although MRI is more sensitive than other methods for the detection of infarction, it has some difficulty distinguishing infarction from other processes, particularly tumor and infection. The diagnosis of infarction is therefore made from the pattern of the edema on MRI and the appropriate clinical history. Gd-DTPA MRI may be specific if gyriform enhancement is seen.

Sodium MRI, MR spectroscopy (MRS), and MR blood flow studies are presently experimental and do

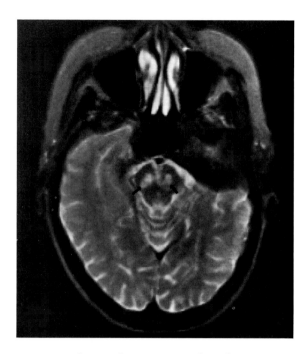

Fig. 2-6 High signal intensity within the pons associated with aging. Frequently there is irregular high signal intensity in the central portion of the pons and mesencephalon (arrows). It probably represents a conglomeration of small microinfarctions, which must not be misinterpreted as acute brain stem infarction.

not have clinical application. Their major use will probably be evaluating the effects of treatment on infarction and selecting patients for surgical intervention.

CT Scanning

Computed tomography is still the most often used imaging technique for a person with a stroke. Although it is less sensitive than MRI for the detection of infarction, it is highly specific for excluding significant disease processes that mimic or complicate ischemic infarction, e.g., hematoma, subarachnoid hemorrhage, chronic subdural hematoma, and tumor.

During the acute stage, CT scanning is dependent on the development of edema for detection of the infarcted tissue. The infarction is seen as a region of hypodensity. The quality and timing of the examination has great effect on the sensitivity of the CT scan for detecting infarction. During the early phase after an infarct (less than 2 days) there is usually insufficient edema for routine detection, and it is after this time that

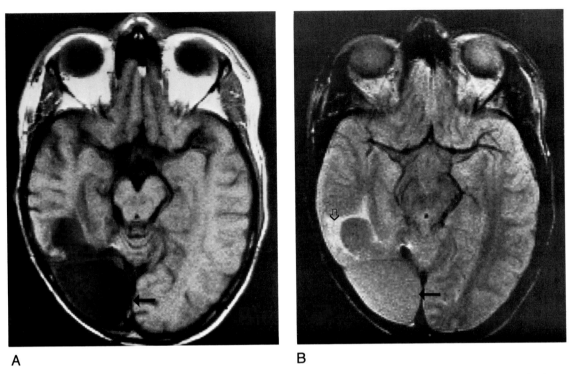

A   B

Fig. 2-7 Old infarction, MRI. (A) T_1-weighted image shows cystic degeneration in the right occipital lobe from prior ischemic infarction (arrow). The region is of CSF intensity. **(B)** Proton density MRI shows isointensity of the cystic cavitation (arrow). Characteristically, there are regions of high signal intensity surrounding the cystic change representing gliosis (open arrow).

most infarctions are seen. Large infarctions are more likely to be detected at an earlier time. Small infarctions less than 2 cm are not consistently seen. Infarctions within the cerebellum or pons are more difficult to image because of the artifacts inherent with CT scans of this region.

The first finding of an infarction is usually a subtle decrease in the density of the gray matter, so it becomes isodense with the underlying white matter (loss of gray–white matter differentiation) (Fig. 2-9). This change represents the cytotoxic edema of the gray matter. At this time there is little mass effect. If contrast enhancement is applied at this stage, there is normal enhancement of the adjacent normal cortex and accentuated hypodensity in the region of infarction because of ischemia (Fig. 2-10). If blood flow into an infarcted region has returned, this pattern may not be seen and the infarcted region may enhance normally.

Over the next few hours the edema increases, so there is more obvious well margined hypodensity of

both the gray matter and the white matter. Typically, the infarction appears trapezoidal or triangular, more or less corresponding with a recognizable vascular territory (Fig. 2-11). Swelling increases and is first seen as a subtle compression of the cerebral sulci when compared with the corresponding opposite side (Fig. 2-9). The mass effect increases to a maximum at 4 to 5 days. Edema tends to become greater with infarctions that are caused by embolization. Lysis of the embolus results in reperfusion of the infarcted tissue, causing greater vasogenic edema and sometimes hemorrhage. The edema may be severe enough to cause herniation of brain (see Fig. 5-34F) or hydrocephalus (Fig. 2-12).

Gradually, encephalomalacia or cystic cavitation develops. With CT scanning it is seen as a gradual decrease in the density of the infarcted tissue until it becomes stable about 2 months after the stroke. At this stage, the infarct becomes sharply demarcated. Encephalomalacia has a density slightly greater than that of CSF. Cystic cavitation is isodense with CSF (Fig.

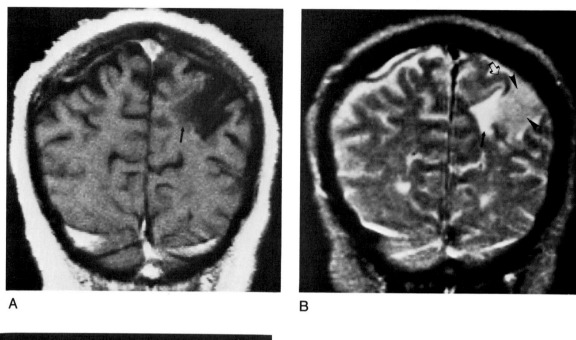

A

B

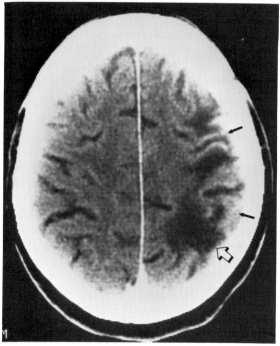

C

Fig. 2-8 Old hemispheric infarction, MRI and CT scans. (A) Coronal T₁-weighted MRI demonstrates a large hypointense region in the left mid-cortex. The cortex in this region has essentially dissolved, and there appears to be a cleft of CSF. Adjacent gliosis is represented by slight hypointensity (arrow). **(B)** T₂-weighted image shows the region of brain dissolution as of nearly CSF intensity (arrowheads). The adjacent gliosis is of greater intensity (arrow). The cortex over the gliotic region is preserved (open arrow). **(C)** Transaxial CT scan through the same region shows the cavitary dissolution as hypodensity (open arrow). There is preservation of cortical stroma through much of the infarction (arrows).

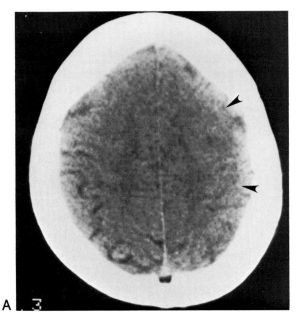

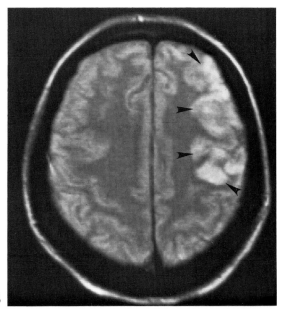

Fig. 2-9 Acute ischemic infarction, CT scan and MRI. (A) Nonenhanced CT scan shows subtle changes of a moderately large infarction of the left hemisphere. There is loss of the normally clear gray-white matter differentiation because of decreased density of the cortical gray matter from edema (arrowheads). There is also minimal swelling with compression of the regional sulci. **(B)** MRI (SE 2500/30) shows hyperintensity of the cortical and subcortical tissues in the region of the infarction (arrowheads).

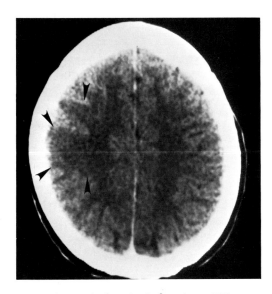

Fig. 2-10 Acute ischemic infarction, CT scan with contrast enhancement. Contrast-enhanced CT scan accentuates the early changes of acute infarction. The normal cortex shows increased density from perfusion with contrast-filled blood. The region of infarction does not show enhancement (arrowheads). The low-density region goes to the cortical surface, a finding characteristic of infarction.

2-13). Because the outer layers of the cortex are more resistant to ischemia, sometimes a cortical ribbon of intact tissue is preserved (Fig. 2-8). Local atrophy is present (Figs. 2-13 and 2-14).

Intravenous contrast enhancement may be used to define a region of infarction not seen with the nonenhanced examination or to differentiate an infarction from tumor. The enhancement with infarction may have many patterns. The principles are similar for both CT and MRI.

1. Ribbon-like cortical gyral enhancement (Fig. 2-15). This pattern is virtually pathognomonic of infarction. It is a result of a combination of loss of the blood-brain barrier and increased capillary filling of the gyri in the region of infarction ("luxury perfusion"). Only rarely does subarachnoid hemorrhage, meningitis, acute seizure, or hemiplegic migraine produce this type of enhancement.

2. Irregular blotchy enhancement (Fig. 2-16). Such enhancement may occur in any region of the infarction. It must be differentiated from the blotchy enhancement seen with grade III astrocytoma.

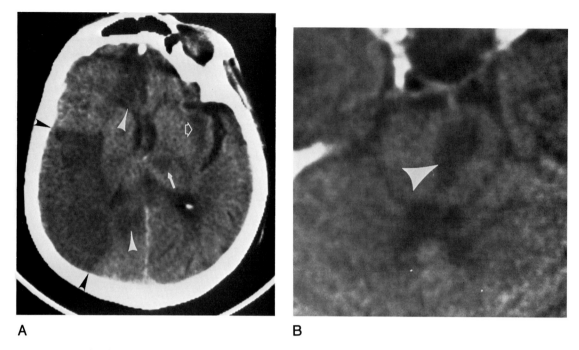

A   **B**

Fig. 2-11 Multiple ischemic infarctions, subacute phase. (A) A large infarction involves the right temporal lobe (black arrowheads). The margins of the infarct are sharp. There is mass effect with compression of the atrium of the right lateral ventricle. Additional infarcts are seen in the right pericallosal distribution (white arrowheads), left insula (open arrow), and left thalamus (arrow). **(B)** Pontine infarction. Well circumscribed low density is seen in the left side of the upper pons (arrowhead). The infarction, sharply demarcated at the midline, is causing slight expansion of the left side of the pons.

3. Homogeneous enhancement throughout the region of the infarction. This picture must be differentiated from the enhancement seen with lymphoma. Slight homogeneous enhancement may render a region of infarction isodense with the surrounding brain and invisible on enhanced CT scans.

4. Small, nonspecific, round, cortical or subcortical enhancement (Fig. 2-17). This picture may be indistinguishable from that produced by a small primary or metastatic tumor. Follow-up scans may be necessary to make the diagnosis.

5. Peripheral enhancement outlining the boundaries of the infarction. This pattern may be impossible to differentiate from a glioma, abscess, or prior hemorrhage. The enhancement may persist for a long time, contracting as the infarction matures. The clinical history, repeat scans, MRI, or a biopsy may be necessary to make the correct diagnosis. This type of enhancement is probably a result of the fibrovascular proliferation

that occurs around infarctions as part of the healing process.

Hemorrhage may be seen as regions of hyperdensity within the hypodense infarcted tissue (Fig. 2-3C). Most commonly they are petechial, although gyral hemorrhage is frequently seen. The small petechial hemorrhages seen on pathologic examination are not often demonstrated with CT scanning. High field MRI is more sensitive for the demonstration of hemorrhage within the infarction, especially during the subacute stage.

Lacunar infarctions are seen as regions of low density in the internal capsule (Fig. 2-13), basal ganglia, or thalamus (Fig. 2-11). CT scanning is not nearly as sensitive as MRI for detecting this type of infarction. Almost all lacunes progress to cystic change. After 2 months they are seen as sharply defined, round or oval, CSF-equivalent-density lesions.

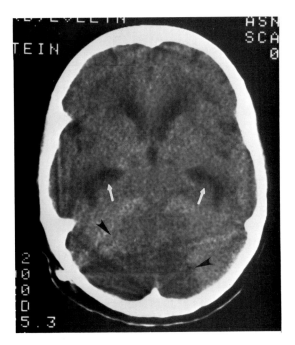

Fig. 2-12 Cerebellar infarction, acute. A large cerebellar infarction (arrowheads) has caused severe edema with obliteration of the basal cisterns and hydrocephalus (white arrows).

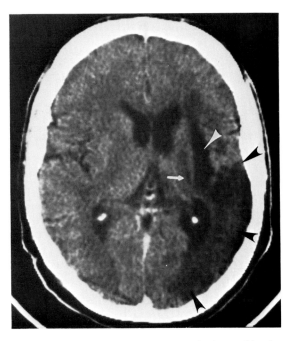

Fig. 2-13 Old infarctions, CT scan. The large old infarction in the region of the putamen (white arrowhead) has a density equivalent with that of CSF, representing cystic encephalomalacia. The large left posterior temporal infarction is hypodense but still has greater density than the CSF (arrowheads). It represents encephalomalacia and gliosis. Considerable atrophy is present, and there is dilatation of the left lateral ventricle and slight shift of the frontal horns to the left. Small lacunar infarctions are seen in the posterior limb of a left internal capsule (white arrow).

Angiography

The most reliable angiographic sign of cerebral infarction is the demonstration of an occluded artery. It usually appears as a gradual tapering of the lumen of the vessel until it is totally occluded. An avascular region appears distal to the occluded vessel and is best seen on the capillary ("brain stain") phase of the angiographic series. The circulation time through the infarcted region is usually slowed, with persistence of contrast in the proximal segments of the occluded vessels (Fig. 2-18).

Collateral circulation is often seen in the region of the infarction, filling the vessels distal to the occlusion in a retrograde fashion. The flow into the infarcted region is delayed, so the retrograde contrast filling of arteries is seen in the capillary or venous phases of the angiography when other arteries have cleared of contrast. The demonstration of collateral circulation is specific for vascular occlusion (Fig. 2-19).

When the vascular occlusion is peripheral to the circle of Willis, the collateral flow is between major vascular territories through the normal leptomeningeal anastomotic channels (Fig. 2-20). For example, with middle cerebral artery branch occlusion, the collateral flow into the peripheral middle cerebral branches beyond the occlusion comes from the ipsilateral pericallosal or posterior cerebral vessels passing through the small anastomotic channels over the convexity. The peripheral occluded branches fill from distal to proximal. Because of anatomic vascular variations and multiple sites of vascular occlusive disease, the collateral patterns are infinite and may become complex. The collateral pattern may become established within a matter of hours.

With occlusions proximal to the circle of Willis, the major vessels of the circle at the base of the brain normally provide the collateral flow (Fig. 2-21). The pat-

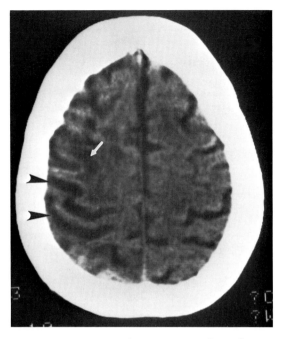

Fig. 2-14 Old parietal infarction. Nonenhanced CT scan shows regional enlargement of cerebral sulci (arrowheads). Hypodensity underneath the cortex represents gliosis (white arrow).

tern depends on the point of obstruction of the major vessel and the configuration of the vascular ring. Variation in the circle of Willis is common (more than 50 percent) (see Ch. 1). Segments of the circle of Willis may not be completely formed. Other rare communications (e.g., a primitive trigeminal artery) and dural anastamoses may also provide collateral flow (see Figs. 1-6 and 2-27A). Dural vessels may contribute to the collateral circulation of peripheral vessels by crossing the meninges to fill cortical arteries.

If blood flow is decreased on one side, collateral unopacified blood may enter at anastomotic points, causing a confusing picture of apparent "filling defects" or "streaming" (Fig. 2-19A). These voids in the contrast column occur at the characteristic entry sites for collateral flow (posterior communicating artery, anterior cerebral artery) and must not be misinterpreted as atherosclerotic narrowing or intraluminal clot.

There may be increased circulation in regions of infarction ("luxury perfusion"), particularly at the periphery (Fig. 2-19B). It is a result of local vasodilation in response to the ischemia. Arteriovenous shunting may be present. These perfusion changes are seen on the angiogram as a regional "blush" during the capil-

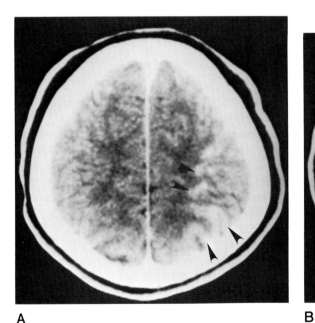

A

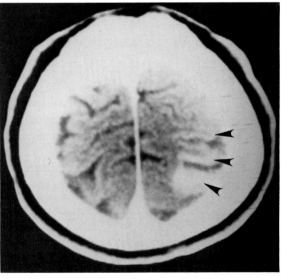

B

Fig. 2-15 Ischemic infarction, gyriform enhancement, CT scans. CT scans show the gyral pattern of enhancement associated with infarction. This pattern is almost pathognomonic of infarction or ischemia (see text).

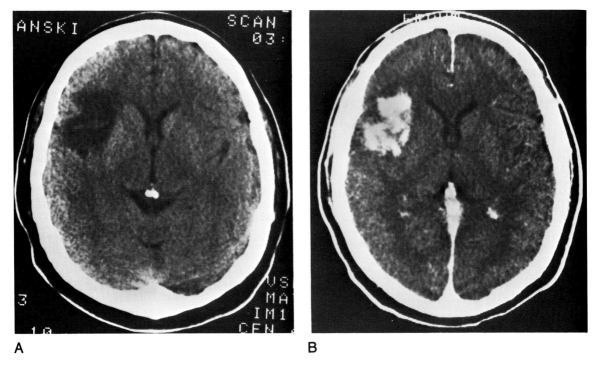

A   B

Fig. 2-16 Ischemic infarction, contrast enhancement. (A) A region of hypodensity is present in the right posterior lateral frontal lobe due to infarction. **(B)** Contrast CT scan shows dense, irregular enhancement throughout the region of infarction. It is difficult to differentiate this pattern of enhancement from that of an anaplastic astrocytoma (grade III).

lary phase commonly associated with one or more early filling veins, as noted below.

ANGIOGRAPHIC SIGNS OF INFARCTION

Specific signs
    Occluded artery
    Collateral circulation
    Delayed washout of contrast from occluded artery
Nonspecific signs
    Avascular region in the brain (capillary phase)
    Early draining vein from "luxury perfusion"
    Local mass effect

Radionuclide Scanning

The conventional radionuclide brain scan is no longer used to detect cerebral ischemia. The test depends on the accumulation of a labeled radiopharmaceutical in regions of blood-brain barrier breakdown. This technique is far less sensitive than CT scanning or MRI and has inferior spatial resolution. Positron emission computed tomography (PET) may be employed to give physiologic information and can define regions of ischemia in the brain. However, it requires the close proximity of a cyclotron for production of the positron-emitting radionuclides, as well as expensive scanning equipment; and, so far, the technique has been generally confined to research institutions. The xenon 133 washout study has been employed to measure regional cerebral blood flow, but it is not practical in the clinical setting.

Single photon emission computed tomography (SPECT) has also been developed. It uses conventional

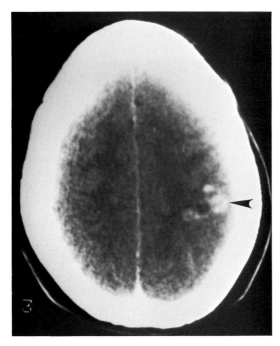

Fig. 2-17 Small infarction, cortical enhancement. A small region of nonspecific cortical enhancement is seen with this infarct. It is impossible to differentiate it from the early change of a peripheral glioblastoma (compare with Figure 5-16).

nuclear cameras modified to rotate about the patient. In a fashion similar to CT scanning, the information is reconstructed into tomographic slices. Spatial resolution is better than that seen with conventional scanning, but it is not nearly as fine as with CT scanning or MRI.

Radionuclide-labeled amines are used as tracers, the most common of which is [123]I-*N*-isopropyl-*p*-iodoamphetamine (^{123}I-IMP). This compound is specifically designed to integrate with the amine metabolism of the neuron. ^{123}I-IMP is lipid-soluble, so it rapidly diffuses across the normal blood-brain barrier and is efficiently extracted into the brain tissue. Although the exact mechanism for uptake into cells is not known, it is thought that the amine first attaches to any one of a number of amine surface receptors. It is then incorporated into the amine metabolism of the cell, remaining within the cell for hours before being broken down to a ketone and excreted. This tracer amine is incorporated only into viable, metabolically active cells. Its distribution is dependent on region cerebral blood flow.

The scan shows the distribution of the radionuclide within the brain. The tracer amine seeks metabolically active neurons. Therefore it is bound by the gray matter predominantly in the cerebral cortex. Less uptake is seen within the basal ganglia. Essentially no uptake is seen within the white matter. There is little or no binding of the tracer in regions where neurons are metabolically inactive. Ischemic and infarcted tissue is seen as a region of photon-deficiency (Fig. 2-22).

The major advantage of ^{123}I-IMP SPECT is its ability to define regions of nonlacunar cerebral infarction and ischemia earlier than with CT scanning. Infarcts may be defined consistently during the first day, whereas this is usually not possible with CT scanning. It may also show ischemic regions when the CT scan is normal. Studies comparing SPECT with MRI are not available at this time. In addition, the ^{123}I-IMP SPECT scan is more sensitive than the CT scan to regions of ischemia (penumbra of ischemia) that may surround the infarction. Thus the region of abnormality may appear larger on the SPECT scan than on the CT scan, giving a better indication of the volume of tissue involved in the ischemic event. The volume often explains symptoms not explained by the distribution of abnormality seen with CT scans. Abnormality extending beyond the boundaries outlined by CT scans suggests that this tissue is ischemic but not infarcted. This finding has prognostic implications for recovery. SPECT scanning may be used to determine the metabolic activity of regions of the brain supplied by stenotic vessels. It may potentially be used to assess the adequacy of collateral circulation and cerebral flow as

---

[123]I IMP SPECT SCANNING

Radionuclide distributed proportionally to
  Regional cerebral blood flow
  Metabolic activity of neurons
Advantages of technique
  Earlier definition of infarction
  Definition of penumbra ischemia
  Definition of infarction when CT scanning
  is negative
  Assessment of metabolic state of brain distal
  to stenotic lesions

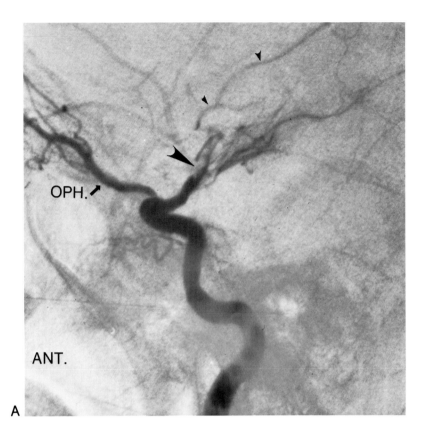

Fig. 2-18 Vascular occlusions from embolizations. (A) Supraclinoid ICA occlusion has occurred in a child secondary to embolization, with the clot outlined in the artery (large arrowhead). A small trickle of contrast has passed by the clot to fill a few middle cerebral branches (small arrowheads). **(B)** Multiple branch occlusions in the middle cerebral and anterior cerebral circulation has occurred secondary to embolization (arrowheads). The occluded vessels are seen as an abrupt termination of the contrast column. A large region of the frontal and parietal lobes is void of contrast-filled vessels because of the occlusions (curved arrow). Multiple occlusions in different vascular territories are characteristic of embolization.

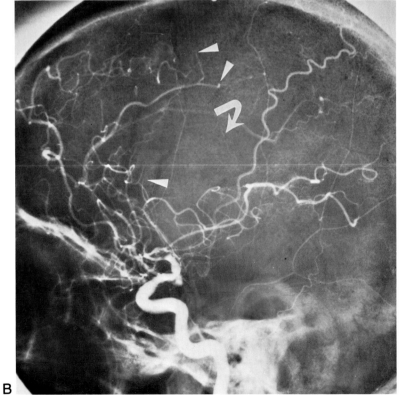

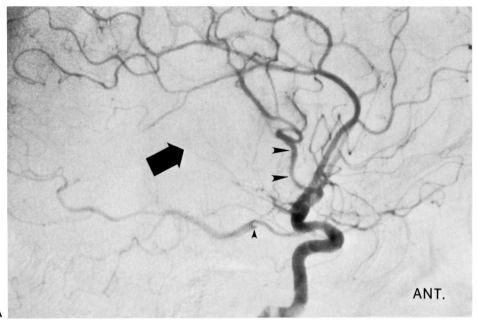

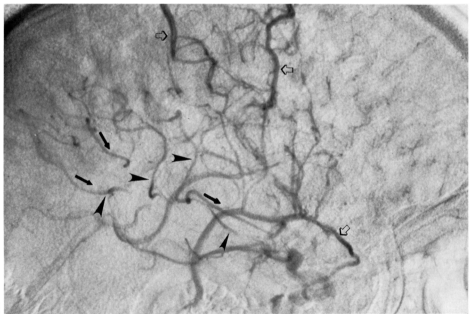

Fig. 2-19 Multiple branch occlusions of the middle cerebral artery. (A) A large vascular void is present in the arterial phase secondary to occlusion of most of the middle cerebral distribution (large arrow). Some anterior branches remain patent but show variation in caliber secondary to vasomotor instability (large arrowheads). It occurs frequently with infarction, particularly from embolization. Note the flow defect in the posterior cerebral artery at its junction with the posterior communicating artery (small arrowhead). It represents unopacified blood entering from the basilar artery. Such defects, particularly at junctions between circulations, must not be misinterpreted as intraluminal clot. **(B)** Collateral circulation. The late capillary phase shows retrograde filling of distal portions of occluded middle cerebral arteries (arrowheads). These vessels have filled through pial anastomoses from the pericallosal vessels. The black arrows indicate the direction of flow. Adjacent regional hyperemia ("luxury perfusion") is indicated by the prominent early draining veins (open arrows). A normal capillary phase is seen in the frontal lobe.

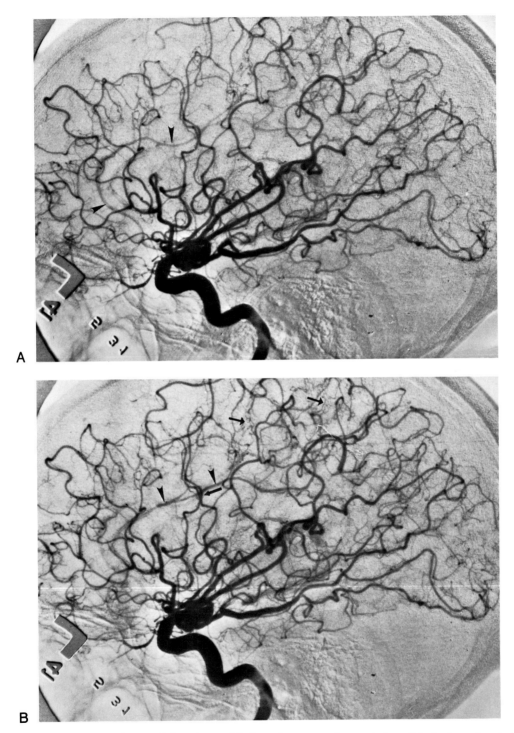

Fig. 2-20 Pericallosal occlusion. (A) Early arterial phase shows complete occlusion of the ipsilateral pericallosal artery. There is faint "flash filling" of the opposite pericallosal artery from cross filling through the anterior communicating artery (arrowheads). **(B)** Delayed arterial phase shows opacification of distal branches of the ipsilateral pericallosal artery from retrograde filling (arrowheads). Note the tangles of vessels representing the pial anastomoses between the middle cerebral and anterior cerebral circulations (arrows). (*Figure continues.*)

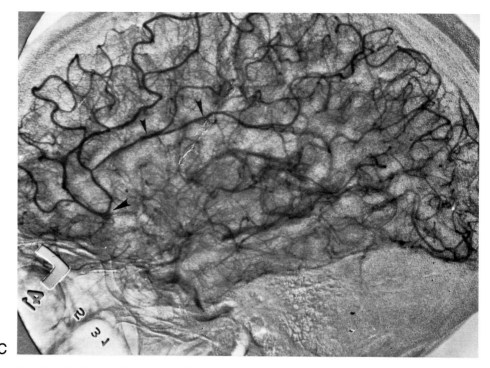

C

Fig. 2-20 (*Continued*) **(C)** Capillary phase demonstrates extensive opacification of the ipsilateral pericallosal branches from retrograde filling (arrowheads). Note the uniform "brain stain," indicating there is no ischemic tissue.

well as the need for surgical correction of stenotic lesions.

Because the amine tracer accumulates within neurons, it has virtually no distribution in the white matter, which means that the technique is of no use for evaluating lacunar infarction. SPECT scanning has been inconsistent in defining regions of transient ischemia in persons with TIA.

ATHEROSCLEROSIS

More than 90 percent of infarctions are caused by atherosclerosis and its complications. The important mechanisms are vessel narrowing and occlusion from the atherosclerotic plaque, platelet emboli from ulcerated plaques and subendothelial hemorrhages, and embolism from endocardial infarction or cardiac arrhythmia.

Atherosclerosis is a diffuse disease with focal accentuations. Most often, it is the focal disease that is the cause of the infarction or cerebral symptoms. The sig-

nificant focal lesion is the atherosclerotic plaque, which consists of subintimal proliferation of smooth muscle cells, excessive connective tissue matrix, and fat deposits in the intima. The plaque may grow large enough to cause complete occlusion of the vessel. Ulcers may form because of subintimal necrosis, resulting in the formation of fibrin-platelet thrombi on the ulcerated surface. Bits of these deposits may break loose and embolize to the cerebral vessels, causing TIA or infarction. Large thrombi may form, causing local occlusion or embolism to a major cerebral vessel.

Almost always, atherosclerotic plaques occur at or near bifurcations of vessels. Less commonly they occur at curves. In the carotid arteries the lesions are most commonly found at the bifurcation of the common carotid artery, at the origin of the common carotid artery from the aortic arch, in the cavernous portion of the internal carotid artery, and at the origin of the vertebral arteries.

Most of the attention is given to the carotid artery bifurcation. Persons with TIA and a more than 80 percent stenosis of the origin of the internal carotid artery

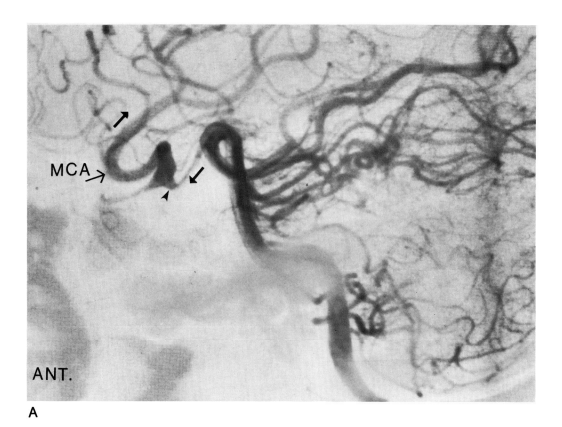

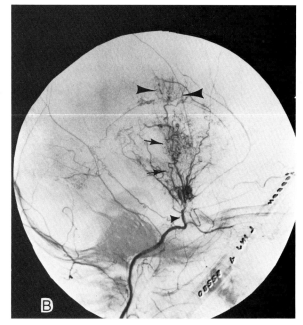

Fig. 2-21 Complete occlusion of the ICA. (A) The supraclinoid ICA fills via retrograde flow through the posterior communicating artery from the basilar circulation. The arrows indicate the direction of flow. Note the small infundibulum at the carotid origin of the posterior communicating artery (arrowhead). **(B)** Supraclinoid ICA occlusion, moyamoya. Gradual occlusion of the supraclinoid carotid artery has allowed development of extensive lenticulostriate collateral vessels that fill into deep medullary arteries. This deep form of collateralization, termed moyamoya, is usually found in children with multiple progressive intracranial arterial occlusions or neurofibromatosis 1. (Fig. B from Drayer, 1984, with permission.)

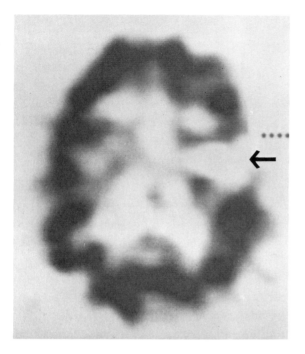

Fig. 2-22 SPECT radionuclide scan, cortical infarction. SPECT scan in the transaxial plane shows a photon-deficient region of the left parietal operculum representing infarcted tissue (arrow).

have been found to have a 5 to 10 percent risk per year of a stroke with permanent residual. Data also suggest that persons with asymptomatic internal carotid stenosis of more than 80 percent also have a much higher incidence of stroke in the distribution of that vessel compared with asymptomatic persons with less than 80 percent stenosis. Successful surgical removal of the plaque by endarterectomy decreases the risk of future stroke to about 2 to 3 percent per year in both groups. Some researchers believe that there is also a positive correlation between surface ulceration and future stroke, but it has not been proved. Data are poor or lacking for other lesions, such as stenosis at the origins of vessels from the aortic arch. About 25 percent of the population of the United States over 60 years of age have an asymptomatic stenosis of 50 percent or greater.

Duplex Ultrasonic Scanning

Noninvasive tests have been developed to detect disease in the extracranial cerebral vessels with the hope that it will lead to effective prophylactic therapy. Duplex scanning—the combination of B-mode imaging and pulsed Doppler flow detection—is now accepted as the standard noninvasive screening test for detection of atherosclerotic disease of the carotid bifurcation. It can reliably differentiate normal from abnormal and define the progression of disease. Oculoplethysmography is of limited value as it depends on a significant decrease in blood flow or blood pressure for the detection of abnormality.

Duplex scanning of the carotid arteries is usually performed to select those patients who may be candidates for carotid angiography. Most commonly this test is performed in those who have an asymptomatic carotid bruit. Patients found to have more than 80 percent stenosis generally go on to angiography for confirmation of the lesion prior to possible carotid endarterectomy. Those found to have less than 80 percent stenosis do not undergo angiography but have follow-up duplex scans at 6-month intervals to detect any progression of disease. Those persons with definite TIAs usually have angiography without prior duplex scanning. The sensitivity of duplex scanning for defining significant stenosis of the carotid arteries approaches 95 percent. The specificity for defining normal arteries is approximately 85 percent.

Most commonly the B-mode scan is performed in both the longitudinal and the transverse planes. The lumen of the vessel is identified as an anechoic channel. The common carotid artery is followed with the transducer along its course until the bifurcation is recognized, usually at the upper margin of the thyroid cartilage. The external carotid artery (ECA) normally branches anteromedially and the internal carotid artery (ICA) posterolaterally. In 5 percent of persons, this relation is reversed. The ICA is normally larger than the ECA. The ECA is reliably identified if the superior thyroid artery is seen to arise from its proximal portion. The waveform produced with the Doppler analysis also helps make this distinction. Because the ICA supplies a low-resistance intracranial circulation, it displays a diphasic pattern; in contrast, the ECA supplies a high-resistance circulation and displays a triphasic pattern.

The anatomic B-mode scan has not proved reliable for the identification of significant stenosis of the ICA. Ironically, the accuracy of the technique decreases as the severity of carotid stenosis increases. Thus it can be particularly difficult to identify severe stenosis or occlusion. Heavy calcification within a plaque may obscure the vessel lumen. Attempts have been made to correlate the texture of the plaque with its composition and clinical prognosis, but the results are inconsistent. The more benign fibrofatty plaque is seen as a relatively homogeneous echogenic deposit with smooth margins bulging into the vessel lumen (Fig. 2-23A & B). Calcific plaques are strongly echogenic with irregular margins and acoustic shadowing (Fig. 2-23C). Ulcerations are seen as niches in the lumen, but they cannot be reliably identified.

Considerable attention has been given to the hemorrhagic plaque. The theory is that ischemia of the vessel wall, produced as part of the atherosclerotic process, damages the vasa vasorum, which then rupture producing an acute hemorrhage. The hemorrhage enlarges the plaque, often causing stenosis or occlusion of the vessel lumen. The hemorrhage may rupture into the lumen, producing distal emboli and a residual ulcer crater. A plaque with a heterogeneous internal echo

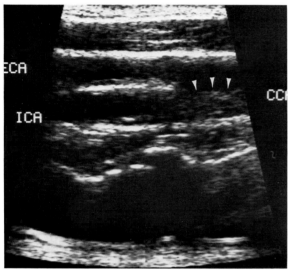

A

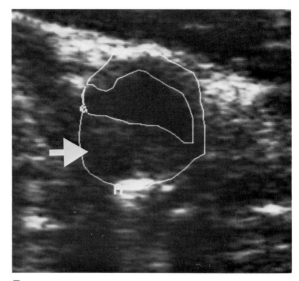

B

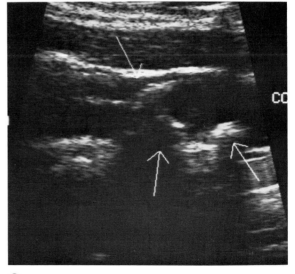

C

Fig. 2-23 B-Mode ultrasound, ICA plaque. (A) Fibrofatty plaque. Longitudinal study demonstrates a smoothly marginated, homogeneous, echogenic mound constricting the lumen of the distal CCA and the proximal ICA (arrowheads). **(B)** Fibrofatty plaque. Transverse view of the distal CCA demonstrates the compromise of the cross-sectional area of the vessel lumen by the posterior plaque (arrow). **(C)** Calcified plaque. Longitudinal study shows highly echogenic calcification within a posterior plaque (arrows). Note the acoustic shadowing from the calcium. (Courtesy of Dr. Howard Raymond, Holyoke Hospital.)

pattern and anechoic regions is thought to have a high probability of containing hemorrhage and surface ulceration.

Useful information is obtained from the pulsed Doppler spectral analysis and blood flow rate calculations. The examination is done with a constant probe angulation. Ideally, the probe angulation is as close to parallel as possible with the vessel to be measured. Practically, about 60 degrees of angulation is possible and adequate. The ultrasound equipment compensates for the angulation when calculating the blood velocity within the vessel lumen. The pulsed technique allows sampling from a small volume of fluid at a specific point within the lumen of the vessel. The B-mode anatomic study is used to set the point of Doppler sampling.

Vessel narrowing results in increased velocity through the region of stenosis. The increase becomes more pronounced with higher grades of stenosis but decreases as the stenosis exceeds 95 percent. The Doppler frequency shift is directly proportional to the change in velocity of the blood cells; that is, the observed peak frequency (in kilohertz) increases with the increase in blood velocity across the narrowed segment.

In addition, stenosis causes turbulence because of disruption of the normal laminar flow. The turbulence produces considerable variation in the speed of flow at different points in the cross section. Sometimes there is even reversal of flow in focal segments. Thus a wide range of frequency shifts is seen, referred to as *spectral broadening.* This broadening generally becomes more pronounced with greater stenosis.

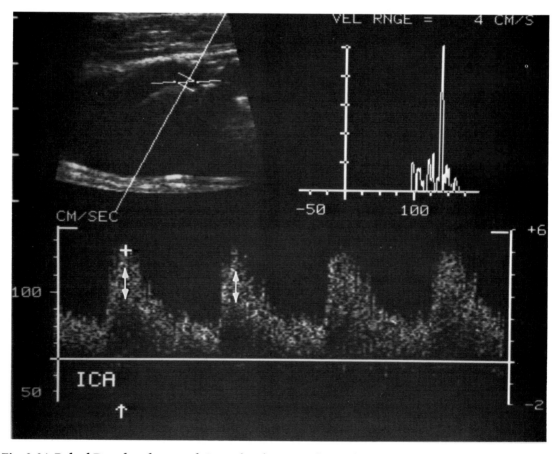

Fig. 2-24 Pulsed Doppler ultrasound. Spectral analysis was taken at the level indicated in the upper left of the figure. The plot shows spectral broadening (opposed arrows), higher peak frequency, and a prolonged peak, characteristic of significant carotid stenosis. (Courtesy of Dr. Howard Raymond, Holyoke Hospital.)

The spectrum of frequency within the vessel lumen is plotted on a graph. By convention, the frequency is along the vertical axis, the time is along the horizontal axis, and the amplitude of echo at each frequency is represented by a gray scale point. The peak frequency increases and the spectral range broadens with carotid stenosis (Fig. 2-24). A color display of the spectral change can make the changes more obvious and easier to recognize (Table 2-1).

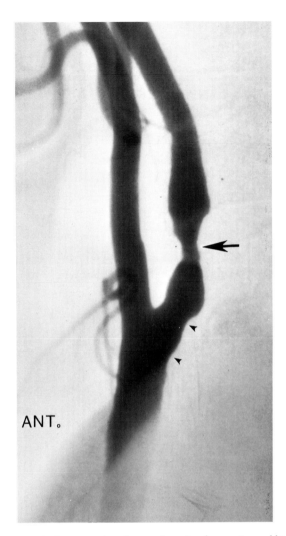

Fig. 2-26 Concentric atherosclerotic plaque. Lateral bifurcation angiography shows significant concentric stenosis of the proximal internal carotid artery just distal to the bifurcation (arrow). A small plaque is seen in the proximal bifurcation (arrowheads).

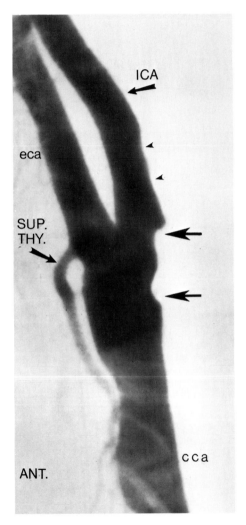

Fig. 2-25 Atherosclerotic plaque. A small atherosclerotic plaque is present that involves the posterior wall of the proximal ICA at the carotid bifurcation (arrows). Minimal plaque is seen more distally (arrowheads). SUP. THY. = superior thyroid artery; cca = common carotid artery; eca = external carotid artery.

Table 2-1 Spectral Analysis Criteria for ICA Stenosis

% Stenosis	Spectral Shift	
	kHz	cm/sec
0–30	< 3.5	< 110
31–50	3.5–4.0	110–125
51–90	4–8	125–250
91–95	> 8	> 250
95–99	Variable, may be < 4	
Occlusion	0	

Adapted from Grant EG, et al: Cerebrovascular ultrasound imaging. Radiol Clin North Am 26:5, 1122, 1988.

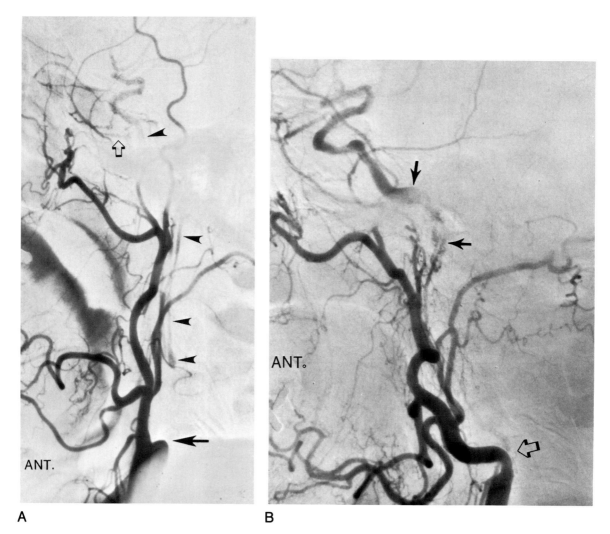

A   B

Fig. 2-27 Complete ICA occlusion with reconstitution. (A) Lateral common carotid arteriography demonstrates the stump of a complete ICA occlusion at its origin (arrow). Distally the cervical ICA is reconstituted (arrowheads), in this case by flow through small collateral vessels from the ECA circulation. Additional collateral flow can be seen through cavernous anastomoses into the cavernous portion of the ICA (open arrow). Patency of the distal portion of the cervical ICA makes endarterectomy technically possible. **(B)** Complete occlusion of the ICA is present (open arrow). There is reconstitution in the petrous portion by way of anastomoses through the ascending pharyngeal artery (arrows).

Angiography

Angiography remains the "gold standard" technique for the detection and evaluation of focal atherosclerotic disease. A plain film rather than the digital technique is preferred, as it provides better spatial resolution. Digital subtraction angiography is also susceptible to artifacts produced by motion and calcium within plaques.

The optimal examination is done with the catheter placed within the common carotid artery about 2 cm proximal to the bifurcation. Care is taken not to pass the guide wire through the region of the bifurcation.

Most lesions are located on the posterior or posterolateral wall of the ICA and are best seen on the lateral projection. Oblique or AP projections are needed to define the true size of the plaque and full extent of ulcerations as the disease process is often asymmetric.

The plaque is seen as a bulge into the vessel lumen (Fig. 2-25). The degree of stenosis of the vessel is determined by measuring the narrowest point seen on the two projections and comparing it with the normal portion of the ICA distal to the carotid bulb. The relation is expressed as the percent stenosis.

$$\frac{\text{Diameter of normal segment} - \text{Diameter of stenotic segment}}{\text{Diameter of normal segment}} \times 100$$

This technique is widely used, although there are some inherent inaccuracies. There is always the problem of which segment of the ICA to choose as a baseline; and with severe stenosis, decreased flow results in a smaller vessel lumen of the normal artery distal to the stenosis.

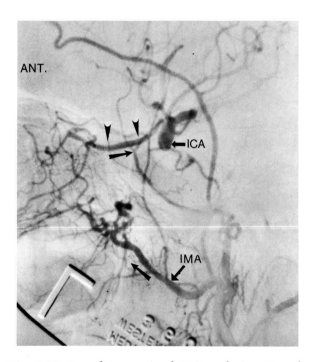

Fig. 2-28 Complete proximal ICA occlusion. Lateral common carotid arteriography demonstrates collateral circulation from the internal maxillary artery (IMA) to the ophthalmic artery (arrowheads) to fill the distal cavernous and supraclinoid portions of the ICA. The arrow below the ophthalmic artery indicates the direction of flow.

A stenosis of 50 percent causes a pressure gradient across the stenosis, but the flow rate remains normal. Stenosis of more than 70 percent causes a proportionally decreased flow rate (Fig. 2-26). The greater the length of the stenosis the greater is the effect on flow for a given degree of stenosis.

Special care must be taken during evaluation of the completely occluded ICA. Subtraction films are done so that a small trickle of contrast into a still patent ICA can be detected (Fig. 2-27). A prolonged injection into the common carotid artery is best in this situation. Chronic occlusion usually shows a blunt "stump." A high grade stenosis that is still patent or a recent occlusion most often shows tapering to the level of occlu-

---

PATTERNS OF COLLATERAL CIRCULATION WITH EXTRACRANIAL VASCULAR OCCLUSIONS

ICA occlusion
  Contralateral ICA – anterior communicating artery – MCA
  Posterior cerebral artery – posterior communicating artery
  Pterygopalatine branches of the internal maxillary artery – ethmoidal branches – ophthalmic artery
  Superficial temporal artery – ophthalmic artery
  Facial artery – inferior cavernous branches – ICA
  Vidian artery – ICA in the petrous portion
  Middle meningeal artery – ophthalmic artery along sphenoid ridge
CCA occlusion
  Vertebral artery – ECA – ICA
  Opposite ECA through midline anastomoses
Vertebral occlusion
  ECA – muscular neck branches – vertebral artery
Proximal subclavian occlusion
  "Subclavian steal" syndrome

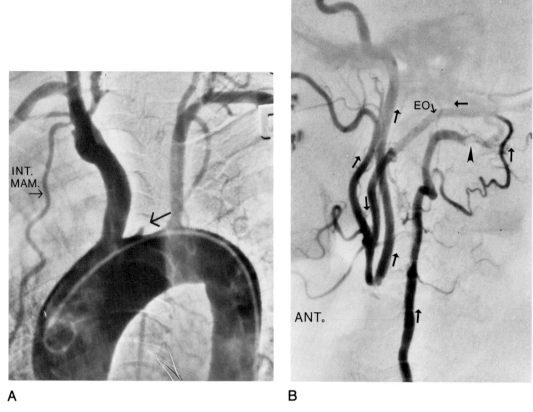

Fig. 2-29 Complete occlusion of the left common carotid artery. (A) Aortic arch examination shows the small "stump" of contrast at the base of a complete occlusion of the left ICA (arrow). INT. MAM. = internal mammary artery. **(B)** Lateral neck view of vertebral injection shows collateral circulation from muscular branches of the distal vertebral artery to the external occipital artery (EO). Retrograde flow in the external occipital artery then fills the internal maxillary and internal carotid arteries. Arrows show the direction of flow. Note the "washout" defect in the distal vertebral artery from unopacified collateral circulation (arrowhead).

sion. Even with the best technique, there is an occasional false-positive diagnosis of complete occlusion.

With complete occlusion, usually there is reconstitution of the distal intracranial ICA through collateral vessels. Mostly it occurs via the ethmoidal branches of the external carotid artery filling the ophthalmic artery in a retrograde fashion, which in turn fills the supraclinoid ICA (Fig. 2-28). Also, the posterior communicating artery allows reversal of flow from the vertebral artery (Fig. 2-21). This situation causes "streaming" of unopacified contrast into the supraclinoid ICA, which must not be interpreted as intraluminal clot or stenosis.

Sometimes there is enlargement of cavernous branches of the external carotid artery filling the "siphon" or small branches from the neck filling the ICA artery within the carotid canal (Fig. 2-27). The site of reentry of contrast into the ICA should be noted. With reentry within the carotid canal or more proximally, endarterectomy is still possible with complete occlusion of the ICA. With reentry at the level of the cavernous portion of the ICA or beyond, endarterectomy is generally considered inadvisable.

Stenosis at the origin of the external carotid artery (ECA) is usually of little hemodynamic importance but

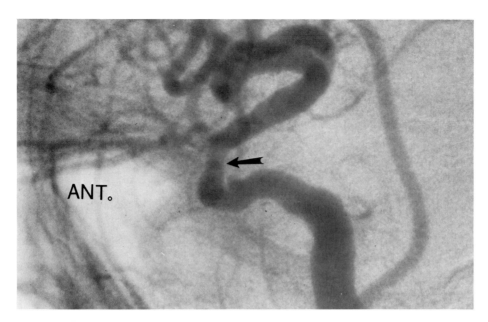

Fig. 2-30 Atherosclerosis, cavernous portion ICA. Atherosclerotic lesions may become severe in the cavernous portion of the ICA (arrow). This lesion is highly associated with death from stroke or myocardial infarction within 5 years.

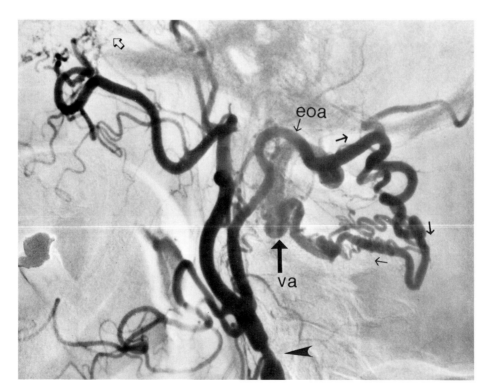

Fig. 2-31 Occlusion of the vertebral artery and ICA. Lateral neck angiography with common carotid injection shows complete occlusion of the ICA and stenosis of the ECA (arrowhead). Cavernous anastomosis branches can be seen from the distal internal maxillary artery (open arrow). Collateral flow occurs through the EOA into the occluded ipsilateral VA (large arrow). The small arrows indicate the direction of flow through the anastomotic muscular branches.

may produce a bruit. It may be important, however, if it interferes with ECA collateral flow when the ICA is occluded.

It is important to recognize "tandem" lesions, as they may be of hemodynamic significance and have bearing on the selection of patients for endarterectomy of a proximal ICA lesion. The most common lesions seen at sites other than the bifurcation appear at the origin of the common carotid artery at the aortic arch (Fig. 2-29) and in the cavernous portion of the ICA (Fig. 2-30).

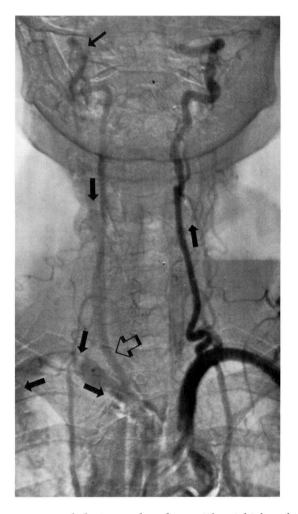

Fig. 2-32 Subclavian steal syndrome. There is high grade stenosis of the innominate artery. Injection into the left subclavian artery shows antegrade flow into the left VA. Retrograde flow occurs down the opposite VA to fill the subclavian artery as well as the right CCA (open arrow). The arrows indicate the direction of flow.

Stenotic atherosclerotic lesions of more than 70 percent often occur at the origins of the brachiocephalic and vertebral arteries (Fig. 2-31). These lesions are generally defined using aortic arch angiography. Severe stenosis of a proximal subclavian artery causes collateral circulation to develop from reversal of flow in the ipsilateral vertebral artery to fill the distal subclavian territory. This disorder is the *subclavian steal syndrome,* with most of the collateral blood supplied by the opposite vertebral artery through the junction at the basilar artery (Fig. 2-32). Subclavian steal is usually well tolerated by the patient, with claudication of the affected arm being the predominant symptom. Only with stenosis of the origin of the opposite vertebral artery or with an inadequate circle of Willis are there signs of vertebrobasilar insufficiency. Patterns of collateral flow with extracranial vascular occlusion are given (see previous box).

Ulceration

Ulceration occurs commonly on the surface of the atherosclerotic plaque. Most ulcers are small and shallow, whereas others are large and extend deeply into the plaque to its base (Fig. 2-33). Platelet and fibrin thrombi form on the surface of the ulceration. It is estimated that more than 50 percent of ulcerations are not detectable with high quality magnification angiography. Moreover, in about 30 percent, surface irregularities thought to be ulcerations are found to be simply surface undulations and not ulcers. Therefore, except for larger craters, the accuracy of the diagnosis of surface ulceration is poor.

Surface fibrin and platelet thrombi are difficult to detect. Sometimes an obvious intraluminal clot can be seen within the vessel lumen (Fig. 2-34). More commonly, however, thrombus cannot be differentiated from the underlying plaque. In general, angiography significantly underestimates the amount of fibrin thrombus present.

Dilatation and Vessel Tortuosity

Atherosclerosis causes ectasia (dilation and elongation) of the vessel. Ectasia is most common in the aorta and the brachiocephalic vessels but may also be seen intracranially (Fig. 2-35). In the extreme, fusiform aneurysms form (see Fig. 3-17). There is a high association with hypertension.

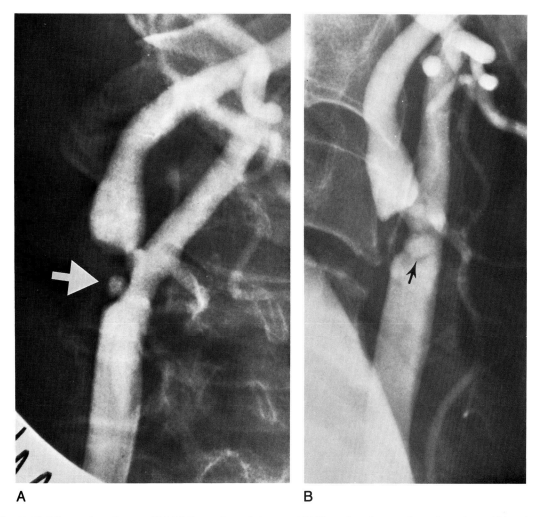

A   B

Fig. 2-33 Ulcerative plaque. (A) Oblique view of the carotid bifurcation shows a deep ulceration within a large posterolateral atherosclerotic plaque (arrow). **(B)** On the direct lateral view it is difficult to identify the ulcer (arrow), as it is seen more "en fasse."

Intracranial Atherosclerosis

Atherosclerosis also involves the intracranial vessels. The most common site is the cavernous portion of the ICA (Fig. 2-30). Severe cavernous segment disease indicates a poor prognosis, as 50 percent of patients die of severe stroke or myocardial infarction within 5 years. Other sites include the supraclinoid carotid artery, the proximal middle cerebral artery, and less commonly any of the peripheral branches (Fig. 2-37) and the basilar artery. Branch narrowings tend to be focal at bifurcations and without intervening regions of dilatation as

seen with vasculitis. At times it is difficult to differentiate atherosclerotic change from arteritis or spasm.

EXTRACRANIAL NONATHEROSCLEROTIC ARTERIOPATHY

Dissection

Dissection (dissecting hematoma) of a major extracranial artery is an uncommon event. It may occur spontaneously or following neck trauma. Because the disease

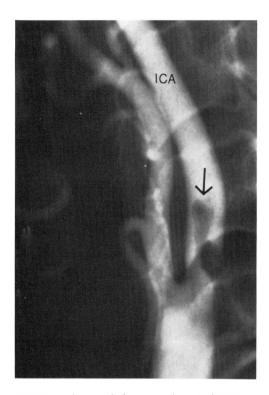

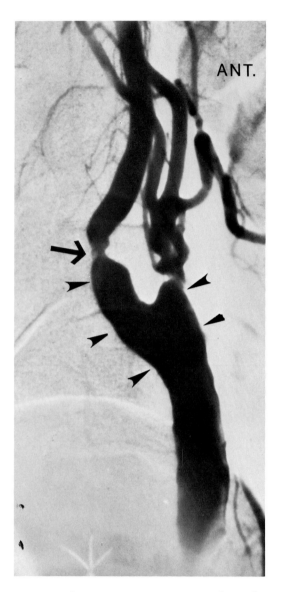

Fig. 2-34 Intraluminal clot. Lateral cervical CCA angiography demonstrates an intraluminal clot arising from a region of minimal disease in the proximal ICA (arrow).

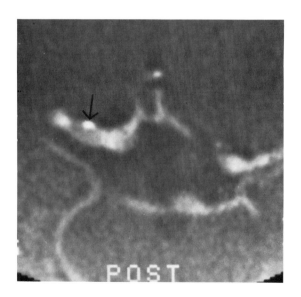

Fig. 2-35 Atherosclerotic ectasia. Contrast-enhanced CT scan through the base of the brain shows ectasia of the supraclinoid ICA and the proximal MCA (arrow).

Fig. 2-36 Endarterectomy, recurrent atherosclerotic stenosis. Following endarterectomy, the vessel lumen becomes larger and has smooth margins (arrowheads). If stenosis recurs, it is usually found at the distal end of the endarterectomy (arrow). Less commonly it is found at the proximal margin.

is generally not recognized unless angiography or MRI of the neck is performed, spontaneous dissection of the extracranial carotid and vertebral arteries is probably more common than is actually perceived. Patients with spontaneous dissection are usually younger than 50 years, and there seems to be a female predilection. It is a

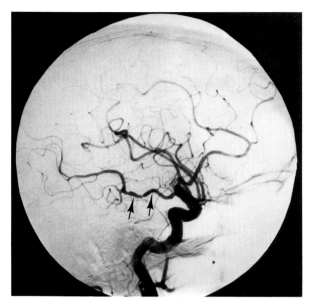

Fig. 2-37 Atherosclerotic narrowing. An irregular narrowing consistent with atherosclerosis (arrows) is seen in the posterior cerebral artery. Such an irregular, nontapered appearance of an artery distinguishes atherosclerosis from vasospasm. (From Drayer, 1984, with permission.)

serious problem that frequently causes permanent neurologic deficits and may cause death from massive hemispheric infarction.

There are two clinical syndromes associated with dissection of the carotid arteries: (1) unilateral headache (hemicrania) and unilateral Horner's syndrome (oculosympathetic palsy) with or without acute contralateral cerebral symptoms; and (2) unilateral headache with delayed contralateral cerebral symptoms. Rarely, cranial nerves 9-11 may be involved. Frequently, the dissection occurs during strenuous exercise, such as marathon running or weight lifting, but it may occur at any time. There may be no predisposing factor, but there is a higher incidence of dissection in patients with connective tissue disorders or fibromuscular hyperplasia.

The dissection is an acute event. It usually regresses without therapy but occasionally progresses to cause permanent, complete occlusion of the vessel. It seldom recurs. Presently, angiography is the most accurate procedure for making the diagnosis and is performed in young patients who have the symptoms outlined above. MRI may supplant angiography in the future.

The most common angiographic finding is a tapered stenosis of the proximal ICA (Fig. 2-38). The stenosis

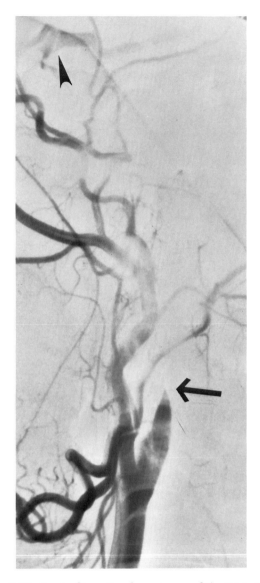

Fig. 2-38 Acute dissecting hematoma of the ICA. Lateral cervical projection of a common carotid injection shows tapered occlusion of the ICA. It is a nonspecific finding of occlusion, but in the appropriate clinical setting it is usually indicative of a dissection. Note the collateral filling into the supraclinoid ICA through the ophthalmic artery.

may be asymmetric and have a "wavy" configuration along one border of the artery (Fig. 2-39). Different projections may be necessary to demonstrate this important finding. The other possible patterns are a long, tapered stenosis and total occlusion with a tapered proximal portion. A false lumen may be filled with

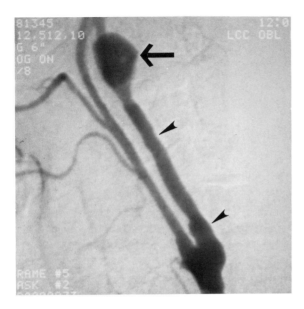

Fig. 2-39 Acute dissecting hematoma, ICA. A dissected segment is patent but shows irregular, wavy "margins" (arrowheads). An aneurysm has developed at the distal end of the dissection (arrow).

contrast, and a saccular-appearing aneurysm may occur at either end of the dissected segment (Fig. 2-39). These saccular aneurysms may enlarge and must be followed with repeat angiography. The termination of the dissection is usually seen as an abrupt return to the normal caliber of the vessel. Distal intraluminal thrombotic emboli may be seen at any level of the intracranial circulation. The dissection may extend into intracranial segments of the vessel and be associated with subarachnoid hemorrhage. It is sometimes possible to identify the hemorrhage in the wall of the ICA with contrast CT scans. MRI may identify the dissecting hematoma in the vessel wall as high signal intensity on both T_1 and T_2 weighted images (Fig. 2-40).

The dissection most commonly involves the cervical and intracanalicular segments of the ICA (60 percent), the cervical segment only (30 percent), or a long segment extending from just above the carotid sinus through to the cavernous portion of the ICA (5 percent). The remaining dissections involve the vertebral artery or the middle cerebral artery. Criteria for surgical intervention are not established. Most patients are treated with anticoagulation to decrease the risk of embolic complication.

Fibromuscular Dysplasia

Fibromuscular dysplasia (FMD) is an arteriopathy of unknown etiology. Segmental overgrowth of fibrous and muscular tissue occurs in the media leading to vessel stenosis. It occurs most frequently in the middle segments of the cervical ICA but may also involve the upper vertebral arteries and the branches of the external carotid arteries. It is bilateral in more than 50 percent. There may be an associated intracranial berry aneurysm or involvement of the renal arteries with FMD, causing renovascular hypertension. The lesions may be found incidentally, but they are also associated with TIAs.

The diagnosis is made with angiography. The characteristic finding is an irregular "string of beads" configuration of the vessel lumen (Fig. 2-41), wherein the lumen is narrowed at multiple levels usually with intervening regions of dilated luminal diameter. There also may be only diffuse smooth narrowing of the vessel, which is difficult to differentiate from spontaneous carotid dissection. Vascular spasm must be differentiated from FMD. Spasm in the extracranial vessels is almost always caused by direct stimulation of the vessel wall by the catheter or the guide wire during the performance of angiography. With spasm, the vessel lumen has no regions of dilatation but does have a more regular pattern of narrowings that change with time.

When associated with CNS symptoms, FMD can best be treated with percutaneous balloon angioplasty, which dilates the narrowed segment and usually stops the CNS symptoms. No treatment is given if the patient is asymptomatic and the lesion is found by chance.

Takayasu's Arteritis

Takayasu's disease is an acute inflammation of the aorta and brachiocephalic vessels that occurs in adolescent and young adult women. Systemic symptoms may be present that are similar to other collagen vascular diseases. Angiography demonstrates smooth, long segments of stenosis in the proximal subclavian and common carotid arteries. The distal portions of these vessels are not affected. Multiple vessel involvement occurs in 80 percent of cases. The stenosis may progress to complete occlusion. Calcification may be seen similar to that which occurs with atherosclerosis. The aorta usually appears normal, but during the later phases of the disease it may become aneurysmal predominantly in the ascending portion.

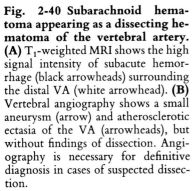

Fig. 2-40 Subarachnoid hematoma appearing as a dissecting hematoma of the vertebral artery. **(A)** T_1-weighted MRI shows the high signal intensity of subacute hemorrhage (black arrowheads) surrounding the distal VA (white arrowhead). **(B)** Vertebral angiography shows a small aneurysm (arrow) and atherosclerotic ectasia of the VA (arrowheads), but without findings of dissection. Angiography is necessary for definitive diagnosis in cases of suspected dissection.

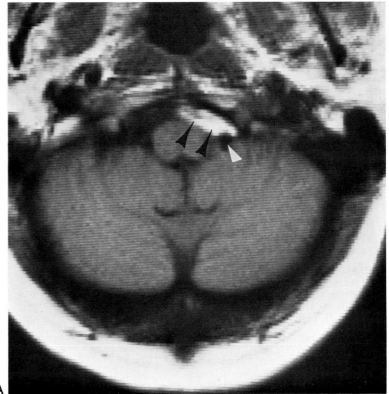

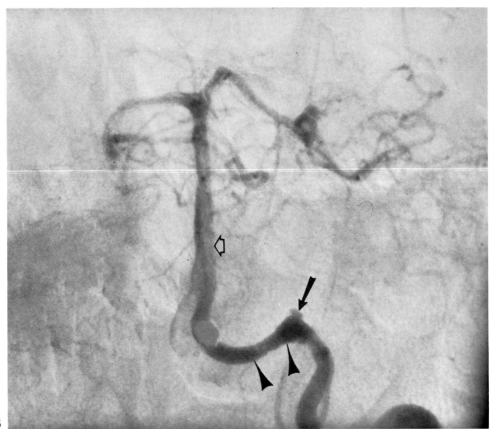

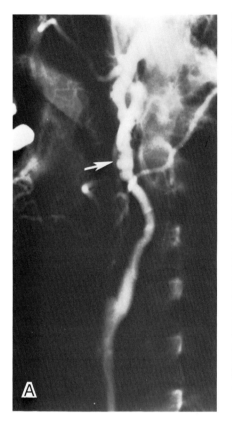 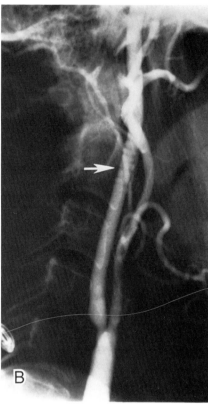

Fig. 2-41 Fibromuscular dysplasia and vascular spasm. (A) Fibromuscular dysplasia. Irregular dilatation and narrowing of the distal cervical segment of the ICA represents fibromuscular dysplasia (arrow). **(B)** Vascular spasm. Regular concentric contractions are demonstrated in the cervical ICA (arrow). The regular spacing and lack of dilatation differentiate spasm from fibromuscular dysplasia. (From Drayer, 1984, with permission.)

INTRACRANIAL NONATHEROSCLEROTIC ARTERIOPATHY

Numerous disease processes can affect the intracranial vessels. These disorders are demonstrated by angiography as luminal narrowings, irregularities, dilatations, and occlusions. The morphologic changes may be localized or diffuse. The vascular changes may be the result of an extrinsic process, such as meningitis or tumor, or an intrinsic process, such as an autoimmune necrotizing angiitis. Because the arterial wall can react in only a limited number of ways to pathologic agents, most of the arteriopathies have similar appearances on angiography. A few have characteristic narrowing patterns, and specific distributions can help to limit the differential diagnosis; but the diagnosis is often made by exclusion of the various known etiologic factors or by biopsy of the meninges or involved vessels. The clinical history is important for defining the diagnosis.

The arteriopathies may cause acute or chronic cerebral symptoms such as headache, fever, personality change, TIAs, infarctions, and hemorrhage. If severe, the resulting ischemia may cause vast regions of brain destruction progressing to a vegetative state or death. Arteriopathies must be differentiated from vascular spasm, atherosclerosis, and dissection. The causes of angiopathy are listed in Table 2-2. Some of the categories are arbitrary, as the etiology and process are often poorly defined.

Hypertensive Arteriopathy; Intracerebral Hematoma

Hypertension is perhaps the major cause of cerebrovascular disease. If affects the middle-aged adult and the elderly. Hypertension has a causative role in extracranial atherosclerotic plaques, lipohyalinosis of the perforating arteries at the base of the brain, and fusiform aneurysms of the aorta and intracranial vessels. The atherosclerotic lesions and their complications have been discussed in previous sections.

Table 2-2 Causes of Arteriopathy in Adults

Extracranial arteriopathy
    Atherosclerosis
    Spontaneous dissection
    Fibromuscular disease
    Takayasu's arteritis
    Temporal arteritis
Intracranial arteriopathy
    Hypertension
        Hematoma (microaneurysms of perforating
            arteries)
        Hypertensive encephalopathy
        Subcortical arteriosclerotic encephalopathy of
            Binswanger
    Infectious arteritis
        Bacteria
        Fungus
        Tuberculosis
        Syphilis
        Mycotic aneurysm
    Collagen vascular disease
        Lupus
        Thrombotic thrombocytopenic purpura
        Scleroderma
        Rheumatoid arthritis
        Dermatomyositis
    Necrotizing and granulomatous arteritis
        Polyarteritis nodosa
        Temporal arteritis
        Isolated intracranial arteritis
        Giant cell arteritis
        Wegener's granulomatosis
    Amyloid angiopathy
    Neoplasia
        Glioma
        Meningeal carcinomatosis
        Meningioma
        Atrial myxoma
    Radiation vasculitis
    Intravenous drug abuse

LOCATION OF HYPERTENSIVE
INTRACEREBRAL HEMATOMA

Lenticulostriate arteries (70%)
    Putamen
    Caudate nucleus
Other sites (30%)
    Thalamus
    Subcortical hemisphere
    Brain stem
    Dentate nucleus

---

percent of all hypertensive hemorrhages are in the distribution of the lenticulostriate arteries (putamen and caudate). Hematomas in these regions in patients over age 50 are almost invariably caused by hypertension, and no further angiographic investigation is necessary. Only rarely does a berry aneurysm rupture into the basal ganglia. When it does, it usually occurs in a young person and is associated with subarachnoid hemorrhage.

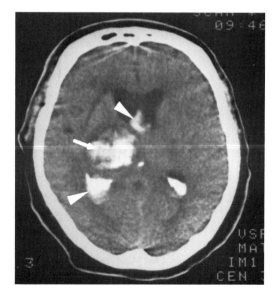

Fig. 2-42 Thalamic hematoma, hypertension. A large hyperdense region is present in the right thalamus representing the hematoma (arrow). There is a minimal amount of surrounding edema. The hemorrhage has ruptured into the ventricular system (arrowheads). Mild hydrocephalus is present.

Hypertension is generally thought to be the cause of small (Charcot-Bouchard) microaneurysms in the perforating arteries of the brain, especially the lenticulostriate group. These aneurysms are occasionally seen with high-magnification selective intracranial angiography. They are prone to rupture, causing hematomas.

The putamen is the most common location of hemorrhage resulting from hypertension. The other common locations are the caudate nucleus, thalamus, pons, dentate nuclei of the cerebellum, and subcortical regions of the cerebral hemispheres (see box). About 70

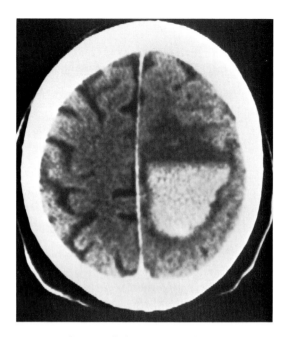

Fig. 2-43 Subcortical hematoma, hypertension. An acute subcortical hematoma is present in the left parietal white matter. The hematoma has not clotted and red blood cells have layered dependently, producing a radiodense fluid level. In older persons, such hematomas are almost always secondary to hypertension or amyloid angiopathy.

Hypertensive subcortical hemispheric hematomas occur in the white matter and have a lateral margin that conforms with the cortical gyri. They usually do not break into the subarachnoid space. In general, among the 50- to 70-year age group these hematomas are considered secondary to hypertension. Contrast-enhanced CT scans and angiography, as well as careful dissection after surgical removal, have almost always failed to identify any underlying structural cause, such as a cryptic tumor or vascular malformation. In the older patients (those over 70), these hematomas may be associated with amyloid angiopathy (see below). It is unusual for hemorrhage to be the presenting feature of a hemispheric tumor.

Computed tomography accurately detects intracerebral hematomas larger than 0.5 cm in diameter. Only the smaller petechial type hemorrhages cannot be seen reliably. The hematoma is represented as a region of nearly uniform increased density in the regions listed above (Figs. 2-42 and 2-43). Initially, during the acute phase, the hematoma is sharply demarcated from the surrounding brain parenchyma. At this time the density

ranges from 50 to 90 Hounsfield units (HU). The high density is from the contraction of the clot increasing the concentration of the blood elements. The mass effect is from the blood volume itself. Within a few hours edema begins to surround the hematoma, becoming maximal after 3 to 4 days and increasing the overall mass effect. The ventricular system may be compressed or shifted, and the sulci are obliterated. Large hematomas may cause herniation and death. The mass effect from large hematomas may last for as long as 4 weeks.

The hematomas have a propensity for dissection centrally into the ventricular system, which may be massive, forming a clot "cast" of the ventricle (Fig. 2-44). Only rarely do they break directly into the subarachnoid space. The prognosis is related to the size of the parenchymal hematoma and to a lesser extent to the amount of blood in the ventricular system. A small amount of blood within the ventricles does not have the grave prognosis that was once thought.

The blood that diffuses from the ventricular system into the subarachnoid space may cause a communicating hydrocephalus. The actual blood in the subarachnoid space is usually not seen on the CT scan. A hematoma in the posterior fossa can compress the fourth ventricle, and rarely a clot plugs the aqueduct resulting in noncommunicating hydrocephalus, which most often resolves spontaneously. The size of the ventricles must be followed by periodic CT scans until the ventricular size is stable or decreasing. Because of the fibrinolysins in the CSF, blood within the ventricular system or subarachnoid space resorbs faster than the blood in the brain parenchyma.

Hematomas show a decreasing density of about 0.7 to 1.0 HU per day. The number of days until the hematoma becomes isodense with the surrounding brain can be predicted from the density of the fresh hematoma. For about 2 to 3 months, the density of the hematoma becomes progressively lower, until it is nearly that of the CSF (Fig. 2-45). During this time the residual hematoma also becomes smaller. At about 6 months the hematoma has completely resorbed, leaving a low density cavity that is smaller than the original hematoma. Small hematomas may leave no focal residual lesion at all. In addition to the focal cavity, the large lesions cause a more generalized regional atrophy, identified by focal dilatation of the adjacent ventricular cavities and the cerebral sulci.

For their size and impressive appearance on the CT scan, hematomas cause relatively little damage to the

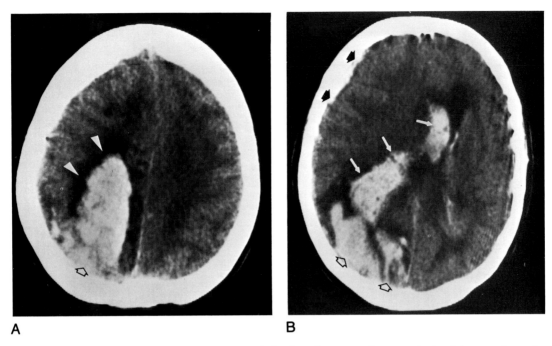

A   B

Fig. 2-44 Subcortical hematoma, hypertension. (A) A large hematoma is present in the right posterior parietal lobe. It is sharply demarcated but surrounded by moderate white matter edema (arrowheads). Hemorrhage has involved the cortical surface (open arrow). **(B)** The hematoma has extended down to the posterior parietal and upper occipital lobes (open arrows) and has dissected into the ventricular system, forming a cast of the right lateral ventricle (white arrows). Blood is also present in the subarachnoid or subdural space (black arrows). There is severe mass effect from hemorrhage and edema as well as subfalcial and craniocaudal herniation with ventricular dilatation.

brain. Hematomas dissect between the white matter fibers, causing compression but little destruction. The brain is able to withstand a considerable amount of compression without subsequent damage.

Approximately 7 to 10 days after the bleed, contrast enhancement may be demonstrated about the periphery of the hematoma (Fig. 2-46). The ring-like enhancement is usually separated from the hematoma and the surrounding parenchyma by a thin rim of low density edema. This pattern is not seen with tumors, and a resolving hematoma may be suspected when such a pattern is recognized. With time, the intensity of the enhancement increases until about 4 to 6 weeks and then gradually subsides over the next 3 to 4 months. The diameter of the ring decreases along with the hematoma. At the final stages, it appears as a small, round or linear density before its complete disappearance (Fig. 2-45). During the period when the enhancement appears ring-like or solid, the lesion may not be differentiated from a tumor or abscess (Fig. 2-46). MRI may

show high signal on the T_1- and T_2-weighted images, indicating prior hemorrhage. In this situation, the clinical history and follow-up scanning may be necessary to make the correct diagnosis.

On MRI, the appearance of hemorrhage and hematoma is complex and time-dependent (Tables 2-3 and 2-4). Multiple factors are involved including the oxidative state of hemoglobin (oxyhemoglobin, deoxyhemoglobin, methemoglobin, and hemosiderin), the location of the hemoglobin (intracellular or extracellular), scan sequences, and the magnetic field strength. The various factors have different effects on proton relaxation. Although based on experimental data, the explanation for the appearance of a hematoma on MRI remains a theory that is not completely satisfactory. What follows is a simplified explanation of the present theory. Changes in the details of the theory may occur in the future.

The time phases of a hematoma can be divided into four periods: hyperacute (first few hours); acute (1 to 5

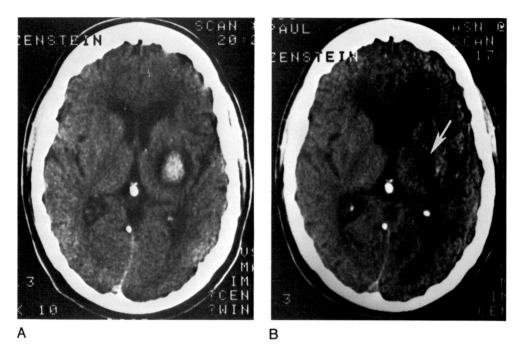

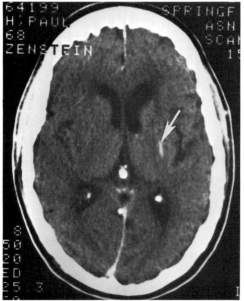

Fig. 2-45 Putaminal hematoma, hypertension (serial study). (A) A classic hypertensive hemorrhage in the left putamen is seen in the subacute phase. The hematoma has decreased slightly in density and is surrounded by a small amount of edema. **(B)** A scan 6 weeks later shows that the hematoma has become hypodense and smaller (arrow), and the surrounding edema has resolved. The left frontal horn has dilated because of regional atrophy. Had contrast been used, ring enhancement about the hematoma would almost certainly be present, which might be misinterpreted as abscess or tumor. **(C)** Contrast-enhanced study performed 1 year later shows that the hematoma has completely resorbed and the cavity has collapsed to a small enhancing slit (arrow).

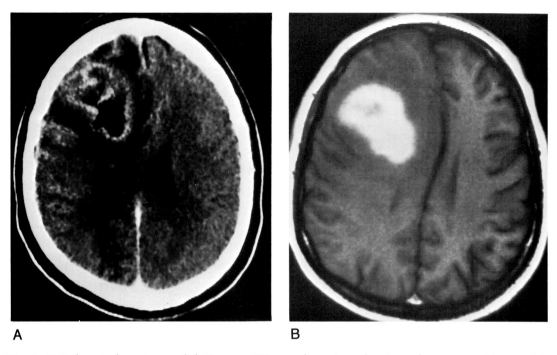

A   B

Fig. 2-46 Subacute hematoma. (A) Contrast CT scan shows irregular ring enhancement with central low density. This pattern is indistinguishable from that of a glioblastoma. There is surrounding edema. **(B)** T_1-weighted MRI shows the high signal intensity of methemoglobin within a resolving hematoma. This picture does not entirely exclude an underlying tumor, and follow-up scans are indicated if there is progression of the patient's symptoms.

days); subacute (5 to 15 days); and chronic (more than 15 days). The borderlines between the phases are not sharp and depend on the environment around the hematoma, particularly the regional tissue oxygen tension. The phases correspond with the various physical states and location of the hemoglobin molecule (Table

Table 2-3 Phases of Hematoma for MRI Purposes

Phase	Time (days)	Condition
Hyperacute	< 12 hours	Intracellular oxyhemoglobin
Acute	1–5	Intracellular deoxyhemoglobin
Subacute	5–15	Methemoglobin — initially intracellular, then extracellular following lysis of RBCs
Chronic	> 15	Hemosiderin within macrophages around the periphery of the hematoma
		Gradual resorption of methemoglobin
		Conversion to cystic cavity
		Resorption of the cyst

2-3). Field strength of the magnet affects the ability to observe magnetic susceptibility effects of intracellular deoxyhemoglobin and hemosiderin. The higher the field strength the more sensitive the scanner is to magnetic susceptibility phenomena.

The hyperacute hematoma consists of oxyhemoglobin within intact red blood cells (RBCs). Oxyhemoglobin is not paramagnetic. Consequently, the hematoma appears as a protein solution with prolonged T_1 and T_2 relaxation times. The hematoma at this stage appears slightly hypointense on T_1-weighted images and hyperintense on T_2-weighted images. At this stage it is nonspecific in appearance and cannot be differentiated from a neoplasm, except by history or the presence of a fluid level (Fig. 2-47). Within 12 hours, oxygen is depleted from the hemoglobin, producing deoxyhemoglobin; the hematoma is now said to have entered the acute phase, and its appearance changes.

During the acute phase the hematoma consists of deoxyhemoglobin within intact RBCs. Deoxyhemoglobin is paramagnetic, but it is not available to interact with regional protons and so it has no effect on the

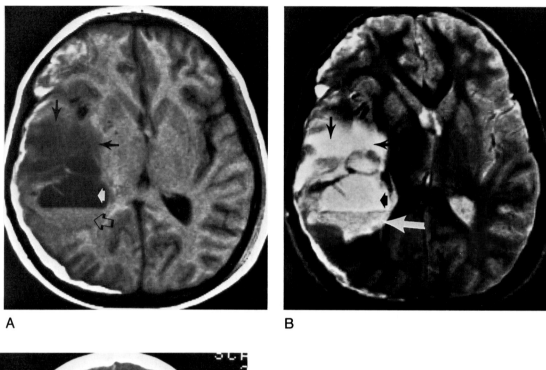

A

B

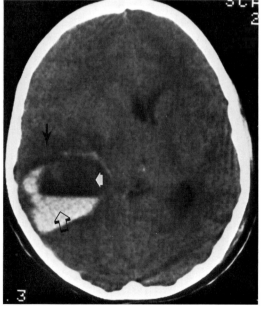

C

Fig. 2-47 Hyperacute hematoma. (A) T_1-weighted MRI shows the hematoma in the posterior right temporal lobe. RBCs with oxyhemoglobin are layered dependently and are nearly isointense with gray matter (open arrow). The serum anteriorly is hypointense but with just slightly greater intensity than that of CSF (white arrow). Edema is present anteriorly (black arrows). **(B)** T_2-weighted MRI shows the layered RBCs as moderately hyperintense (white arrow). The serum is very hyperintense (fat black arrow), as is the edema anteriorly (black arrows). **(C)** CT scan shows the dependent RBCs as high density (open arrow). The serum is low density, just slightly higher than that of CSF (white arrow). The edema anteriorly is just slightly hypodense and is difficult to see (black arrow). Note the subdural hemorrhage and right frontal contusion seen with MRI, but not with CT.

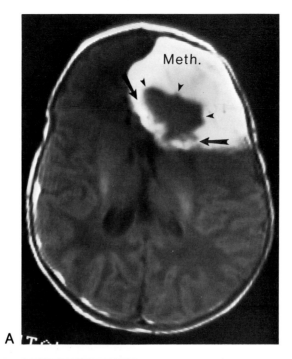

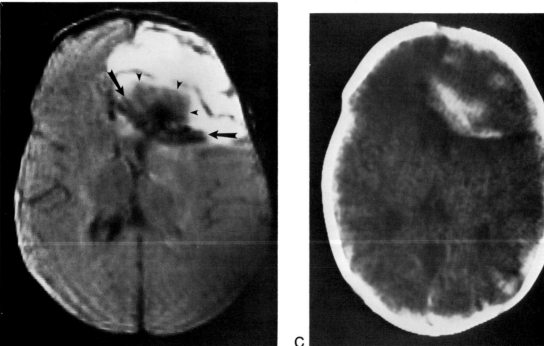

Fig. 2-48 Subacute hematoma, MRI and CT scan. The MRI scans are of a 10-day-old infant whose hemorrhage occurred at birth. **(A)** T$_1$-weighted (SE 600/15) scan shows a large hemorrhagic region in the left frontal lobe. The circumferential high signal intensity region represents extracellular methemoglobin (Meth.). The posteromedial hypointense region (arrowheads) represents persisting deoxyhemoglobin. Note that behind this region there is high signal from methemoglobin formation (arrows). **(B)** T$_2$-weighted (SE 2500/90) scan shows high signal intensity anteriorly, representing methemoglobin and edema. The posteromedial region of hypointensity represents deoxy-hemoglobin (arrowheads). The far posterior region of hypointensity represents intracellular methemoglobin (arrows). Compare this region with the high signal intensity on the T$_1$-weighted study. **(C)** CT scan performed 1 day after the MRI shows patchy hemorrhagic contusion of the left frontal lobe with a more consolidated hematoma in the posteromedial aspect. It is this hyperdense region of hematoma that shows persisting deoxyhemoglobin and methemoglobin in the intracellular state.

Table 2-4 MRI of Hematoma, High Field Strength (> 1.0T)

Phase	Appearance
Hyperacute	*IC deoxy*
T_1	Isointense or slightly hypointense
T_2	Hyperintense
Acute	*EC deoxy*
T_1	Isointense or slightly hypointense
T_2	Hypointense hemorrhage surrounded by hyperintense edema
Subacute	*Met Hb*
T_1	Hyperintensity of periphery of hematoma with gradual filling in of the center
T_2	Hyperintensity of periphery of hematoma with gradual filling in of the center — but all somewhat delayed compared with T_1 changes.
	Thin peripheral rim of hypointensity from early hemosiderin deposition
Chronic	
T_1	Gradual decrease in signal intensity and size of the hematoma; will become near CSF intensity
T_2	Persistent high signal intensity until hematoma is completely resorbed
	Residual hypointensity of hemosiderin deposition

T_1-weighted images. The hemorrhage remains of slightly low intensity, as during the hyperacute phase. However, the intracellular paramagnetic deoxyhemoglobin produces local variations (inhomogeneity) in the magnetic field within the hematoma. This causes both T_2 and T_2^* dephasing, resulting in a markedly shortened T_2 relaxation time. The actual hematoma or hemorrhage appears hypointense on the T_2-weighted images during this phase (Fig. 2-3; see also Fig. 7-3). Edema develops around the hematoma, and clot retraction extrudes serum peripherally so the tissue surrounding the hematoma appears of high intensity on the T_2-weighted images.

The subacute phase is complex. It begins with the conversion of deoxyhemoglobin to methemoglobin, which usually occurs about 5 days after the bleed. The periphery of the hematoma converts first and the process progresses inward toward the center (centripetal) at a variable rate until the entire hematoma is converted to methemoglobin. Methemoglobin is strongly paramagnetic and is available for proton interaction. This effect is especially strong when methemoglobin is free

after cell lysis, but it has a moderately strong effect when methemoglobin remains within intact RBCs. Therefore it produces a strong T_1 shortening effect, which is seen as high signal intensity on the T_1-weighted images. On T_1-weighted images, the hematoma becomes bright on the periphery and gradually fills in with brightness as the hematoma converts to all methemoglobin (Fig. 2-48).

On the T_2-weighted images, the hematoma becomes of high intensity during the subacute phase. This change occurs primarily because of the strong T_1 shortening effect of methemoglobin and its carryover to T_2-weighted imaging. The net result is apparent T_2 prolongation. In fact, methemoglobin has little direct effect on T_2 relaxation. This T_1 shortening effect is strongest when methemoglobin is extracellular and is less strong when the methemoglobin remains within intact RBCs. Therefore on the T_2-weighted images, the hematoma becomes of high signal intensity (bright) where cell lysis has occurred and remains of relative low intensity (dark) where RBCs remain intact (Fig. 2-48). The hematoma gradually fills in with high intensity throughout as RBC lysis becomes complete, but this pattern usually lags behind the centripetal progression seen on the T_1-weighted images. The peripheral edema continues to be imaged as high signal intensity surrounding the hematoma nidus, although edema decreases during the late subacute phase.

After this point the hematoma is considered to enter the chronic phase. A rim of low signal intensity appears around the hematoma and is thought to represent hemosiderin within macrophages (Fig. 2-49). The intracellular hemosiderin distorts the local magnetic field in a manner similar to the effect of intracellular deoxyhemoglobin. Therefore it causes regional dephasing and a strong reduction of the T_2 and T_2^* relaxation time wherever hemosiderin is taken up within the macrophages. As the hematoma nidus becomes smaller, the thickness of the ring generally becomes thicker, filling in the region previously occupied by the hematoma. The finding of residual hemosiderin after the hemorrhage has resorbed can be useful for determining prior episodes of bleeding, as with an arteriovenous malformation.

On the T_1-weighted images the hematoma gradually loses methemoglobin, resulting in gradual diminution of the T_1 signal intensity within the hematoma nidus. The nidus becomes isointense with the brain and eventually nearly isointense with the CSF as the hema-

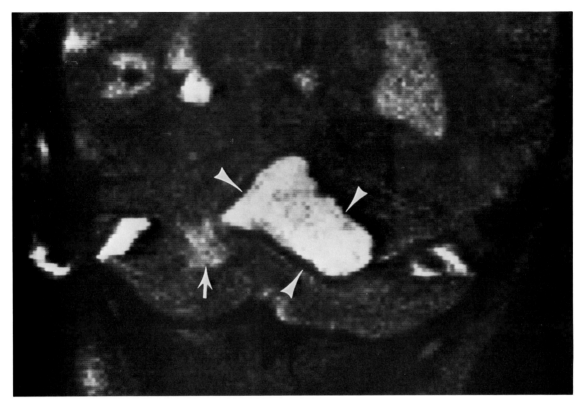

Fig. 2-49 Late subacute hematoma. T_2-weighted MRI shows the hyperintense hematoma in the central portion of the cerebellum. The hematoma has filled in almost completely with high signal as RBC lysis has become complete. A surrounding rim of low signal intensity is developing and represents hemosiderin within macrophages (arrowheads). A small amount of edema persists in the right cerebellar hemisphere (arrow). Other small hemorrhages are present more laterally.

toma resorbs and converts to a cystic cavity containing proteinaceous fluid. It may eventually disappear completely.

The central high T_2 signal intensity of the hematoma produced by methemoglobin persists for some time and becomes true T_2 prolongation as the hematoma liquefies into a high protein cystic cavity (Fig. 2-50). It may decrease in intensity slightly to become nearly isointense with the CSF, depending on the amount of protein within the cystic fluid. The high T_2 signal disappears only with complete obliteration of the hematoma cavity. The low intensity hemosiderin ring collapses with the residual cyst and may ultimately be seen as a small "slit". This may be the only indication that a hemorrhage has been present. GRE sequences are the most sensitive for detection of hemosiderin deposits because of their greater sensitivity to magnetic susceptibility effects.

Angiography is necessary only if there is a reasonable probability that the hematoma may have been caused by an aneurysm, vascular malformation, or tumor. Etiologies other than hypertension are considered if the hematoma is inhomogeneous, has central low density on CT scans, occurs in a noncharacteristic location, or has calcium associated with it. Hematomas in the temporal region may be a result of intraparenchymal bleeding from rupture of an aneurysm at the middle cerebral artery bifurcation, and angiography is generally indicated. A blood-fluid level may occur with acute hematomas of any etiology, although this sign was once thought to represent hemorrhage into a tumor.

The angiographic signs of intracerebral hematoma depend on the location of the hemorrhage. Local mass effect is seen, which is nonspecific and cannot be differentiated from other avascular mass lesions. Hemorrhages within the basal ganglia usually arise laterally in

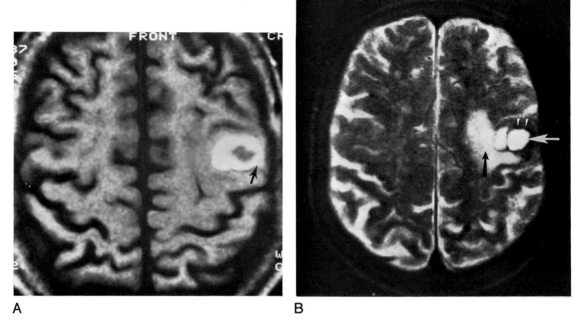

A   B

Fig. 2-50 Hemorrhagic infarction. (A) T_1-weighted image shows a hemorrhage in the subacute phase with peripheral high signal intensity of methemoglobin and central low density of persistent deoxyhemoglobin. The hemorrhage goes right to the cortical surface in what was thought to be hemorrhagic infarction. **(B)** In this case the T_2-weighted MRI shows diffuse homogeneous central high T_2-signal intensity (white arrow), which persists until the hematoma is completely resorbed. A minimal amount of peripheral hemosiderin is seen (arrowheads). The white matter high signal intensity represents subcortical edema and later gliosis from the infarction.

the putamen and external capsule, and therefore they almost always displace the lenticulostriate group of vessels medially. Aneurysm, vascular malformations, and tumors are recognized by their characteristic angiographic findings. Early draining veins may also be present in the region of the hematoma and do not specifically indicate a vascular lesion.

In cases of suspected hematoma or in patients with hypertension and the stroke syndrome, a nonenhanced CT examination is performed as the first imaging procedure. MRI may be used and provides equal sensitivity but is generally unnecessary.

Contrast-enhanced CT or MRI may be used to define an underlying tumor, but it is often difficult to distinguish abnormal enhancement from the hematoma density until the hematoma has matured. On MRI, the usual temporal evolution of hemorrhage within tumor is often delayed. The intracellular deoxyhemoglobin phase may persist for weeks, and there may be little peripheral hemosiderin deposition. Hem-

orrhage within tumor may appear less homogeneous than nontumoral hemorrhage because of the underlying structure of the tumor and changes from prior hemorrhages. A Gd-DTPA enhanced MRI with T_1-weighted sequence may define a tumor during the hyperacute and acute phases as a region of high signal intensity within the low signal hemorrhage.

Hypertensive Encephalopathy

Hypertensive encephalopathy is an acute neurologic syndrome consisting in severe hypertension initially associated with headache, nausea and vomiting, and later seizures, stupor, and coma. Papilledema, retinal hemorrhages, and cardiac and renal failure are usually present. Complete or partial recovery may occur with the lowering of the blood pressure.

The pathogenesis of the syndrome is unproved. Probably the disorder is a result of a breakdown of autoregulation of cerebral blood flow in the face of the extremely high blood pressure. The latter appears to cause intermittent regions of vasodilatation (regions of lost autoregulation) alternating with regions of preserved autoregulation (vasospasm). The loss of the autoregulation of the flow results in hyperemia, cerebral edema, petechial hemorrhages, and infarction. These changes occur predominantly in the deep cerebral white matter, basal ganglia, and brain stem. Pregnancy-induced hypertension (preeclampsia/eclampsia) is essentially the same process.

The CT findings correlate well with pathologic studies. Diffuse, symmetric, well demarcated, low density regions in the white matter occur with the syndrome and resolve after the blood pressure is lowered. The diffuse brain swelling causes ventricular compression with sulcal and cisternal obliteration. The central cerebellum is involved in the most severe cases, and hydrocephalus may occur. MRI shows high T_2 signal in the white matter, often with patchy signal void from petechial hemorrhage. Angiography sometimes shows the varying caliber of the vessels.

Migraine

Migraine is a common clinical constellation that has headache as the central feature. It affects up to twenty-five percent of the adult population and may occur in adolescents. It is more frequent in women. The cause is unknown.

The syndrome is subclassified as classic migraine, complicated migraine, and common migraine. Classic migraine consists of focal CNS abnormalities (prodromes) preceding and blending into the onset of severe headache which is most often unilateral and throbbing. The prodromes usually are various scotomata but may include aphasia, hemiparesis and hemisensory deficits as well. The focal symptoms last only a short time, up to thirty minutes. If the focal symptoms last longer, or result in permanent residua, the syndrome is called complicated migraine. Common migraine refers to a migraine type headache without the prodromes. Vertebrobasilar migraine refers to prodromes involving structures within the posterior fossa. Ophthalmoplegic migraine refers to oculomotor palsy that occurs during the time of the headache.

Migraine is thought to be caused by a cerebrovascular disturbance. The present theory states that the process begins with vasoconstriction of both the intracranial and extracranial vessels. The vasoconstriction phase may produce significant and measureable cerebral ischemia resulting in the prodromes or focal CNS deficits. The following vasodilatation phase is associated with the headache. A decrease in glucose metabolism and cerebral blood flow has been documented with PET scanning and Xenon-133 blood flow studies.

In general, patients with migraine do not need CT or MR scanning for diagnosis or management. However, certain abnormalities have been seen with inmaging. On MRI, focal high T_2 signal white matter abnormalities have been demonstrated in up to forty-one percent of those with classic or common migraine, and even more commonly in those with complicated migraine. The abnormalities vary from a few small punctate high signal lesions to more extensive confluent involvement in both the periventricular and subcortical regions. The lesions resemble those seen with multiple sclerosis or Binswanger's subcortical arteriosclerotic encephalopathy. Less commonly, cortical infarction may be seen. Mild diffuse atrophy is common, especially with migraine that has been present for more than five years. Very rarely migraine has been associated with a cerebral arteriovenous malformation.

Cerebral angiography has on rare occasion demonstrated cerebral vasospasm with migraine. However, it should not be performed for diagnosis as cerebral angiography poses a significant risk to the patient with migraine, especially during the prodromal phase. Cerebrovasospasm may be triggered or exacerbated and result in permanent CNS deficits. The test should be avoided when possible, and never performed during the migraine attack. If the angiography is essential for evaluation of an unrelated problem, pretreatment with 40 mg of propranolol may decrease the risk of iatrogenic vasospasm.

Subcortical Arteriosclerotic Encephalopathy of Binswanger

Binswanger's encephalopathy is discussed in Chapter 10.

Bacterial Arteritis

Intracranial arteries are susceptible to surrounding inflammatory reaction or pus particularly meningitis. An arteritis occurs from without, with edema, inflammatory cells, and bacteria traversing inward across the vessel wall to the intima. The vessel lumen is narrowed by the effects of the swelling in the vessel wall, and thrombosis may occur on an inflamed intima. The arteries at the base of the brain are usually the most severely affected, probably because pus tends to accumulate in the basal cisterns. *Hemophilus influenzae* and *Staphylococcus* cause the most severe changes of arteritis and often involve the cortical vessels as well.

There is a general correlation between the severity of the meningitis and the arteritis; but even in relatively mild infections or infections that are treated early and appropriately, the arteritis may be severe and cause extensive brain damage from infarction. Venous occlusive disease may also occur. Inflammatory arteritis cannot be differentiated from other types of arteritis by angiography. The infarctions and subsequent encephalomalacia may be imaged with MRI and CT (Fig. 8-2).

Fungal Arteritis

Arteritis may be seen after a large number of fungal infections of the meninges. Rarely, arteritis occurs from hematogenous intraluminal spread. Today, fungal infections are seen more commonly because of the relatively large number of people who are immunodeficient and thus susceptible to these "opportunistic" infectious agents. The mechanism of the arteritis is the same as for the bacterial infections described above. The most common infectious agents are *Cryptococcus, Nocardia, Coccidioides, Aspergillus, Candidia, Mucor,* and rarely *Actinomyces* and *Histoplasma.* The angiographic findings are nonspecific and similar to those of bacterial arteritis.

Tuberculous Arteritis

Tuberculous meningitis is generally seen in children and is associated with a primary infection outside the intracranial structures. The CSF contains high levels of protein, mononuclear leukocytes, and low glucose and chloride levels. The disease primarily involves the basal cisterns (pontine and suprasellar cisterns), where a thick, gelatinous, inflammatory exudate forms. In time, the exudate becomes hard and often calcifies. The engulfed vessel walls are involved with the inflammatory process and are mechanically constricted by the fibrosis. The vessel lumens are severely narrowed, and the obliterative endarteritis leads to total occlusions. The supraclinoid portions of the internal carotid, the proximal middle cerebral arteries, the lenticulostriate arteries, and the basilar artery are most severely involved (Fig. 2-51). Vascular insufficiency syndromes and stroke may occur. Peripheral involvement of the cortical vessels has not been seen following tuberculosis.

Syphilitic Arteritis

A severe arteritis may result from tertiary meningovascular syphilis. CNS symptoms may occur within months or may not become apparent for up to 5 years. There is a predilection for involvement of the proximal portions of the middle cerebral artery, although any vessel, large or small, may be affected. The angiographic picture is that of arteritis, although there is a greater tendency for aneurysm formation, particularly if the large vessels (i.e., basilar artery) are involved. The CSF serology is always positive.

Mycotic Aneurysm

Mycotic aneurysms result from septic embolizations, usually associated with subacute bacterial endocarditis. They are rarely associated with acute bacterial endocarditis. Almost all of the aneurysms occur in the more peripheral branches of the intracranial vessels, most often the middle cerebral artery (MCA). They may be small or large; and they may rupture, often with lethal consequences. Because there is usually an inflammatory reaction adjacent to the aneurysm, adhesions form, directing the extravasated blood into either the brain parenchyma or the subdural space. The hemorrhages may be small or large. Free subarachnoid hemorrhage is unusual.

Rarely, a mycotic aneurysm occurs in the thoracic aorta, particularly after thoracic cardiovascular surgery. These aneurysms are frequently associated with infections, especially those caused by *Aspergillus* or *Salmonella.* Large vegetations may form on the intima of the proximal aorta and result in distal septic embolization to the brain, causing arteritis and occasional aneurysm formation.

It is usually not possible to directly diagnose an intracranial mycotic aneurysm with CT scanning or MRI. The findings are nonspecific: infarction, hemorrhagic infarction, intracerebral hematoma, subdural hematoma, and sometimes subarachnoid hemorrhage.

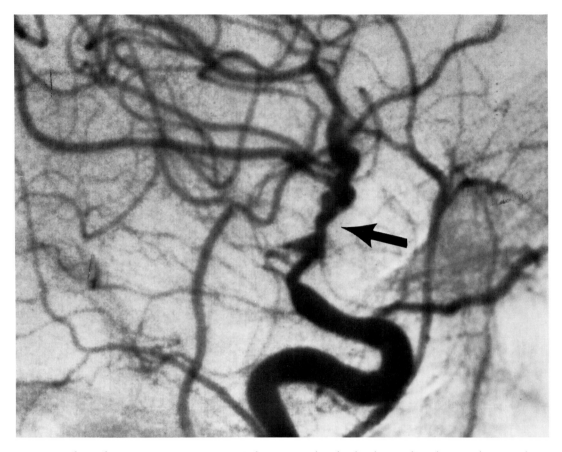

Fig. 2-51 Tuberculous arteritis. Constriction is demonstrated in the distal supraclinoid ICA and proximal MCA (arrow). This pattern may also be seen with syphilitic or fungal arteritis.

When found in the presence of subacute bacterial endocarditis, a mycotic aneurysm is strongly considered and angiography performed (Fig. 8-12).

Collagen-Vascular Disease

Systemic lupus erythematosus is the most common collagen-vascular disorder. It is a generalized disorder predominantly affecting women (8:1), most commonly between the ages of 15 and 40. As many as 50 percent of persons with the disease have lesions in the CNS, although not all of them are symptomatic.

A diffuse vasculitis occurs that involves both intracranial and extracranial vessels. Angiography shows the typical although nonspecific narrowings and dilatations of the involved vessels (Fig. 2-52). Symptoms include seizures, mental changes, headache (migraine type), and focal neurologic signs from small infarctions. Large infarctions are rare.

Most commonly, CT scans and MRI show generalized cerebral volume loss, which results from atrophy caused by microinfarctions and from the effects of steroid therapy. MRI is more sensitive than CT scanning for detecting focal abnormalities of the brain in patients with lupus. The lesions have prolonged T_1 and T_2 relaxation times. Three patterns are usually seen: (1) cerebral infarction with a relatively small area of increased intensity; (2) multiple small regions of increased intensity, probably representing microinfarctions; and (3) focal ribbon-like areas of increased intensity involving the cortical gray matter that regress in about 2 weeks. These lesions may represent areas of

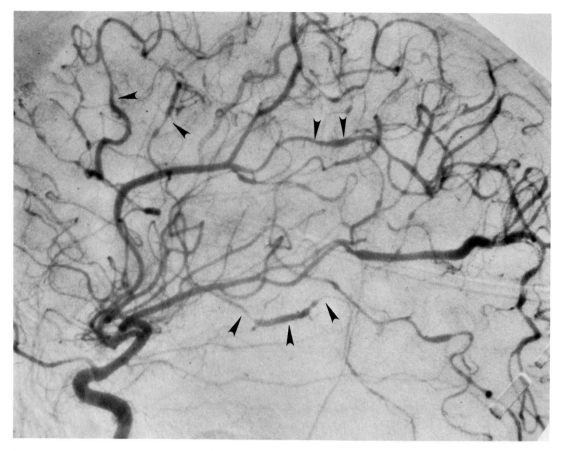

Fig. 2-52 Arteritis. ICA angiography shows diffuse segmental narrowing and dilatation of multiple intracranial vessels (arrowheads). This pattern is typical of arteritis, whatever the cause.

ischemia without actual infarction. Only the larger lesions may be seen on high-resolution CT scanning. Contrast enhancement may show lesions that would otherwise be occult.

Necrotizing Angiitis

The vascular changes of necrotizing angiitis are similar to those of collagen diseases, although they tend to be somewhat more severe and there is more necrosis within the vessel walls. Polyarteritis nodosa is the characteristic disease, but similar necrotizing changes occur with thrombotic thrombocytopenic purpura, isolated intracranial arteritis, temporal arteritis, and Wegener's granulomatosis.

Angiography may show regions of focal narrowing, but biopsy is necessary for a precise diagnosis. When

possible, the biopsy is performed on these narrowed regions, as the diseases have a multifocal distribution with skip areas. The ophthalmic artery is frequently involved in temporal arteritis (Fig. 2-53). The erythrocyte sedimentation rate is almost always elevated in the presence of active arteritis.

Amyloid Angiopathy

Cerebral amyloid angiopathy is becoming recognized as a common cause of subcortical hematomas in the elderly. The disease is generally not seen in persons under 60 years of age. Over this age, the incidence proportionately increases, with as many as 50 percent of people over the age of 80 years having the amyloid changes. These changes are not related to the effects of hypertension, and the cause is unknown.

Fig. 2-53 Necrotizing angiitis; temporal arteritis. (A)
Common carotid arteriography in the neck shows diffuse
changes of arteritis involving the ECA and its branches (arrowheads). Change in the ECA distribution may be the only
finding with arteritis. **(B)** Lateral intracranial view shows the
changes of arteritis in the ophthalmic and internal maxillary
arteries (arrowheads).

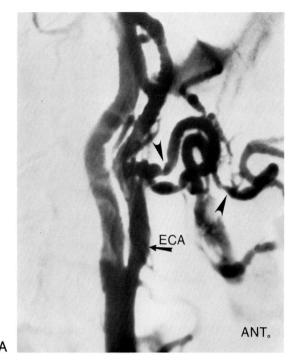

A

B

The amyloid infiltration affects only medium-sized and small arteries in the cerebral cortex and leptomeninges. The involved vessels rupture easily after minor trauma or mild elevations of blood pressure. They may also rupture spontaneously. CT scanning easily demonstrates the usually large peripheral subcortical hematomas, which occur most often in the more posterior parts of the brain, particularly the occipital lobes. Multiple hematomas may occur, sometimes simultaneously. Changes of arteritis and occlusion are unusual on angiography. Definitive diagnosis is made by biopsy of the meninges, usually at the time of hematoma removal.

Neoplasia

In certain situations tumors severely affect the vessels in the brain. Most commonly, vessel damage is secondary to constriction by a meningioma at the base of the brain (see Fig. 5-34). Parasellar meningiomas may constrict or totally occlude the cavernous portion of the internal carotid artery, its supraclinoid portion, or the proximal portions of the middle cerebral arteries. In these instances it is usually impossible for the neurosurgeon to remove the tumor without causing either rupture or occlusion of the major vessel involved. The diagnosis of meningioma is usually clear from the characteristic vascular blush of the tumor. Rarely, an exceptionally virulent glioblastoma multiforme invades a cortical vessel, resulting in its occlusion and the stroke syndrome. Atrial myxomas embolize to the peripheral cortical branches, particularly at bifurcations, invade the vessel wall, and cause a focal aneurysm. Sporadically, other tumors follow this sequence as well.

Radiation Arteriopathy

High doses of radiation (more than 5,000 R) may cause an obliterative arteritis. The risk of radiation-induced angiopathy increases in an exponential fashion with

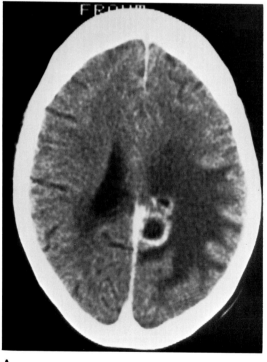

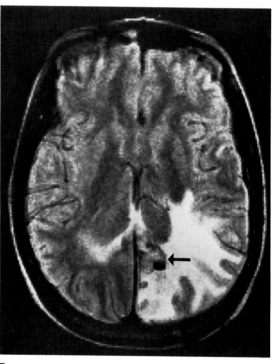

A

B

Fig. 2-54 Radiation necrosis. (A) Contrast-enhanced CT scan shows ring-like enhancement deep in the posterior left hemisphere surrounded by considerable white matter edema. This material was removed and was found to be entirely necrotic tissue. **(B)** T$_2$-weighted MRI shows the necrotic region as one of hypointensity (arrow). It is surrounded by high signal intensity, representing edema and gliosis. Slight white matter changes are seen on the opposite side. This patient had radiation implantation. Postirradiation changes are confined to the field of exposure.

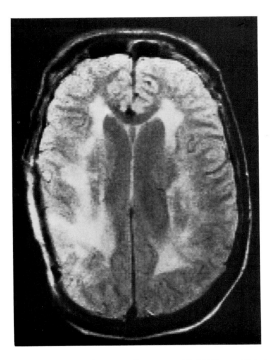

Fig. 2-55 Postirradiation change, MRI. Bilateral high T_2 signal intensity is seen in the white matter, representing demyelination. This patient had undergone whole-brain irradiation.

doses over 6,000 R. On angiography, the vessels may show diffuse narrowing of the lumen within the fields of irradiation. The vasculopathy usually occurs 1 to 3 years after cessation of irradiation, but the latent period may be as long as 10 years. Mild involvement causes demyelination. More severe involvement produces focal tissue necrosis. Tissue necrosis causes striking and confusing changes on the CT scan with large regions of intense, irregular contrast enhancement, edema with mass effect, and increased intracranial pressure (Fig. 2-54). MRI shows high T_2 signal within white matter from demyelination (Fig. 2-55). Only by biopsy can the nidus of radiation necrosis be differentiated from recurrent tumor, especially glioblastoma. The symptoms of the increased intracranial pressure are greatly relieved by removal of the enhancing necrotic tissue, which causes the edema.

Drug Abuse

Intravenous amphetamines may cause the typical changes of arteritis described earlier in the chapter. Mycotic aneurysms may occur, not always associated with subacute bacterial endocarditis. Both of these processes, along with the induced hypertension, may cause intracranial hemorrhages of almost any type. Today's mercurial fashion in the use of drugs means that any combination of agents may be encountered, and so the changes seen must be considered in the appropriate clinical setting. Chronic use of foreign substances of almost any type can produce brain cell loss and atrophy that is visible on the CT scan. Cocaine use is associated with cerebral hematomas and infarctions. Changes consistent with vasospasm but not vasculitis have been seen on angiography. Subarachnoid hemorrhage after cocaine use is usually due to rupture of a preexisting berry aneurysm.

THROMBOSIS OF THE CEREBRAL VEINS AND DURAL SINUSES

Cerebral venous thrombosis is usually not an independent disease but occurs as the result of various pathologic factors.

1. Local effects of infection, particularly sinusitis
2. Trauma, including surgical trauma
3. Hypercoagulable states, as with pregnancy
4. Congestive heart failure
5. Local tumor, particularly meningioma

The symptoms depend on the location and extent of the brain infarctions that result. Headache is almost always present, and there may be papilledema from increased intracranial pressure. Hemiparesis, the most common deficit, frequently fluctuates in severity. Seizures may occur. These symptoms are somewhat different from those usually associated with arterial occlusion and so help with the differential diagnosis.

The infarctions caused by venous thrombosis are often hemorrhagic. The hemorrhages are almost always confined to the cortical areas in the region of the thrombosis and vary in size from small, punctate collections to widespread cortical involvement. When the superior sagittal sinus is thrombosed, the hemorrhages are frequently located bilaterally in the high parasagittal convexities. Deep vein thrombosis can cause symmetric deep hemorrhagic necrosis.

On the noncontrast CT examination, a linear increased density within a cortic vein *(cord sign)* or within a sinus is sometimes seen, probably representing a clot.

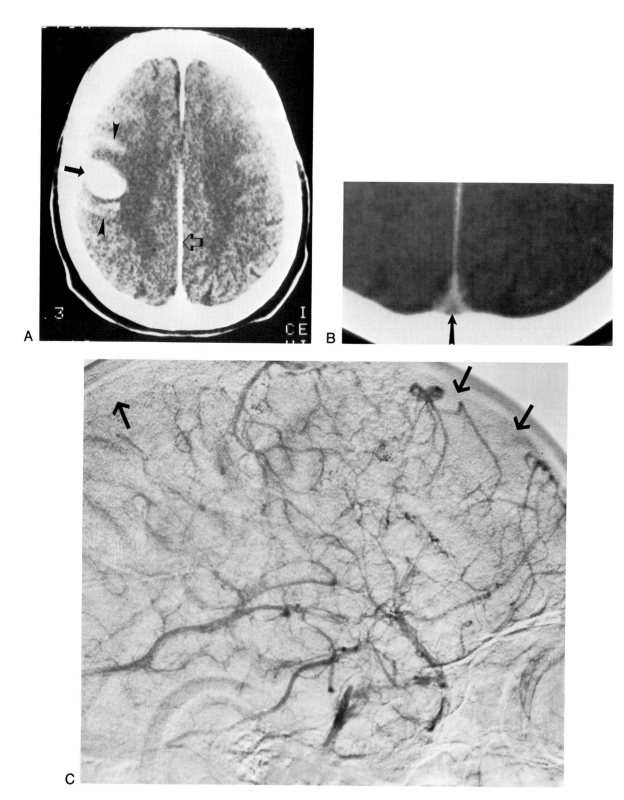

Fig. 2-56 Sagittal sinus thrombosis. (A) Contrast-enhanced CT study shows hemorrhagic cortical infarction over the right parietal lobe (arrow) with adjacent cortical gyral enhancement (arrowheads). The falx shows striking enhancement (open arrow). **(B)** Wide window view of the posterior sagittal sinus shows the delta sign with nonopacification of the sinus cavity (arrow). Wide windows are necessary to observe this sign. **(C)** Venous phase angiography demonstrates nonopacification of the entire sagittal sinus (arrows). There is prominent opacification of the inferior cortical veins draining to patent basal sinuses.

There can be considerable swelling of the brain from hyperemia. Subarachnoid hemorrhage is frequent, but the amount of blood is small and is not usually seen on the CT scan.

Abnormal contrast enhancement occurs in the cortical "ribbon" pattern. A defect in the contrast-filled sagittal sinus may represent a clot and can best be seen in the region of the torcula *(delta sign)* (Fig. 2-56). Tentorial or falx enhancement may be unusually prominent. Ischemic infarct, without hemorrhage, occurs in up to 40 percent, and the diagnosis of venous thrombosis is suggested only by the clinical symptoms listed above. MRI may show the clotted sinus with absent flow-void. However, care must be taken to be certain that the increased intensity within a sinus is not flow-related enhancement.

Angiography remains the definitive diagnostic test (Fig. 2-56C). The diagnosis is made when a sinus or vein is not opacified. The occluded vein may be seen, although a single cortical vein thrombosis is almost impossible to recognize because of the great variation in venous anatomy. The circulation is slowed in the region of the occlusion, and there is prolongation of the "brain blush" of the capillary phase of the angiogram. Irregular and tortuous, almost corkscrew-like, collateral veins may be seen, and the direction of the flow in these veins is reversed from normal. Enlarged deep medullary veins can be seen with extensive sagittal sinus thrombosis. To best visualize the sagittal sinus, slightly oblique lateral and AP projections are used to distinguish the sinus from the density of the inner table of the calvarium and eliminate superimposition. Most angiography is done with a unilateral injection of contrast, and there is unopacified blood from the opposite side flowing into the sinuses, which may be misinterpreted as thrombosis. If there is any question about the diagnosis, bilateral simultaneous carotid injection is done.

GLOBAL ISCHEMIA AND HYPOXEMIA

Global ischemia or hypoxemia occurs when either the cerebral perfusion falls below the critical level or the blood is not adequately oxygenated. Both factors may be present simultaneously. In adults, global ischemia or hypoxia results most commonly from the circulatory arrest that occurs with hemorrhagic or cardio-

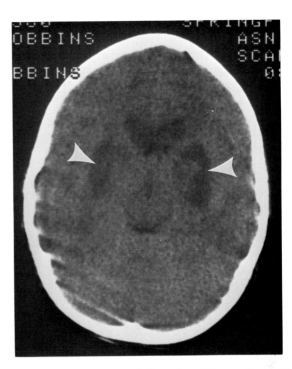

Fig. 2-57 Hypoxic encephalopathy. CT scan of a child in a near-drowning accident shows bilateral symmetric regions of hypodensity involving the lentiform nuclei (arrowheads). This pattern is characteristic after pure hypoxemia.

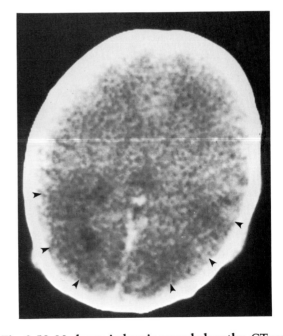

Fig. 2-58 Moderate ischemic encephalopathy. CT scan shows hypodensity in the posterior parietal lobes representing ischemic change (arrowheads).

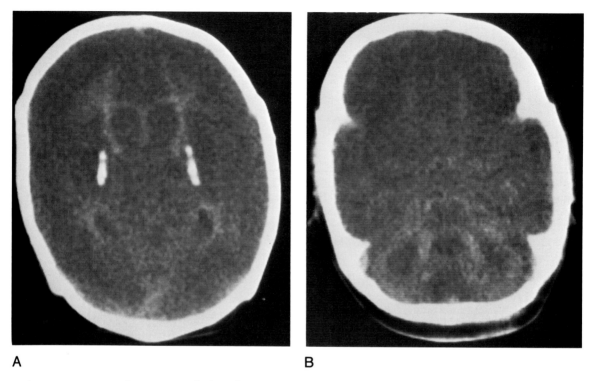

Fig. 2-59 Severe ischemic encephalopathy. (A) Scan through the level of the ventricles shows hypodensity involving all portions of both cerebral hemispheres including the basal ganglia and the thalamus. The ependyma shows preserved density. Calcifications developed in the globus pallidus nuclei bilaterally. **(B)** Scan through the posterior fossa shows preservation of cortical and periventricular tissue density in the cerebellum. Only the most severe ischemic events produce changes in the cerebellum and thalamic nuclei.

genic shock, carbon monoxide poisoning, and respiratory arrest. In newborns and children, it is most commonly the result of prematurity, status epilepticus, near-drowning, and child abuse. The effects on the brain vary with the age of the patient and whether deoxygenation or low perfusion is predominant.

When deoxygenation is the primary factor (global hypoxemia), the major abnormality is seen in the putamen and hippocampal gyri. These regions have high metabolic rates and are the most sensitive to anoxia. On CT scans the cytotoxic edema is seen as bilateral hypodensity in the lentiform nuclei (Fig. 2-57). With MRI, the edema is hypointense on T_1- and hyperintense on T_2-weighted images. This pattern is most commonly seen with near-drowning and carbon monoxide poisoning but can be produced by any purely hypoxic event.

When global low perfusion is the major factor, the findings are predominantly within the "watershed" regions (Fig. 2-58), particularly with older individuals whose cerebral circulation is compromised. The abnormalities are seen on CT scans as hypodensity in the deep frontal and parietal white matter. With more severe ischemia, the cortex becomes hypodense as well (Fig. 2-59). Later, atrophy develops with dilatation of the lateral ventricles, particularly the atria. MRI shows high T_2 signal within the deep white matter (Fig. 2-60). The thalami and cerebellum are typically spared unless extreme ischemia has occurred. The region along the course of the main branches of the middle cerebral artery tend to be less affected than other portions of the hemispheres. Mild damage from global ischemia may not be seen during the acute phase but only after 1 to 2 months, when slight dilatation of the atria of the lateral ventricles indicates the mild deep posterior parietal lobe injury.

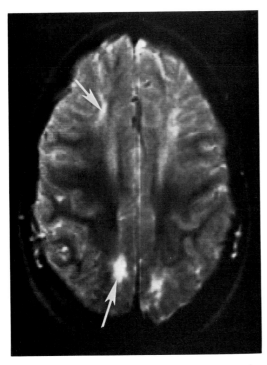

Fig. 2-60 Paraventricular leukomalacia, mild hypoxic ischemic encephalopathy. T$_2$-weighted MRI examination shows high signal in the frontal and parietal white matter. The white matter is also atrophic in these regions (arrows), a residual of mild hypoxic/ischemic encephalopathy.

BRAIN DEATH

Brain death is the result of irreversible global cerebral circulatory arrest. Most of the time such arrest is the result of a marked increase in the intracranial pressure from brain edema or hemorrhage so that the pressure is higher than the circulatory perfusion pressure. Clinical criteria have been established to define brain death, including the absence of cerebral electrical activity as defined by electroencephalography. When there is any doubt about meeting the clinical criteria, definite proof of absent cerebral circulation is considered equivalent to brain death. There must be absent flow in both internal carotid and vertebrobasilar circulations.

Selective cerebral angiography is the most accurate test. The demonstration of absent cerebral blood flow with preservation of normal extracranial circulation is accepted as proof of brain death. All the cerebral vessels must be studied.

Because of the cost and difficulty of performing cerebral angiography, other methods have been used to define brain death. The radionuclide brain scan is most commonly employed and can be done with portable equipment. Brain death is diagnosed when there is no evidence of intracranial tracer but normal tracer is seen in the superficial scalp tissues. Dynamic contrast-enhanced CT scans may also be used. After contrast infusion, there is no measured increase in density of the brain, whereas there is normal increase in density of the soft tissues over the calvarium.

SUGGESTED READING

Barkovich AJ, Atlas SW: Magnetic resonance imaging of intracranial hemorrhage. Radiol Clin North Am 26:801, 1988

Barnett HJM, Mohr JP, Stein BM, Yatsu FM (eds): Stroke: Pathophysiology, Diagnosis and Management. Churchill Livingstone, New York, 1986

Bluth EI, Wetzner SM, Stavros AT, et al: Carotid duplex sonography: a multicenter recommendation for standardized imaging and Doppler criteria. Radiographics 8:487, 1988

Braffman BH, Zimmerman RA, Trojanowski JQ, et al: Brain MR: pathologic correlation with gross and histopathology. 1. Lacunar infarction and Virchow-Robin spaces. AJNR 9:621, 1988

Brant-Zawadzki M: Ischemia. In: Stark DD, Bradley WG Jr (eds): Magnetic Resonance Imaging. CV Mosby, St. Louis, 1988

Brant-Zawadzki M, Weinstein P, Bartowski H, et al: MR imaging and spectroscopy in clinical and experimental cerebral ischemia: a review. AJNR 8:39, 1987

Brooks RA, Di Chiro G, Patronas N: MR imaging of cerebral hematomas at different field strengths: theory and applications. J Comput Assist Tomogr 13:194, 1989

Brown JJ, Heslink JR, Rothrock JF: MR and CT of lacunar infarcts. AJNR 9:477, 1988

Erickson SJ, Middleton WD, Mewissen MW, et al: Color Doppler evaluation of arterial stenoses and occlusions involving the neck and throacic inlet. Radiographics 9:389, 1989

Fishman MC, Naidich JB, Stein HL: Vascular magnetic resonance imaging. Radiol Clin North Am 24:485, 1986

Golden GS: Stroke syndromes in children. Neurol Clin 3:59, 1985

Gomori JM, Grossman RI: Head and neck hemorrhage. p. 71. In Kressel HY (ed): Magnetic Resonance Annual. Raven Press, New York, 1987

Gomori JM, Grossman RI, Hackney DB, et al: Variable appearances of subacute intracranial hematomas on high-field spin-echo MR. AJNR 8:1019, 1987

Gonzalez CF, Doan HT, Han SS, et al: Extracranial vascular angiopathy. Radiol Clin North Am 24:419, 1986

Hayman LA, Taber KA, Jhingran SG, et al: Cerebral infarction: diagnosis and assessment of prognosis by using ^{123}IMP-SPECT and CT. AJNR 10:557, 1989

Hecht-Leavett C, Gomori JM, Grossman RI, et al: High-field MRI of hemorrhagic cortical infarction. AJNR 7:581, 1986

Holman BL (ed): Radionuclide Imaging of the Brain. Churchill Livingstone, New York, 1985

Houser OW, Campbell JK, Baker HL Jr, et al: Radiologic evaluation of ischemic cerebrovascular syndromes with emphasis on computed tomography. Radiol Clin North Am 20:123, 1982

Jacobs IG, Roszler MH, Kellt JK, et al: Cocaine abuse: neurovascular complications. Radiology 170:223, 1989

Kilgore BB, Fields WS: Arterial occlusive disease in adults. p. 2310. In Newton TH, Potts DG (eds): Radiology of the Skull and Brain: Angiography. CV Mosby, St. Louis, 1974

Kissel JT: Neurologic manifestations of vasculitis. Neurol Clin 7:655, 1989

Lande A, Berkman YM: Aortitis. Radiol Clin North Am 14:219, 1976

Savoiardo M, Bracchi M, Passerini A, et al: The vascular territories of the cerebellum and brainstem: CT and MRI study. AJNR 8:199, 1987

Smullens SN: Surgical treatable lesions of the extracranial circulation, including the vertebral artery. Radiol Clin North Am 24:453, 1986

Soges LJ, Cacayorin ED, Petro GR: Migraine: evaluation by MR. AJNR 9:425, 1988

Tsuruda JS, Kortman KE, Bradley WG Jr: Radiation effects on cerebral white matter: MR evaluation. AJNR 8:431, 1987

3

Intracranial Aneurysm and Subarachnoid Hemorrhage

An aneurysm is an abnormal focal bulge of the vessel wall. More than 99 percent arise from arteries. Intracranial aneurysms occur in 5 to 10 percent of the population of the United States. More than 90 percent of them are congenital or "berry" aneurysms that occur in characteristic sites around the circle of Willis. Atherosclerotic fusiform aneurysms of the larger intracranial arteries account for 5 percent. The remaining rare types are infectious (mycotic), post-traumatic, dissecting, or neoplastic. Venous aneurysms occur as part of arteriovenous malformations (AVMs).

CONGENITAL ("BERRY") ANEURYSMS

Congenital aneurysms are thought to result from a structural weakness in the media of the arterial wall, usually small fenestrations at the junctions of arteries. Hypertension and atherosclerosis may contribute to the process. A familial tendency is present. The incidence of aneurysms occurring at similar sites is twice that of the remaining population.

Ninety-five percent of aneurysms occur in the internal carotid distribution; only 5 percent occur in the vertebrobasilar system. The junction of the anterior cerebral artery with the anterior communicating artery (ACA) is the most common site. The next most common sites are the internal carotid artery at the level of

the posterior communicating artery (PCA) and the middle cerebral artery (MCA) at the bifurcation (see below). Aneurysms are multiple in about 20 percent of cases. Most of the aneurysms are small (less than 1 cm). Giant aneurysms (more than 2.5 cm) occur and are most common in the extradural segments of the ICA, the bifurcation of the MCA, or at the tip of the basilar artery. Intracranial "berry" aneurysms may also be associated with AVMs and other vascular anomalies, e.g., primitive trigeminal artery, fibromuscular hyperplasia, coarctation of the aorta, polycystic kidney disease, and sickle cell anemia. The smaller aneurysms primarily

---

LOCATION OF BERRY ANEURYSMS

Common (90%)
   Anterior communicating (35%)
   Posterior communicating (30%)
   Middle cerebral artery (25%)
Less common (10%)
   Bifurcation of the ICA
   Tip of the basilar artery
   Origin of the PICA
   Supraclinoid ICA
   Miscellaneous sites

---

present with subarachnoid hemorrhage. The giant aneurysms act as mass lesions and have a low incidence of rupture. The onset of a unilateral third nerve (CN III), palsy may be an indication of the presence of an expanding internal carotid aneurysm at the level of the posterior communicating artery.

Subarachnoid Hemorrhage

Subarachnoid hemorrhage is the hallmark presentation of the small congenital "berry" aneurysms. It usually occurs in patients 40 to 50 years old. Seventy-five percent of adults with nontraumatic subarachnoid hemorrhage (SAH) have a demonstrable aneurysm by angiography; 10 percent have a primary intracerebral hemorrhage as the cause without a demonstrable aneurysm; and only 3 to 5 percent have an AVM. Other rare causes make up 1 to 2 percent. About 10 percent have no demonstrable cause—presumably an occult (nonimaged) aneurysm or AVM. Subarachnoid hemorrhage in persons under 25 years of age is more likely to be secondary to an AVM. Aneurysms are infrequent in children.

Subarachnoid hemorrhage presents with the abrupt onset of a severe headache, usually the worst ever experienced by the patient. Nausea, vomiting, and a decrease in mental status and consciousness frequently occur. Prior to a major hemorrhage, the patient may experience small "sentinel" hemorrhages that cause relatively mild headache that may be dismissed.

In addition to the subarachnoid bleeding, about 25 percent of patients have an intraparenchymal hematoma. It occurs most commonly in the deep medial temporal lobe due to rupture of an MCA aneurysm at its bifurcation and in the medial inferior frontal lobes, the corpus callosum, and the septum pellucidum due to rupture of an ACA aneurysm. When large, the hematomas are surgically removed to control intracranial pressure and herniation. Small focal perianeurysmal clots may form.

Intraventricular hemorrhage also occurs after rupture of aneurysms, most commonly from rupture of an ACA aneurysm through the adjacent thin lamina terminalis into the third ventricle. Less commonly, aneurysms in other locations rupture into the ventricles. Intraventricular bleeding may leave hemosiderin deposits along the ependymal lining.

The prognosis after subarachnoid hemorrhage can be related to the "grade" of the patient at the time of initial

---

SUBARACHNOID HEMORRAGE PROGNOSTIC GRADING SYSTEM

Grade 1: Either no symptoms or only mild signs of meningeal irritation. The patient is fully alert and the headache is mild.
Grade 2: The patient is still alert but has a moderate or severe headache. A minimal neurologic deficit may be present.
Grade 3: Mental function changes are present such as lethargy or confusion. A mild to moderate degree of neurologic deficit may be present.
Grade 4: Patient is stuporous.
Grade 5: Coma is present with or without signs of decerebration.

---

evaluation by a physician. The most common grading system has five categories, listed above.

The grading system is useful for defining the prognosis for the patient or evaluating surgical or medical therapeutic regimens. Patients in the grade 1 or 2 category have a good prognosis for successful corrective surgery, whereas those with grade 4 or 5 disease have a poor prognosis, with mortality approaching 100 percent. Grade 3 is intermediate, with about 30 to 40 percent overall mortality. There is general correlation with the amount of subarachnoid hemorrhage and the clinical grade of the patient.

Complications After Subarachnoid Hemorrhage

Delayed complications have a strong effect on the eventual outcome after subarachnoid hemorrhage. The most important are given below. There is a 35 percent risk of major rebleeding during the first 3 weeks after a

---

DELAYED COMPLICATIONS OF SAH

Vasospasm and infarction
Rebleeding
Hydrocephalus

subarachnoid hemorrhage due to aneurysm. Afterward, this risk gradually decreases. Rebleed significantly worsens the prognosis. To decrease this risk for rebleed, some neurosurgeons recommend early aneurysm surgery, especially in patients of low clinical grade. The use of antifibrinolysis therapy has been discontinued.

Delayed vasospasm is an additional significant risk factor. This complication occurs in more than 50 percent of persons with subarachnoid hemorrhage. It is known that the degree of spasm correlates positively with the amount of the subarachnoid hemorrhage, but the mechanism of its production is unknown. Most likely, it is caused by the chemical breakdown products of the subarachnoid blood. Vasospasm is not present immediately but becomes evident 5 to 10 days after the hemorrhage. The vascular narrowing may last for weeks. In the case of severe spasm, inflammatory changes develop in the walls of the affected arteries so the narrowing becomes fixed for some time. These narrowed segments have been dilated with some success using small balloon angioplasty catheters.

The vasospasm may become severe enough to cause brain ischemia and infarction, although the relation between the spasm and ischemia is not proved conclusively. Additionally, with vasospasm the intima may be affected, so there is secondary formation of local thrombus and distal embolization. If surgery is performed in the presence of spasm, there is a high rate of subsequent infarction and a poor outcome. Multiple angiographies or transorbital ultrasonographies are used to define the status of the vasospasm prior to surgery. Calcium channel blockers have been used with some success in an attempt to decrease the amount of vasospasm after subarachnoid hemorrhage.

Some degree of communicating hydrocephalus almost always accompanies a subarachnoid hemorrhage no matter how small the bleed. It is thought to be caused by decreased resorption of CSF by mechanical "plugging" of the arachnoid villi by the subarachnoid red blood cells. The hydrocephalus occurs almost immediately and can usually be seen on the initial CT or MRI scan. Mostly it resolves spontaneously, but occasionally the ventricular system becomes large so that surgical ventricular decompression becomes necessary. Rarely, a large amount of blood within the ventricular system blocks the ventricular foramina, resulting in an "entrapped" ventricle or noncommunicating hydrocephalus.

CT Scanning

The CT scan is the most useful imaging technique for defining subarachnoid hemorrhage. It has greater sensitivity than MRI. When the nonenhanced CT examination is performed within 48 hours of the hemorrhage, the subarachnoid blood can be defined about 90 percent of the time. The CT scan is negative only in those patients with low clinical grade and a small amount of subarachnoid blood.

The hemorrhage is seen as high density within the basal cisterns and the cerebral sulci (Fig. 3-1). Specific patterns of bleeding frequently make it possible to locate the aneurysm that has bled (Figs. 3-2 and 3-3). This ability may be of great importance when multiple aneurysms are found by subsequent angiography. The patterns are given in Table 3-1. When a large subarachnoid hemorrhage has occurred, blood diffusely floods the subarachnoid space, and localization is not possible

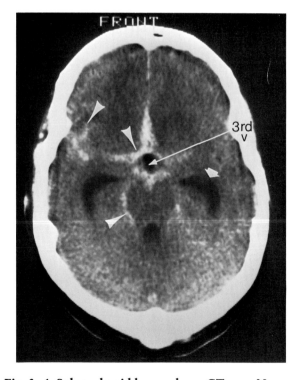

Fig. 3–1 Subarachnoid hemorrhage. CT scan. Nonenhanced transaxial CT scan shows diffuse increased density in the suprasellar cistern, the right sylvian fissure, and the perimesencephalic cisterns (arrowheads). It represents the subarachnoid blood. Moderate hydrocephalus is present with dilatation of the temporal horns (arrow).

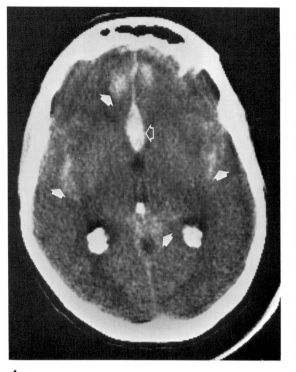

A

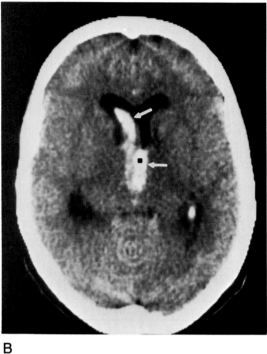

B

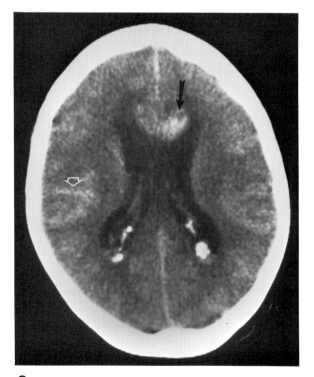

C

Fig. 3–2 Anterior communicating artery aneurysm rupture. (A) CT scan shows a focal rounded clot in the posterior frontal interhemispheric fissure, possibly extending into the base of the septum pellucidum (open arrow). Subarachnoid hemorrhage is also seen diffusely within the cerebral sulci and basal cisterns (solid arrows). **(B)** Intraventricular rupture has occurred with blood clot seen in the right frontal horn and third ventricle (arrows). Mild hydrocephalus is present. Subarachnoid blood might not be present when the aneurysm ruptures directly into the ventricular system. **(C)** ACA aneurysm has ruptured into the corpus callosum with blood dissecting through the genu (arrow). Minimal subarachnoid blood is seen in the sylvian fissue (open arrow).

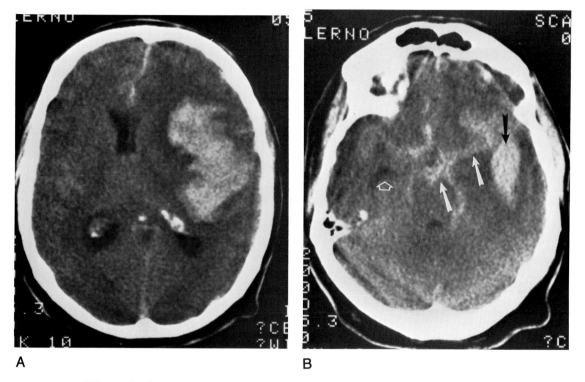

A   B

Fig. 3–3 Middle cerebral artery aneurysm rupture. (A) Large blood clot is seen in the region of the left sylvian fissure and temporal lobe. It could also represent a subcortical intraparenchymal spontaneous hemorrhage. Mass effect is present with subfalcial herniation and mild hydrocephalus of the right lateral ventricle. **(B)** CT scan at a lower level shows the base of the hematoma within the left sylvian fissue (black arrow). In addition, there is subarachnoid blood in the horizontal sylvian fissure, suprasellar cistern, and perimesencephalic cisterns (white arrows). The left perimesencephalic cistern is larger than the right one because of the contralateral shift of the pons from the temporal hematoma. The right temporal horn is slightly dilated from hydrocephalus (open arrow).

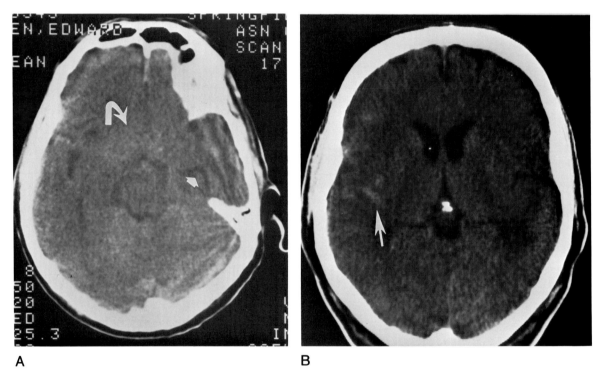

Fig. 3–4 Subtle subarachnoid hemorrhage. (A) Transaxial view through the basal cisterns shows isodensity of the cisterns from a small subarachnoid hemorrhage (curved arrow). Minimal hydrocephalus is present, indicated by slight dilatation of the left temporal horn (arrow). **(B)** Subtle increased density is seen in the right sylvian fissue from subarachnoid hemorrhage (arrow).

Table 3-1 Characteristic Patterns of Hemorrhage with Location of Aneurysm

Site	Hemorrhage
ACA	Frontal interhemispheric fissure
	"Flame shape" into frontal lobe
	Anterior suprasellar cistern
	Corpus callosum
	Intraventricular blood
PCA	Ipsilateral suprasellar cistern
MCA	Ipsilateral sylvian fissure
	Medial temporal lobe/sylvian fissure
Basilar artery	Posterior suprasellar cistern
	Prepontine cistern
PICA	Foramen magnum

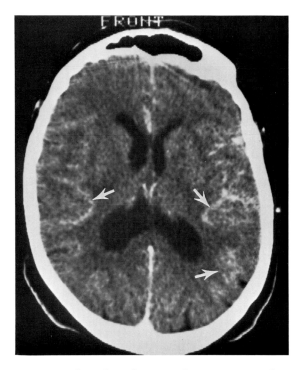

Fig. 3–5 Subarachnoid Hemorrhage, meningeal enhancement. Contrast-enhanced CT scan of a patient with no demonstrable SAH shows diffuse "smudgy" enhancement of the meninges (arrows). It is a nonspecific finding and may also be seen with meningitis or meningeal carcinomatosis.

(Fig. 3-1). Small hemorrhages may raise the density of the basal cisterns just enough that they become isodense with the brain, and the diagnosis may be difficult to make (Fig. 3-4). In this situation contrast infusion may show diffuse enhancement of the meninges (Fig. 3-5). Contrast enhancement may also demonstrate the aneurysm itself, although only large aneurysms (more than 1 cm) are routinely seen (Figs. 3-6 and 3-7). Because patients with subarachnoid hemorrhage undergo angiography, it is not necessary to try to demonstrate aneurysms. CT scanning cannot be used to screen for aneurysm.

Communicating hydrocephalus may be subtle but is almost always present (Fig. 3-1). Sometimes it can be recognized on CT scans only by the slight dilatation of the temporal horns of the lateral ventricles (Fig. 3-4A). If hydrocephalus is moderate, serial scans are performed every few days until the ventricles stabilize or become smaller. Hydrocephalus can become a significant problem and causes an increase in the intracranial pressure, which can further compromise the cerebral blood flow in the patient with vasospasm. There are no CT criteria for deciding at what point the ventricular enlargement becomes significant. The decision for shunting is a matter of clinical judgment.

Focal regions of low density, mostly conforming to known vascular patterns, are indicative of cerebral ischemia or infarction. These low density regions usually appear after 1 week and are considered to be a consequence of vasospasm. When a low density region is first seen, it is impossible to determine if it represents reversible ischemia or infarction. Regions of ischemic edema without infarction regress in time, whereas a com-

pleted infarction shows persistent hypodensity. The severity of the ischemic change on CT and the vasospasm seen on angiography generally correlate with the severity of clinical cerebral dysfunction.

MRI

Magnetic resonance imaging is not as useful as CT scanning for the diagnosis of subarachnoid hemorrhage, which is much more difficult to demonstrate with MRI; a possible explanation is the high PO_2 of the CSF, which delays the formation of deoxyhemoglobin. Although MRI can define infarction and hydrocephalus, it does not have any clinical advantage in this setting. If a clot forms within the cisterns it may be imaged with MRI (Fig. 3-8).

The aneurysm itself may be identified with MRI as a round region of abnormal flow-void adjacent to a major artery at the base of the brain (Fig. 3-9). However, the technique is not reliable for the detection or definition

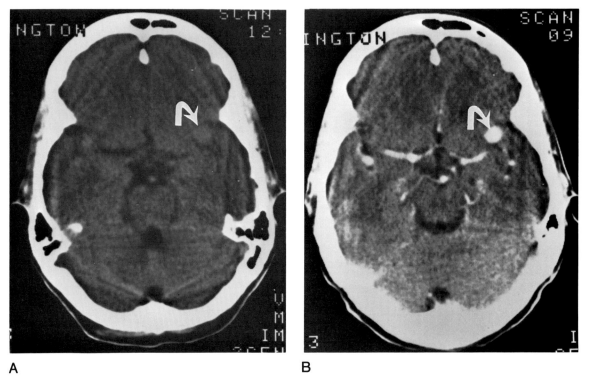

A   B

Fig. 3–6 MCA aneurysm. (A) Nonenhanced CT scan shows the moderate-sized left MCA aneurysm as a focal found region of slight hyperdensity within the sylvian fissure (curved arrow). **(B)** Contrast-enhanced examination shows the aneurysm lumen as a homogenous dense contrast collection (curved arrow). A clotted aneurysm would not fill with contrast, which is common with giant aneurysms. Small aneurysms cannot be routinely detected with a contrast CT scan.

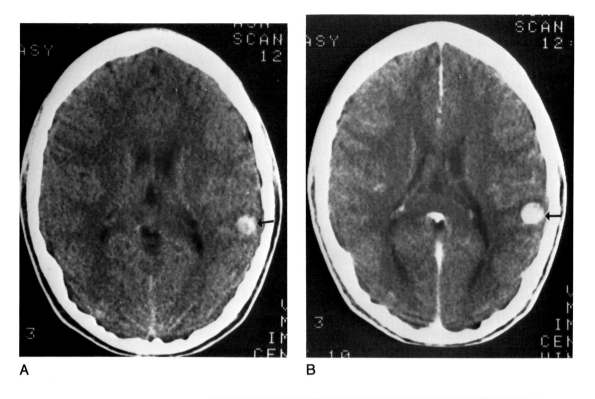

A   B

Fig. 3–7 Peripheral aneurysm of MCA. **(A)** Nonenhanced CT scan shows a round hyperdense lesion in the region of the left posterior sylvian fissure (arrow). The hyperdensity represents either a small amount of calcium or acute clot. **(B)** Contrast-enhanced study shows the densely enhancing lumen of the aneurysm. **(C)** ICA angiography demonstrates the aneurysm sac on the angular branch of the middle cerebral artery (open arrow). Peripheral aneurysms may due to infection (mycotic) or trauma, or they may be idiopathic.

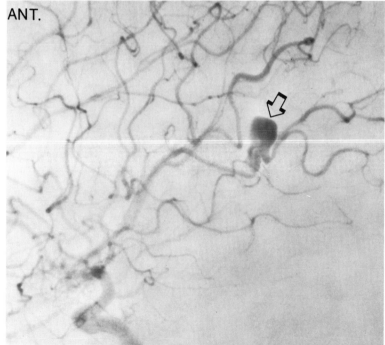

C

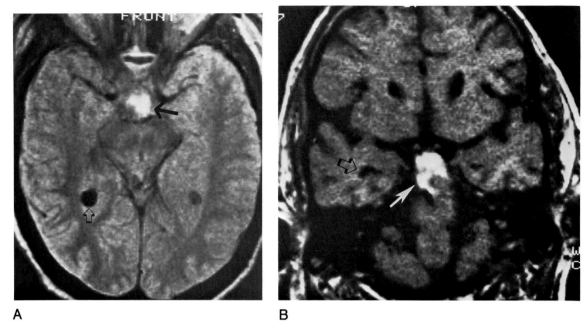

A   B

Fig. 3–8 Subarachnoid hemorrhage, with clot; MRI. (A) Transaxial proton density MRI through the supra-sellar cistern shows a hyperintense blood clot (arrow). A calcified glomus is seen in the atrium of the right lateral ventricle (open arrow). **(B)** Coronal T_1-weighted MRI demonstrates the hyperintense clot in the suprasellar cistern extending inferiorly on the right in the prepontine cistern (arrow). It was from a rupture of a posterior communicat-ing artery (PCA) aneurysm. The right temporal horn is slightly dilated from hydrocephalus (open arrow).

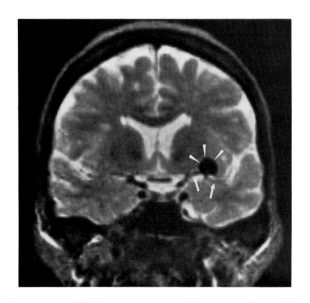

Fig. 3–9 Left MCA aneurysm, MRI. T_2-weighted MRI shows a rounded region of flow-void, representing a moder-ately large aneurysm of the bifurcation of the left MCA (ar-rowheads). The MCA can be seen within the sylvian fissure because of the flow-void within the hyperdense cisterns (arrows).

of small aneurysms and cannot be used as a screening examination or in place of angiography prior to sur-gery. The changes of subacute or chronic hemorrhage are sometimes seen adjacent to an aneurysm that has bled. The ventricles or brain surface may be outlined by a rim of very low signal intensity from hemosiderin deposited in the ependyma following intraventricular hemorrhage.

Angiography

Cerebral angiography remains the only reliable means of identifying cerebrovascular aneurysms. The angiog-raphy is performed with selective ICA and vertebral injections using magnification filming technique when possible. The injection rate is reduced slightly (4 to 5 ml/sec) to decrease the potential for aneurysm rupture due to pressure changes. The study can be performed at any time after the aneurysm rupture. Oblique and sub-mental-vertex views are frequently necessary to define the details of the aneurysm. When possible, a complete angiogram is performed to identify all potential aneu-rysms. Both vertebral arteries may need to be injected to

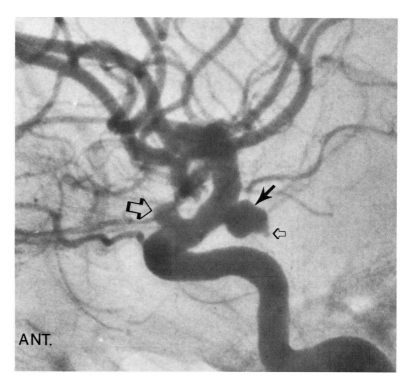

Fig. 3–10 Aneurysms: PCA, supraclinoid ICA. Lateral ICA angiogram shows a typical aneurysm of the ICA at the level of the PCA (black arrow). Note the small "daughter" bulges at the apex of the aneurysm (small open arrow), which is a sign highly associated with recent bleeding or expansion of the aneurysm. A smaller aneurysm is present just distal to the ophthalmic artery (large open arrow). Note that the contrast density within the aneurysm is similar to that of the adjacent vessel.

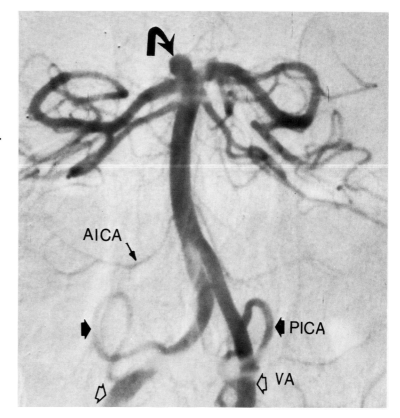

Fig. 3–11 Aneurysm of the tip of the basilar artery. A small aneurysm is seen at the tip of the basilar artery (curved arrow) on a Water's projection of vertebral angiography. This view shows the entire basilar artery to good advantage and is excellent for aneurysm detection. Both vertebral arteries need to be opacified either by bilateral selective injection or by reflux from unilateral injection.

sufficiently opacify the origin of the PICAs. If no aneurysm or other source of the subarachnoid hemorrhage can be found, selective external carotid angiography is performed to search for dural AVMs. Occasionally, an aneurysm is seen on follow-up angiography that was not seen initially. The goals of angiography are as follows:

1. Identification of an aneurysm or multiple aneurysms
2. Determination of which aneurysm has bled
3. Definition of the neck of the aneurysm
4. Relation of the aneurysm to the surrounding vessels and brain structures
5. Detection of vasospasm
6. Definition of the flow patterns of the circle of Willis

The aneurysm is identified as a rounded, contrast-filled bulge originating from the adjacent artery at characteristic sites (Figs. 3-10 and 3-11). The density of the contrast within the aneurysm is the same as that within the normal arteries. A vessel seen "on end" or a tortuosity of a normal vessel may simulate an aneurysm but has observed contrast density that is greater than the adjacent normal vessels. Oblique views are almost always necessary to better define the aneurysm.

When multiple aneurysms are present, the size of the aneurysm is the most reliable sign for determining which aneurysm has bled. In 95 percent of cases with multiple aneurysms, it is the largest one that has bled. Aneurysms smaller than 5 mm almost never bleed. Because ruptured aneurysms have almost always expanded near the apex of the dome and bleed from this expansion, the dome usually shows a focal, rounded, secondary bulge or at least some irregularity of the margin (Fig. 3-10). There may be multiple rounded focal expansions, appearing as either a segmented worm or a small cluster of berries. Local vasospasm also points to the nearest aneurysm as the source of the subarachnoid hemorrhage but is less reliable (Fig. 3-12). Demonstration of extravasation of contrast from

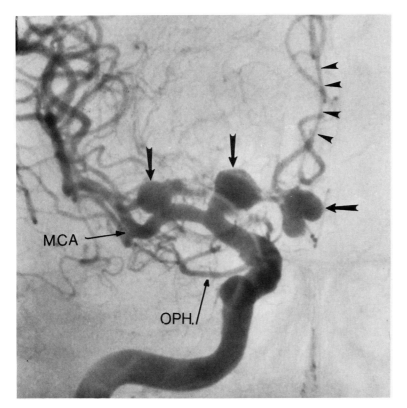

Fig. 3-12 Multiple aneurysms. Aneurysms are present at the right MCA, the proximal anterior cerebral artery, and the level of the anterior communicating artery (arrows). The aneurysms are similar in size. However, the lobular shape of the ACA aneurysm and the regional spasm of the pericallosal artery (arrowheads) make it likely that this aneurysm is the one that has ruptured.

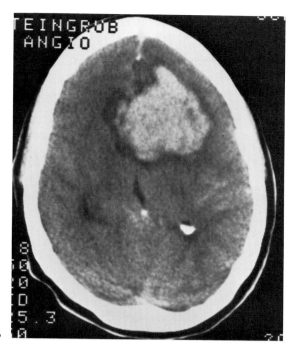

Fig. 3–13 Intraparenchymal hemorrhage from peripheral aneurysm rupture. (A) CT scan shows a large hematoma involving the corpus callosum and extending into the deep frontal white matter. This hemorrhage is deeper than the average subcortical hemorrhage associated with hypertension. Angiography should be performed for hemorrhages such as this one to detect a possible aneurysm or vascular malformation. **(B)** Lateral ICA angiography demonstrates an aneurysm of the pericallosal artery at the origin of the callosal marginal artery (large arrow). The pericallosal artery is stretched. The hematoma has depressed the sylvian vessels (small arrows) and is stretching a posterior frontal opercular branch (open arrow).

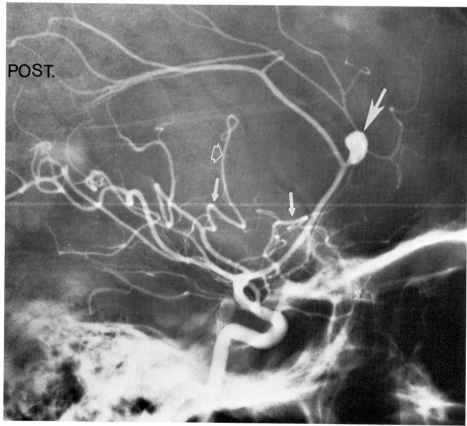

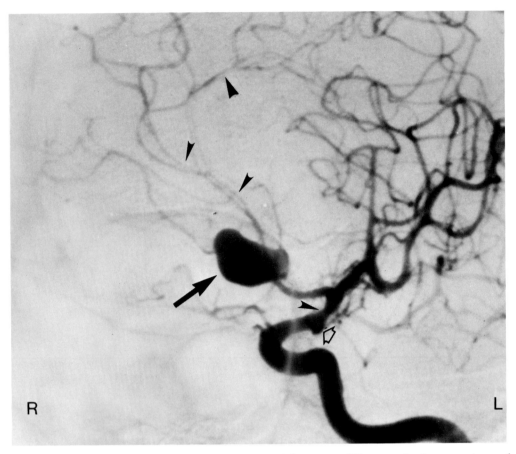

Fig. 3–14 Anterior communicating artery aneurysm, with spasm; oblique projection anteriography. A large aneurysm is present at the anterior communicating artery (arrow). There is diffuse severe spasm of the supraclinoid ICA and the pericallosal vessels (arrowheads). Spasm is multifocal with varying degrees of vasoconstriction along the vessel. A small aneurysm is present at the PCA (open arrow).

the aneurysm is clearly definitive of rupture, but this problem almost never presents. A local hematoma may indicate the site of rupture (Figs. 3-2, 3-3, and 3-13).

A small aneurysm in the region of the PCA must be differentiated from an infundibulum of the PCA itself. An aneurysm is more than 3 mm and has a rounded, dome-like configuration. An infundibulum is smaller than 3 mm, is triangular in shape, and frequently has a visible vessel emerging from the dome (see Fig. 2-21A).

Vasospasm is represented by narrowing of the vessel lumen. It has a multifocal distribution (Fig. 3-14). Vasospasm usually occurs near the region of the aneurysm but may be seen at some distance. When severe, it causes a demonstrable decrease in the cerebral circulation. It begins 5 to 10 days after the subarachnoid hemorrhage but may persist for weeks.

GIANT ANEURYSM

Only 2 percent of intracranial aneurysms are "giant aneurysms." These lesions are arbitrarily defined as those more than 2.5 cm in diameter. Giant aneurysms seldom rupture but, rather, become apparent because of local mass effect. They are predominantly recognized in the older age groups. About 75 percent have peripheral calcification that can be seen on plain films and CT scanning. Thick walls and mural thrombus are common. They may cause bone erosion particularly in the region of the sella turcica.

Most giant aneurysms arise in the intracavernous portion of the ICA (Fig. 3-15) and are at least partially extradural. These lesions may cause compression of cranial nerves (CN) III to VI, which course in the lateral

Fig. 3–15 Giant aneurysm of the ICA. (A) A giant aneurysm is present arising from the cavernous portion of the right ICA (arrowheads). A small amount of calcification is present in the wall (arrow). Erosion of the dorsum and the right side of the sella has occurred (open arrowhead). This aneurysm shows nearly uniform contrast enhancement. **(B)** Lateral common carotid angiography demonstrates a contrast-filled giant aneurysm of the cavernous segment.

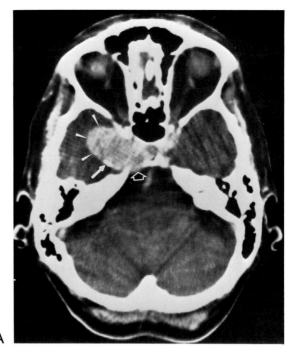

A

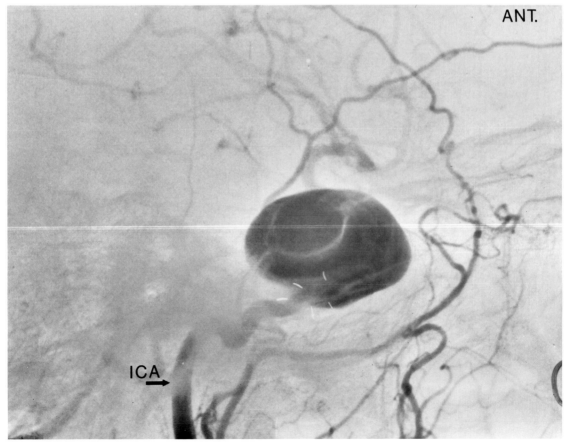

B

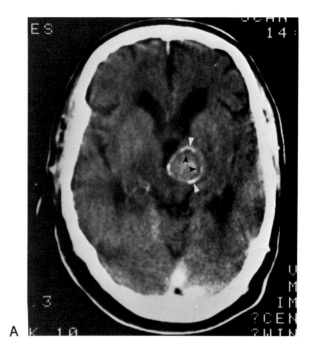

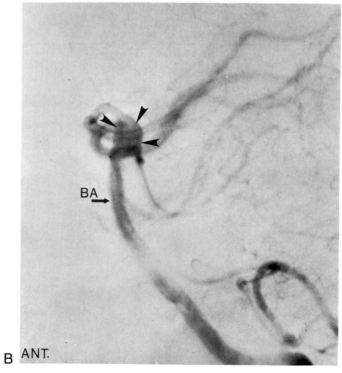

Fig. 3–16 Giant aneurysm from the tip of the basilar artery. (A) Transaxial contrast-enhanced CT scan shows a spherical mass extending up into the base of the thalamus, distorting the posterior third ventricle. The rim of the mass has irregular calcification (white arrowheads). The central portion of the sphere has inhomogeneous hyperdensity with only minimal if any contrast enhancement. This aneurysm has caused mild hydrocephalus. Such aneurysms are often misdiagnosed as tumor. The concentric ring of hypodensity just inside the calcified wall represents chronic clot (black arrowheads). **(B)** Lateral vertebral angiography demonstrates contrast filling only the base of the aneurysm (arrowheads). The remainder of the aneurysm is filled with clot. BA = basilar artery.

dural wall of the cavernous sinus. When they are very large, the aneurysm erodes and enlarges the sella from the side. The predominant unilateral expansion indicates an aneurysm rather than an intrasellar tumor. Proptosis can occur with expansion forward into the posterior orbit.

The next most common location is the basilar artery, from either the tip (Fig. 3-16) or along the main portion. These lesions can compress the posterior third ventricle or the brain stem. Rarely, giant aneurysms arise from the middle cerebral artery at the bifurcation or from the anterior cerebral artery. Intradural giant aneurysms present with subarachnoid hemorrhage about 40 percent of the time. Peripheral embolization can occur from the mural thrombus. The parent vessel may be atheromatous and friable in the region from which the aneurysm arises and may be incorporated into the wall of the aneurysm sac. The neck of the aneurysm is usually small.

Angiography demonstrates most giant aneurysms as large abnormal collections of contrast (Fig. 3-15). A swirling effect of the contrast is often seen at the time the contrast bolus reaches the aneurysm. However, the actual size of the aneurysm is often underestimated because of the large amount of clot lining the periphery of the cavity. Occasionally, only a small part of the aneurysm fills with contrast (Fig. 3-16).

The CT scan better demonstrates the size of the aneurysm, as the entire structure can be visualized (Fig. 3-16). The appearance of the aneurysm depends on the amount of clot within the lumen. If the entire lumen is patent, on the nonenhanced CT scan the lesion appears as a slightly hyperdense mass often with rim density representing the calcification in the wall. The contrast-enhanced CT scan shows uniform hyperdensity of the opacified blood within the aneurysm (Fig. 3-15). The homogeneity and hyperdensity may be identical to some tumors, especially pituitary adenomas and parasellar meningiomas. In this instance, angiography or MRI may be necessary to make the correct diagnosis.

Partially thrombosed aneurysms have a different appearance. On the nonenhanced CT scan, the lesion appears as a mass with a central or eccentric round region of slight hyperdensity with peripheral hypodensity representing the chronic clot (Fig. 3-16). With contrast enhancement, the central region becomes very hyperdense owing to opacified flowing blood. Little

change occurs in the other portions of the lesion except the wall, which may enhance.

A completely thrombosed aneurysm is nearly homogeneously isodense because of the lumen-filled clot. Slight peripheral contrast enhancement may occur. These lesions may be difficult to diagnose and are often mistaken for a tumor, particularly meningioma or craniopharyngioma.

The characteristic signs of a giant aneurysm can be seen with MRI. If the cavity is patent, there is almost always a central flow-void, although inhomogeneity of signal or even hyperintensity may occur because of turbulence, flow-related enhancement, or the echo rephasing phenomenon. The peripheral clot shows inhomogeneous hyperintensity. Calcium in the rim is not reliably seen with MRI. There may be a small amount of subacute hemorrhage adjacent to the aneurysm and sometimes edema of adjacent brain parenchyma. The finding of flow-void reliably differentiates giant aneurysm from tumor. Thrombosed aneurysms show varying intensity depending on the age of the clot.

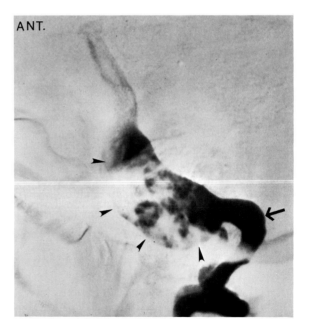

Fig. 3-17 Atherosclerotic giant basilar artery aneurysm. Lateral vertebral angiogram shows a giant fusiform atherosclerotic aneurysm of the basilar artery (arrowheads). Atherosclerotic ectasia of the distal vertebral artery is present (arrow).

ATHEROSCLEROTIC FUSIFORM ANEURYSMS

Fusiform aneurysms represent the progression of atheroectasia of the vessel. The aneurysms may become large with a diameter of more than 2.5 cm so that they are classified as a form of giant aneurysm. Most commonly they involve the basilar artery (Fig. 3-17), but they may also involve the upper terminal portion of the ICA, with extension into the proximal segments of the middle and anterior cerebral arteries. The vessel is not only dilated but elongated and tortuous. The aneurysms may compress cranial nerves, and occasionally a basilar artery aneurysm compresses the posterior third ventricle and aqueduct, causing hydrocephalus. They seldom rupture. Because small perforating branches arise from the aneurysmal sac, they are almost impossible to resect safely. Except for the shape of the aneurysm, both the CT and angiographic findings follow the same principles of diagnosis as described above for giant saccular aneurysms.

MYCOTIC ANEURYSM

Mycotic aneurysms are discussed in Chapters 2 and 8.

SUGGESTED READING

Alcock JM: Aneurysms. p. 2435. In Newton TH, Potts DG (eds): Radiology of the Skull and Brain: Angiography. CV Mosby, St. Louis, 1974

Atlas SW: Intracranial vascular malformations and aneurysms. Radiol Clin North Am 26:821, 1988

Davis KR, Kistler JP, Heros RC, et al: A neuroradiologic approach to the patient with a diagnosis of subarachnoid hemorrhage. Radiol Clin North Am 20:87, 1982

Drayer BP: Diseases of the cerebrovascular system: aneurysms. In Heinz ER (ed): The Clinical Neurosciences: Neuroradiology. Churchill Livingstone, New York, 1984

Silver AJ, Pederson ME Jr, Ganti SR, et al: CT of subarachnoid hemorrhage due to ruptured aneurysm. AJNR 2:13, 1981

4

Arteriovenous Malformations

Congenital cerebrovascular malformations have been classified by Rubinstein into four groups: (1) arteriovenous malformation (AVM); (2) cavernous hemangioma (angioma); (3) venous angioma; and (4) capillary telangiectasis. The AVM is by far the most common type, occurring in about 3 percent of persons with subarachnoid hemorrhage or intracerebral hematoma. AVMs are uncommon in the general population, occurring in about 0.1 percent. The other groups are rare. Even more rare are the malformation syndromes listed below. Overall, AVMs account for less than 1 percent of all strokes.

ARTERIOVENOUS MALFORMATION

An AVM is a developmental anomaly of blood vessels consisting of a tortuous tangle of arteries and veins that are abnormal in caliber and length. The malformation may be small, with a single feeding artery-to-vein fistula, or large, with multiple feeding arteries from multiple vascular territories feeding large varicose deep and superficial veins. The arteries and veins communicate directly without an intervening capillary network, allowing the shunting of blood from artery to vein. They occur predominantly in the parietal lobe but may be found in any region of the brain. The malformations are further subclassified according to their vascular supply. Pial malformations (75 percent) are supplied solely by cerebral or cerebellar cortical arteries. Dural malformations (10 percent) are supplied solely by dural meningeal arteries. Mixed malformations (15 percent) are supplied by both pial and dural arteries. Posterior fossa malformations are of the mixed type 50 percent of the time.

The brain parenchyma in and around the malformation degenerates, resulting in atrophy and gliosis so that the vessels of the malformation become compact. Calcification occurs in almost all malformations and may be minimal or heavy. Chronic changes from small sub-

---

CEREBRAL VASCULAR MALFORMATIONS

Common
    Arteriovenous malformation—pial, dural, mixed
Uncommon
    Venous angioma
    Cavernous hemangioma
    Capillary telangiectasis
Rare
    Carotid–cavernous fistula
    Vein of galen aneurysm
    Traumatic A-V fistulas
    Encephalofacial angiomatosis (Sturge-Weber)
    Hereditary telangiectasis (Osler-Weber-Rendu disease)
    Wyburn-Mason syndrome

119

clinical hemorrhages are seen both within the lesion or in the adjacent brain. Hemosiderin deposits are found particularly around the periphery. Areas of cerebral infarction may be found outside the region of the lesion and are thought to result from ischemia caused by a "steal" of blood flow to larger AVMs. The draining veins may become large with the development of deep venous varices. It is generally accepted that AVMs hemorrhage from rupture of these dilated thin-walled veins.

The initial clinical presentation is varied in persons with an AVM. Fifty percent present with either an intraparenchymal hematoma or subarachnoid hemorrhage. The peak incidence is during the 20- to 30-year age period. Ironically, it seems to be the smaller AVMs that have the greater risk of hemorrhage. In contrast to subarachnoid hemorrhage due to berry aneurysms, the mortality rate from the first bleed is relatively low, about 10 percent, probably because the hemorrhage is of venous origin. A few persons present with a subdural hematoma near the region of the malformation, which is most likely due to dural malformations. When all malformations are considered as a group, there is a yearly risk of hemorrhage of 1 to 4 percent and a yearly rebleed risk of 3 percent.

About 33 percent of persons with an AVM present with a seizure disorder that may be either focal or generalized. Headache resembling migraine is the presenting symptom in 9 percent. In later life, presenile dementia may occur, the cause of which is unknown.

The consensus is that AVMs should be resected if they have bled at least once and are in a location where they can be totally resected without causing neurologic damage. Incomplete resections are of limited value. Rarely, an AVM is removed in an attempt to relieve intractable seizures, but the results have been inconsistent. Headache is generally not an indication for surgical removal. AVMs that have not bled are usually not removed.

Various methods are used to treat AVMs. Surgical removal is the most common and most successful treatment for lesions near the cortical surface limited to one arterial vascular distribution. For the AVM to be completely treated, the actual tangle ("sponge") must be obliterated. If an AVM is incompletely removed or obliterated and a fistula remains, new vessels contribute to the lesion and the AVM again grows. It may be possible to partially or sometimes completely obliterate the nidus of the AVM by embolization using a small (2 French) superselective catheter and embolic occlusive materials. Following this procedure, it is said that 30 percent of AVMs initially thought to be surgically unresectable can subsequently be totally resected.

Skull Radiography

About one-third of persons with an intracranial AVM show some characteristic skull abnormality, most commonly evidence of large feeding arteries or veins causing erosion of the bone. They include enlargement of the carotid groove in the paracavernous region, enlarged meningeal grooves on the inner table, enlarged or increased numbers of holes for perforating vessels (particularly in the region of a dural AVM), and inner table thinning from dilated cortical draining veins. Calcification is seen in only 20 percent with plain film skull radiography, whereas it is seen in most AVMs with CT scanning.

CT Scanning

The CT appearance of an AVM is characteristic. On the nonenhanced CT scan the lesion is most commonly seen as a region of mixed high and low density (Fig. 4-1A). The margins are poorly defined, calcifications are frequently observed, and there is almost always some degree of local atrophy, which may be indicated by subtle focal dilatation of the nearby ventricular cavities or sulci. Minor degrees of focal encephalomalacia may be seen adjacent to the nidus. It is rare to see large regions of ischemia or infarction. When close observation is made of these findings, most AVMs that are larger than about 1 cm can be suspected on the nonenhanced CT examination.

The contrast-enhanced CT examination shows nonhomogeneous increased density of the lesion and better demonstrates the malformation. The enhanced regions represent contrast-filled vessels with flowing blood, and the lower density indicates clotted channels and atrophic tissue. Large feeding arteries and veins are shown as serpiginous linear channels (Fig. 4-1). It is important to recognize the vascular territories involved and the location of large draining veins. If there is recent hemorrhage or excessive calcification, the abnormal enhancement may not easily be seen. However, the recognition of dilated arteries at the base of the brain and large draining veins allow one to make the diagnosis of AVM.

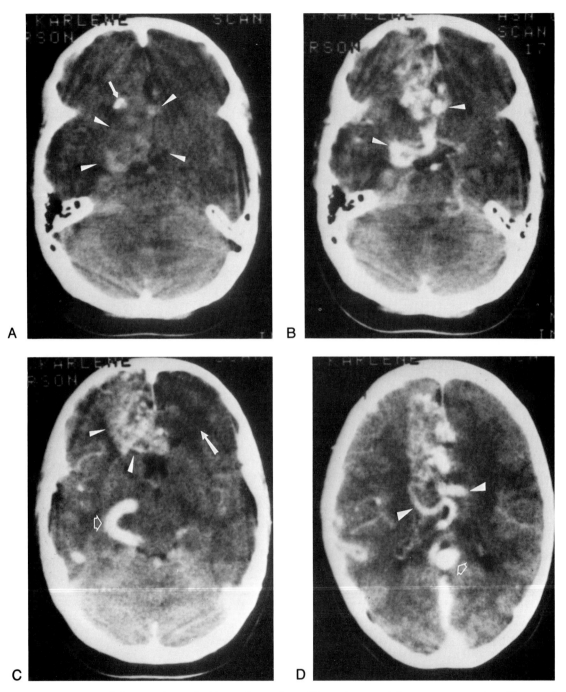

Fig. 4-1 AVM, CT. (A) Nonenhanced CT scan shows the malformation as an inhomogeneous region of increased density representing blood-filled vascular channels and adjacent gliosis (arrowheads). Calcification is present (arrow). **(B)** Contrast-enhanced CT scan at the same level as the scan in Fig. A shows the contrast-filled, grossly dilated vessels, mostly enlarged veins (arrowheads). **(C)** Scan at a higher level shows the "sponge" of the malformation (arrowheads). It extends across the corpus callosum but causes little mass effect. There is a huge draining vein on the right, probably the basal vein (open arrow). A region of hypodensity in the left frontal lobe represents ischemia or infarction from "steal" (arrow). **(D)** Scan through a higher level shows that the malformation is large and extends posteriorly in the corpus callosum and cingulate gyrus. There are large dilated draining veins (arrowheads) and a moderately enlarged vein of Galen (open arrow).

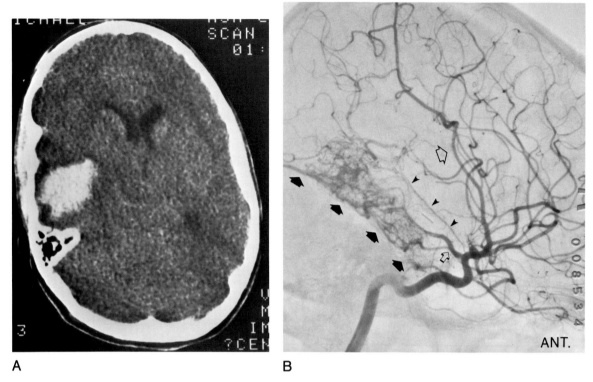

A   B

Fig. 4-2 AVM, intraparenchymal hematoma. (A) Moderate-sized subcortical hemorrhage is present in the right middle temporal lobe. There is mild mass effect. The basal cisterns and sulci are not well seen, possibly indicative of a small subarachnoid hemorrhage making the CSF isodense with the brain. **(B)** Lateral ICA angiography demonstrates a large vascular malformation involving the medial and inferior temporal lobe (black arrows). It is supplied by the temporal branches of the posterior cerebral artery, which has a fetal type communication with the ICA (bottom open arrow). The temporal hematoma has caused elevation of the sylvian vessels (top open arrow) and delayed filling of temporal opercular arteries over the lateral cortex. The anterior choroidal artery is stretched because of the temporal lobe mass (arrowheads).

Computed tomography remains a primary means of detecting the complications associated with vascular malformations of the brain. Subarachnoid hemorrhage is recognized by the increased density in the subarachnoid cisterns (see Ch. 3). There is more likely to be blood within the sulci over the convexities than in the basal cisterns. A brain hematoma is more likely to be seen with a ruptured AVM than with a ruptured aneurysm (Fig. 4-2). The hematoma may be large and cause brain herniation. Small hematomas may cause little permanent damage, as the bleed may occur into the already atrophied brain tissue. The hematoma may be indistinguishable from hematomas of other causes such as hypertension or tumor. The hemorrhage may be the only indication of a cryptic (nonvisible) vascular malformation.

Hydrocephalus may occur after rupture of an AVM, caused acutely by the mass of the hematoma, subarachnoid hemorrhage, or intraventricular blood. The size of the ventricles must be followed, as shunting may be required. An entrapped ventricle is also possible.

MRI

Routine spin echo MRI distinguishes a vascular malformation from other abnormalities, primarily by the recognition of flow-void within the serpiginous abnormal feeding and draining vessels of the malformation. The dilated vascular channels of the AVM appear dark on the MRI image (Fig. 4-3). When there is difficulty determining whether low signal is representative of blood flow or paramagnetic effect, GRE imaging may

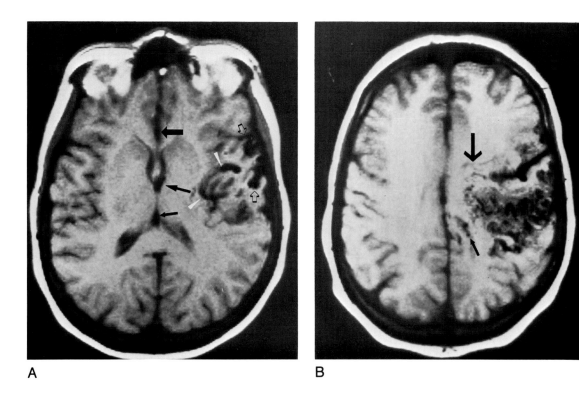

A   B

Fig. 4-3 AVM, MRI. (A) T_1-weighted MRI through the
ventricular system shows the flow-void hypointensity of enlarged sylvian vessels (white arrowheads) and large cortical
veins over the temporal lobe (open arrows). The pericallosal
arteries are enlarged (large arrow), indicating that they also
supply the malformation. Enlargement of the internal cerebral vein (small arrows) indicates that the malformation has
deep venous drainage as well. There are no changes of hemorrhage. **(B)** Scan through the hemisphere shows the main
nidus of the large parietal malformation with irregular dilated vascular channels. Enlarged deep medullary veins drain
to the deep venous system (large arrow). Enlarged cortical
arteries in the pericallosal distribution also feed the malformation (small arrow). **(C)** T_2-weighted MRI shows the high
intensity regions of gliosis within the malformation (arrow).
There is no hemosiderin deposition associated with this
AVM.

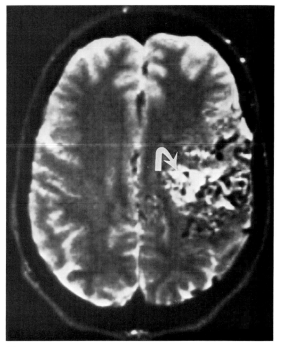

C

be used. Most commonly, vessels with flow-void on the SE images appear hyperintense with GRE sequences. Calcium or hemosiderin remain of low intensity. Gd-DTPA shows variable enhancement of the vessels depending on the speed of flow. Slower flow shows greater enhancement. In general, contrast enhancement is not necessary for the diagnosis. As with CT scanning, a large hematoma may obliterate visualization of the AVM.

The MRI scan shows changes of subacute and chronic hemorrhage, as well as variable hemosiderin deposition within and near the AVM. A thin hemosiderin deposit may be seen over the ventricular and cortical surfaces. Calcium is poorly recognized and may be difficult to differentiate from hemosiderin within the malformation. Local gliosis surrounding the AVM appears as high signal intensity on the T_2-weighted images (Fig. 4-3C). Usually there is no mass effect or edema with an AVM unless there has been recent hemorrhage. Focal atrophy may be seen.

Angiography

Cerebral angiography remains the most precise technique for the anatomic definition of the AVM. The study must be complete and of high technical quality. It is essential to selectively opacify all the vessels that may be contributing to the malformation (Fig. 4-4). Rapid serial filming must be done through the venous phase to determine the flow patterns of both the arteries and the veins. In some cases, three or four films per second are required. Selective bilateral external carotid angiography is routinely performed when the AVM is of the posterior fossa or in the peripheral portion of the cerebral hemispheres so as to detect dural vascular supply (Fig. 4-4C). Contralateral contribution from the exter-

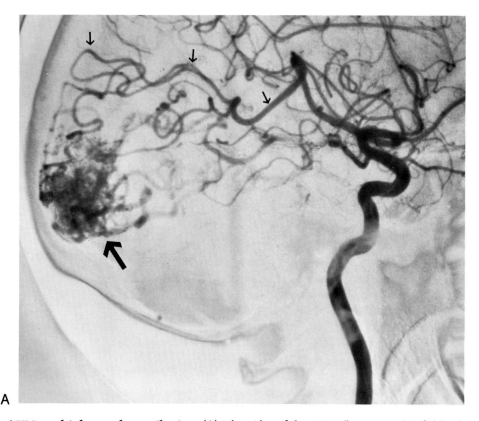

A

Fig. 4-4 AVM, multiple vessel contribution. (A) The nidus of the AVM (large arrow) is fed by the angular branch (small arrows) and posterior temporal branches of the middle cerebral artery. *(Figure continues.)*

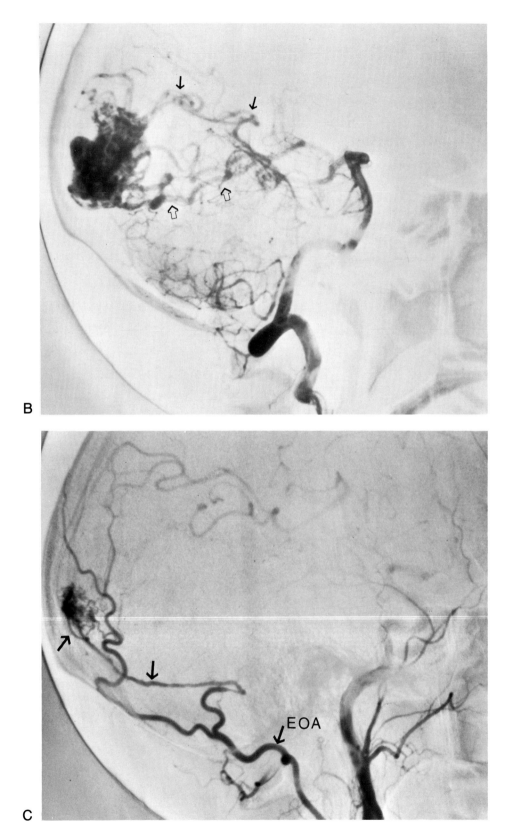

B

C

Fig. 4-4 *(Continued)*. **(B)** Vertebral angiography shows that the malformation is also supplied by the parieto-occipital branches (arrows) and the medial temporal branches (open arrows) of the posterior cerebral artery. **(C)** Selective external carotid angiography. The AVM also receives supply from a dural vessel rising from the external occipital branch of the external carotid artery (arrows). EOA = external occipital artery.

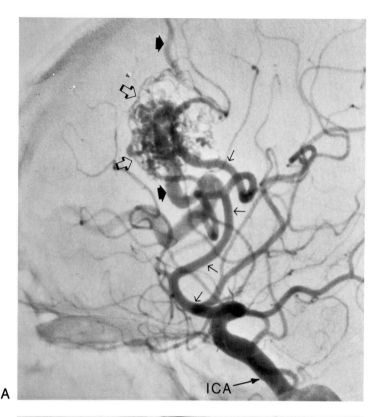

A

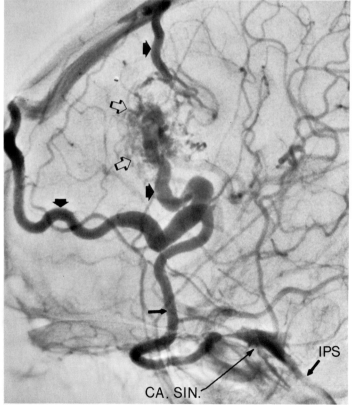

B

Fig. 4-5 AVM, arteriography. (A) Lateral
ICA angiography in the early arterial phase
shows a large feeding middle cerebral vessel
(small arrows) supplying the nidus of the
malformation (open arrows). The vessel
shows uniform enlargement throughout. Extremely early draining veins are already seen
in this early arterial phase (large black
arrows). Note that the nidus appears compact. **(B)** Late arterial phase shows large superficial draining veins (large black arrows).
A vein drains inferiorly (small arrow) into the
cavernous sinus (CA. SIN.) and the inferior
petrosal sinus (IPS).

nal or internal carotid arteries to the malformation can be seen in up to 30 percent. Large doses of contrast may be necessary to adequately visualize a large malformation. This method can be done safely as most of the contrast passes through the AVM, not the normal cerebral vascularity.

The angiographic criteria of an AVM are as follows (Figs. 4-4 to 4-6).

1. A "sponge" of abnormal vessels, representing the nidus of the malformation. The vessels are tightly packed together as the intervening brain tissue is atrophic. Tumor neovascularity is not packed nearly as tightly as with an AVM.

2. Large feeding arteries, with uniform enlargement from their origin. Vessels feeding tumors may enlarge, but more peripherally near the tumor and not from the origin of the vessel.

3. Large rapidly filling veins with frequent varix formation. Early draining veins are also seen with high grade tumors, but the veins tend to be of normal size and do not fill as early as with the AVM.

4. Mass effect if the AVM has recently ruptured. This effect also occurs with tumors. When the AVM is small, it may be difficult to distinguish from a tumor by angiography.

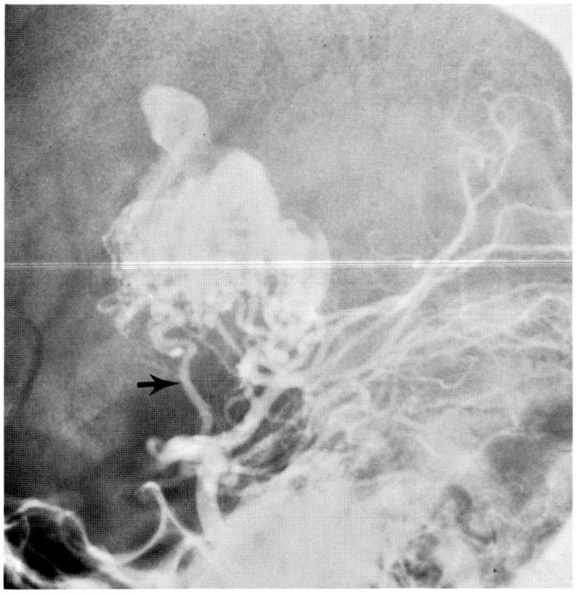

Dural Vascular Malformations

A dural vascular malformation may be confined entirely to the dura and fed by dural vessels, or it may involve both the dura and the brain and be fed by both dural and pial vessels. A pure dural malformation tends to have a direct arteriovenous (A-V) communication, so it is, in essence, a dural A-V fistula. The most frequent type is a direct arterial feeder into a dural sinus, a carotid-cavernous fistula being a striking example. Multiple arterial feeders may contribute to the malformation. The most common sites for dural A-V malformations are at the cavernous sinus and the lateral or sigmoid sinus of the posterior fossa (Fig. 4-7). Selective internal (ICA) and external (ECA) carotid artery arteriography is usually necessary to define the vascular supply of these unusual malformations.

The malformations may be a cause of a subarachnoid hemorrhage, although they are most frequently found incidentally. Angiography is the only means for their diagnosis, as the lesions cannot be seen with CT scans or MRI.

Vein of Galen Aneurysm

The vein of Galen aneurysm is a rare type of vascular malformation that is almost always diagnosed during the newborn period. It is comprised of direct fistulous communications of arteries with the deep veins. A large single feeding artery may be the cause. There is high flow into the vein, resulting in the aneurysmal dilatation. The high flow may cause congestive heart failure and a loud intracranial bruit. The vein of Galen aneurysm may compress the aqueduct, causing hydrocephalus (Fig. 4-8).

VENOUS ANGIOMA

Cerebral venous angioma is an uncommon form of vascular malformation that is composed solely of veins. On angiography, it is characterized by a group of enlarged deep medullary veins that converge to drain into a large intraparenchymal vein that usually courses through the central white matter to the cortical surface to drain into a dural sinus (Figs. 4-9 and 4-10). The

Fig. 4-6 AVM, within the thalamus. Lateral vertebral angiography shows a large vascular malformation within the thalamus. It is fed by enlarged thalamoperforate branches (arrow).

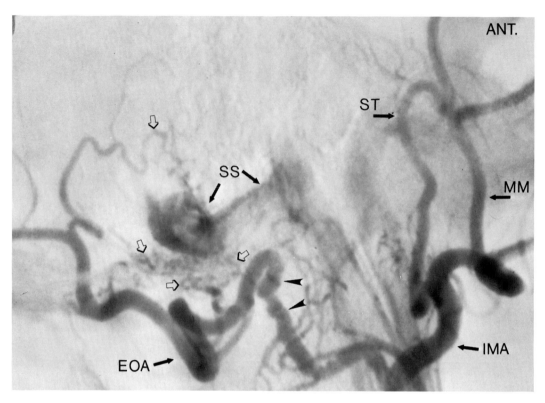

Fig. 4-7 Dural AVM. Lateral selective ECA angiography demonstrates a dural vascular malformation into the sigmoid sinus (SS). There are multiple feeders supplying the fistula (open arrows). These feeders arise from the external occipital artery (EOA). The irregularity of the EOA most likely represents fibromuscular dysplasia (arrowheads). IMA = internal maxillary artery; ST = superficial temporal artery; MM = middle meningeal artery.

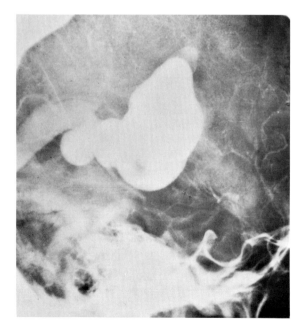

Fig. 4-8 Vein of Galen aneurysm. A huge aneurysm of the vein of Galen is filled with contrast. It empties into a large, straight sinus posteriorly. This aneurysm is a result of the thalamic vascular malformation demonstrated in Figure 4-6.

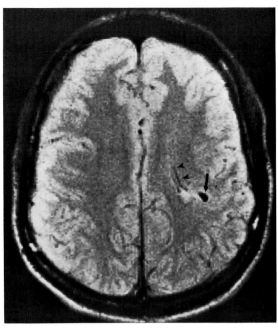

Fig. 4-9 Venous angioma. (A) Proton density MRI in the transaxial plane shows the anomalous medullary veins (arrowheads) draining into a large vein (arrow), which traverses the white matter to the cortical surface. **(B)** AP angiography of the same patient shows the medullary veins (arrowheads) converging to drain into the large anomalous vein (arrow), which courses through the white matter to the cortical surface. SAG = posterior sagittal sinus; TORC = torcula; TRANS = transverse sinus.

A

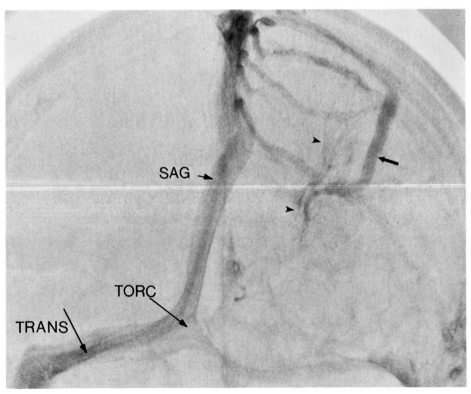

B

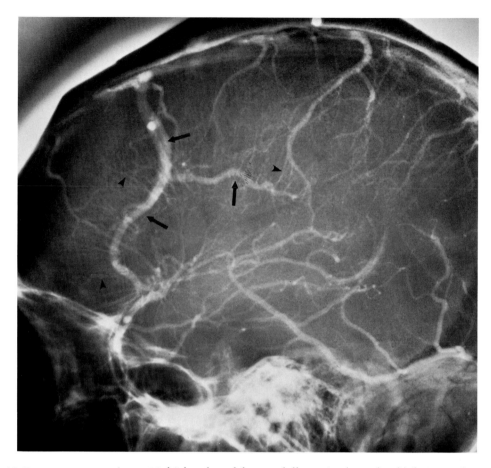

Fig. 4-10 Large venous angioma. Multiple enlarged deep medullary veins (arrowheads) drain into large anomalous veins coursing through the white matter to the cortical surface (arrows). This "angioma" is the predominant drainage of the entire frontal lobe in this patient. The subependymal veins of the lateral ventricles are underdeveloped.

veins fill at the normal time, and there is no shunting. It sometimes has a "head of Medusa" pattern (Fig. 4-9B). It occurs most often in the frontal portions of the cerebral hemispheres but may be seen in any location, including the cerebellum, brain stem, and spinal cord. Venous angioma is considered to be an anomalous venous drainage pattern rather than a true angioma.

On the contrast-enhanced CT scan the large intracerebral vein is often seen as a curvilinear density coursing through the brain to the cortical surface. There is no edema, and the lesion does not calcify. The nonenhanced examination is almost always normal. On MRI, the large anomalous vein is seen as tubular structure with flow-void (Fig. 4-9). Rarely, there are some associated adjacent parenchymal intensity changes, both high and low signal, that possibly represent local ische-

mia and gliosis. The clinical significance of these changes is unknown.

The clinical presentation is varied. Most of the lesions are asymptomatic and are found incidentally at CT scanning or angiography. They have, however, been associated with hemorrhage, seizures, headaches, or ataxia, although their causal role in these processes is unknown.

CAPILLARY TELANGIECTASIS

Capillary telangiectases are composed of dilated capillaries that vary in caliber. Most commonly seen as incidental findings at autopsy, they are occasionally associated with a small intracerebral hemorrhage.

These lesions are "cryptic," as they cannot be demonstrated by CT scans, MRI, or angiography.

CAVERNOUS HEMANGIOMA

The cavernous hemangioma is the rarest type of vascular malformation, but it is clinically important because it can hemorrhage or cause seizures. It is potentially totally resectable. These lesions most commonly occur in the subcortical regions of the cerebral hemispheres, but they may also lie deep within the brain, particularly near the region of the pineal. Calcification is present in 30 percent of lesions.

The CT scan demonstrates a well circumscribed, slightly hyperdense, often calcified lesion that shows minimal homogeneous contrast enhancement (see Fig. 6-21). There is no mass effect or surrounding edema. A hematoma may be present; and in this situation the lesion usually cannot be recognized. The lesion has

characteristics of a meningioma or lymphoma; and depending on the location of the malformation, it may be difficult to differentiate between these possibilities. Because the blood flow is so slow through the hemangioma, it is almost never detected with angiography. With MRI, the lesion is slightly hypointense on both T_1- and T_2-weighted images, but there may be circumferential changes of low intensity from hemosiderin and high T_2 signal representing gliosis and chronic hemorrhage (Fig. 4-11).

"CRYPTIC" VASCULAR MALFORMATION

A "cryptic" malformation is defined as one that cannot be observed with angiography. It is thought to be small, possibly obliterated by hemorrhage or thrombosis. The lesion may be suspected with MRI or CT scanning. The subacute and chronic changes of multiple

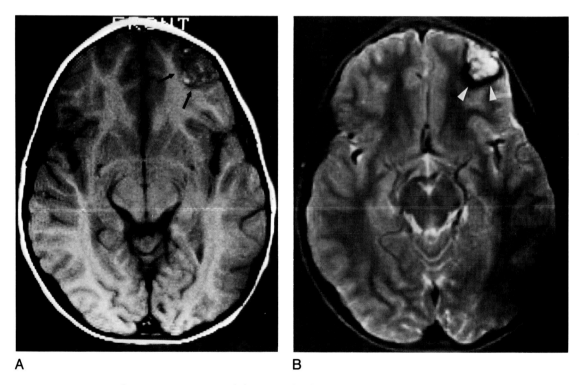

A   B

Fig. 4-11 Cavernous hemangioma, MRI. (A) T_1-weighted MRI shows the cavernous hemangioma as a generally low-intensity lesion on the cortical surface of the left frontal lobe (arrows). A few focal high signal intensity regions represent chronic hemorrhage. **(B)** T_2-weighted MRI shows high signal intensity through the lesion representing gliosis. The lesion is surrounded by a rim of extreme hypointensity representing hemosiderin deposition.

hemorrhages are detected, and it is assumed that they are due to an underlying occult vascular malformation.

With MRI, the T_2-weighted image is the most useful, particularly with high field strength units. The lesion is seen as inhomogeneous with a "target" configuration. Characteristically, there is a peripheral rim of low signal intensity thought to represent hemosiderin deposits within macrophages. Centrally, there is mixed high signal from chronic hemorrhage and low signal from calcium and iron. MRI is more sensitive than the CT scan for detecting "cryptic" AVMs. In the literature, few of the lesions described as "cryptic" AVMs have been histologically proved.

The CT scan generally displays "cryptic" malformations as foci of calcium or iron without mass effect.

There may be minimal contrast enhancement, but it is inconsistent. On CT scans the lesion cannot be differentiated from the early changes of a calcified glioma or the rare calcified infarction.

MALFORMATION SYNDROMES

Encephalofacial (Trigeminal) Angiomatosis (Sturge-Weber Syndrome)

Sturge-Weber syndrome is a congenital anomaly usually associated with a hemangioma or nevus of the face, most commonly in the distribution of the trigeminal

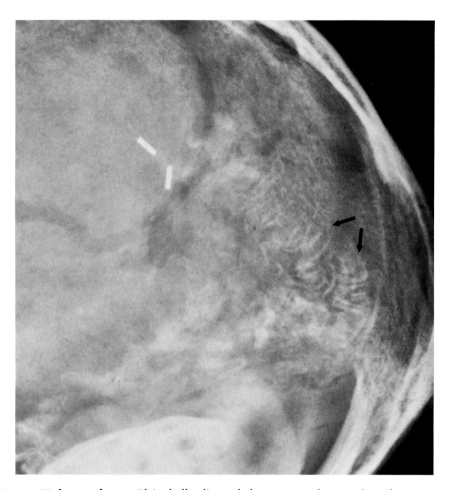

Fig. 4-12 Sturge-Weber syndrome. Plain skull radiograph demonstrates the typical gyriform pattern of cortical calcification (arrows) indicative of the angiomatous malformation.

nerve. Persons affected may have seizures, hemiparesis, and mental retardation. Intracranially, there is a complex venous and capillary malformation of the leptomeninges that occurs over the cortex of a hemisphere. Calcification occurs in the cortex of the brain underneath the malformation and creates a typical gyriform pattern that can be seen on skull radiography (Fig. 4-12) and CT scans. Local atrophy is present that may be severe enough to cause calvarial changes of the Dyke-Davidoff-Mason syndrome (thickening of the calvarium and unilateral volume loss of the cranial cavity). Angiography demonstrates occluded arteries and veins in the region of the malformation. The CT scan shows the calcium and atrophy but little or no contrast enhancement. GRE MRI sequences show the cortical calcifications as serpiginous signal dropout.

Wyburn-Mason Syndrome

In its complete form, the Wyburn-Mason syndrome consists in cutaneous, retinal, cerebral, and mandibular or maxillary AVMs. Any portion of the brain may be involved, but most often it is the optic pathways. The malformations may be large and appear as typical AVMs, as described above. The facial malformations may cause serious bleeding into the nasal cavities or mouth.

SUGGESTED READING

Atlas SW: Intracranial vascular malformations and aneurysms: current imaging applications. Radiol Clin North Am 26:821, 1988

Eskridge JM: Interventional neuroradiology: state of the art. Radiology 172:991, 1989

Fults D, Kelly DL Jr.: Natural history of arteriovenous malformations of the brain: a clinical study. Neurosurgery 15:658, 1984

Lemme-Plaghos L, Kucharczyk W, Brant-Zawadzki M, et al: MR imaging of angiographically occult vascular malformations. AJNR 7:217, 1986

Pelz DM, Fox AJ, Viñuela F, et al: Preoperative embolization of brain AVMs with isobutyl-2 cyanoacrylate. AJNR 9:757, 1988

Rubinstein LJ: Tumors of the central nervous system. p 241. Armed Forces Institute of Pathology, Washington, DC, 1972

Smith HJ, Strother CM, Kikuchi Y: MR imaging in the management of supratentorial intracranial AVMs. AJNR 9:225, 1988

5

Cranial Tumors

Tumors of the brain and its linings account for about 1 percent of all deaths, and for about 9 percent of all neoplastic disease. The tumors are generally classified according to cytogenetic lines. The classification system presented here is a compilation of those proposed by the World Health Organization and by Rubinstein in the Armed Forces Institute of Pathology fascicle *Tumors of the Central Nervous System.* The tumor types and approximate frequency of occurrence are given on page 136. The frequency of tumor types actually observed varies according to referral pattern.

Nearly 95 percent of tumors are accounted for by glioma, metastasis, meningioma, pituitary adenoma, and acoustic neurinoma. All the others are uncommon. Brain tumors characteristically occur within given age ranges and have strong predilections for certain intracranial regions (Table 5-1). Although some tumors have specific imaging characteristics, it may be impossible to correctly identify a specific tumor type solely with imaging. The imaging factors used to identify specific tumors are given on page 136.

IMAGING OF TUMORS

The main diagnostic imaging modalities for evaluation of neoplastic disease of the brain are MRI, CT scanning, and angiography. MRI has the greatest sensitivity for detection of tumors and is the preferred initial examination. CT scanning is best for defining bone destruction or sclerosis associated with metastatic tumors, pituitary adenomas, meningiomas, acoustic neurinomas, adjacent carcinomas from the sinuses or pharynx, and glomus tumors. Radionuclide scanning has little diagnostic role here.

Contrast Enhancement

Intravenous contrast enhancement is basic to the evaluation of neoplastic disease with both MRI and CT scanning. Gd-DTPA is presently used with MRI and aqueous iodinated agents for CT scans.

Most tumors show contrast enhancement. This abnormal accumulation of contrast in the tumor results primarily from leakage of contrast into the tumor interstitium because of the absence of a blood-brain barrier within the tumor neovascularity. Contrast enhancement is seen as hyperdensity on CT scans (Fig. 5-1) and hyperintensity on T_1-weighted MRI (Fig. 5-2).

The region of contrast enhancement corresponds well with the main tumor mass. However, malignant tumor cells are commonly found beyond the enhanced portion of the tumor, particularly with glioma. Enhancement correlates with tumor grade (degree of malignancy) only for glial tumors.

Contrast enhancement indicates tumor viability. Therefore whenever a biopsy is to be performed, it is done in a region of the tumor that demonstrates contrast enhancement. Ring enhancement implies central necrosis, cyst formation, or abscess. In some tumor types there is characteristic enhancement, which is discussed below. The diagnostic implications of contrast enhancement in tumors is the same for both CT scanning and MRI.

MRI

On MRI, neoplastic lesions are detected because of their long T_1 and T_2 relaxation times compared with those for brain parenchyma. This prolongation is be-

FREQUENCY OF CEREBRAL
NEOPLASMS ACCORDING TO
TUMOR TYPE

Neuroglial tumors (40%)
  Glioblastoma (55%)
  Astrocytoma (22%)
  Ependymoma (6%)
  Medulloblastoma (6%)
  Oligodendroglioma (5%)
  Mixed and gliosarcoma (4%)
  Others (2%)
Metastatic tumor (35%)
  Lung (adenocarcinoma, small cell carcinoma) (40%)
  Breast carcinoma (40%)
  Others (kidney, colon, prostate, melanoma) (20%)
Mesodermal tumors (10%)
  Meningioma (common)
  Sarcoma (rare)
    Hemangiopericytoma
Pituitary tumors (5%)
  Microadenoma
  Macroadenoma
Cranial nerve tumors (3%)
  Schwannoma (neurinoma): CN VIII (common), CN V (uncommon)
Lymphoreticular system tumors (2%)
  Lymphoma
  Leukemia (chloroma)
Others (5%)
  Pineal region tumors
  Craniopharyngioma
  Hemangioblastoma
  Embryonic tumors
  Neuronal tumors
    Gangliocytoma
    Ganglioglioma
    Ganglioneuroblastoma
    Neuroblastoma
  Chordoma
  Dermoid, epidermoid, teratoma

FACTORS USEFUL FOR
IDENTIFICATION OF BRAIN TUMORS

Location
  Site
  Surface of brain
  Gray-white junction
  White matter
Age
Imaging characteristics of the tumor
  Relative CT density
  Intensity of MRI signal
  MRI signal change with T_1 and T_2
Contrast enhancement
  Presence
  Pattern
Edema
  Pattern
  Amount
Calcification
Cystic change
Shape
Pattern of growth
Adjacent bone changes
Number of lesions

cause of the increased water content of the neoplastic tissue. Therefore the tumor is seen as low signal intensity of the T_1-weighted images and as high signal intensity on the T_2-weighted images. Similarly, MRI is particularly sensitive to the detection of surrounding vasogenic edema, which also exhibits prolonged T_1 and T_2 relaxation times and is apparent as low intensity on T_1-weighted images and high intensity on T_2-weighted images.

At times the tumor nidus is difficult to differentiate from the surrounding edema, as both regions exhibit prolonged T_1 and T_2 relaxation times. Commonly, however, there is less prolongation of T_1 and T_2 in the tumor than in surrounding edema. Therefore on the T_1-weighted images, the tumor is differentiated by its slightly greater intensity than the surrounding edema and on the T_2-weighted images by its slightly less intensity than the surrounding edema (Fig. 5-3).

Contrast enhancement is done with intravenously

Table 5-1 Neoplasm Type According to Age and Location

Site	Adults	Children
Cerebral hemispheres	**Glioma**	**Astrocytoma**
	Metastasis	**Ependymoma**
	Neuronal tumors	Mixed tumor
	Mixed tumors	Metastasis
		Primitive neuronal tumor
Meninges	**Meningioma**	**Leukemia**
	Metastasis	**Metastasis**
Sella, juxtasellar area	**Pituitary adenoma**	**Craniopharyngioma**
	Meningioma	Optic glioma
	Craniopharyngioma	Hypothalamic glioma
	Hypothalamic glioma	
	Epidermoid, teratoma	
	CN V neurinoma	
	Chordoma	
	Sphenoid sinus carcinoma	
	Nasopharyngeal carcinoma	
Pineal Region	**Metastasis**	**Dysgerminoma**
	Glioma, usually tectal	Pinealoma
	Subependymoma	Pineoblastoma
		Embryonal yolk sac tumor
		Teratoma
		Glioma
Intraventricular area	**Meningioma**	**Ependymoma**
	Exophytic glioma	Choroid plexus papilloma
	Colloid cyst of third ventricle	
	Ependymoma	
	Choroid plexus papilloma	
	Epidermoid	
	Metastasis	
	Xanthogranuloma	
Cerebellar hemisphere	**Metastasis**	**Astrocytoma**
	Hemangioblastoma	Medulloblastoma ($>$12 years of age)
	Astrocytoma (rare)	
	Neuronal tumors	
Midline cerebellum	**Metastasis**	**Medulloblastoma**
	Meningioma of fourth ventricle	**Ependymoma**
		Astrocytoma
Brain stem	**Metastasis**	**Astrocytoma**
	Glioma	
Cerebellar pontine angle	**Acoustic neurinoma**	Epidermoid
	Meningioma	Acoustic neurinoma (NF-2)
	Epidermoid	Meningioma
	Metastasis	
Skull	**Metastasis**	Metastasis
	Chordoma	Epidermoid
	Sinus carcinoma	Histiocytosis X
	Direct invasion	Sarcoma
	Glomus tumor	
	Sarcoma	

Bold letters indicate the most common tumors.
Adapted from Dubois PJ: p. 365. In Heinz ED (ed): *The Clinical Neurosciences: Neuroradiology.* Churchill Livingstone, New York, 1984.

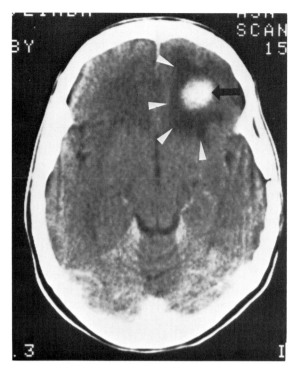

Fig. 5-1 Metastatic adenocarcinoma of the lung, CT scan with contrast enhancement. Note the typical features of a cerebral neoplasm. There is dense contrast enhancement of the tumor nidus (black arrow) that is surrounded by white matter vasogenic edema (white arrowheads).

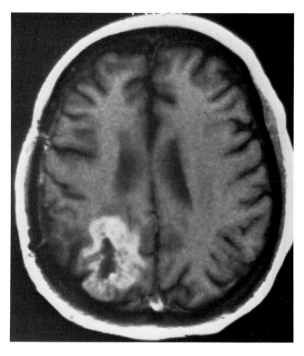

Fig. 5-2 Glioblastoma multiforme. MRI with Gd-DTPA contrast enhancement shows the striking hyperintensity of the tumor nidus on T_1-weighted images.

administered gadolinium-DTPA/dimeglumine (Gd-DTPA). The present recommended dose is 0.1 mmol/kg body weight. MRI is best performed immediately after the injection but may be performed anytime up to 1 hour later. T_1-weighted technique is used to visualize contrast enhancement. It clearly distinguishes the high intensity enhancement from the surrounding lower intensity edema and brain tissue.

Contrast-enhanced MRI is the most sensitive imaging technique for the detection of almost all intracranial tumors, particularly glioblastoma, metastasis, meningioma, and acoustic neurinoma and those in the posterior fossa in children. Enhanced MRI provides accurate localization of the tumor nidus.

The specific identification of tumor type with MRI is often difficult. Specific diagnosis is based primarily on the statistics of location, image pattern, clinical history, and age of the patient. Specific T_1 and T_2 relaxation rates have been of little use for defining specific tumor

types. Some helpful additional signal characteristics are discussed under specific subsections.

CT Scanning

The contrast-enhanced scan in the transaxial plane is the most common CT examination for the evaluation of tumors. A bolus or bolus–drip infusion of contrast is given using 27 to 42 g of iodine. When subtle metastatic disease is sought as part of staging, the high dose (80 g of iodine) drip technique followed by a 1.0- to 1.5-hour delayed scan is the most sensitive CT technique for the detection of the lesions. Other projections, particularly the coronal view, are useful for evaluating tumors at the base of the skull (sella, planum sphenoidale) and those near the tentorium. Thin sections (less than 5 mm) through the posterior fossa and temporal regions reduce the artifact due to bone asymmetry.

Tumors that do not enhance are recognized (1) directly by their different absorption density compared with the surrounding brain or (2) indirectly by peritu-

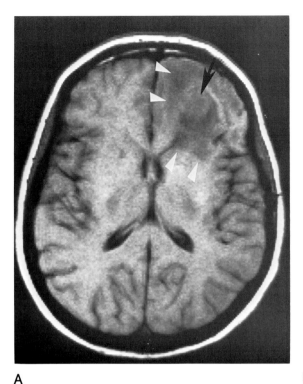
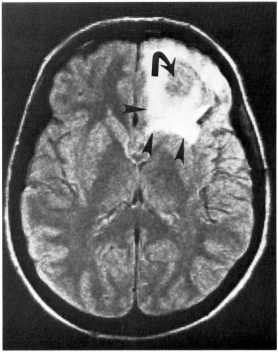

A   B

Fig. 5-3 Metastasis, carcinoma of the lung. (A) T_1-weighted image shows the tumor nidus (black arrow) slightly hyperintense to the surrounding hypointense edema (white arrowheads). **(B)** Lightly T_2-weighted image shows the tumor nidus (curved black arrow) to be relatively hypointense to the surrounding hyperintense edema (black arrowheads). The CT scan of this patient is shown in Figure 5-1.

moral edema and mass effect. Additional differential diagnostic information is sometimes gained with a nonenhanced scan (calcium, tumor density). The terminology for nonenhanced lesions is as follows.

Hyperdensity: Tumors that have a generally homogeneous greater absorption density compared with the surrounding brain (Fig. 5-4). It may result from fine calcification, hemorrhage, or a high nuclear/cytoplasmic ratio, as seen in box.

Hypodensity: Tumors that have a lower absorption density than the surrounding brain. It is accounted for by the water content of the tumor tissue, cysts, necrosis, or fat (extreme hypodensity). Low grade astrocytoma is a common example.

Isodensity: Tumors that have the same absorption density as the surrounding brain and therefore are at the same gray scale density as the brain. This pattern is the most common one for a tumor nidus.

HYPERDENSE TUMORS, NONENHANCED CT SCANS

Adults
  Meningioma
  Metastatic tumors
    Melanoma
    Colon
    Kidney
    Choriocarcinoma
    Osteogenic sarcoma
  Lymphoma
  Colloid cyst
  Cavernous hemangioma
Children
  Medulloblastoma
  Hamartoma

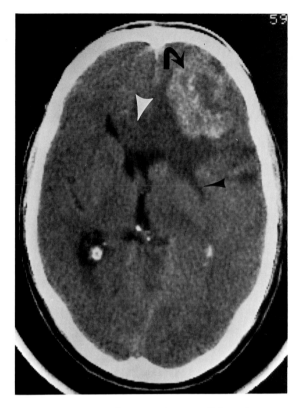

Fig. 5-4 Metastatic adenocarcinoma of the colon. Nonenhanced CT scan shows a hyperdense tumor nidus in the left frontal lobe (curved black arrow). Note the extensive white matter edema extending into the external capsule (black arrowhead) and across the corpus callosum (white arrowhead). There is subfalcial herniation and compression of the frontal horns of the ventricular system.

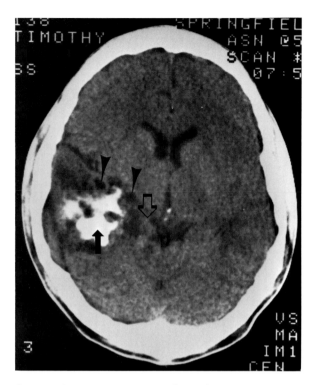

Fig. 5-5 Astrocytoma. Nonenhanced CT scan shows a mixed density tumor in the right posterior temporal lobe. There is dense calcification (black arrow), isodense solid tumor (open black arrow), and low density cysts (black arrowheads). An oligodendroglioma or ganglioneuroma could have this same appearance.

Mixed density: Tumors that are inhomogeneous with regions of hyperdensity and hypodensity, resulting from a mixture of necrosis, hemorrhage, cysts, calcification, and viable tumor nidus (Fig. 5-5).

Angiography

The role of angiography in the evaluation of brain tumors has decreased immensely. The technique is now used primarily to: (1) differentiate tumor from infarction in difficult cases; (2) differentiate glioma from metastasis when a biopsy cannot be performed; (3) define vascular anatomy for large meningiomas prior to surgical removal and preoperative embolization; (4) differentiate an aneurysm from a pituitary tumor; and (5) topographically localize a small metastasis prior to surgical excision. Specific angiographic signs are discussed in the following sections.

BRAIN EDEMA

One of the most serious side effects of brain tumors is cerebral edema. Brain tumors produce varying amounts of edema, usually related to their speed of growth and neovascularity. The edema is of the vasogenic type; that is, it results from the absence of the blood-brain barrier in tumor neovascularity, which allows leakage of proteins and other solutes into the surrounding extracellular space of the white matter. The edema may spread along white matter tracts far away from the tumor mass, sometimes crossing the midline (Fig. 5-4). As a rule, tumors cause relatively little edema in gray matter.

Brain edema may occur with both intracerebral and

extracerebral tumors, although the extracerebral tumors (meningiomas) tend to produce less. Edema is particularly frequent and severe with metastatic carcinomas and may be excessive from a small, sometimes invisible focus. As edema is a primary cause of increased intracranial pressure and mass effect with tumors, it should be quantified in the report. On CT scans edema is seen as a region of hypodensity (Fig. 5-4). On MRI it is hypointense on T_1-weighted images and hyperintense on T_2-weighted images (Fig. 5-3). Brain edema will usually decrease following glucocorticoid therapy.

CYST FORMATION

Cysts occur within tumors and may be small (microcysts) or large. Large cysts are most often seen with low grade astrocytomas and craniopharyngiomas but may also be seen with a pituitary adenoma, meningioma, acoustic neurinoma, and hemangioblastoma. Microcysts are most commonly seen in the more malignant primary gliomas. Cystic cavities may result from necrosis or hemorrhage, and they may be difficult to differentiate from true cysts.

Cysts may contain nearly pure water or considerable protein or other debris, often from prior hemorrhage. Usually, large cysts have homogeneous contents whereas solid tumor tends to be more inhomogeneous. At times cysts and solid tumors will have similar imaging characteristics and cannot be differentiated. A fluid level caused by the heavier, dependent proteinaceous material is diagnostic of a cyst when seen on CT scans or MRI.

On MRI the signal characteristics of cysts are determined predominantly by the characteristics of the contained water. The water may be "pure" and free of protein, and therefore "unbound." In this state, the cyst fluid has the same signal characteristics as CSF. With increased protein content, protons become "bound" in a hydration layer adjacent to the protein, significantly decreasing the T_1 relaxation time of the water solution. The net effect is to increase the signal intensity of the cyst on both the T_1- and T_2-weighted images so that the contents of the cyst appear brighter than the CSF on both sequences (see Fig. 5-9). In general, the most benign tumors have cyst fluid whose intensity is near that of CSF. MRI is the most accurate imaging study to differentiate a cyst from a solid tumor. Intraoperative ultrasonography may also be used.

On CT scans cysts appear as a low density area, resembling CSF. Higher protein density is reflected in greater CT density of the cyst (compared with CSF) and may appear the same as solid tumor. Because of decreased contrast resolution, the CT scan is not as accurate as MRI for defining the contents of a cyst or for differentiating a cyst from a solid or necrotic tumor (see Fig. 5-9).

HEMORRHAGE

A large hemorrhage from a tumor is unusual; and when it does occur, it is usually impossible to immediately identify a tumor as the cause. Only later does the tumor become apparent on MRI or contrast-enhanced CT scans. However, small hemorrhages are frequently seen within tumors (most commonly metastasis from melanoma, hypernephroma, and choriocarcinoma). They cause a slight hyperdensity of the tumor on CT scans. Because the changes of hemorrhage are usually chronic, on MRI there is focal hyperintensity within the tumor on T_1- and T_2-weighted images. Paramagnetic effects of hemosiderin sometimes produce focal low signal within or around hemorrhagic sites on T_2-weighted SE or GRE images.

CALCIFICATION

Calcification occurs within many tumors and has diagnostic significance (see box below). It may be punctate or diffuse and is best seen as high density with CT scanning. Calcium produces signal void on MRI and so

---

TUMORS THAT COMMONLY CALCIFY

Meningioma
Craniopharyngioma
Oligodendroglioma
Astrocytoma
Ependymoma
Choroid plexus papilloma
Ganglioneuroma
Dysgerminoma (pineal)
Chordoma
All tumors after irradiation

is more difficult to identify by that technique. GRE images are somewhat more sensitive to calcium and may define the deposits when SE MRI cannot. Calcium cannot be differentiated from hemosiderin by MRI. Calcification frequently occurs within tumors after radiation therapy and this must not be mistaken for contrast enhancement on CT scans.

METASTASIS OF PRIMARY CNS TUMORS

Metastasis of primary intracerebral tumors is relatively unusual. The most frequent mode of spread is through the CSF to the leptomeninges or into the ventricular system. Tumor contact with the surface of the brain or ependyma is necessary for spread through the CSF. Medulloblastoma is the tumor most likely to spread in this fashion, although it can occur with other types, particularly ependymoma, germinoma, neuroblastoma, glioblastoma, and hemangioblastoma.

Distant somatic metastasis from hematogenous seeding may occur rarely. Metastasis outside the CNS almost always occurs after a surgical procedure that allows the tumor access to the vascular system or other body cavities. Glioma is the most likely to metastasize in this fashion, being found most often in the regional lymph nodes or lungs. Medulloblastoma most frequently goes to the bones. Tumors may metastasize through shunt catheters into distant body cavities.

SPECIFIC TUMORS

The specific cranial tumors discussed here are organized into broad anatomic categories. For adults, the anatomy has been divided into the supratentorial region (cerebrum, meninges, calvarium), the sella and base of the skull, and the posterior fossa. Tumors more common to children and adolescents are discussed in Chapter 6.

Supratentorial Tumors

TUMORS OF NEUROGLIAL ORIGIN

Glial tumors are the most common primary brain neoplasms. Present concepts ascribe the origin of glial tumors to the three types of neuroglial cell normally found in the brain and spinal cord: astrocytes, oligodendrocytes, and ependymal cells. These cells constitute the supporting stroma of the brain. The medulloblastoma, generally considered a glial tumor, arises from a primitive cell with potential to differentiate along multiple cell lines.

The grading of glial tumors is somewhat confused because of the inherent inhomogeneity of the tumor and the use of two nosologic systems (Kernohan 1952, Rubinstein 1972). Table 5-2 gives a simplified classification that compares the two commonly used systems.

The histologic determination of malignancy is made by quantifying the mitotic figures, necrosis, and vascular proliferation. The grade of the tumor is assigned according to the most malignant portion of the tumor. Glial tumors are notoriously pleomorphic, and grading errors can occur with biopsy if only small portions of the tumor are sampled. A glial tumor may also change with time, so a once-benign-appearing tumor may change into a more malignant variety. When there are nearly equal numbers of two cell lines (i.e., astrocytoma and oligodendroglioma) the tumor is designated "mixed." Also, adjacent mesenchymal tissue may be induced to malignant change and incorporated within the glial tumor (i.e., glioma and fibrosarcoma). This type of tumor is called *gliosarcoma*. Lesser amounts of mixing of cell types is common, and glial tumors rarely demonstrate a pure cell line.

Table 5-2 Glial Tumors, Grading* and CT/MRI Characteristics

Histology	Contrast enhance	Edema	Angiography
"Benign"			
Grade I (astrocytoma)	No	No	Avascular mass
Grade II (astroblastoma)	No	No	Avascular mass
"Malignant"			
Grade III (anaplastic astrocytoma)	Usually (80%)	Yes	Avascular mass or sometimes "blush"
Grade IV (glioblastoma)	Yes	Yes	Highly vascular mass

*Grading according to Kernohan (1952). Corresponding classification according to Rubinstein (1972) is within parentheses.

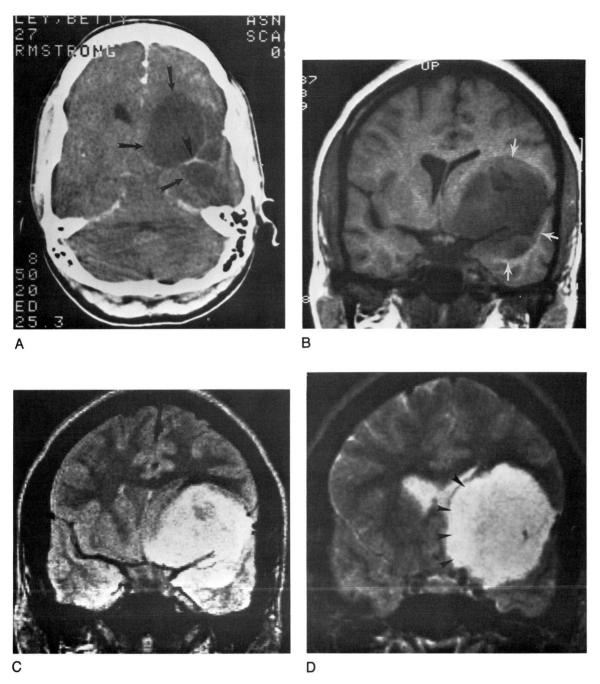

Fig. 5-6 Astrocytoma, grade I. (A) Contrast-enhanced CT study shows a hypodense mass in the left posterior frontal and anterior temporal regions (arrows). The density of the tumor is greater than that of the CSF. There is no contrast enhancement. The mass surrounds the left middle cerebral artery (arrowhead). **(B)** Coronal T_1-weighted image shows the tumor mass in the left posterior frontal lobe extending into the superior medial portion of the temporal lobe (arrows). The mass had greater intensity than CSF and is inhomogeneous, indicating that it is solid rather than cystic. **(C)** Lightly weighted T_2-weighted image shows the mass to be inhomogeneous and of greater signal intensity than CSF, which is typical for solid astrocytomas. **(D)** Heavily T_2-weighted image shows the mass to be nearly isointense with the CSF. There is slightly greater intensity along the medial margin of the tumor (arrowheads). *(Figure continues.)*

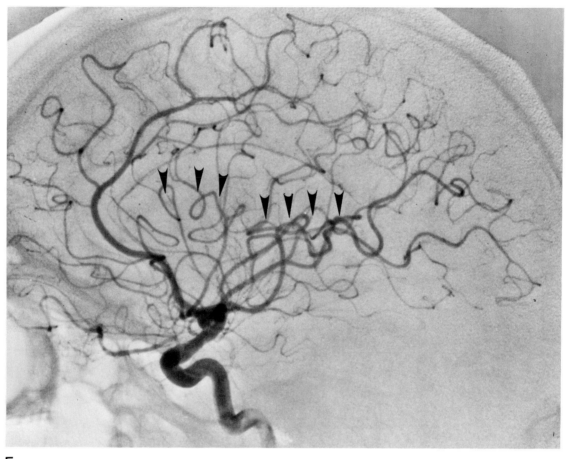

E

Fig. 5-6 *(Continued).* **(E)** Left ICA angiography shows a subtle avascular mass distorting the anterior sylvian vessels (arrowheads). The posterior frontal cortical branches are stretched.

In general, the higher the malignant grade of glioma, the greater is the amount of abnormal vascular proliferation within the tumor nidus. This situation results in greater contrast enhancement and greater surrounding vasogenic edema. The neovascularity can be seen with angiography. As a rule, grade III and grade IV gliomas demonstrate abnormal contrast enhancement, surrounding vasogenic edema, and neovascularity on angiography. Grade I and grade II tumors show no enhancement, little edema, and no neovascularity on angiography (Table 5-2).

Glial tumors most commonly arise within the white matter of the cerebral hemispheres but may be deep within the internal capsule, thalamus, or brain stem. Rarely, glial tumors arise within the gray matter or the subpial space and reach the cortical surface. Character-istically, glial tumors occur within the cerebral hemispheres in adults and in the cerebellum, pons, hypothalamus, and optic chiasm in children. The tumors tend to be varied in shape and often resemble the structures they replace. Although the contrast-enhanced margin may appear relatively sharp, there is always a gradual histologic transition from tumor to normal brain. Even the most benign gliomas do not have a true tumor capsule, although some have a pseudocapsule of compressed gliotic brain. Concurrent malignant degeneration may take place at distant sites within the brain, creating multicentric gliomas. The most extreme example of this pattern of growth is gliomatosis cerebri, where nearly the entire brain exhibits low grade neoplastic transformation. Delayed development of other gliomas may occur after removal of the initial tumor.

This pattern of growth has grave implications for the treatment of glioma and explains the seemingly inevitable recurrence of the tumor after resection.

ASTROCYTOMA (GRADES I AND II)

In the adult, low grade astrocytoma is nearly always a solid tumor of the cerebral hemispheres. Cystic astrocytomas are much less common. When discovered, the tumors may be any size, superficial or deep. Diffuse growth may occur within the white matter, especially extending from the frontal into the temporal lobe, a characteristic location. Little or no surrounding edema is present, although the tumor itself has a markedly increased water content when compared with normal brain tissue. The mass effect may be slight and is a direct result of the tumor itself. Neovascularity is minimal (Fig. 5-6).

Calcification may occur within the tumor in either small flecks or dense hunks (Fig. 5-5). Occasionally, these inclusions are the only indication that a tumor is present. Similar calcification occurs within oligodendrogliomas and gangliogliomas. Long-term serial examination at yearly intervals may be necessary to distinguish the calcification of tumor from focal benign idiopathic calcification, sometimes called a *brain stone* (Fig. 5-7).

Gliomatosis cerebri is the term applied to the rare diffuse infiltration of a cerebral hemisphere with low grade astrocytic cells. The CT or MRI scan usually shows an isodense expansion of one entire hemisphere, with no contrast enhancement. The diagnosis can be made only by biopsy.

Because of increased water content, low grade astrocytomas exhibit relatively low intensity on T_1- and high intensity on T_2-weighted MRI. Most often the tumor is well circumscribed but may be poorly marginated. Most solid tumors demonstrate some internal inhomogeneity (Fig. 5-6). Cystic tumors are homogeneous, with MRI signal characteristics of pure or proteinaceous water (see section above). At times it is impossible to differentiate a cystic tumor from a solid tumor. Low grade astrocytomas do not enhance with Gd-DPTA. Calcifications may be seen as regions of signal dropout.

With CT scanning, low grade astrocytomas appear as well circumscribed regions of hypodensity (18 to 24 HU) (Fig. 5-6). Calcification occurs in 10 percent of tumors and may have any appearance. Contrast uptake

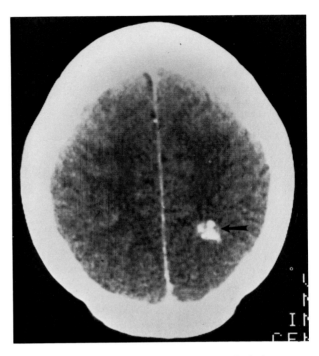

Fig. 5-7 "Brain stone". CT scan shows a calcific lesion in the left parietal subcortical region (arrow). It is impossible to determine the nature of such a lesion. However, this finding could be the only sign of a low grade glioma, and serial scanning is necessary to detect possible change.

does not occur with grade I and II astrocytoma, except for rare exceptions. However, the lack of tumor enhancement is no guarantee of low grade histology, as 20 percent of anaplastic (grade III) astrocytomas also show no enhancement. Sometimes there is increased density after contrast in the compressed brain tissue or gyri adjacent to the tumor, but it must not be misinterpreted as abnormal enhancement of the tumor itself.

At best, angiography demonstrates a nonspecific mass effect, and it may show no abnormality (Fig. 5-6). Low grade astrocytoma does not demonstrate neovascularity or early draining veins. Angiography has little role in the evaluation of low grade glioma, except perhaps in difficult cases, where it may differentiate tumor from infarction with vascular occlusion.

ANAPLASTIC ASTROCYTOMA (GRADE III)

Anaplastic astrocytoma contains any number of cells displaying more malignant change but falls short of the high grade malignancy of glioblastoma. It exhibits mi-

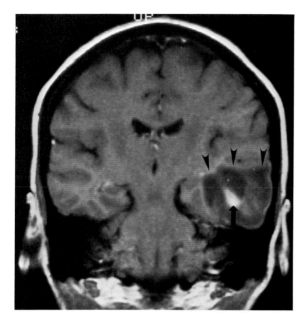

Fig. 5-8 Anaplastic astrocytoma, grade III. Gd-DTPA contrast-enhanced T_1-weighted MRI shows an inhomogeneous low intensity tumor mass in the left temporal lobe (arrowheads). There is a focal region of enhancement within the tumor (arrow). Note that the tumor extends to the cortical surface.

About 80 percent of anaplastic astrocytomas demonstrate contrast enhancement. Some tumors have such a small region of anaplasia that contrast uptake is nondetectable, and the tumor appears identical to a low grade astrocytoma. The pattern of contrast uptake varies considerably and may show any of the following patterns.

1. Small blotch of enhancement at the periphery of a cyst or within the solid portion of the tumor (Fig. 5-8)
2. Fine rim enhancement of a cyst with or without an enhancing tumor nodule (Fig. 5-9)
3. Several somewhat thick ring-enhancing structures
4. Homogeneous enhancement throughout the entire solid portion of the tumor
5. Dense, thick, irregular enhancement, with a ring-like pattern indistinguishable from that of glioblastoma

In glial tumors the slightest amount of contrast enhancement is enough to make the diagnosis of anaplasia (malignancy) likely.

On angiography a mass lesion can be seen that may be avascular or show a small vague tumor "blush." Discrete neovascularity is generally not seen (see Fig. 1-12).

GLIOBLASTOMA (GRADE IV)

Glioblastoma is the most common primary tumor of the brain. It accounts for up to 20 percent of all intracranial tumors and 50 percent of glial tumors. The tumor is highly anaplastic and grows in an infiltrative and destructive manner. It induces striking neovascularity. Central necrosis is an almost constant feature. Multiplicity of tumor sites is present about 5 percent of the time. Untreated, the usual survival is 3 to 5 months after diagnosis. With surgical decompression followed by radiation treatment, the survival may be extended 6 to 12 months. Presently, the tumor is almost always fatal.

The tumor is most commonly found in the cerebral hemispheres but may also be within the deep structures and the brain stem. Cerebellar glioblastoma is rare. It typically grows as an irregularly shaped mass in the white matter but may reach the cortical surface where it invades surface arteries and produces infarction. The tumor frequently involves the corpus callosum, crossing the midline and producing the characteristic "but-

tosis, necrosis, vascular proliferation, and cyst formation, particularly microcysts. Significant edema is usually present around the tumor. These tumors are inhomogeneous, with regions of both low and high grade change. Clinically, the tumors are moderately aggressive but not as much as the glioblastoma.

On MRI, the tumor shows hypointensity on T_1-weighted images and hyperintensity on T_2-weighted images but usually with considerable inhomogeneity. Surrounding edema is usually present. Gd-DTPA enhancement occurs in a large number of the tumors and is indicative of anaplasia (Fig. 5-8). The patterns are similar to those observed by CT scanning (see below). It is usually not possible to specifically identify microcystic change and necrosis within the tumor. Large cysts may be seen (Fig. 5-9).

As expected from the histology, these tumors also have a variable CT appearance. Solid tumors may be hypodense, isodense, or hyperdense. Inhomogeneity is common. Sharply outlined cysts occur that have a CT density of about 12 to 25 HU. Calcification is rare. It may be impossible to differentiate tumor from edema.

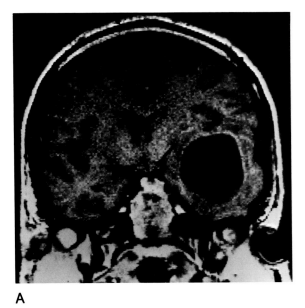

A

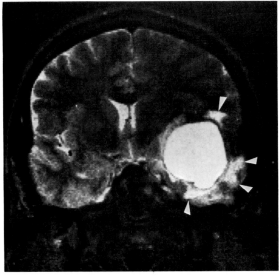

B

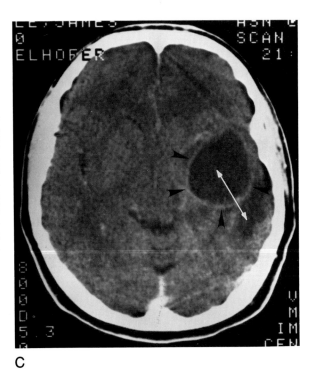

C

Fig. 5-9 Anaplastic astrocytoma, grade III, cystic. (A) Coronal T_1-weighted MRI shows the well circumscribed left temporal lobe mass. It is uniformly hypointense but of slightly greater intensity than the CSF. This picture is typical of a cyst with proteinaceous fluid. **(B)** T_2-weighted MRI showing a hyperintense cystic mass in the left temporal lobe. Note that the cyst fluid has higher signal intensity than the surrounding edema (arrowheads). **(C)** Contrast-enhanced CT scan shows enhancement of the cyst capsule (arrowheads). Note that the cyst fluid is of lower density than the edema fluid (opposing arrows). For an angiogram of a temporal lobe mass, see Figure 1-12.

terfly" pattern. White matter edema occurs with more than 90 percent of the tumors, and in 75 percent it is extensive. The edema significantly adds to the mass effect produced by the tumor. It may be diminished by systemic glucocorticoid therapy.

The diagnosis is based on the pattern of contrast enhancement, the shape of the lesion, its location within the white matter (especially the corpus callosum), and the presence of central necrosis.

On MRI the tumor shows varying degrees of hypointensity on T_1- and hyperintensity on T_2-weighted images (Fig. 5-10). There is inhomogeneity of the

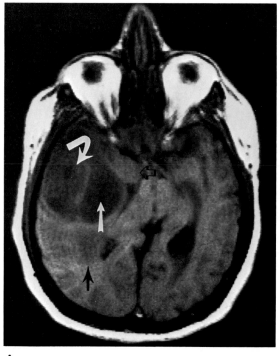

A

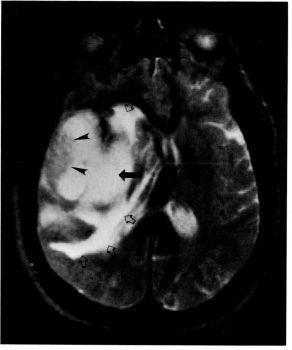

B

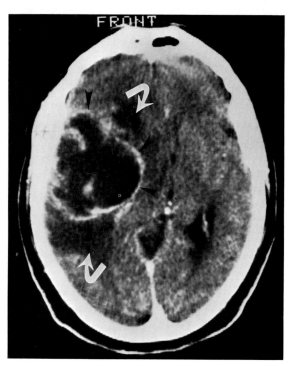

C

Fig. 5-10 Glioblastoma, grade IV. (A) T$_1$-weighted MRI shows an inhomogeneous hypointense mass in the right temporal lobe. The more medial portion of the mass (white arrow) is of lower intensity than the lateral portion (curved arrow), indicating greater necrosis. Surrounding edema is seen as slight hypointensity (black arrow). Note the uncal herniation (open arrow). **(B)** T$_2$-weighted MRI showing the medial portion of the tumor as high intensity (arrow) and a lower intensity, more solid portion laterally (arrowheads). The surrounding white matter edema is of greater intensity than the necrotic portion of the tumor (open arrows). **(C)** Contrast-enhanced CT scan shows the typical irregular ring-like enhancing mass with central low density necrosis (arrowheads). Edema is seen as low density in the white matter surrounding the contrast-enhanced tumor nidus (curved arrows).

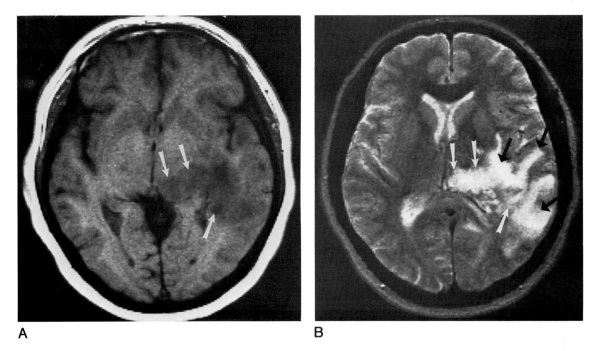

Fig. 5-11 Glioblastoma, thalamic. **(A)** T$_1$-weighted MRI shows a hypointense lesion within the posterior left thalamus and appearing to extend into the medial left temporal lobe (arrows). **(B)** T$_2$-weighted image shows the tumor in the thalamus to be of high intensity (white arrows) but slightly less intense than the surrounding edema (black arrows).

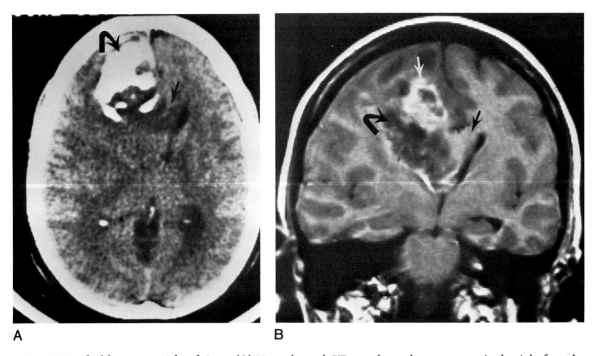

Fig. 5-12 Glioblastoma, with calcium. **(A)** Nonenhanced CT scan shows the tumor mass in the right frontal lobe with a large amount of dense calcification (curved arrow). Noncalcified hypodense tumor is seen crossing the corpus callosum (arrow). **(B)** T$_1$-weighted MRI with Gd-DTPA shows the typical enhancement pattern of a glioblastoma (white arrow). More homogeneous enhancement is seen in the portion of the tumor that crosses the corpus callosum (black arrow). The calcium is seen as regions of signal loss (curved arrow). This growth pattern is typical for glioblastoma. The presence of calcium suggests that originally this tumor was a predominantly lower grade astrocytoma or oligodendroglioma. The tumor is invading the ventricular cavity.

tumor mass, representing necrosis, cystic change, hemorrhage, and neovascularity. The high T_2 signal of vasogenic edema is striking and extends far beyond the margin of the main tumor mass. On the T_2 images, the tumor mass is usually slightly less intense than the surrounding edema (Fig. 5-11). Focal low intensity on T_2-weighted images usually represents acute hemorrhage but may rarely be due to calcium (Fig. 5-12).

Gd-DTPA enhancement is almost always present. It is usually ring-like, with thick, irregular walls that have a garland-like inner pattern (Fig. 5-2). The central nonenhancing region represents necrosis or less commonly cyst formation. The enhancement clearly outlines the main tumor mass, distinguishing it from low intensity surrounding edema on T_1-weighted images. Contrast enhancement is often necessary to help differentiate glioblastoma from other tumors, abscess, and infarction.

On CT scans, contrast uptake in demonstrated in more than 95 percent of glioblastomas, and the use of contrast is essential for the evaluation of this tumor (Fig. 5-10). With early tumors the enhancement is minimal and nonspecific (Fig. 5-13) or even absent. The contrast outlines the region of neovascularity of the tumor and indicates accurately the size of the main tumor mass. However, there is always tumor beyond the perimeter of the enhancement. Similar to Gd-DTPA enhanced MRI, glioblastomas almost always appear as irregular ring-enhancing lesions with a variable shape and ring thickness. Homogeneous tumor enhancement is rare. The central low density nonenhancing segment of the tumor represents necrosis 95 percent of the time. It may fill in somewhat with contrast over time. Rarely, contrast accumulates in the dependent portion of a cyst. Calcification is rare.

On angiography, a typical vascular pattern is demonstrated about 50 percent of the time (Fig. 5-14). When present it is accurate for the diagnosis, differentiating glioma from metastasis or abscess. Therefore angiography is still useful for confirming the diagnosis of glioblastoma when biopsy cannot be done. The typical diagnostic pattern is as follows.

1. Abundant irregular neovascularity, with sites of dilatation and narrowing of the vessels. There is contribution from multiple cortical branches. Meningeal contribution is rare.
2. Large early-appearing draining veins, representing arteriovenous shunting.
3. Drainage by way of enlarged deep medullary veins to the subependymal veins.

Drainage by deep medullary veins reflects the white matter location of the tumor. The deep veins of the white matter can be identified by their characteristic straight radial course toward the subependymal veins of the lateral ventricles. Normally, these veins are seen late in the venous phase as fine vessels, visible no more than 1 cm into the paraventricular white matter. When they are enlarged, they are strong evidence for glioblastoma. These veins may also be enlarged with other white matter pathology, such as lymphoma, multifocal leukoencephalopathy, fulminant multiple sclerosis, and deep arteriovenous malformations. However, the clinical setting and the type of neovascularity usually allows distinction of these other entities. Deep medullary vein enlargement is not seen with metastasis, an important differential angiographic finding.

The combination of the characteristic findings on MRI or CT scans and angiography is essentially pathognomonic for the diagnosis of glioblastoma.

Differential Diagnosis

1. *Metastasis.* It is important to differentiate metastasis from glioblastoma. Occasionally, on MRI or CT scanning a metastatic tumor has a configuration and enhancement pattern similar to the classic pattern of glioblastoma described above. The differential points are given below. It is important to emphasize that it may be impossible to differentiate a glioblastoma from a metastasis by imaging, and biopsy may be required (Fig. 5-15).

2. *Brain abscess.* The pattern of a brain abscess may mimic that of a glioblastoma. The diagnosis of abscess must be strongly considered when there is a relatively thin, regular rim of contrast enhancement around a central cavity, although a glial tumor occasionally has this pattern (see Fig. 8-11). An abscess may also have a characteristic capsular blush on angiography. A thick enhancing wall with the inward curving garland pattern is generally not present with abscess.

3. *Infarction.* Rarely, a peripheral glioblastoma is examined during its early stage of development. There may be only edema of the gray matter or a small ring or gyral enhancement on MRI or CT scans (Fig. 5-16). It may resemble infarction, and only the history or repeat scanning in a few weeks can ensure the correct diagnosis.

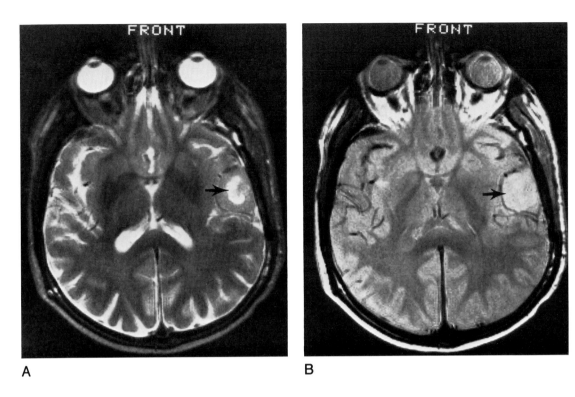

A

B

Fig. 5-13 Early glioblastoma. (A) T$_2$-weighted MRI shows a high signal intensity tumor nidus in the left temporal lobe. **(B)** Lightly T$_2$-weighted image shows a nearly homogeneous region of high signal intensity in the left middle temporal lobe (arrow). **(C)** Contrast-enhanced CT scan shows a small ring-enhancing tumor nidus in the left temporal subcortical region (arrow).

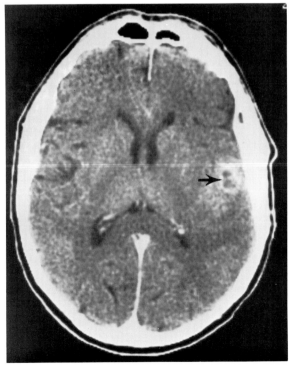

C

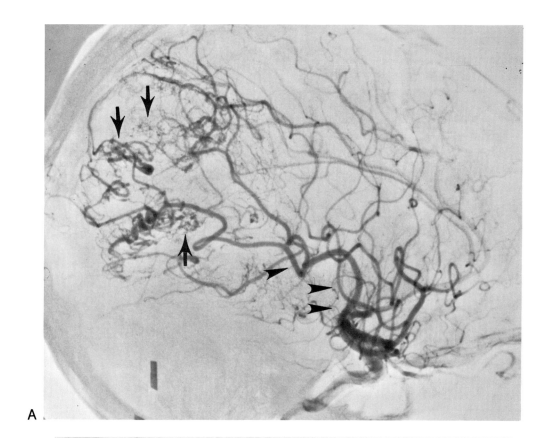

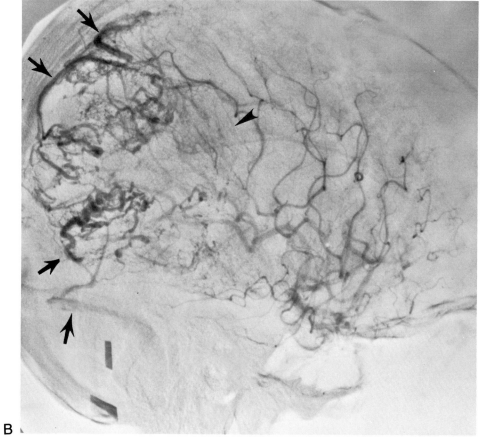

Fig. 5-14 Glioblastoma, right posterior parietal lobe. Legend on page 153.

Fig. 5-14 Glioblastoma, right posterior parietal lobe.
(A) ICA angiography shows a large right posterior parietal mass with irregular neovascularity (arrows). The sylvian vessels are displaced forward (arrowheads). **(B)** Late arterial phase shows multiple early cortical veins draining into sinuses (arrows). Small straight medullary arteries and veins are seen (arrowhead). **(C)** Contrast-enhanced CT scan shows the typical irregular enhancing tumor nidus in the right posterior parietal lobe (black arrow). There is surrounding edema and "pseudoenhancement" of compressed gyri (arrowheads). A second glioma shows early development in the left hemisphere (open arrow).

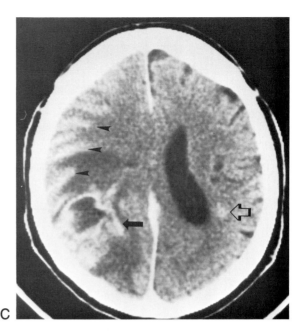

C

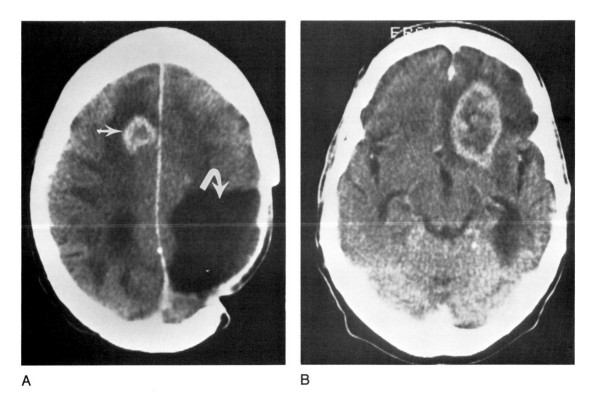

A   B

Fig. 5-15 Multicentric glioma. (A) Contrast-enhanced CT scan shows a large region of porencephaly from prior excision of a glioblastoma (curved arrow). Now, a year later, the patient has a new lesion in the right posterior frontal lobe (arrow), which proved to be a glioblastoma. **(B)** A second, larger glioblastoma is present in the left frontal lobe. Without biopsy, it would be impossible to differentiate these lesions from metastasis.

DIFFERENTIAL DIAGNOSIS OF
SOLITARY RING ENHANCING BRAIN
LESIONS

Metastasis
    Clinical findings
        Known primary malignancy that frequently metastasizes to the brain
    CT/MRI findings
        Multiple enhancing lesions of varying size; may be solitary in 50 percent
        At corticomedullary junction
        Excessive surrounding edema
    Angiography
        Drainage to single cortical vein
        Single feeding artery
        Well organized neovascularity or diffuse "stain"
Glioblastoma
    CT/MRI finding
        Single, irregularly shaped enhancing lesion, central necrosis
        Located within white matter
    Angiography findings
        Grossly irregular neovascularity
        Large multiple early draining veins
        Deep medullary venous drainage
Abscess
    Clinical findings
        Fever
    CT/MRI findings
        Thin-walled homogeneous ring-enhancing lesion
    Angiography findings
        Faint, round "blush" from uptake by the abscess capsule
    Radionuclide study
        Indium-111-labeled leukocytes uptake

Uncommon Glial Tumors

OLIGODENDROGLIOMA

Oligodendroglioma is a rare tumor that accounts for about 5 percent of intracranial gliomas. Its peak incidence is in persons 30 to 55 years of age. These tumors most often occur in the frontal lobes and rarely in the occipital lobes. Calcification is characteristic of the tumor, occurring in about 75 percent. Most of these tumors are low grade and exhibit no contrast uptake and only minimal if any peritumoral edema (Fig. 5-17). Their imaging characteristics are the same as those of low grade astrocytoma, described above. Noncalcified oligodendroglioma cannot be differentiated from low grade astrocytoma. As with all gliomas, contrast enhancement indicates anaplasia.

EPENDYMOMA

Ependymoma is primarily a tumor of childhood and is discussed in that section. However, cerebral hemispheric ependymoma does occur rarely in the young adult, usually at the level of the junction of the parietal, temporal, and occipital lobes. They are characteristically located adjacent to the lateral ventricle and may have an intraventricular component (see Fig. 6-6). Cysts, calcification, and surrounding edema are common. The tumor shows variable contrast uptake on CT scans. When there is no calcification, ependymoma appears similar to anaplastic astrocytoma or glioblastoma, although it occurs in a younger age group.

MIXED GLIOMA

Mixed gliomas account for about 5 percent of the glial tumors and, except for the gliosarcoma, are usually low grade. They are indistinguishable from the other glial tumors, particularly the oligodendroglioma. Gliosarcoma appears as a peripheral tumor with an imaging pattern of glioblastoma. Angiography usually shows some meningeal vascular contribution to the tumor. Mixed low grade tumors are common in the region of the hypothalamus in children and tend to display uniform contrast enhancement.

COLLOID CYST

A colloid cyst is a rare benign tumor that originates from the ependyma (neuroepithelium) of the roof of the anterior third ventricle at the level of the foramen of Monro. It is composed of a dense fibrous capsule filled with a fluid that varies from a thick mucoid material with debris to clear fluid. It commonly appears on CT scans as a round, hyperdense lesion less than 2 cm in diameter (Fig. 5-18); uncommonly, it is isodense or hypodense. On MRI, it is usually isointense on the T_1- and T_2-weighted images but may be hyperintense or

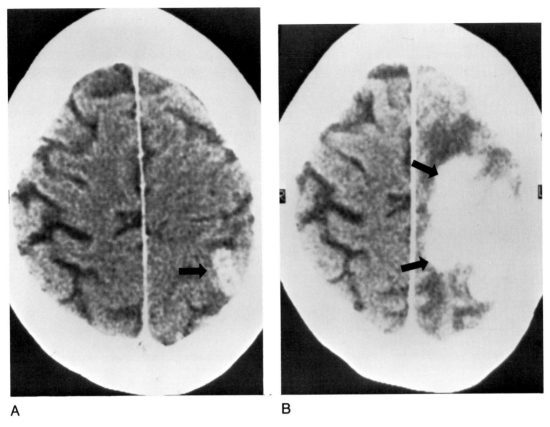

A   B

Fig. 5-16 Early peripheral glioblastoma. (A) A small cortical enhancing lesion is present in the left posterior parietal lobe. At this stage it is indistinguishable from the gyral enhancement of infarction (arrow). **(B)** CT scan 6 weeks later shows gross enlargement of the tumor (arrows).

hypointense on T_2. Sometimes there is contrast enhancement of the capsule, but contrast is not necessary or useful in the diagnosis if the characteristic findings are present.

The cysts are congenital but grow slowly. Therefore they usually do not cause symptoms until adulthood. They may obstruct the foramina of Monro and cause hydrocephalus, which is sometimes intermittent. Meningioma and ependymoma rarely occur in this region and may be differentiated from a colloid cyst by their more uniform contrast enhancement or hypointense T_1 signal on MRI.

SECONDARY NEOPLASMS— METASTASIS

Cerebral metastatic tumor is the second most common type of intracerebral neoplasm, accounting for about 35 percent of all intracranial tumors. Most are hematoge-

nous metastases. The most common types are bronchogenic carcinoma (small cell carcinoma, adenocarcinoma) and breast carcinoma. Less frequent metastatic tumors arise from renal cell carcinoma, colon carcinoma, and melanoma. However, any advanced or aggressive tumor may metastasize to the brain. The meninges of the brain or spine are only rarely involved and then most commonly with breast carcinoma or small cell carcinoma of the lung. Metastasis to the spinal cord is rare.

Most commonly, hematogenous metastases are seen as multiple lesions located at the gray-white corticomedullary junction. The lesions are usually spherical but may assume any shape. Some appear to be entirely cystic. Neovascularity is present, accounting for vasogenic white matter edema and contrast enhancement of the tumor. The amount of edema is variable, but characteristically it is extensive for the size of the tumor nidus. In general, the specific histology of the metas-

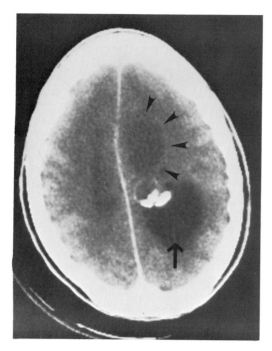

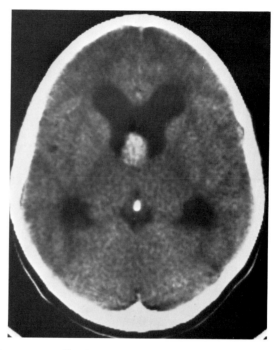

Fig. 5-17 Oligodendroglioma. Contrast-enhanced CT scan shows the typical findings of oligodendroglioma. There is no contrast enhancement. Dense calcification is present in the central portion of the tumor. There is a large cystic lesion posteriorly (arrow). A barely identifiable solid portion of the tumor is seen more anteriorly (arrowheads). The faintly identifiable rim represents a "pseudocapsule."

Fig. 5-18 Colloid cyst. Nonenhanced CT scan shows a homogeneously dense, round lesion at the level of the foramina of Monro. The formina are obstructed, causing hydrocephalus.

tasis cannot be determined from its shape or pattern of contrast enhancement.

Cerebral metastasis is the initial presentation of neoplasia in about 10 percent of patients. The metastatic tumor deposit is solitary 30 to 50 percent of the time, depending on the tumor type. Carcinoma of the lung is the most likely to be solitary. Headache, seizures, and progressive focal neurologic symptoms are the most common presenting complaints. Ninety percent of patients with cerebral metastasis have a history of a carcinoma known to metastasize to the brain. Differentiation of a solitary metastasis from a primary brain tumor may not be possible without biopsy or discovery of the likely primary tumor.

Gd-DTPA contrast-enhanced MRI is the most sensitive examination for the detection of metastatic disease in the brain. Additional lesions may be seen with enhancement that were not apparent on the nonenhanced scan.

With nonenhanced MRI the lesions are ordinarily hypointense on T_1- and hyperintense on T_2-weighted images (Fig. 5-3). However, melanoma characteristically shows high intensity on T_1- and hypointensity on T_2-weighted images because of the paramagnetic effects of both melanin and the acute and chronic hemorrhage that is almost always present in these tumors (Fig. 5-19). Some mucinous cystadenocarcinomas and choriocarcinoma may also show this pattern. Edema is a prominent accompaniment to metastasis and is strikingly seen with MRI. Sometimes with small tumors only the edema is seen on the scan, and the edema may be difficult to differentiate from infarction when it involves the cortical surface.

The postcontrast CT scan detects about 95 percent of metastatic tumors in the brain that are 5 mm or larger. It is sometimes possible to detect the presence of smaller lesions by the observation of surrounding edema or by the use of very high dose contrast enhancement and delayed scanning. Characteristically, the metastatic tumor deposits are seen as multiple spherical contrast

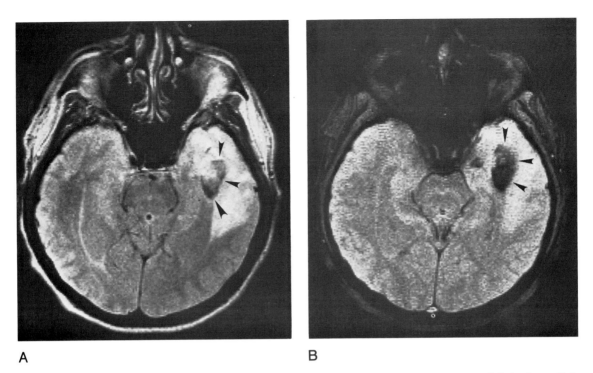

A   B

Fig. 5-19 Metastatic melanoma. (A) T$_2$-weighted SE MRI shows the hypointense tumor nodule in the medial left temporal lobe (arrowheads). The surrounding high intensity signal represents edema. **(B)** Fisp 20;300/20 GRE MRI shows extreme hypointensity of the tumor nodule because of accentuation of paramagnetic effects with the gradient echo images (arrowheads).

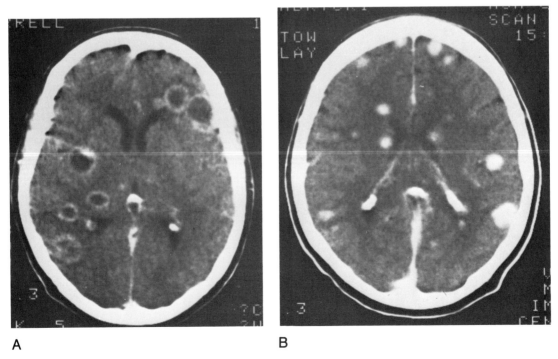

A   B

Fig. 5-20 Metastasis, adenocarcinoma of the lung. (A) Multiple metastases with ring-like contrast enhancement. **(B)** Multiple metastases with homogeneous contrast enhancement. Multiple metastases tend to have varying sizes of lesions, whereas multiple abscesses tend to be more uniform in size.

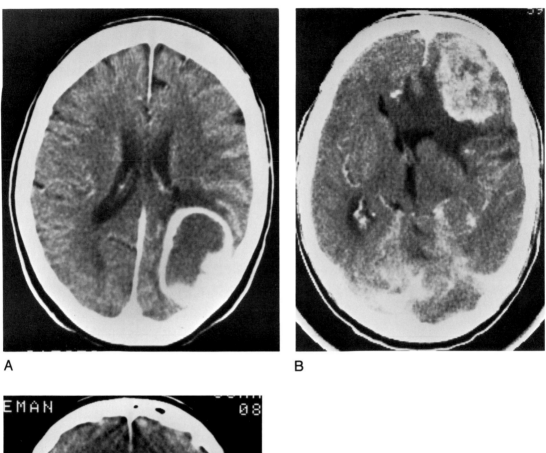

A

B

C

Fig. 5-21 Large solitary metastasis. (A & B) It is impossible to reliably differentiate a large solitary metastasis from a glioblastoma. **(C)** This contrast-enhanced lesion in the pons represents a metastasis (arrow). Although less common, a glioma could also have this appearance.

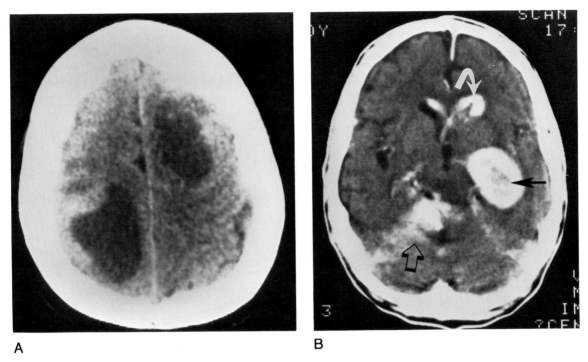

A   B

Fig. 5-22 Metastatic tumor. (A) Metastases sometimes appear entirely hypodense with little if any contrast enhancement. They can mimic cerebral infarction. **(B)** Small cell carcinoma of the lung. Contrast-enhanced CT scan shows metastatic tumor deposits in the parenchyma (black arrow), along the ependyma of the ventricular cavities (curved arrow), and in the meninges of the cisterns (open arrow).

enhancing lesions with sharp outlines (Fig. 5-20). Edema is present about 90 percent of the time. Small lesions tend to have uniform complete enhancement, whereas larger lesions are often ring-like with central necrosis.

In general, it is not possible to determine the type of tumor metastasis from the appearance on CT. Hyperdensity from either hemorrhage or calcium suggests that the tumor is a melanoma, hypernephroma, choriocarcinoma, mucinous cystadenocarcinoma (Fig. 5-4), or lymphoma. A large solitary metastatic lesion may be indistinguishable from a glioblastoma (Fig. 5-21). Some large cystic-appearing lesions with focal contrast enhancement are identical to anaplastic (grade III) astrocytoma. In a small percentage (less than 5 percent), only the edema or necrosis of a tumor situated on the cortex is seen (Fig. 5-22), and the differentiation from infarction is sometimes difficult. CT scanning for metastatic disease includes bone window images. CT scanning is generally superior to MRI for the evaluation of osseous metastasis.

Meningeal carcinomatosis can be suggested with CT scans and MRI by the presence of diffuse contrast enhancement of the meninges or ependyma (Fig. 5-23). There may be obliteration of the sulci or enhancing nodules in the cisterns. Mild hydrocephalus is usually present. The diagnosis is confirmed with CSF cytology. Meningeal metastatic tumor cannot be seen without enhancement. Contrast-enhanced MRI seems to be more sensitive than CT scanning for the detection of meningeal carcinomatosis (Fig. 5-24). In adults, carcinoma of the breast and small cell carcinoma of the lung account for most cases of meningeal carcinomatosis.

Cerebral angiography is no longer used for the detection of cerebral metastasis, but it can be helpful for differentiation of metastasis from primary tumor infarction or abscess and for localization prior to surgical excision. Almost all metastatic tumors produce enough mass effect to be visualized with angiography. About 50 percent exhibit some hypervascularity.

Four patterns of hypervascularity have been described.

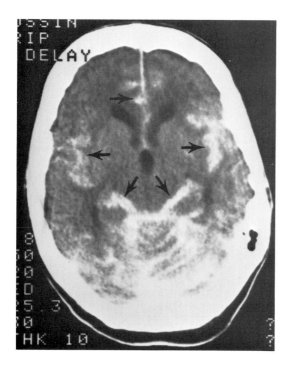

Fig. 5-23 Meningeal carcinomatosis. Contrast-enhanced CT study shows intense contrast enhancement of the meninges of the basal cisterns, sylvian fissures, and interhemispheric fissure (arrows). Communicating hydrocephalus is also common because of cisternal blockage.

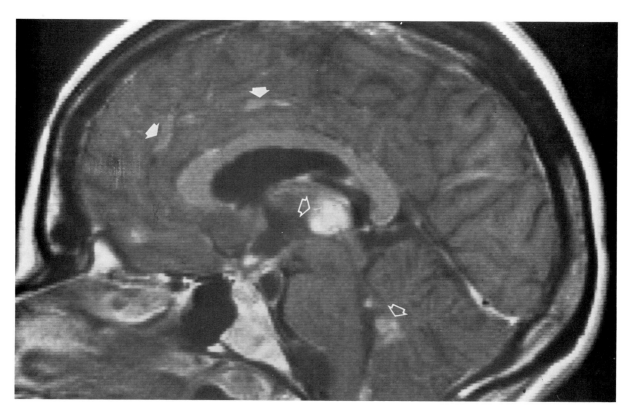

Fig. 5-24 Meningeal metastasis, astrocytoma of the spinal cord. Parasagittal Gd-DTPA-enhanced MRI demonstrates multiple enhancing lesions along the meningeal surface of the interhemispheric fissure (solid arrows). Deposits are also present within the ventricles (open arrows). Gd-DTPA-enhanced MRI is the most sensitive technique for the detection of meningeal metastasis.

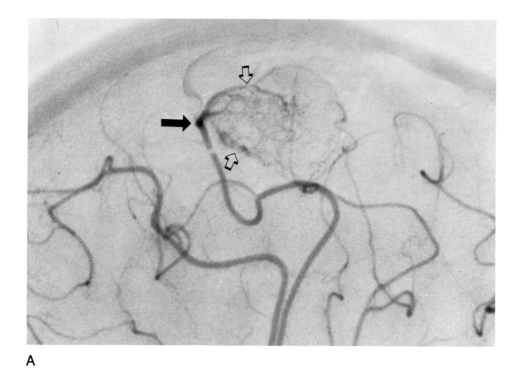

A

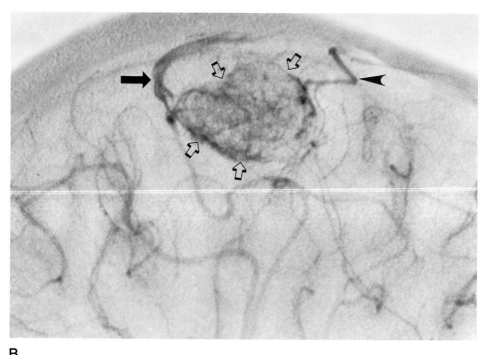

B

Fig. 5-25 Metastatic adenocarcinoma. (A) Early arterial phase shows the fine tumor neovascularity (open arrows) being filled primarily by a single feeding artery (solid arrow). **(B)** The tumor nodule is well circumscribed with uniform neovascularity (open arrows). There is a primary early filling cortical draining vein (solid arrow) and a small secondary cortical draining vein (arrowhead). This pattern is typical for cerebral metastasis.

1. The tumor has a network of thin, regular, tortuous vessels, with early venous filling. Frequently, there is a single feeding artery and one, or perhaps two, cortical draining veins. This pattern is essentially pathognomonic for a metastatic tumor (Fig. 5-25).
2. The tumor shows a diffuse blush, simulating a meningioma but without supply from meningeal vessels and a shorter duration of the "stain" than a meningioma.
3. The tumor appears as a ring-shaped lesion, formed by a vascular periphery and an avascular central region of necrosis.
4. The tumor shows irregular, "wild" neovascularity with prominent early draining veins, indistinguishable from glioblastoma.

The histology of these tumors correlates poorly with the pattern of neovascularity, except for the hypernephroma, which is highly vascular with a generally homogeneous persisting stain; it mimics hemangioblastoma when seen in the posterior fossa. Metastatic tumors almost always drain to the surface cortical veins, whereas glioblastomas nearly always have at least some of their drainage deep into the ventricular system, often with demonstrable enlargement of the deep medullary veins.

Radionuclide brain scanning has been supplanted by contrast CT scanning or MRI. The sensitivity of radionuclide scanning of the brain is about 85 percent — less than that of contrast-enhanced CT scanning and MRI. The radionuclide study is performed with the chelates of technetium, DTPA, or glucoheptinate. Metastatic tumors are detected as regions of radionuclide accumulation and are generally round and discrete, sometimes with a doughnut pattern. Single lesions are nonspecific, and identical patterns may be seen with primary tumors, abscess, and sometimes infarction. However, an indium-111-labeled white blood cell examination may be used to differentiate an abscess from a tumor.

Calvarial metastasis occurs but with less frequency than cerebral metastasis. Focal head pain is common, caused by the lesion. By far the most common calvarial metastasis is carcinoma of the breast (see box). Most commonly, these metastatic lesions are lytic (Fig. 5-26), but blastic lesions or a combination of the two forms (mixed) may occur. On skull radiographs the margins of metastatic lesions are usually irregular and lack definition. A small central bone sequestrum may remain. Beveled margins may be present, particularly

when only one table of the calvarium is involved. Blastic metastasis does not cause skull thickening, differentiating it from Paget's disease. Calvarial metastatic tumor may grow inward into the epidural space, or through the dura to involve the subdural space and sometimes the cortical surface of the brain (Fig. 5-27). Skull lesions may also be seen with bone windows on CT scans or with MRI (Fig. 5-26).

When multiple and small, lytic metastasis may not be distinguishable from multiple myeloma. Myeloma lesions involve the diploë, are usually small and generally uniform in size, and have rather sharp margins compared with metastatic tumors. The clinical history, age, and evaluation of the serum protein are important for making the differential diagnosis. The small lytic lesions of hyperparathyroidism must be differentiated from metastatic disease, but they tend to be uniform in size and relatively sharply demarcated.

Isolated metastatic deposits must be differentiated from the lucency produced by *venous lakes,* which are normal dilatations of the diploic veins. They do not cause erosion of the inner or outer tables, which may be evaluated by tangential radiography. Also, a draining diploic vein may be seen entering the region of lucency. The radionuclide bone scan is negative.

Secondary neoplasm may involve the base of the skull as well. Most commonly this is from carcinoma of the prostate (usually blastic) or breast. Bone destruction

---

MULTIPLE LYTIC LESIONS OF THE CALVARIUM

Metastatic carcinoma
    Adults
        Breast
        Lung
        Kidney
        Thyroid
    Children
        Neuroblastoma
        Leukemia
        Histiocytosis X
Myeloma (other macroglobulinemias)
Hyperparathyroidism
Sarcoidosis and other granulomas
Venous "Lakes"

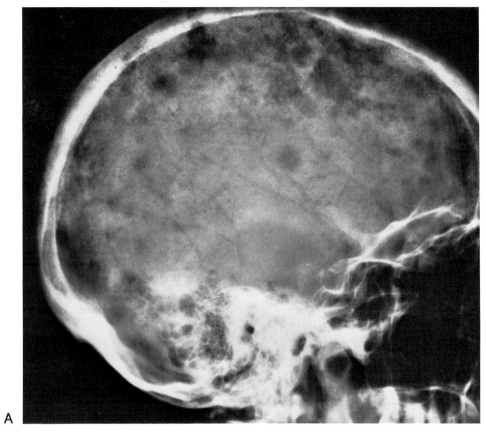

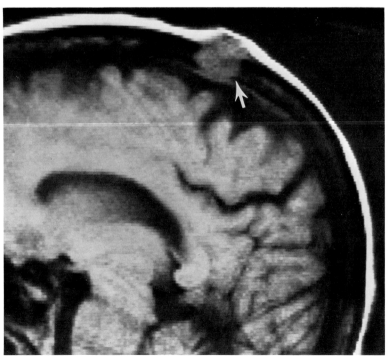

Fig. 5-26 Calvarial metastases, breast carcinoma. (A) Multiple lytic metastases are seen in the calvarium. The lesions are of many sizes with indistinct margins. **(B)** MRI demonstrates an isodense mass within the calvarium (arrow). It displaces the marrow and has grown outward into the subcutaneous fat of the scalp.

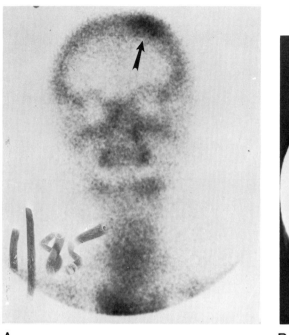

A

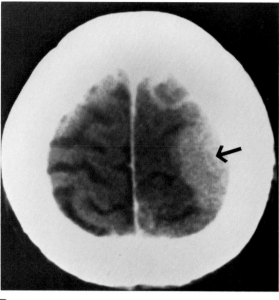

B

Fig. 5-27 Metastatic carcinoma to the calvarium. (A) Radionuclide bone scan showing a region of hyperactivity in the left parietal bone (arrow). **(B)** Contrast-enhanced CT scan shows an enhancing extracerebral mass underneath the left calvarium, causing compression of the cerebral cortex (arrow). This presentation mimics that of a meningioma. *(Figure continues.)*

from direct invasion occurs from carcinoma of the nasopharynx and sphenoid sinus and glomus tumors. CT with bone windowing is the best modality to visualize these lesions.

MENINGIOMA

Meningioma is the third most common intracranial tumor, accounting for about 10 percent of tumors involving the central nervous system. It is the most common extracerebral tumor. The tumor originates from cell elements within the meninges, usually those packing the arachnoid villi. As a result, the tumor is usually attached to the dura. The preferential sites for meningioma correspond with the distribution of the arachnoid villi along the major dural sinuses and at the exits of the spinal nerves from the meningeal sleeves. However, because meningioma may arise from any arachnoidal site (see box), it is seen over the convexities or at sites of infolding of the arachnoid into the brain

SITES OF CRANIAL MENINGIOMA
(IN ORDER OF FREQUENCY)

1. Parasagittal, falx, or sagittal sinus
2. Cerebral convexity
3. Sphenoid ridge
4. Subfrontal, olfactory groove
5. Parasellar
6. Tentorial
7. Posterior fossa (CPA cistern and foramen magnum)
8. Temporal fossa
9. Intraventricular
10. Intraorbital, along the optic nerve sheath

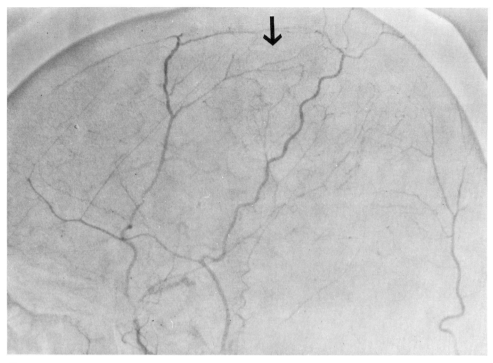

C

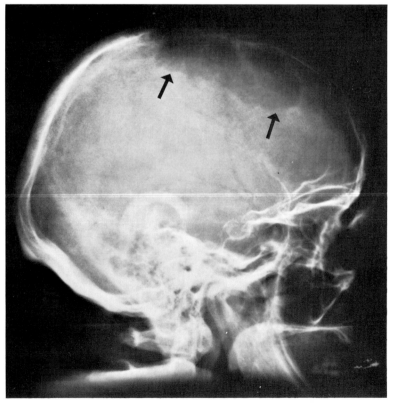

Fig. 5-27 *(Continued).* **(C)** Selective external carotid arteriography shows the tumor to be essentially avascular, differentiating it from a meningioma (arrow). Metastasis was to the calvarium with secondary inward growth. **(D)** Osteoporosis circumscripta. An extensive lytic process involves the calvarium. It may be indistinguishable from metastatic or primary tumor without biopsy. *(Figure continues.)*

D

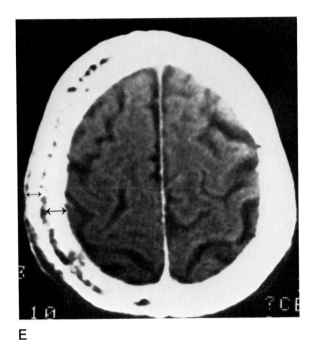

E

Fig. 5-27 *(Continued)*. **(E)** Paget's disease. CT shows the typical changes of thickening of the outer and inner tables with overall enlargement of the calvarium (opposed arrows). There is irregular density within the diploic space. Blastic metastasis would cause increased bone density but not thickening.

(choroid plexus). Rarely, it occurs entirely within the brain along the pia extension around cortical vessels.

Most meningiomas are benign, slowly growing, well encapsulated tumors that cause symptoms by indentation of the brain or compression of cranial nerves. About 5 percent show signs of aggressive growth or malignancy (sarcoma) and may actually invade brain tissue. Meningiomas may infiltrate and destroy adjacent bone. True hyperostosis with an increase in the thickness of bone is common adjacent to the tumor and has diagnostic importance. The bone expansion may cause compression of exiting cranial nerves.

Meningioma may grow as a diffuse sheet of tumor over the brain or the base of the skull. Such development is referred to as *en plaque growth*. These tumors are difficult to image and sometimes are suspected only because of the presence of hyperostosis of the adjacent bone.

Calcification is common within meningiomas. It is usually diffuse and fine but may occur in large, focal clumps. Small, densely calcified meningiomas are slow-growing and may remain the same size for years. Necrosis and cyst formation is rare. Multiple meningiomas occur about 2 percent of the time, most often in association with neurofibromatosis (NF-2).

In general, the prognosis for meningioma is excellent. Many tumors can be completely removed; however, local tumor recurrence is a problem. Periodic follow-up imaging is essential for the timely detection of tumor recurrence, and the tumor may be much more aggressive after recurrence. Contrast-enhanced scans are essential. MRI may better show tumor recurrence when multiple surgical clips are present.

Stroke may result from arterial occlusion, when large tumors encase major vessels. Venous sinus thrombosis may result from local tumor invasion, particularly at the sagittal sinus. Rarely, a meningioma erodes into a paranasal sinus, causing pneumocranium or CSF fistula. Meningioma is sought when certain characteristic clinical findings are present (Table 5-3).

The diagnosis of meningioma is generally made with contrast-enhanced MRI or CT scanning. The tumor always exhibits strong contrast enhancement because the neovascularity derived from the meninges is somatic in nature. Only heavily calcified tumors will not show enhancement. Angiography also has an important role in the evaluation of meningioma: It is used to confirm the diagnosis by demonstrating the characteristic meningeal vascular supply. It is also important for mapping the vascular supply and demonstrating the relation of the tumor to major cerebral vessels prior to surgery or preoperative embolization.

With MRI, meningioma characteristically appears as a slightly hypointense or isointense extracerebral mass on T_1-weighted images (Fig. 5-28). It is moderately

Table 5-3 Characteristic Clinical Symptoms Produced by Meningioma

Symptom	Location
Spastic paraparesis	Large parasagittal
Spastic monoparesis of the leg	Unilateral, parasagittal
Seizure, focal	Convexity
Anosmia	Subfrontal
Cranial nerve paresis	Parasellar, sphenoid ridge, tentorium, CPA
Exophthalmos	Sphenoid ridge
Medullary compression with focal neck pain	Foramen magnum
Organic brain syndrome	Large frontal tumor

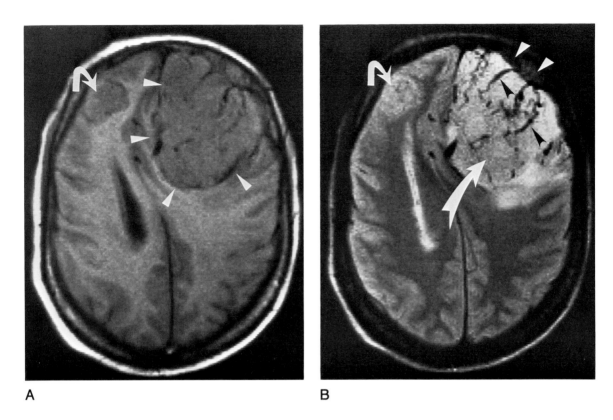

A

B

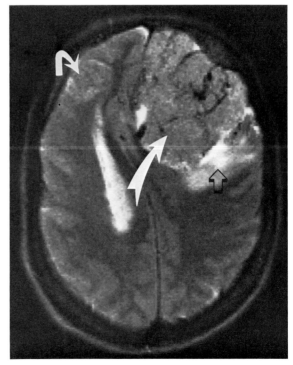

C

Fig. 5-28 Meningioma. (A) T_1-weighted MRI shows a large, slightly hypointense mass in the left frontal fossa (arrowheads). The brain is compressed and displaced away from the mass. A second, smaller meningioma is present in the right frontal region (curved arrow). **(B)** Lightly T_2-weighted MRI shows the meningioma as hyperintense (large white arrow). Flow voids of large vascular channels are present within the tumor (black arrowheads). The smaller, right frontal meningioma is also hyperintense (curved white arrow). Note the thickened calvarium (white arrowheads). **(C)** Heavily T_2-weighted image shows the meningioma as being less intense, a characteristic finding (large white arrow). Right frontal meningioma shows the same signal change (curved white arrow). Also note the slight edema in the adjacent brain (open arrow). *(Figure continues.)*

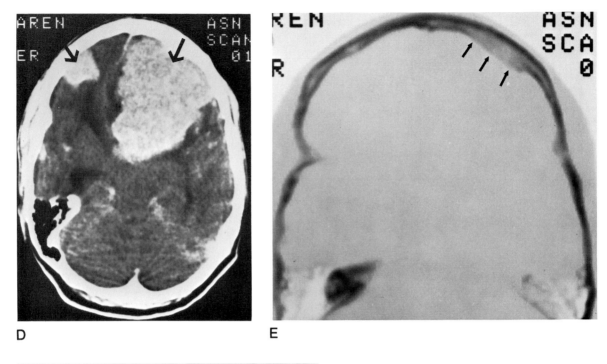

D

E

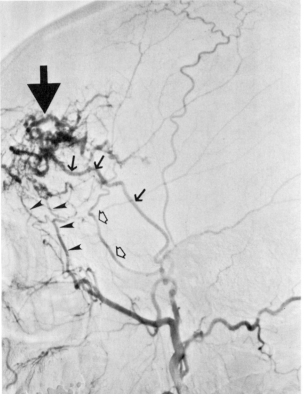

F

Fig. 5-28 *(Continued).* **(D)** Contrast-enhanced CT scan shows the homogeneously enhancing meningiomas (arrows). **(E)** Bone windows show local hyperostosis of the inner table of the left frontal bone (arrows). **(F)** Selective left external carotid angiography shows the marked hypervascularity of the tumor (large arrow). It is supplied by anterior branches of the superficial temporal artery (small arrows), ethmoidal branches of the internal maxillary artery (arrowheads), and (minimally) the middle meningeal artery (open arrows).

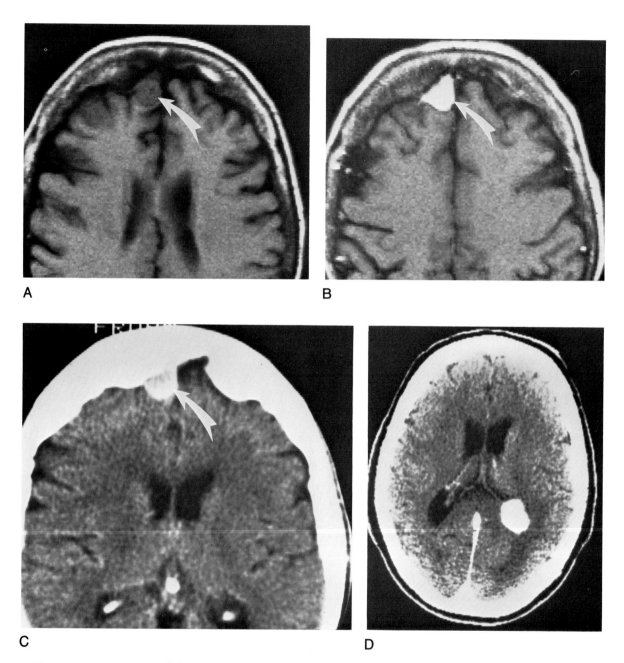

A

B

C

D

Fig. 5-29 Meningioma. (A) T_1-weighted MRI shows the subtle changes of a small meningioma (arrow). **(B)** Gd-DTPA contrast enhancement of the meningioma shows strong enhancement on T_1-weighted images (arrow). **(C)** Contrast-enhanced CT study easily identifies the strongly enhancing meningioma (arrow). **(D)** Intraventricular meningioma. A densely enhancing round mass is present within the atrium of the left lateral ventricle attached to the glomus. A benign xanthogranuloma of the glomus would have the same appearance.

hyperintense on the lightly T_2-weighted (proton density) images but decreases in intensity on the heavily T_2-weighted images. A thin rim of water density may outline the mass and is thought to represent entrapped CSF. After Gd-DTPA injection, meningioma shows strong hyperintensity on the T_1-weighted images. Small meningiomas are easily seen after enhancement (Fig. 5-29). Without Gd-CTPA enhancement small tumors may be difficult to recognize and then often only by a subtle distortion of the adjacent brain anatomy. Bone invasion is seen as loss of the normally high marrow signal at the tumor site. Cysts are sometimes seen within the tumor. Calcium is more difficult to recognize than with CT scans and is represented by signal void within the mass. MRI is generally not as reliable as angiography for determining the patency of adjacent venous sinuses, although gradient echo imaging sometimes helps by showing increased intravascular signal in patent vessels.

Most meningiomas exhibit a characteristic pattern on CT scans (Fig. 5-30). On the precontrast CT scan, 80 percent of the tumors are identified as a homogeneous, slightly hyperdense mass with its base on a dural surface. Isodense tumors occur about 15 percent of the time. Rarely, the tumor is hypodense or cystic and mimics an anaplastic astrocytoma. Cysts may be within or adjacent to the tumor. Occasionally, there is a thin rim of CSF trapped between the tumor and the cortical surface.

There may be fine or conglomerate calcification (20 percent). Edema is common (60 percent) and occasionally severe. In general, for the size of the tumor, the edema is less severe than that seen with glioma or metastasis. Infarction may be seen in the distribution of vessels occluded by the tumor.

Bone window images are essential for the CT evaluation of meningioma and identify hyperostosis or bone destruction of the adjacent calvarium. The hyperostosis may be just a small region of enostosis (Fig. 5-28), or it may cause gross enlargement over a large region of the bone (Fig. 5-31). Tumor is usually present within hyperostotic bone.

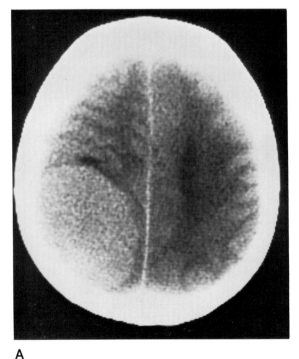

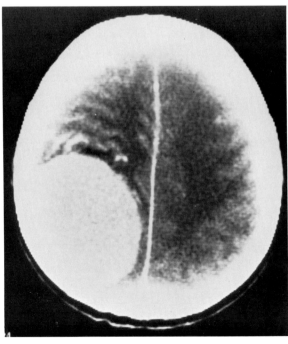

A

B

Fig. 5-30 Meningioma, CT scans. These scans show the classic appearance of a large meningioma. **(A)** Nonenhanced CT scans shows the large right posterior parietal convexity meningioma as being hyperdense. **(B)** With contrast enhancement there is intense homogeneous enhancement of the meningioma.

Fig. 5-31 Meningioma; hemangioma.
(A) Extensive hyperostosis of the frontal and parietal bones from a large meningioma. Note the enlarged vascular grooves in the calvarium caused by both meningeal and superficial vessels (arrowheads). **(B)** The hyperostosis of meningioma must be distinguished from other lesions that expand or thicken the inner table. The typical hemangioma expands the calvarium without causing hyperostosis (open arrows). The diploic space is replaced with enlarged vascular channels and intervening radially oriented bone trabeculae (arrow). *(Figure continues.)*

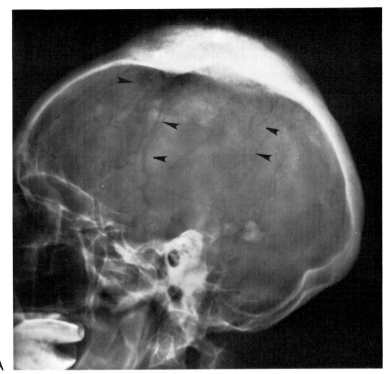

A

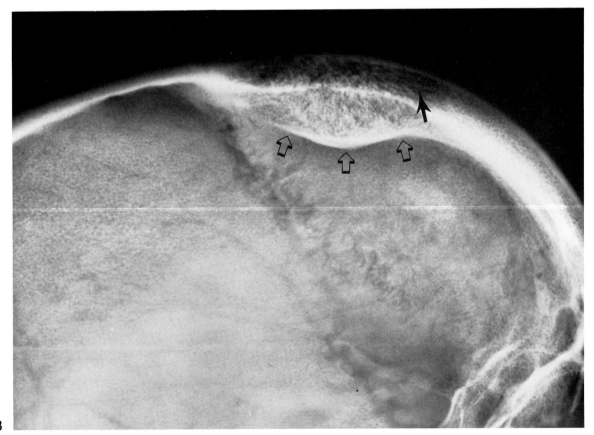

B

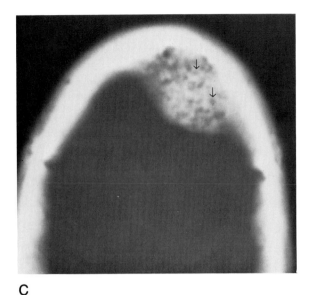

C

Fig. 5-31 *(Continued).* **(C)** CT scan of the hemangioma demonstrates the radially oriented vascular channels (arrows) with intervening bone trabeculae.

Table 5-4 Characteristic Meningeal Vascular Supply to Meningioma

Location	Arteries
Convexity, parasagittal	Middle meningeal artery
Falx	Superficial temporal artery
	Anterior falx artery
Subfrontal	Penetrating dural arteries from the ethmoidal branches
Parasellar	Meningohypophyseal vessels
	Cavernous dural branches
Tentorial	Tentorial branch of meningo-hypophyseal trunk
CPA	Penetrating branches from the ascending pharyngeal artery
	Tentorial and clival branches
Posterior fossa	Posterior meningeal branches from the vertebral artery
Intraventricular	Choroidal artery (anterior, posterolateral, PICA)

Except those that are entirely calcified, almost all meningiomas (98 percent) demonstrate intense and generally homogeneous contrast uptake. Uptake may not be identifiable in tumors that are thin (en plaque) or obscured by adjacent bone artifact. The contrast-enhanced region represents the actual tumor.

Malignant sarcomatous change is suggested by blurred borders, inhomogeneous enhancement due to regressive changes within the tumor, and adjacent satellite lesions. In these cases it may be impossible to differentiate the malignant meningioma from a glioblastoma or gliosarcoma.

Angiography is useful for the diagnosis and mapping of the vascular supply prior to surgery. The angiographic hallmark of meningioma is the meningeal vascular supply of the tumor. It is normally demonstrated by selective cerebral angiography, particularly selective external carotid injection. The tumor receives vascular supply from regional meningeal vessels at the site of its attachment to the dura (Fig. 5-32). Intraventricular tumors are supplied by the regional choroidal arteries. When the tumor is large, its inner portion may receive additional vascular supply from the pial vessels of the cerebral arteries, but most of the tumor is still supplied by the meningeal vessels. The superficial temporal ar-

tery or other scalp vessels may contribute to tumors, especially those that have grown through the calvarium (Fig. 5-28F). The location of meningiomas and their characteristic vascular supplies are given in Table 5-4.

The meningeal vascular supply is more or less radially oriented from the base into the tumor. The tumor shows an intense homogeneous blush that begins in the later arterial phase and persists throughout the venous phase (Fig. 5-33). The mass is sharply outlined. Early venous drainage is rare. Except those that are small and calcified, all meningiomas show significant meningeal vascular supply and blush. If the meningeal supply is little or absent, the diagnosis of meningioma is unlikely (see differential diagnosis below, and Fig. 5-27).

Selective angiography is preferred. For convexity tumors, external and internal carotid angiographic runs are appropriate to clearly differentiate the meningeal and cortical supply to the tumor. Bilateral studies are performed, as frequently there is important supply from contralateral vessels. Subtraction films are basic. Special note is made of the patency of the dural venous sinuses (Fig. 5-34), the position of major vessels relative to the tumor, and any vascular constriction or occlusion. The last point is particularly important for tumors at the base of the brain near the internal carotid and middle cerebral arteries.

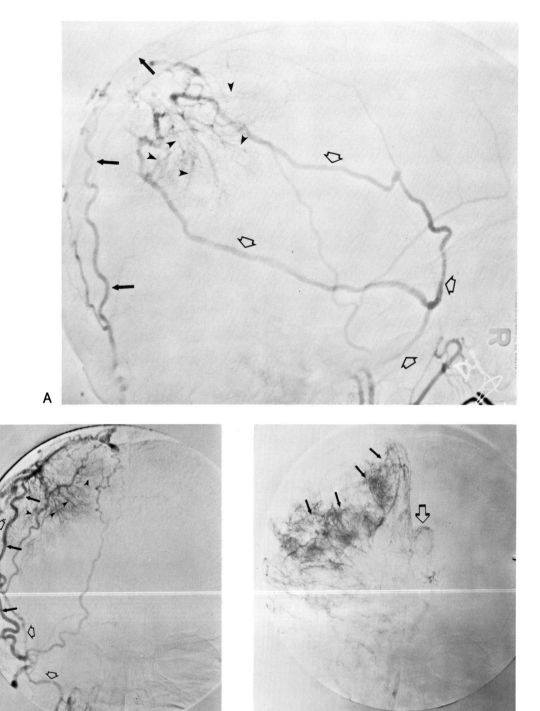

Fig. 5-32 Meningioma. The CT scan of this case is shown in Figure 5-30. **(A)** Selective right external carotid artery (ECA) arteriography shows gross enlargement of the posterior branches of the middle meningeal artery (open arrows). This artery is the primary supply to the fine radial vessels of the tumor (arrowheads). The posterior occipital scalp branch also supplies the tumor (arrows). **(B)** AP view of Fig. A. The vessels are labeled with the same types of arrow. **(C)** Internal carotid artery (ICA) injection in the AP projection. It shows the pial vascular supply to the inner portion of this large meningioma (black arrows). Note the subfalcial herniation (open arrow). *(Figure continues.)*

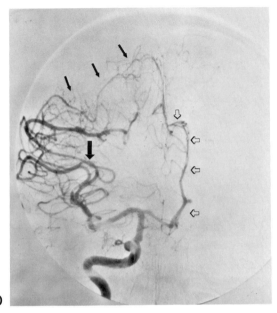

D

Fig. 5-32 *(Continued).* **(D)** ICA injection in the AP projection. The arterial phase shows the displacement of the cortical vessels away from the inner table (small black arrows), downward displacement of the sylvian point (large black arrow), and subfalcial herniation with a "square" type shift of the pericallosal artery (open arrows). The square shift is commonly seen with posterior masses. **(E)** Skull radiograph showing abnormal vascular channels corresponding to the enlarged meningeal vessels demonstrated in Fig. A (arrowheads).

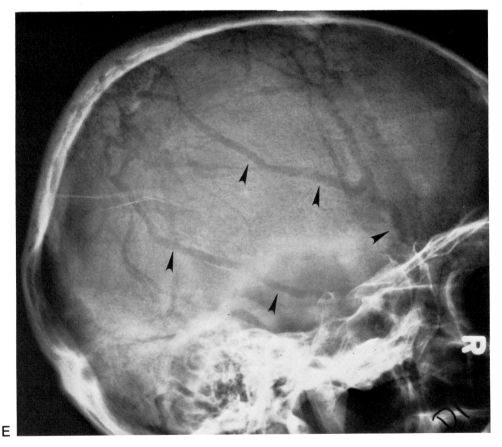

E

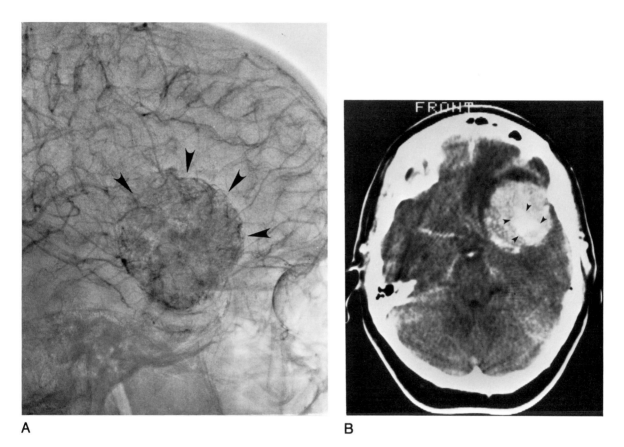

A

B

Fig. 5-33 Meningioma, sphenoid ridge. (A) The angiographic stain of the meningioma normally becomes homogeneously hyperintense during the capillary and venous phases (arrowheads). **(B)** Contrast-enhanced CT scan. Note the dense calcium that is barely seen within the enhanced tumor (arrowheads).

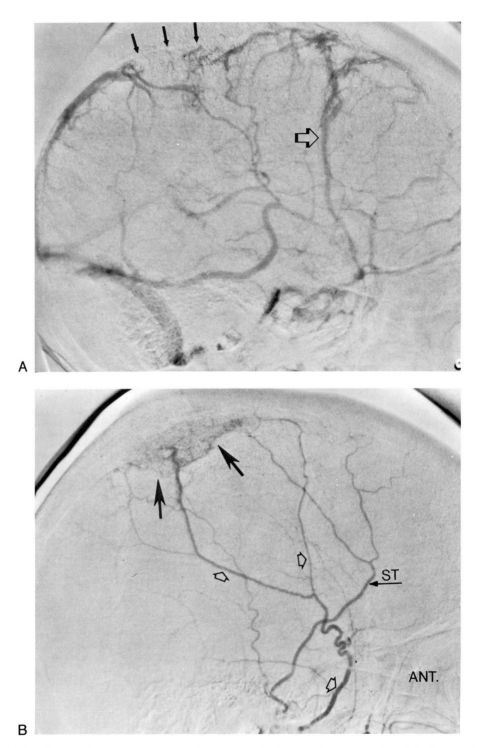

Fig. 5-34 Vessels occluded by meningioma. (A) A parasagittal meningioma has occluded the dural sagittal sinus (black arrows). Note the collateral veins draining the frontal region (open arrow). **(B)** Lateral selective ECA arteriography. The parasagittal meningioma (black arrows) is supplied by branches of the middle meningeal artery (open arrows). The "blush" outlines the tumor. ST = superficial temporal artery. *(Figure continues.)*

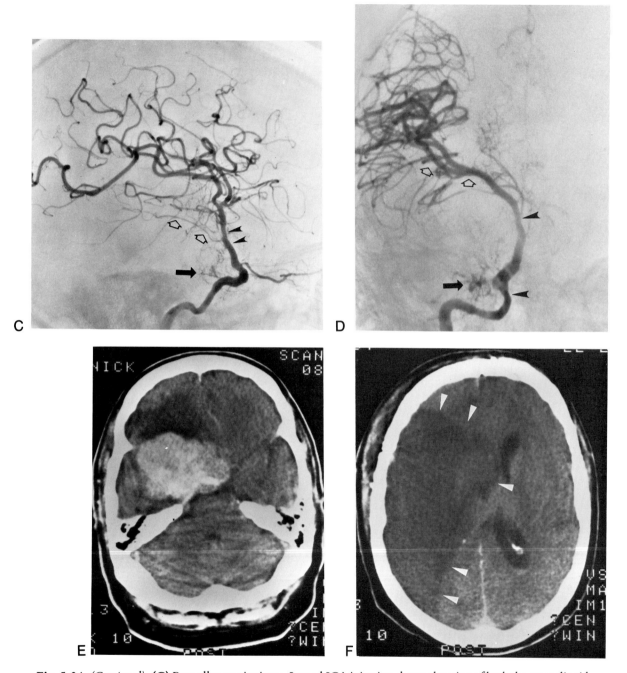

Fig. 5-34 *(Continued).* **(C)** Parasellar meningioma. Lateral ICA injection shows elevation of both the supraclinoid ICA and horizontal MCA. Vessel irregularity indicates tumor encasement (arrowheads). Hypertrophied branches from the meningohypophyseal trunk supply the tumor (arrow). There is gross elevation of the sylvian vessels and the anterior choroidal artery (open arrows). **(D)** AP view of the same injection showing constriction of the ICA (arrowheads), elevation of the MCA (open arrows), and hypertrophy of the meningohypophyseal vessels (black arrow). **(E)** Contrast-enhanced CT scan of the meningioma of the right sphenoid wing and parasellar region. **(F)** Postoperative infarction of the right hemisphere from right MCA occlusion (arrowheads). Infarctions may result from thrombosis caused by the tumor constriction or by manipulation at the time of surgical excision.

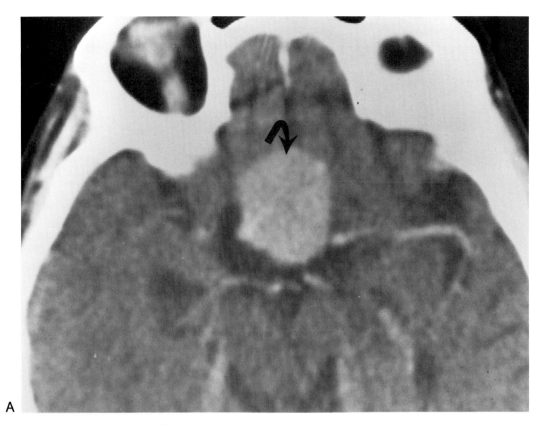

A

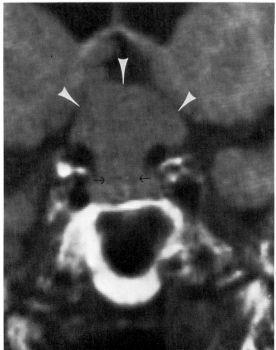

B

Fig. 5-35 Meningioma, suprasellar. (A) Transaxial CT scan shows a homogeneously enhancing mass within the suprasellar cistern (arrow). This mass cannot be differentiated from a pituitary adenoma with suprasellar extension. **(B)** Coronal T_1-weighted MRI through the sella turcica demonstrates the homogeneous isointense mass within the suprasellar cistern (arrowheads). The mass is separated from the slightly more hyperintense normal pituitary gland by the diaphragma sellae (arrows). The sella is normal in size. In this case, MRI makes the correct diagnosis. With a pituitary macroadenoma with suprasellar extension, the sella is almost always enlarged.

Large vascular tumors may be embolized prior to surgical removal to decrease the vascularity of the tumor so that surgical removal is easier. Gelfoam or other material is injected into the external carotid artery or branches supplying the tumor. Balloon occlusion catheters must be used to avoid inadvertent backflow embolization into the internal carotid circulation.

Differential Diagnosis

Although most meningiomas are obvious, at times the tumor appears similar to other neoplastic masses. It may be especially difficult to differentiate a meningioma from a peripheral lymphoma, as the two tumors often have similar MRI and CT scanning characteristics. Some cerebral metastases and gliomas have an appearance similar to that of meningioma, especially small peripheral enhancing lesions or cystic masses. If the dura is invaded, these tumors may have slight meningeal vascular supply, seen with angiography, but it is always less than with meningioma. It may be particularly difficult to differentiate blastic calvarial metastasis (prostate or breast carcinoma) from meningioma especially if there has been inward tumor invasion through the dura (Fig. 5-27).

A suprasellar meningioma must be differentiated from a pituitary macroadenoma. Both tumors show homogeneous enhancement and have similar characteristics on MRI and CT scans. Meningioma usually arises from the posterior planum sphenoidale and lies entirely above the sella within the suprasellar cistern (Fig. 5-35). Meningeal vascular supply is seen with angiography. Pituitary adenoma is almost always an intrasellar tumor, enlarging the sella and secondly extending into the suprasellar cistern. Coronal MRI and CT scans usually differentiate between the two tumors. Pituitary adenoma does not ordinarily show significant neovascularity on angiography.

A cerebellopontine angle meningioma (see Fig. 5-59) must be differentiated from an acoustic neurinoma, exophytic pontine astrocytoma, and metastatic tumor, particularly melanoma. The acoustic neurinoma enlarges the internal auditory canal; a meningioma does not. Meningioma also shows meningeal vascular supply on angiography, whereas an acoustic neurinoma shows little neovascularity. On CT scans, large aneurysms occasionally simulate a meningioma in the suprasella region or cerebellar pontine angle cistern. MRI or angiography makes the correct diagnosis.

Lymphoma

Non-Hodgkin's lymphoma is unusually found in the CNS, accounting for about 2 percent of all intracranial tumors, although the incidence is increasing. Primary CNS lymphoma is much more common than metastatic lymphoma. Its peak incidence is at about 50 years of age, although the tumor may occur at any age after 10. Persons who are immunodeficient have a much greater risk for CNS lymphoma (e.g., those with AIDS, allograft recipients, cancer victims, those undergoing cancer chemotherapy).

Most primary lymphomas involve the deep structures (basal ganglia, thalamus, corpus callosum) and the deep white matter of the cerebrum, although the tumor may be found anywhere in the brain. Paraventricular location is characteristic. Single and multiple lesions are present with about equal frequency. With multiple lesions, the deep structures are almost always involved. There is usually less mass effect than would be expected for the size of the tumor because of relatively little surrounding edema. Response to glucocorticoid therapy and radiation may be dramatic, the tumor disappearing within days. However, considerable clinical disability remains despite apparent disappearance of the tumor. Guided needle biopsy is excellent for diagnosis and immunologic typing for therapy.

On the nonenhanced CT scan, the tumors are usually seen as large (more than 4 cm), homogeneous, slightly hyperdense, often well demarcated lesions. There is intense, homogeneous enhancement with contrast (Fig. 5-36). Sometimes ring-like enhancement occurs and is identical to that of glioblastoma, metastasis, or abscess. Surrounding edema is variable but is often little or absent. The tumor may diffusely infiltrate the subependymal regions, outlining the lateral ventricles.

The full extent of the edema is shown better on MRI than on CT scanning. The tumor is slightly hypointense on T_1- and slightly hyperintense on T_2-weighted images (Fig. 5-36). It may be difficult to define the tumor within the edema without Gd-DTPA enhancement.

Metastatic non-Hodgkin's lymphoma from somatic sites occurs only rarely. It tends to have a peripheral location, having infiltrated the brain from the meninges. Hodgkin's lymphoma almost never involves the brain parenchyma, although it may involve the meninges. When peripheral, lymphoma in the brain resem-

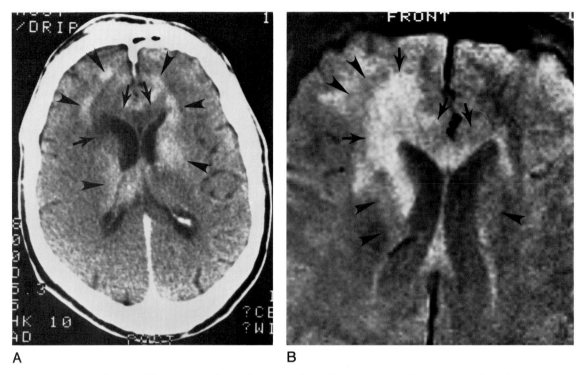

A

B

Fig. 5-36 Lymphoma. (A) Contrast-enhanced CT scan shows homogeneous enhancement of lymphoma involving the deep paraventricular structures bilaterally, including the basal ganglia and thalamus (arrowheads). Edema is present in the corpus callosum and adjacent to the right frontal horn (arrows). **(B)** Lightly T_2-weighted MRI shows the edema in the corpus callosum and adjacent to the right frontal horn as regions of high signal (arrows). The tumor itself shows only minimally increased T_2 signal and is difficult to identify (arrowheads).

bles meningioma. Biopsy or angiography may be necessary to differentiate between the two tumors.

Primary Nerve Cell Tumors

Primary nerve cell tumors arise from neurons within the brain or ganglion cells outside the brain. They account for fewer than 0.5 percent of brain tumors and are found most commonly in individuals under 30 years old. Seizures are the most common clinical symptom, and neurologic deficit is rare. Most tumors grow slowly and may be present for years prior to presentation. The tumors have been named according to an ascending grade of malignancy: *gangliocytoma, ganglioglioma, ganglioneuroblastoma,* and *neuroblastoma.*

Most of these tumors arise within the medial portion of the temporal lobe adjacent to the atrium of the lateral ventricle, although a few may also be found within the cerebellum or deep structures. Characteristically, the tumor is moderately large with large cysts, calcifica-

tion, and a peculiar tendency to produce local atrophy and adjacent ventricular dilatation (Fig. 5-37). Contrast enhancement may be seen within the solid portions of the tumor, but it does not correlate with the degree of malignant change. The tumor may appear similar to oligodendroglioma and ependymoma. A calcified tumor in the cerebellum in an adult is usually one of the neuronal series.

Epidermoid Tumor

An epidermoid tumor is a congenital lesion. It is a cyst lined by squamous epithelium and filled with the debris of desquamation. Most commonly it occurs in the cerebellopontine angle cistern, the suprasellar cistern, and the temporal fossa. It may also occur, however, within the calvarium, where it appears on a skull radiograph as a well outlined, round, lytic lesion with a slightly sclerotic margin (Fig. 5-38).

On CT scans, epidermoid is a well circumscribed

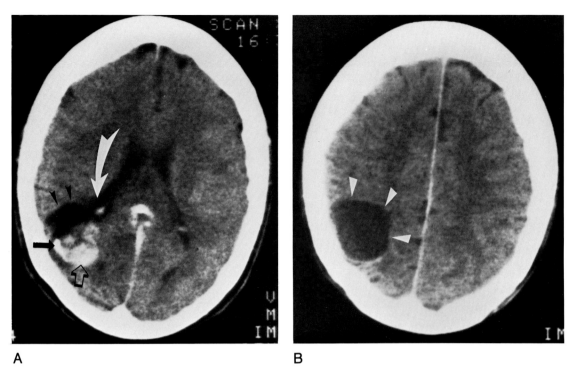

A   B

Fig. 5-37 Ganglioglioma. (A) Tumor is present in the medial posterior temporal lobe. There is a cyst (arrowheads), contrast enhancement (open arrow), calcification (black arrow), and local atrophic change with dilatation of the atrium of the right lateral ventricle (large white arrow). **(B)** With neuronal tumors, the cyst is characteristically large (arrowheads).

mass that is usually hypodense and shows no contrast enhancement. It is occasionally isodense or even hyperdense (Fig. 5-38). It may resemble an arachnoid cyst. Rarely, there is a rim of calcification.

With MRI, it is hypointense (near CSF intensity) on T_1-weighted images and moderately hyperintense to CSF on the T_2-weighted images. Inhomogeneity within the cyst is common. The T_2-weighted MRI characteristics differentiate the lesion from an arachnoid cyst. The tumor may become large without causing symptoms.

Sella and Juxtasella Tumors

PITUITARY ADENOMA

Pituitary adenoma is the most common tumor of the sella turcica and suprasellar cistern. It is a benign, slow-growing tumor that arises from the adenohypophysis (anterior lobe). Only rarely is it invasive or malignant.

In adults, pituitary tumors account for about 10 percent of primary intracranial tumors. The tumor is rare in children. Seventy percent of the tumors produce a hormone. Small tumors (less than 10 mm) are called *microadenomas.* Large tumors (more than 10 mm) are called *macroadenomas.* The sella turcica is usually normal with a microadenoma but is expanded with a macroadenoma.

A small pituitary tumor, i.e., confined within the sella, is usually suspected by the clinical syndrome of hormone excess. A prolactin-secreting adenoma *(prolactinoma)* is the most common; it produces amenorrhea, galactorrhea, and decreased libido in women and hypogonadism and decreased libido in men. The tumor is ten times more common in women. Hyperprolactinemia with the serum prolactin level more than 100 ng/ml indicates a high probability of a pituitary tumor. Excessive growth hormone production produces acromegaly in the adult and gigantism in adolescents. Excessive adrenocorticotropic hormone (ACTH) or

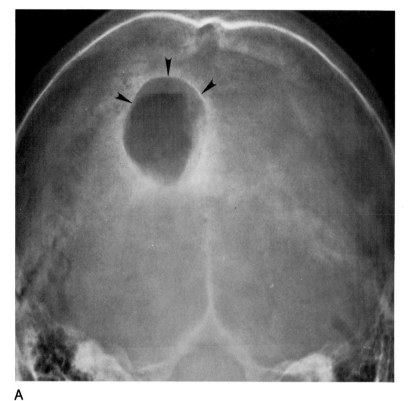

Fig. 5-38 Epidermoid. (A) Skull radiograph demonstrates a purely lytic lesion of the calvarium with sharply defined sclerotic margins. It is a characteristic picture. Compare with Figure 6-22B. **(B)** Epidermoid within the left sylvian fissure. CT scan typically shows an epidermoid as very hypodense. There is minimal mass effect, as with most slowly enlarging tumors or cysts. **(C)** Epidermoid. Rarely, an epidermoid has high density contents. This one extends through the tentorium into the cerebellopontine angle (CPA) cistern (arrow). (Fig. B from Dubois, 1984, with permission.)

A

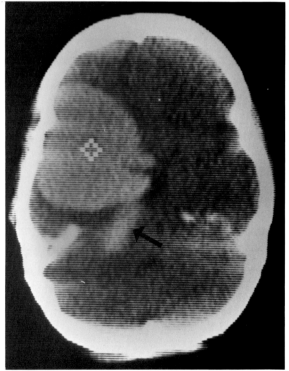

B

C

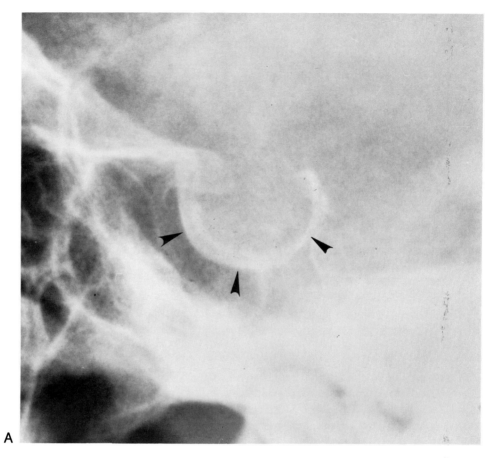

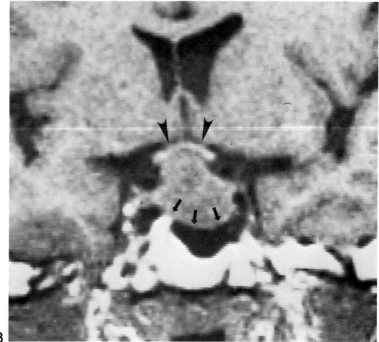

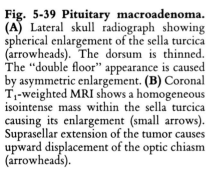

Fig. 5-39 Pituitary macroadenoma.
(A) Lateral skull radiograph showing spherical enlargement of the sella turcica (arrowheads). The dorsum is thinned. The "double floor" appearance is caused by asymmetric enlargement. **(B)** Coronal T_1-weighted MRI shows a homogeneous isointense mass within the sella turcica causing its enlargement (small arrows). Suprasellar extension of the tumor causes upward displacement of the optic chiasm (arrowheads).

A

B

183

thyroid-stimulating hormone produces Cushing's syndrome or hyperthyroidism. Small nonsecreting tumors are clinically unrecognized.

Nonsecreting tumors are almost always large at the time of diagnosis, expanding the sella (Fig. 5-39) and frequently extending into the suprasellar cistern. Within the suprasellar cistern the tumor may compress the optic chiasm, producing variable visual field deficits, bitemporal hemianopsia being the most common. Much less commonly there may be CN III, IV, V, and VI abnormalities from lateral invasion or extension into the cavernous sinus. Rarely, there is sudden hemorrhage into the tumor, causing severe headache, often with acute chiasmal compression or ocular nerve palsy from rapid expansion of the tumor. This condition is referred to as *pituitary apoplexy.* Large tumors may extend high in the brain to obstruct the foramina of Monro and cause hydrocephalus. Headache is common and may be the only presenting symptom with pituitary tumor.

Highly aggressive tumors erode the floor of the sella and infiltrate the dural sinuses or upper clivus. Some break through the dura into the temporal or posterior fossa. These "invasive adenomas" are refractory to definitive treatment by either surgery or irradiation.

The previous histologic classification of the tumor as chromophobic, eosinophilic, or basophilic has generally been replaced by classification based on the presence and type of hormonal secretion. Classification is not important for prognosis. Metastasis or spread into the subarachnoid spaces has been reported, but it is rare.

Macroadenoma

The preferred imaging technique for evaluation of macroadenoma is MRI. T_1-weighted images are the most useful. The tumor is usually isointense to brain on T_1-weighted images and is slightly hyperintense on T_2-weighted images (Fig. 5-40). MRI is especially useful for evaluating any suprasellar or parasellar extension. Displacement of the optic chiasm or indentation of the hypothalamus is well seen. Coronal and sagittal planes are the most informative. A slice thickness of 5 to 7 mm is adequate. Gd-DTPA is usually not necessary for evaluating macroadenomas.

Cysts occur within macroadenomas and are seen on MRI as pockets of CSF-equivalent signal intensity. Hemorrhage is usually chronic when found and displays high signal intensity on both T_1- and T_2-weighted images (Fig. 5-41). Invasions of the clivus, somewhat difficult to identify with MRI, may be seen as replacement of the normal fat signal of the marrow.

Invasion into the cavernous sinus is common with macroadenoma, although it is often difficult to diagnose with either MRI or CT scanning. The most reliable MRI finding is encasement of the carotid artery by the tumor. Other signs are asymmetric enlargement and asymmetric signal intensity of the cavernous sinus (Fig. 5-42). At best, MRI is only about 50 percent accurate for detection of cavernous sinus invasion.

With MRI the location of the cavernous segment of the internal carotid arteries is well seen and the presence of aneurysm easily determined. MRI eliminates the need for angiography in the evaluation of pituitary macroadenoma.

Computed tomography adequately demonstrates the important features of macroadenoma. Coronal contrast-enhanced thin section imaging is the most useful. On the noncontrast CT scan, a pituitary macroadenoma usually appears as a sharply marginated, homogeneous, moderately hyperdense (35 to 50 HU) mass within the sella and suprasellar cistern. The sella is enlarged. Ten percent of the tumors are hypodense or of mixed density because of the presence of cysts or old hemorrhage within the tumor. Density greater than 50 HU implies recent hemorrhage (apoplexy). Calcification within the tumor is rare but may occur as either a thin rim along the tumor margin or diffusely within the tumor.

Most commonly, there is uniform contrast enhancement of the adenoma, with characteristics similar to those of a meningioma. Mixed density enhancement may occur (Fig. 5-41). The nonenhancing regions within the tumor usually are cysts or regions of resolving hemorrhage. There is no correlation between enhancement and hormonal function or malignancy of the tumor.

Invasive tumors cause either erosion of the floor of the sella or more diffuse destruction of the clivus, simulating a sphenoid sinus carcinoma (Fig. 5-43). CT scanning with bone window imaging is superior to MRI for detecting invasion of the clivus. Invasion of the cavernous sinus is difficult to define with CT scans, but it can be diagnosed when there is enlargement of a cavernous sinus or obvious tumor beyond the lateral or posterior wall of the cavernous sinus (Fig. 5-42).

After surgical resection of a pituitary macroadenoma there is often considerable nonneoplastic tissue re-

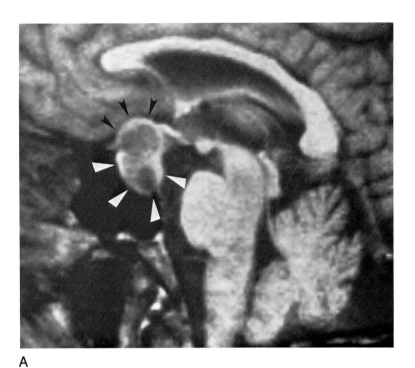

A

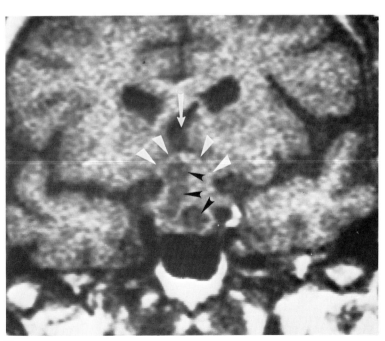

Fig. 5-40 Pituitary macroadenoma, cystic. (A) Sagittal T_1-weighted MRI shows a cystic pituitary mass. There is enlargement of the sella turcica (white arrowheads) and suprasellar extension (black arrowheads). **(B)** Coronal T_1-weighted MRI shows the suprasellar extension of the tumor (white arrowheads) indenting the anterior third ventricle (white arrow). Cysts within the tumor are represented by low signal intensity (black arrowheads). *(Figure continues.)*

B

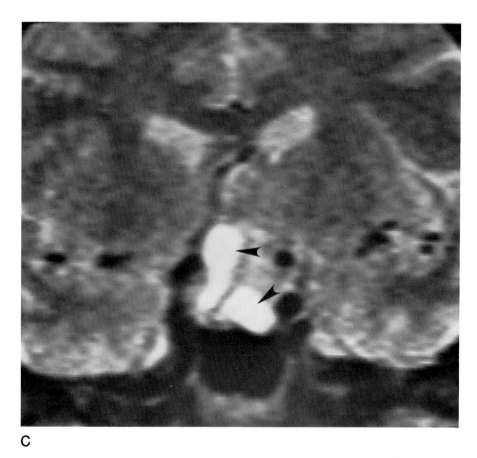

C

Fig. 5-40 *(Continued).* **(C)** T_2-weighed MRI shows the cyst as high signal intensity (arrowheads).

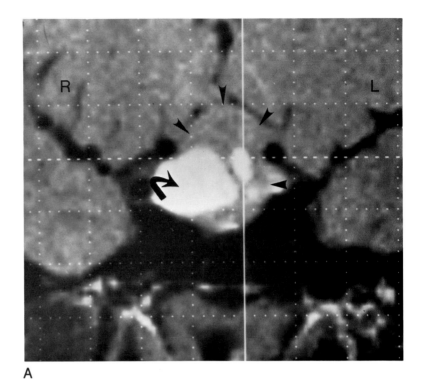

A

Fig. 5-41 **Pituitary adenoma with chronic hemorrhage.** (A) T$_1$-weighted MRI in the coronal plane shows a pituitary macroadenoma with suprasellar extension (arrowheads). The remains of a hemorrhage into the tumor or cyst is seen as high signal intensity (curved arrow). (B) Contrast-enhanced CT scan of the same patient shows the suprasellar extension of the contrast-enhancing tumor (arrowheads). The low density region represents the old hemorrhage or hemorrhagic cyst (curved arrow). The floor of the sella has resorbed and is expanded downward. Laterality is reverse of MRI image.

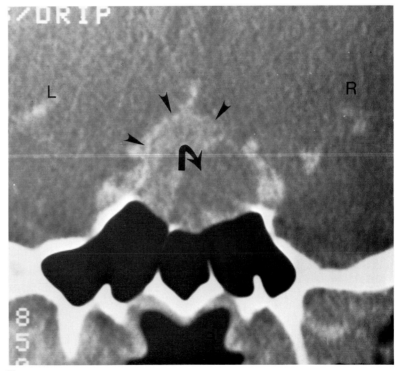

B

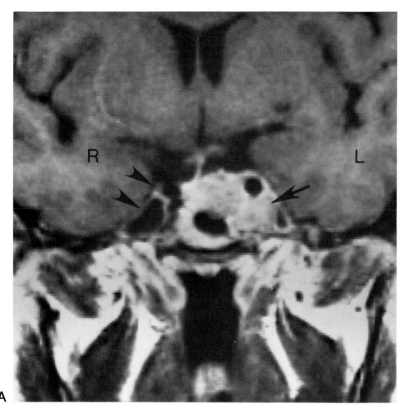

Fig. 5-42 Pituitary adenoma, invasion of the cavernous sinus and upper clivus. (A) Gd-DTPA contrast-enhanced T$_1$-weighted MRI shows an enhancing adenoma invading laterally into the cavernous sinus. The sinus is enlarged, and the tumor surrounds the ICA (black arrow). The right cavernous sinus (black arrowheads) is normal. **(B)** Contrast-enhanced CT scan in the coronal plane also shows the tumor invading and enlarging the right cavernous sinus (black arrows) surrounding the contrast-filled ICA (white arrow). The normal size and enhancement of the right cavernous sinus is seen (arrowheads). This lesion is an invasive adenoma with inferior extension and destruction of the upper portion of the left side of the clivus (open arrow). Laterality of CT is reverse of MRI.

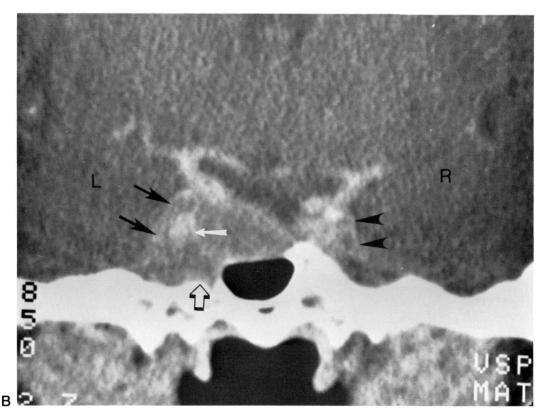

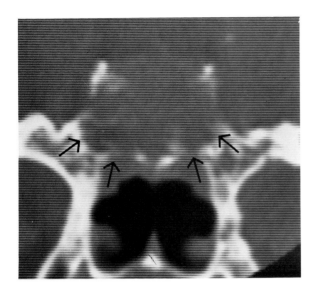

Fig. 5-43 Invasive pituitary adenoma. Coronal CT scan with a wide window shows that the tumor has extended inferiorly to fill the sphenoid sinus and cause destruction of the base of the skull (arrows). A sphenoid sinus carcinoma might produce the same findings.

maining in the region of the original tumor that slowly resolves over 2 to 3 months (Fig. 5-44). Therefore the amount of residual tumor cannot be accurately evaluated until after this period.

Tumor recurrence is seen in about 12 percent of patients and usually becomes apparent after 4 to 8 years. The sella is often packed with fat or muscle at the time of surgery, making recognition of recurrent tumor more difficult. Initially the fat displays high intensity on MRI; the intensity decreases with time, however, so that after 1 year it is isointense with other intrasellar tissues and cannot be differentiated from recurrent tumor. Baseline postoperative scans are obtained 3 months after surgery so that future changes in the amount of intrasellar tissue will be apparent.

Microadenoma

The preferred technique for detecting a microadenoma is MRI. The examination is performed in the coronal plane using thin section (3 mm) T_1-weighted imaging

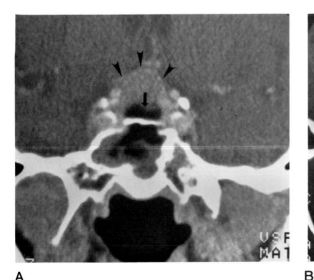

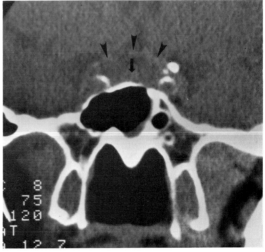

A B

Fig. 5-44 Pituitary adenoma, postoperative evaluation. (A) Postoperative contrast-enhanced CT scan in the coronal plane 2 weeks after transsphenoidal hypophysectomy shows considerable abnormal enhancing tissue remaining within the sella and suprasellar cistern (arrowheads). Fat packing is seen in the inferior sella turcica (arrow). There are postsurgical changes within the sphenoid sinus. **(B)** CT scan without contrast done 3 months after surgery shows that the tissue mass has decreased considerably in size without treatment (arrowheads). The density of the fat has increased (arrow). The changes within the sphenoid sinus have resolved.

or T_1-weighted Gd-DTPA enhanced imaging. T_2-weighted images are not as sensitive for this lesion.

The normal pituitary gland has signal intensity approximating that of cerebral white matter. The gland is seen in the inferior sella turcica, 4 to 8 mm in height but it may appear slightly larger in young women. Its upper border may be straight or with slight upward or downward convexity. The pituitary stalk is seen as a thin midline structure extending downward from the infundibulum of the hypothalamus into the posterior portion of the gland. It may normally angulate slightly away from the midline. Fat intensity may be seen in the posterior sella, probably within the neurohypophysis (posterior lobe).

A pituitary microadenoma is seen as a small (less than 10 mm), round region of hypointensity within the pituitary gland. It is usually positioned posterolaterally, often enlarging the ipsilateral portion of the gland. It may displace the pituitary stalk contralaterally.

Gd-DTPA contrast enhancement may be used to increase the sensitivity of the MRI when the T_1-weighted images are nondiagnostic. The scan is performed as soon as possible after infusion of contrast. The normal gland and the cavernous sinus show increased signal intensity. The tumor is seen as a small, round region of nonenhanced low signal intensity within the intensely enhancing gland (Fig. 5-45).

Microadenomas frequently invade the dura of the medial margin of the cavernous sinus. However, this dural membrane is so thin that it is not reliably imaged with MRI and the invasion cannot be defined.

Computed tomography is an acceptable technique for evaluating microadenomas, although compared with MRI it is slightly less sensitive for detection of the tumor. Thin section (2 mm), high resolution coronal imaging is used. It is usually done with the patient prone and the neck extended as far as possible. The gantry is angled so the plane of the scan is as close as possible to true coronal. The scan sections must fall away from any dental hardware. Bone images are also obtained. High dose (40 to 60 g of iodine) intravenous contrast is essential and is best given as a rapid bolus just before rapid sequence scanning. This method densely opacifies the pituitary gland, cavernous sinus, and internal carotid arteries.

Microadenoma most commonly appears as a focal, low density, nonenhancing region within the densely enhancing pituitary gland (Fig. 5-46). There may be

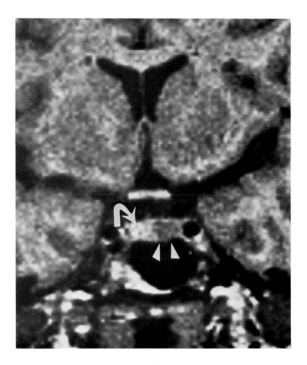

Fig. 5-45 Pituitary microadenoma. Coronal Gd-DTPA-enhanced T_1-weighted MRI shows the nonenhancing adenoma (arrowheads) displacing the intensely enhanced normal pituitary gland (curved arrow).

enlargement of the gland so that it is more than 9 mm in height, with displacement of the infundibulum away from the side of the tumor. A small, focal, downward bulge of the sella floor is sometimes seen adjacent to the tumor but by itself cannot be used to indicate a microadenoma. Rarely, microadenomas calcify, resulting in a "pituitary stone." The sensitivity of CT scanning is reported to be 40 to 90 percent, depending on the study. The criteria and approximate correlation with surgical findings are given in Table 5-5.

Because most prolactin-secreting pituitary adenomas are successfully treated with bromocriptine, identification of the adenoma is often not necessary. The imaging is done primarily to exclude a macroadenoma. The diagnosis and follow-up can be done by clinical measurements. There is no longer any indication for plain film tomography in the diagnosis of macroadenoma, and angiography is of no use.

When surgical excision of a microadenoma is being considered, it becomes important to identify the location of the microadenoma. For ACTH-secreting

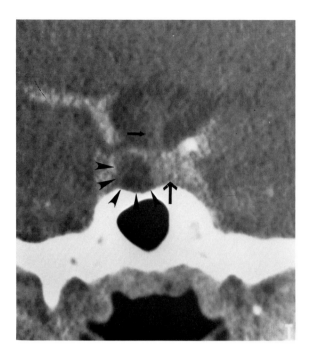

Fig. 5-46 Pituitary microadenoma, CT scan. Coronal contrast-enhanced CT scan shows the nonenhancing hypodense adenoma (arrowheads) displacing the normally enhanced pituitary gland (arrow). The height of the gland is increased. The pituitary stalk is displaced to the opposite side (small arrow).

CRANIOPHARYNGIOMA

Craniopharyngioma has a peak incidence during childhood and adolescence, with a second peak in adults about 40 to 50 years old. It is discussed in Chapter 6.

DIFFERENTIAL DIAGNOSIS

Meningioma

Meningioma occurs in the sella region, arising from the dura of the posterior portion of the planum sphenoidale, tuberculum sellae, diaphragma sellae, dorsum sellae, and lateral dura of the cavernous sinus. Meningioma in the suprasellar region may mimic a pituitary adenoma (Fig. 5-35). However, with meningioma the sella is not enlarged and there is often characteristic sclerosis of the adjacent bone. Angiography shows the characteristic meningeal vascular supply.

Aneurysm

A giant aneurysm of the internal carotid artery may expand into the sella and suprasellar cistern. It may mimic a pituitary adenoma or meningioma. Contrast enhancement on CT scans is intense and occurs early.

tumors, bilateral simultaneous inferior petrosal sinus blood sampling for ACTH often defines the laterality of the tumor when it cannot be imaged with either MRI or CT scans.

Table 5-5 Criteria for CT Diagnosis of Microadenoma

Finding	Frequency of Finding (%)	% Correlation with Histology
Discrete hypodense lesion	50	90
Focal floor erosion or bulge	40	70
Focal upward convexity of gland	30	80
Pituitary height > 9 mm	10	100
Infundibular displacement	20	80

LESIONS OF THE SELLA AND JUXTASELLA REGION

Common lesions
    Pituitary adenoma
    Meningioma
    Empty sella
    Giant aneurysm
    Invasive tumors of the sphenoid sinus and nasopharynx
Uncommon lesions
    Arachnoid cyst (suprasellar)
    Epidermoid
    Rathke's pouch cyst
    Metastasis
    Trigeminal schwannoma (Meckel's cave)
    Chordoma/chondrosarcoma
    Granuloma
    Cysticercosis (common in endemic regions)

On MRI, flow void is usually seen within the aneurysm. However, the signal intensity within an aneurysm may be inhomogeneous because of high signal clot or slow related enhancements. The sella is usually eroded and enlarged from one side, rather than the more central enlargement seen with a pituitary adenoma. Rim calcification is common with giant parasellar aneurysms. When there is any question of an aneurysm, MRI or bilateral carotid angiography is performed (See Chapter 3, Fig. 3-15).

"Empty Sella" Syndrome

The empty sella refers to herniation of the suprasellar arachnoid into the sella turcica through an opening in an incompletely formed diaphragma sellae. The sella then becomes filled with CSF. The CSF pulsations may enlarge the sella, so that on plain film radiography it mimics the changes of a pituitary adenoma. CT scanning and MRI can identify the fluid within the sella. Defining the pituitary stalk within the fluid is diagnostic of empty sella. The stalk is not seen with an intrasellar cyst or cystic tumor. If necessary, CT positive-contrast cisternography can differentiate between cyst and empty sella: The empty sella fills with the contrast; the intrasellar cyst does not.

An empty sella is common (10 to 20 percent of the general population) and is usually asymptomatic. Rarely, there is minor hypopituitarism due to posterior compression of the gland, visual field deficit due to "falling" of the optic chiasm into the sella, and a CSF fistula into the sphenoid sinus. Because it is so common, an empty sella may be found in association with other lesions, e.g., pituitary microadenoma.

Rathke's Pouch Cyst

Rathke's pouch cyst is a rare congenital cyst within the sella turcica or suprasellar cistern. It may be of any size and has the typical appearance of simple cystic lesions on both MRI and CT scans. When large, these cysts are impossible to differentiate from a cystic macroadenoma.

Meckel's Cave Tumor (Trigeminal Neurinoma)

Meckel's cave is an invagination of the dura at the posterior cavernous sinus, adjacent to the posterior sella turcica. It contains the gasserian ganglion of the trigeminal nerve (CN V). Trigeminal neurinoma (schwannoma) is a rare tumor that occurs most often in the gasserian ganglion within Meckel's cave. The tumor may become large, erode the lateral sella, and anteriorly displace the proximal cavernous portion of the internal carotid artery (ICA). On MRI the tumors are hypointense on T_1-weighted images and hyperintense on T_2-weighted images. CT scans show intense homogeneous enhancement typical of a neurinoma. Angiography shows forward displacement of the posterior segment of the cavernous portion of the ICA as well as neovascularity and blush in the tumor fed by vessels from the meningohypophyseal trunk (Fig. 5-47). It may be impossible to differentiate this tumor from a meningioma in the same region.

Metastasis

Metastasis to the pituitary gland is rare, with the posterior lobe being more frequently involved. Breast and lung carcinomas are the most frequent tumor to metastasize to the pituitary gland. The lesion appears similar to a macroadenoma on CT scanning and MRI. Metastasis to the sphenoid bone is more common, sometimes simulating an invasive adenoma; it is most commonly from breast or prostate carcinoma (Fig. 5-48A). Pain and cranial nerve abnormalities may result from metastatic tumor to the base of the skull. Blastic metastasis must be differentiated from fibrous dysplasia, which tends to thicken the bone (Fig. 5-48B).

Sphenoid sinus carcinoma and nasopharyngeal carcinoma may spread into the sella and sphenoid bone. Lytic bone destruction occurs, which may be difficult to differentiate from a large invasive adenoma. A retropharyngeal or sinus mass suggests the correct diagnosis (Fig. 5-49).

Chordoma/Chondrosarcoma

Chordoma is a rare tumor that arises from notochord remnants in the middle clivus, just below the sella turcica. The tumor is slow-growing, but there is always extensive bone destruction and often invasion upward into the sella and cavernous sinuses. Calcification within the tumor is common. On MRI the tumor shows prolonged T_1 and T_2 relaxation times. Calcium is less reliably demonstrated. MRI is excellent for defining associated carotid artery constriction or invasion into the posterior fossa. The tumor cannot be differen-

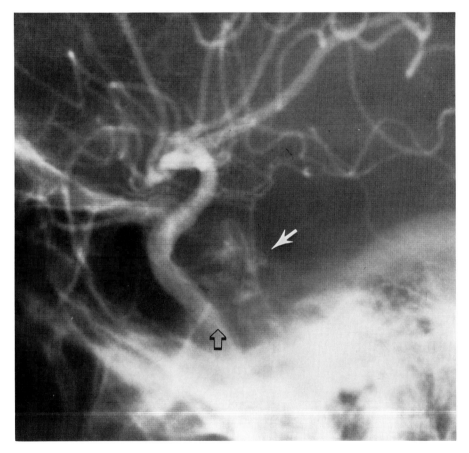

Fig. 5-47 Trigeminal neurinoma within Meckel's cave. Lateral ICA angiography demonstrates the characteristic anterior displacement of the proximal cavernous segment of the ICA (open arrow). Meningohypophyseal vessels supply the tumor (arrow).

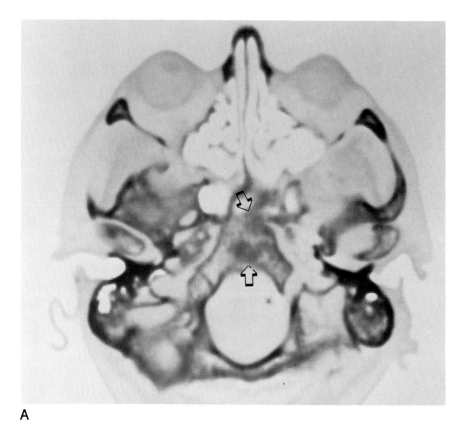

A

Fig. 5-48 Metastatic carcinoma; fibrous dysplasia. (A) Metastatic prostate carcinoma to the clivus. CT scan with bone windowing and reversed gray scale demonstrates the blastic reaction to the metastatic deposits (arrows). This technique is the most sensitive one for demonstrating metastatic disease to the base of the skull. Prostatic carcinoma frequently involves the base of the skull but only rarely involves the calvarium. *(Figure continues.)*

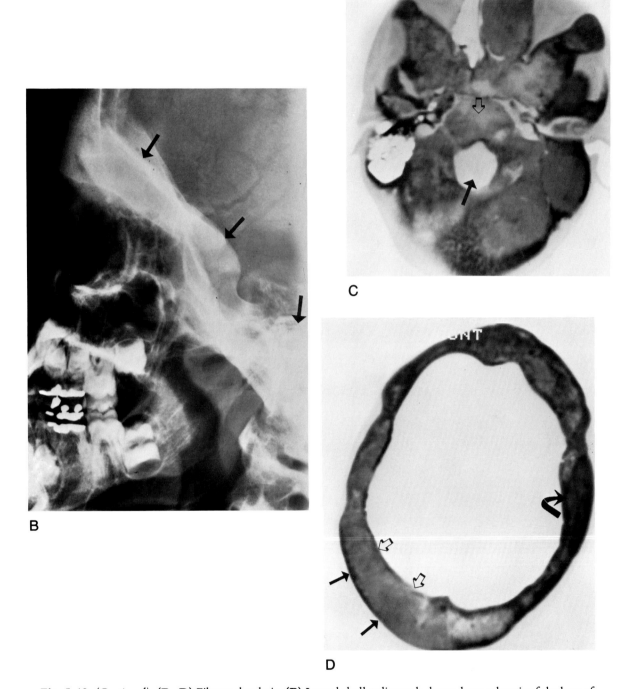

Fig. 5-48 *(Continued).* **(B–D)** Fibrous dysplasia. **(B)** Lateral skull radiograph shows dense sclerosis of the base of the skull (arrows). Such sclerotic density may also be found with meningioma and prostatic metastasis. **(C)** Transaxial CT scan through the skull base shows the diffuse involvement. The bone is thickened, causing constriction of the foramen magnum (arrow). Typical "ground glass" increased medullary density is present with fibrous dysplasia (open arrow). **(D)** CT scan through the calvarium shows the typical features of fibrous dysplasia. The calvarium is thickened. The external table is expanded outward (arrows), but there is little change of the internal table (open arrows). The tables are not thickened. Between the tables the dysplasia produces fine bone spicules, which create the homogeneous increased density. Some regions may show greater density (curved arrow).

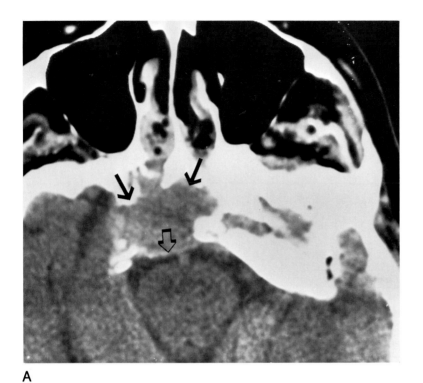

A

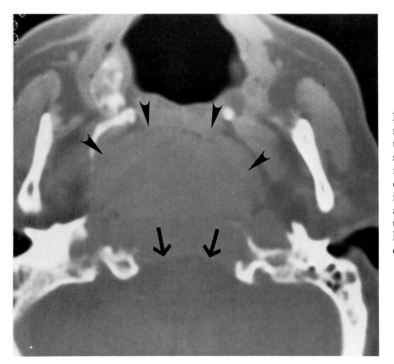

B

Fig. 5-49 Nasopharyngeal carcinoma. (A) Transaxial CT scan through the upper clivus and sphenoid sinus shows a large soft tissue tumor mass (black arrows). The mass has eroded posteriorly through the clivus into the prepontine cistern (open arrow). **(B)** Scan at a lower level shows the large nasopharyngeal mass (arrowheads). It has completely eroded the clivus posteriorly (arrows).

tiated from the even more rare chondrosarcoma, although chondrosarcoma tends to arise more laterally (See also Chapter 13).

Granuloma and Cysticercosis

Sarcoid, tuberculosis, and giant cell granuloma may occur within the sella and extend into the suprasellar cistern, but these lesions are rare. The lesions show uniform contrast enhancement on CT and may be indistinguishable from an adenoma. Cysticercosis appears as any cystic lesion of the sella and is suspected only in the appropriate clinical context.

Posterior Fossa Tumors in Adults

CEREBELLAR (INTRA-AXIAL) TUMORS

Metastasis

Metastasis is by far the most common neoplastic lesion seen in the posterior fossa in adults. It occurs primarily within the cerebellar hemispheres (Fig. 5-50) but is also seen within the pons (Fig. 5-21C) and subarachnoid space. Hydrocephalus may result from compression of the fourth ventricle. The characteristics of a metastasis are the same as described in the section on metastasis above.

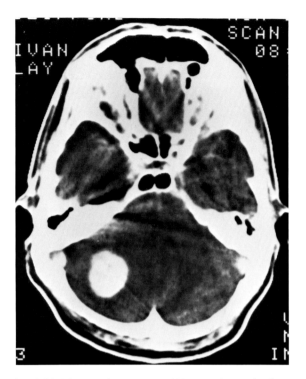

Fig. 5-50 Metastasis, contrast CT scan. A round enhancing lesion in the cerebellum in an adult is almost always a metastasis.

INTRA-AXIAL POSTERIOR FOSSA
LESIONS IN ADULTS

Common tumors
    Metastasis
    Hemangioblastoma
Uncommon tumors
    Glioma
    Neuronal tumors
    Choroid plexus papilloma
    Fourth ventricular meningioma
Other lesions
    Infarction
    Abscess
    Arteriovenous malformation
    Cysticercosis

Hemangioblastoma

Hemangioblastoma, a low grade tumor arising from blood vessels, almost always occurs in the cerebellar hemispheres. It is histologically similar to hemangiopericytoma (angioblastic meningioma). Accounting for only about 7 percent of posterior fossa tumors in adults, hemangioblastoma is the most common primary cerebellar tumor. The peak incidence is at age 30 years. There is a 2:1 male predominance. The tumor may be found in the spinal cord but almost never in the cerebral hemispheres. About 10 percent of hemangioblastomas are seen as part of the Von Hippel-Lindau (VHL) syndrome (see Ch. 12). Erythrocythemia is commonly produced by the tumor and may serve as a marker for recurrence.

On CT scans the tumor most commonly appears as a hypodense cyst, with one or more solid, intensely enhancing mural nodules or regions of cyst wall thickening. Prominent feeding arteries may be seen. Sometimes the tumors are more solid with multiple cysts

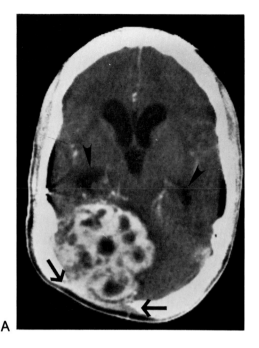

A

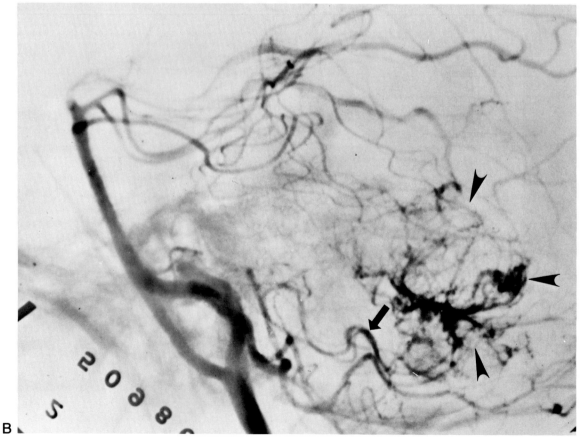

B

Fig. 5-51 Hemangioblastoma. (A) Contrast-enhanced CT scan shows an intensely enhancing large mass in the right cerebellar hemisphere. Multiple cysts are within the tumor. The mass has caused hydrocephalus with dilatation of the lateral ventricles and temporal horns (arrowheads). An occipital craniectomy defect is present from prior surgery (arrows). **(B)** Lateral vertebral angiography demonstrates the very hypervascular mass with large irregular vessels (arrowheads). The PICA is displaced downward and forward (arrow). *(Figure continues.)*

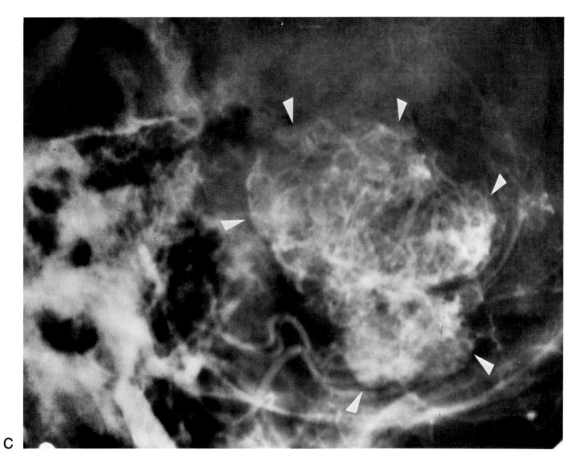

C

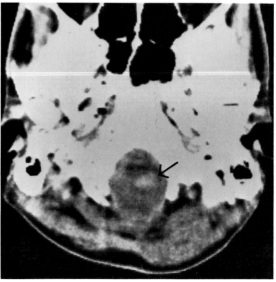

D

Fig. 5-51 *(Continued)*. **(C)** There is an intense delayed stain (arrowheads). Often there are prominent early draining veins. **(D)** Small tumor is present at the foramen magnum, representing a meningeal metastasis (arrow).

(Fig. 5-51) or ring-like in appearance with low density central necrosis. Small tumors show homogeneous contrast enhancement. In these instances the tumor is difficult to differentiate from metastasis or glioma by CT scanning. Because the tumor is highly vascular, a dynamic contrast examination through the lesion shows rapid uptake of contrast followed by a rapid decrease, while remaining hyperdense. Multiple lesions may occur, particularly with the VHL syndrome or as recurrent tumor after surgical excision.

The MRI procedure has a slightly greater sensitivity than CT scanning for the detection of these tumors. The cyst is isointense with CSF on both T_1- and T_2-weighted images. On the T_2-weighted images, the mural nodule is slightly hyperintense to brain but hypointense to the cyst fluid. Prominent vascular channels with flow-void are characteristic in the solid portions.

Angiography demonstrates the vascular component of the tumor as a homogeneously dense nodule surrounded by mass effect representing the cyst. Occasionally, there is a tangle of vessels with rapid shunting to early draining veins, simulating a vascular malformation or vascular metastasis, e.g., renal carcinoma

(Fig. 5-51). Angiography may detect lesions that cannot be seen with CT scans (Fig. 5-52). At this time it is not clear whether angiography or MRI is more sensitive for the detection of multiple tumors.

Other Intra-axial Tumors

All other posterior fossa intra-axial tumors are rare. Glioma occurs most commonly within the pons and almost never in the hemispheres in adults. Tumors of the neuronal series (ganglioglioma) occur within the hemispheres and are often cystic and calcified, producing little or no mass effect.

TUMORS OUTSIDE THE CEREBELLUM (EXTRA-AXIAL TUMORS)

Most of the extra-axial tumors in the posterior fossa occur in the cerebellopontine angle (CPA) cistern. These tumors produce tinnitus, unilateral neurosensory hearing loss, and sometimes vertigo. Large tumors produce hydrocephalus, cerebellar dysfunction, or contralateral hemiparesis.

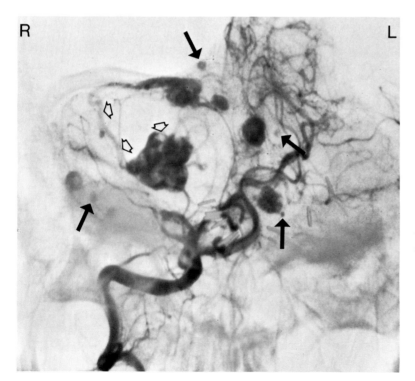

Fig. 5-52 Hemangioblastoma, recurrent, with metastasis. Right vertebral angiography in the Towne projection demonstrates a typical hemangioblastoma nodule with intense stain, early draining vein, and surrounding mass from cyst formation (open arrows). Small metastatic nodules (arrows) are best demonstrated with angiography because of the high spatial resolution of the technique.

EXTRA-AXIAL POSTERIOR FOSSA
LESIONS IN ADULTS

Common lesions
    Acoustic neurinoma (80%)
    Meningioma (10%)
    Epidermoid (4%)
Uncommon lesions
    Metastasis
    Invasive nasopharyngeal carcinoma
    Trigeminal neurinoma
    Chordoma/chondrosarcoma
    Glomus tumor (Fig. 5-60)
    Arachnoidal cyst
    Sarcoma of the petrous pyramid
    Aneurysm
    Basilar artery ectasia

Schwannoma (Neurinoma)

Neurinomas arise from the Schwann cells that envelop the cranial nerves. Sensory nerves are involved much more frequently than motor nerves. Most originate from the eighth (acoustic) nerve (CN VIII), particularly the vestibular branch. Acoustic neurinoma is the most common extra-axial tumor of the posterior fossa.

Less commonly, a neurinoma arises from the trigeminal nerve at the entrance to Meckel's cave. Tumors of the other cranial nerves are rare. The peak age range is 35 to 60 years, but rarely it is found in adolescents, especially those with neurofibromatosis (NF-2). The female/male ratio is 2:1. Multiple tumors of the cranial nerves, including bilateral acoustic neurinomas, are found with neurofibromatosis (NF-2).

At the time of discovery an acoustic neurinoma may be small and entirely within the internal auditory canal (intracanalicular), or it may be large, indenting the pons and cerebellar hemisphere. Rarely, it produces hydro-

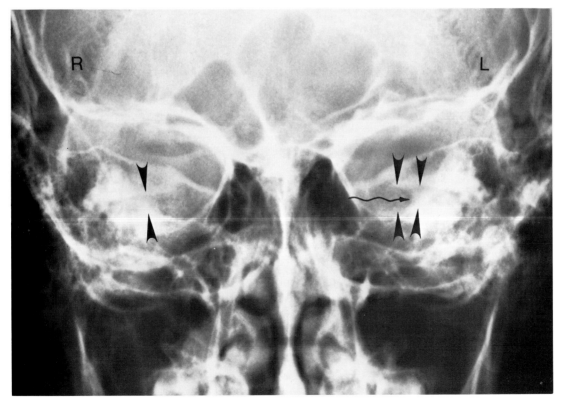

Fig. 5-53 Acoustic neurinoma. AP skull radiograph shows enlargement of the porus acusticus on the left compared with that on the right (arrowheads). There is erosion of the posterior wall of the internal auditory canal (IAC) (arrow).

cephalus owing to compression of the fourth ventricle. The tumor may have considerable cystic change but no calcification. Enlargement of the internal auditory canal is almost always present with larger tumors and is a hallmark of the diagnosis (Fig. 5-53).

The most sensitive imaging technique for the detection of an acoustic neurinoma is MRI. Thin-section transaxial slices are preferred. Most tumors can be seen on the nonenhanced T_1-weighted images but are better defined after Gd-DTPA enhancement (Fig. 5-54). The tumor obliterates the normal outline of the acoustic nerve within the internal auditory canal. The mass is hyperintense to the CSF and slightly hypointense to the adjacent pons. Lightly weighted T_2 (proton density) images may show the tumor as slightly hyperintense to CSF, especially if there is cystic change. On the late echo T_2-weighted images, the tumor is slightly hypointense to CSF. In large tumors there is consider-

A

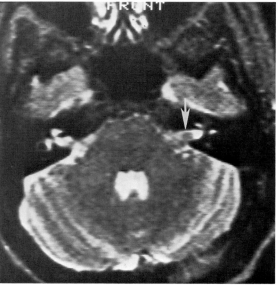

B

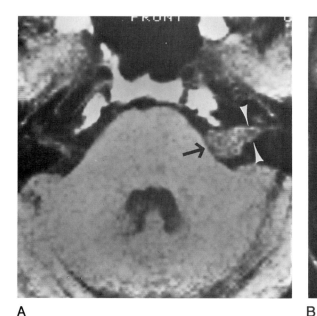

C

Fig. 5-54 Acoustic neurinoma. (A) T_1-weighted MRI shows a small acoustic neurinoma on the left (arrow) that extends into the IAC (arrowheads). **(B)** Heavily T_2-weighted MRI shows the tumor to be hypointense relative to the CSF (arrow). **(C)** Gd-DTPA-enhanced T_1-weighted MRI shows intense enhancement of a small right-sided acoustic neurinoma with intracanalicular extension. This method is the best imaging technique for demonstration of small acoustic neurinomas.

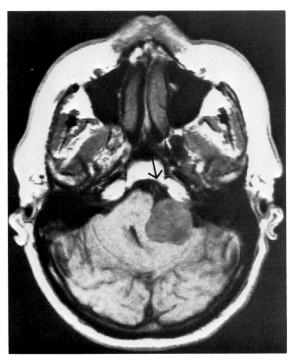
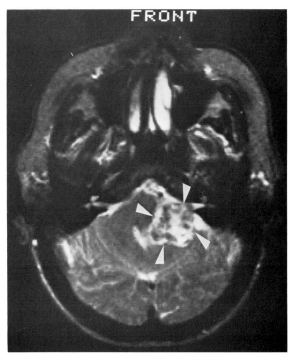

A   B

Fig. 5-55 Large acoustic neurinoma. (A) T_1-weighted MRI shows the slightly hypointense mass in the left CPA cistern. There is sharp demarcation from the distorted pons. The ipsilateral peripontine cistern is widened, confirming the extra-axial position of the tumor (arrow). **(B)** Heavily T_2-weighted MRI shows considerable inhomogeneity within the tumor (arrowheads).

able signal inhomogeneity, sometimes with demonstrable cysts (Fig. 5-55). There is almost never any edema produced in the adjacent pons.

On the nonenhanced CT scan, these tumors are almost always isodense and, unless large, difficult to identify. Almost all neurinomas require contrast enhancement for visualization (Fig. 5-56). The tumors show characteristically intense, usually homogeneous enhancement. Inhomogeneity occurs with central cystic change. Only tumors that are larger than 1 cm are routinely detectable on 5-mm transaxial scans of the posterior fossa. Bone window images show enlargement of the internal auditory canal with all but the smallest tumors.

Small intracanalicular tumors present a special problem for diagnosis with CT scanning. A contrast CT cisternogram must be performed if these tumors are to be seen; the safest and easiest is the air cisternogram. It is performed by introducing about 5 cc of air into the lumbar subarachnoid space with the patient horizontal and the side of interest up. The air is manipulated blindly into the CPA cistern and internal auditory canal by slightly elevating the upper torso. A small tumor is seen as a filling defect in the internal auditory canal, sometimes bulging slightly into the adjacent cistern (Fig. 5-57). Occasionally, adhesions prevent the air from entering the canal, resulting a false-positive diagnosis of tumor. Gd-DTPA-enhanced MRI is the more accurate technique for the diagnosis of these small tumors.

Angiography is no longer necessary for the diagnosis of acoustic neurinoma, although sometimes it is requested by the neurosurgeon to identify the position of the regional arteries. Usually, the anterior inferior cerebellar artery (AICA) is displaced upward and anteriorly over the tumor, and the petrosal vein is often compressed or occluded. Large tumors displace the basilar artery (Fig. 5-58).

Thin-section tomography is no longer used for the diagnosis of acoustic neurinoma. This technique relies

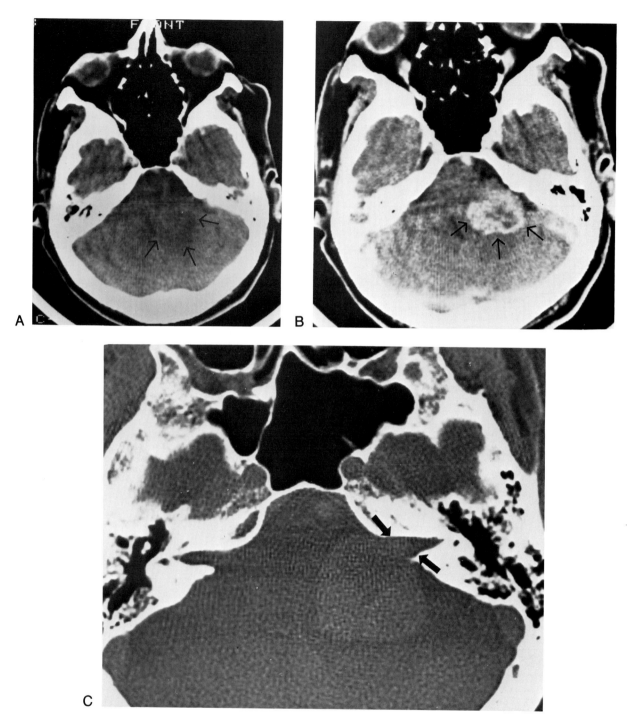

Fig. 5-56 Large acoustic neurinoma. (A) The tumor is nearly isodense with the brain and is difficult to identify on the nonenhanced CT scan (arrows). **(B)** Contrast-enhanced CT scan shows intense enhancement of the tumor, with the central nonenhanced regions most likely representing cysts (arrows). **(C)** High resolution bone window study shows characteristic enlargement of the left IAC (arrows).

Fig. 5-57 Intracanalicular acoustic neurinoma. CT air cisternogram shows the small tumor mass within the IAC (arrowheads). A normal IAC would completely fill with air.

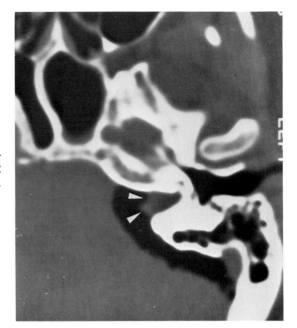

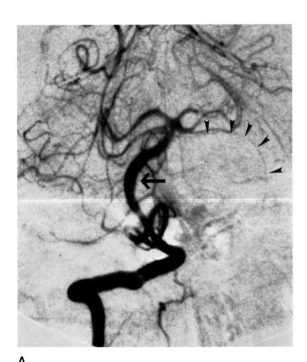

A

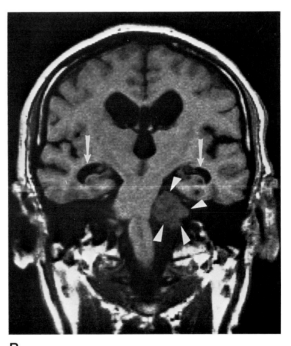

B

Fig. 5-58 Acoustic neurinoma. (A) AP vertebral angiography shows a large left-sided acoustic neurinoma. There is elevation of the AICA (arrowheads), and the basilar artery is displaced to the right (arrow). **(B)** Coronal T_1-weighted MRI showing the left-sided tumor (arrowheads) with displacement of the pons. Note the hydrocephalus and dilatation of the temporal horns (arrows).

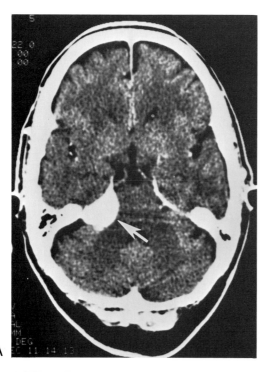

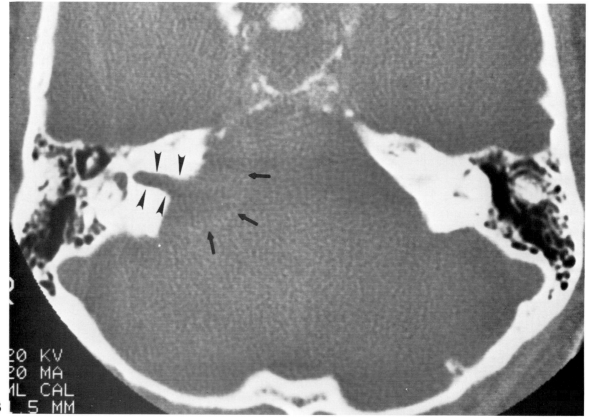

Fig. 5-59 Meningioma within CPA cistern. (A) Contrast-enhanced CT scan shows homogeneous enhancement of the tumor in the right CPA cistern (arrow). It lies slightly higher than the usual acoustic neurinoma. **(B)** High resolution bone window CT scan shows a normal IAC (arrowheads). The outline of the tumor can barely be seen (arrows). *(Figure continues.)*

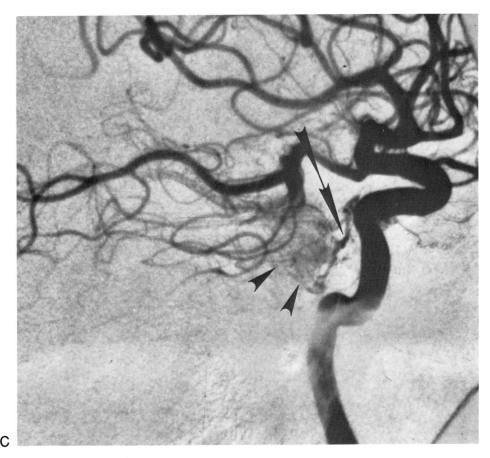

C

Fig. 5-59 *(Continued).* **(C)** ICA angiography shows the characteristic blush of the meningioma (arrowheads) supplied by meningohypophyseal vessels (arrow). An acoustic neurinoma shows minimal if any neovascularity on angiography.

on enlargement of the internal auditory canal to indicate the presence of tumor. A more than 2-mm difference in the diameter of the porus acousticus (medial entrance to the canal) is strongly suggestive of the diagnosis in the appropriate clinical setting. The posterior wall of the canal may be shortened (Fig. 5-53). The test is much less sensitive than MRI or CT scanning.

A neurinoma of the trigeminal nerve is rare. It most often occurs at the level of the gasserian ganglion within Meckel's cave but it can be seen in the posterior fossa along the nerve adjacent to the pons. It has the same imaging characteristics as an acoustic neurinoma but is more superior and anterior in location. It may be difficult to differentiate from a meningioma (Fig. 5-47).

Meningioma

Meningioma is the second most common extra-axial tumor of the posterior fossa. It occurs within the CPA cistern, along the clivus, or at the level of the foramen magnum. The imaging characteristics are described in a section above.

Meningioma may appear similar to an acoustic neurinoma (Fig. 5-59). However, the internal auditory canal does not enlarge. There are almost never any bone changes with meningioma in the posterior fossa. Calcification may be present. Angiography usually shows enlargement of regional meningeal vessels and a "blush" that is much more intense than with the usual acoustic neurinoma. The common carotid injection

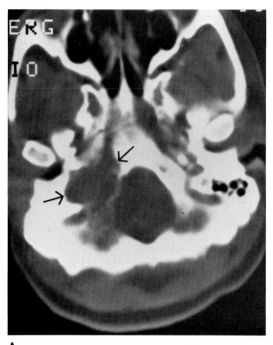

A

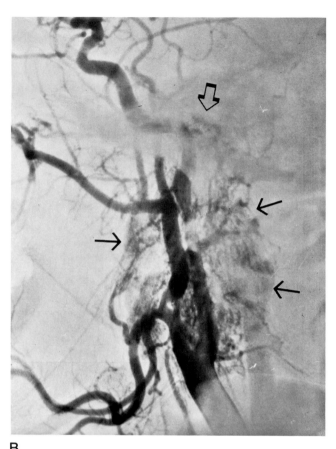

B

Fig. 5-60 Glomus vagale tumor. (A) CT scan through the base of the skull shows bone destruction on the right (arrows). **(B)** A large hypervascular glomus vagale tumor is present within the neck (arrows). It has extended superiorly to erode the base of the skull (open arrow). Glomus tumors may be found within the tympanic cavity, at the jugular bulb, in the upper neck, or in the carotid body.

most commonly demonstrates the meningeal vascular supply to CPA tumors.

Epidermoid

Epidermoid tumors may be found in the posterior fossa, particularly within the CPA cistern. They are discussed in a previous section.

Metastasis

Metastasis occurs in the region of the CPA. It is usually a result of meningeal involvement with carcinoma of the breast, small cell carcinoma of the lung, and melanoma. Metastasis may rarely involve the petrous pyra-

mid. Tumors from the nasopharynx can invade the posterior fossa and enter the CPA after having eroded through the base of the skull.

Other uncommon extra-axial tumors (Fig. 5-60) that can extend into the posterior fossa are listed above. Their characteristics are the same as discussed in their respective sections elsewhere in the text.

SUGGESTED READING

Chakeres DW, Curtin A, Ford G: Magnetic resonance imaging of pituitary and parasellar abnormalities. Radiol Clin North Am 27:265, 1989

Curnes JT: MR imaging of peripheral intracranial neoplasms: extraaxial vs intraaxial masses. J Comput Assist Tomogr 11:932, 1987

Davis JM, Zimmerman RA, Blaniuk LT: Metastasis to the central nervous system. Radiol Clin North Am 20:417, 1982

Destian S, Sze G, Krol G, et al: MR of hemorrhagic intracranial neoplasms. AJNR 9:1115, 1988

Dorne HL, O'Gorman AM, Melanson D: Computed tomography of intracranial gangliogliomas. AJNR 7:281, 1986

Dropcho EJ: The remote effects of cancer on the nervous system. Neurol Clin 7:579, 604, 1989

Ganti SR, Hilal SK, Stein BM, et al: CT of pineal region tumors. AJNR 7:97, 1986

Hasso AN, Fahmy JL, Hinshaw DB: Tumors of the posterior fossa. In Stark DD, Bradley WG (eds): Magnetic Resonance Imaging. CV Mosby, St. Louis, 1988

Haughton VM, Daniels DL: The posterior fossa. In Williams AL, Haughton VM (eds): Cranial Computed Tomography. CV Mosby, St. Louis, 1985

Jack CR, Bhansali DT, Chason JL, et al: Angiographic features of gliosarcoma. AJNR 8:117, 1987

Kazner E, Wende S, Grumme T, et al: Computed Tomography of Intracranial Tumors. Springer-Verlag, Berlin, 1982

Kernohan JW, Sayre GP. Tumors of the central nervous system. Fascicle 35, Atlas of tumor pathology. Armed Forces Institute of Pathology, Washington, DC, 1952

Kortman KE, Bradley WG: Supratentorial neoplasms. In Stark DD, Bradley WG (eds): Magnetic Resonance Imaging. CV Mosby, St. Louis, 1988

Kulkanni MV, Lee KF, McArdle CB, et al: 1.5-T MR imaging of pituitary microadenomas: technical considerations and CT correlation. AJNR 9:5, 1988

Lee SR, Sanches J, Mark AS, et al: Posterior fossa hemangioblastomas: MR imaging. Radiology 171:463, 1989

Lee Y-Y, Bruner JM, VanTassel P, Libshitz HI: Primary central nervous system lymphoma: CT and pathologic correlation. AJNR 7:599, 1986

Lee Y-Y, VanTassel P: Intracranial oligodendrogliomas: imaging findings in 35 untreated cases. AJNR 10:119, 1989

Manelfe C, Lasjaunias P, Ruscalleda J: Preoperative embolization of intracranial meningiomas. AJNR 7:963, 1986

Naheedy MH, Haag JR, Azar-Kia B, et al: MRI and CT of sellar and parasellar disorders. Radiol Clin North Am 25:819, 1987

Oct RF, Melville GE, New PFJ, et al: The role of MR and CT in evaluating clival chondromas and chondrosarcomas. AJNR 9:715, 1988

Press GA, Hesselink JR: MR imaging of cerebellopontine angle and internal auditory canal lesions at 1.5T. AJNR 9:241, 1988

Rubinstein LJ. Tumors of the central nervous system. Second series, fascicle 6, Atlas of tumor pathology. Armed Forces Institute of Pathology, Washington, DC, 1972

Russell EJ, Geremia GK, Johnson CE, et al: Multiple cerebral metastasis: detectability with Gd-DTPA enhanced MR imaging. Radiology 165:609, 1987

Schwaighofer BW, Hesselink JR, Press GA, et al: Primary intracranial CNS lymphomas: MR manifestations. AJNR 10:725, 1989

Tampieri D, Melanson D, Ethier R: MR of epidermoid cysts. AJNR 10:351, 1989

Teng MMH, Huang C, Chang T: Pituitary mass after transsphenoidal hypophysectomy. AJNR 9:23, 1988

VanTassel P, Lee Y-Y, Bruner JM: Symchronous and metachronous malignant gliomas. AJNR 9:725, 1988

Whelan MA, Reede DL, Meisler W, et al: CT of the base of the skull. Radiol Clin North Am 22:177, 1984

Williams AL: Tumors. In Williams AL, Haughton VM: Cranial Computed Tomography. CV Mosby, St. Louis, 1985

Yuh WTC, Wright DC, Barloon TJ, et al: MR imaging of primary tumors of trigeminal nerve and Meckel's cave. AJNR 9:655, 1988

6

Cranial Tumors in Children and Adolescents

Of all neoplasia in children, brain tumors are second in frequency only to leukemia. Twenty percent of all brain tumors occur in persons less than 20 years old, with the peak age range in this group 5 to 10 years. About 50 percent of the tumors occur in the posterior fossa. There is a definite tendency for childhood tumors to occur toward the midline, which accounts for the associated high incidence of hydrocephalus. Headache, vomiting, and ataxia are the usual presenting symptoms. Skull radiography usually shows changes of increased intracranial pressure (Fig. 6-1).

In general, MRI is preferred for the detection of childhood tumors. The tumors exhibit prolonged T_1 and T_2 relaxation times. The anatomic location and spread of the tumor is well demonstrated. Transaxial and parasagittal planes are most useful in the posterior fossa, and the coronal plane often helps in the supratentorial region. Hydrocephalus is easily identified. However, most of the tumors have similar MRI characteristics so histologic diagnosis is often not possible. The pattern on CT scans, without and with contrast enhancement, often gives more information about the specific tissue type. Plain films are of little specific use, except for calvarial lesions.

Angiography is seldom required for diagnosis or presurgical evaluation. Virtually all tumors except the rare choroid plexus papilloma or meningioma are avascular and are seen only indirectly as mass effect. The angiographic principles are given in Figure 6-2.

INFRATENTORIAL TUMORS

Cerebellar Astrocytoma

Cerebellar astrocytoma is one of the two most common posterior fossa tumors. It is usually the pilocytic type and has a generally benign clinical course. It grows slowly and is often large at the time of clinical recognition. Almost invariably, the presenting signs and symptoms are those of hydrocephalus, caused by compres-

---

INFRATENTORIAL TUMORS IN CHILDREN

Cerebellar astrocytoma (33%)

Medulloblastoma (33%)

Pontine astrocytoma (20%)

Ependymoma (10%)

Others (4%)
    Choroid plexus papilloma
    Dermoid, epidermoid
    Neuroectodermal tumor
    Meningioma
    Neurinoma

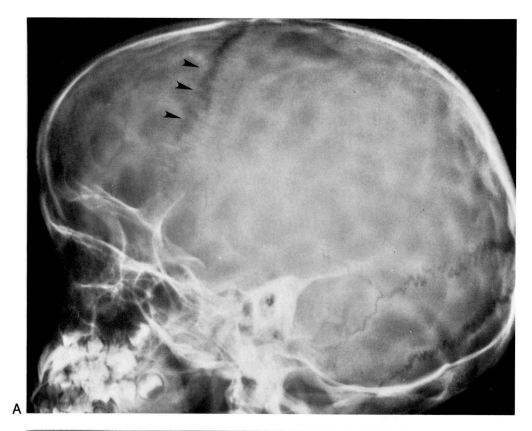

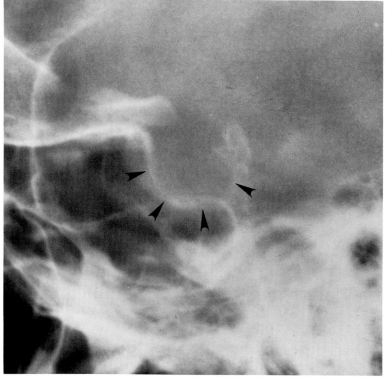

Fig. 6-1 Increased intracranial pressure. (A) Plain skull radiograph shows separation of the intracranial sutures (arrowheads) and increased convolutional markings. **(B)** Lateral view of the sella shows demineralization of the floor of the sella (arrowheads), which has occurred as a result of increased intracranial pressure.

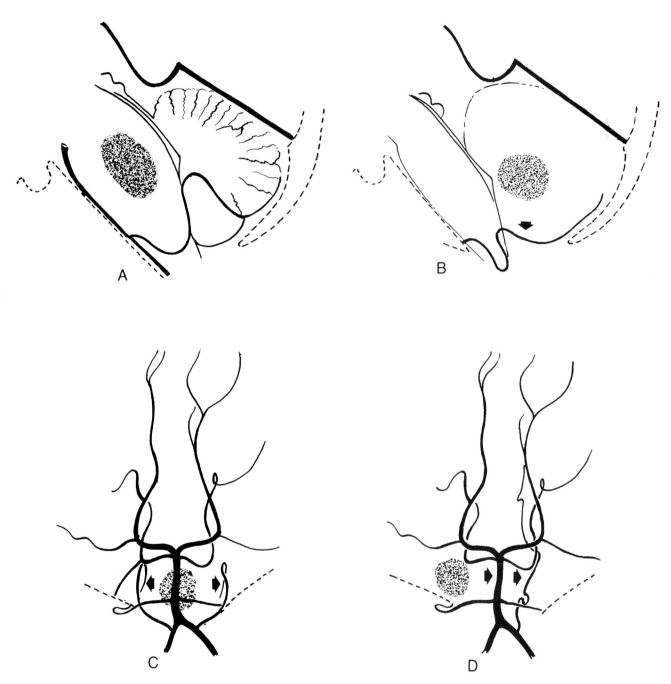

Fig. 6-2 Angiographic principles. The four typical posterior fossa tumors of childhood. **(A)** Intrapontine tumor (pontine glioma). The patient presents with progressive cranial nerve palsies. **(B)** Midline mass just at or behind the apex of the fourth ventricle (medulloblastoma). Note the caudal displacement of the PICA. The patient presents with hydrocephalus, increased intracranial pressure and usually has truncal ataxia. **(C)** Intraventricular tumor in the fourth ventricle. Note the separation of the choroidal loops (ependymoma or choroid plexus papilloma). The patient presents with hydrocephalus. **(D)** Hemispheric tumor. A lateral hemispheric tumor is usually an astrocytoma. Note the displacement of the choroidal loop and inferior vermian artery off the midline. The patient has incoordination on the side of the tumor. Hydrocephalus is common. (From Yock, 1984, with permission.)

Table 6–1 CT Differential Diagnosis of Common Posterior Fossa Tumors in Children

Parameter	Medulloblastoma	Astrocytoma	Ependymoma
CT Density	Hyperdense	Hypodense	Isodense
Enhancement	Homogeneous (except for necrosis)	Homogeneous (in solid portion)	Heterogeneous
Cysts	Microcysts	Common, large	No
Necrosis	Common	Uncommon	Sometimes
Calcification	Rare	Sometimes	Common

See also Table 5–1, page 137.

sion of the fourth ventricle. The peak age of occurrence is 5 to 10 years; there is no sex preference. Most tumors straddle the boundry between the vermis and the adjacent cerebellum, although some are entirely within the vermis, cerebellar hemisphere, or fourth ventricle. Fifty percent have a large central cyst with a peripheral thin rim of tumor tissue, often with a focal mural nodule. The remaining 50 percent are solid or partially cystic. Anaplasia sometimes occurs, particularly within the more solid or centrally located tumors. When anaplastic tumors occur in the midline, they are difficult to differentiate from medulloblastoma and ependymoma using either MRI or CT scanning (Table 6-1).

On MRI the tumor is hypointense on T_1- and hyperintense on T_2-weighted images. Solid tumors are relatively homogeneous. Cysts are recognized as round regions of CSF intensity within the tumor mass. Peripheral edema is uncommon. Enhancement with Gd-DTPA often occurs in the solid portions but adds little diagnostic information.

On CT scans the solid tumors are slightly hypodense (Fig. 6-3). Only rarely are they hyperdense or of mixed density. Calcification is seen in 10 percent, usually as a conglomeration. When calcification is seen in a childhood posterior fossa tumor that is eccentrically positioned, the diagnosis of astrocytoma is virtually certain.

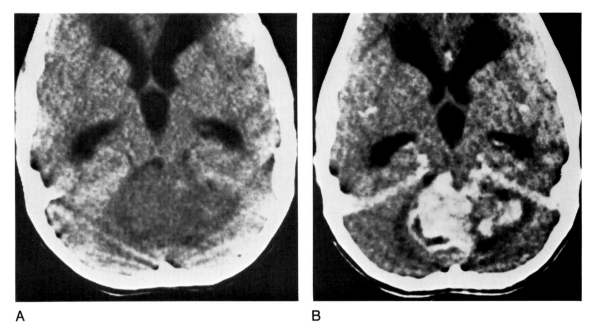

A   B

Fig. 6-3 Pilocytic astrocytoma. (A) Nonenhanced CT scan shows a large hypodense mass involving the medial left cerebellar hemisphere and vermis. There is secondary hydrocephalus. **(B)** Contrast-enhanced study shows enhancement throughout the solid portions of the tumor. There is minimal surrounding edema.

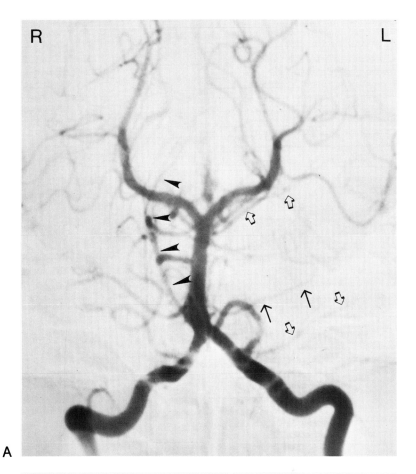

A

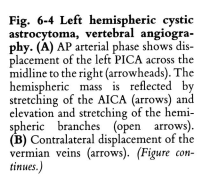

Fig. 6-4 Left hemispheric cystic astrocytoma, vertebral angiography. (A) AP arterial phase shows displacement of the left PICA across the midline to the right (arrowheads). The hemispheric mass is reflected by stretching of the AICA (arrows) and elevation and stretching of the hemispheric branches (open arrows). (B) Contralateral displacement of the vermian veins (arrows). (Figure continues.)

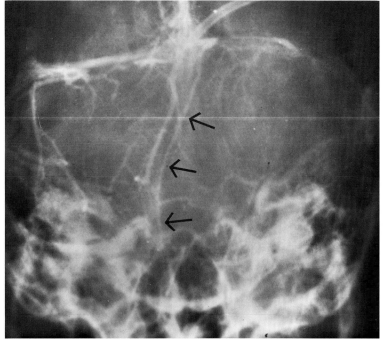

B

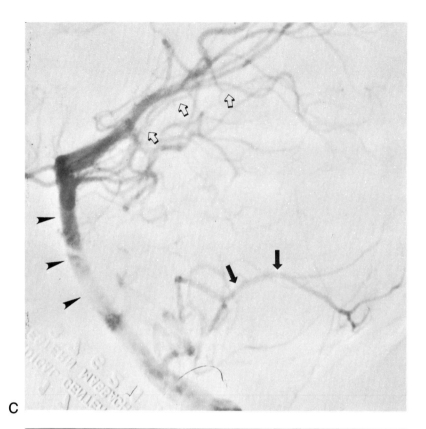

C

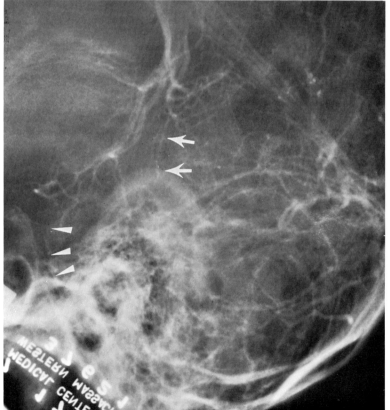

D

Fig. 6-4 *(Continued)*. **(C)** Lateral arterial phase shows anterior displacement of the basilar artery, widening and stretching of the PICA from lateral displacement (arrows), and upward bowing of the SCAs (open arrows). **(D)** Lateral venous phase shows anterior displacement of the precentral cerebellar vein (arrows) and the anterior pontomesencephalic vein (arrowheads). The angiogram demonstrates a posterior compartment hemispheric mass.

Contrast enhancement may be intense and is usually homogeneous within the solid portions, or mural nodule. Enhancement does not correlate with the histologic grade of the tumor. Angiography shows the tumor as an avascular mass (Fig. 6-4).

Medulloblastoma

The medulloblastoma is a highly malignant, devastating tumor of the midline of the posterior fossa. It is classified as grade IV. Its peak incidence is between 5 and 10 years of age, but it may occur in newborns and adolescents. In adolescents the tumor tends to be more peripheral in the cerebellar hemispheres. The male/female ratio is 2:1.

The tumor arises from the velum of the fourth ventricle and spreads in all directions. It frequently occupies the fourth ventricle, spreads through the foramina into the pericerebellar cisterns, and into the aqueduct. Hydrocephalus is common. The tumor can metastasize, most commonly by seeding, to the entire subarachnoid space, including the ventricular system and spinal region. Shunting of hydrocephalus into the abdomen may spread tumor to the peritoneum. Occa-

sionally, hematogenous metastases occur in the lungs or bones.

On MRI, medulloblastoma appears as a well defined midline vermian and fourth ventricular mass of low intensity on T_1- and high intensity on T_2-weighted images. Hemorrhage, necrosis, and microcysts are common. Surrounding edema is often seen. Enhancement occurs after Gd-DTPA and may help define meningeal metastasis about the brain and spinal cord.

On CT scans, most medulloblastomas appear as well delineated, slightly hyperdense tumors in the midline of the posterior fossa, occupying the region of the vermis and fourth ventricle (Fig. 6-5). Mixed density is a result of cysts, necrosis, and hemorrhage within the tumor. Isodense and hypodense medulloblastomas are unusual. Calcification is rare and, if present, is of the diffuse, fine variety. Frequently, there is surrounding edema.

Contrast enhancement, a constant feature, may be slight to intense. Focal regions of necrosis and microcysts create defects in the otherwise uniform enhancement pattern. Metastatic tumor in the meninges also enhances. Angiography shows an avascular midline mass.

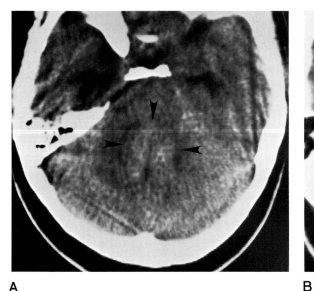
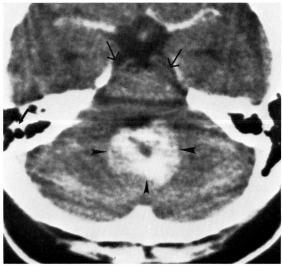

A   B

Fig. 6-5 Medulloblastoma. (A) Nonenhanced CT scan shows a slightly hyperdense midline mass within the vermis and posterior fourth ventricle (arrowheads). **(B)** There is blotchy enhancement of the solid tumor (arrowheads). Note the anterior displacement of the pons and obliteration of the prepontine cistern (arrows). Hydrocephalus is present. *(Figure continues.)*

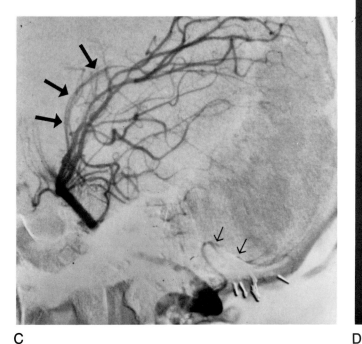

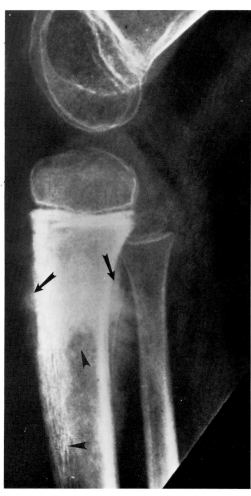

C   D

Fig. 6-5 *(Continued).* **(C)** Lateral vertebral angiogram shows downward and forward displacement of the PICA by the vermian mass (small arrows). There is upward herniation through the tentorium as shown by superior displacement of the SCAs (large arrows). **(D)** Metastatic medulloblastoma to bone. The metastatic deposit has caused permeative change (arrowheads) and periosteal new bone formation (arrows). Pure lytic lesions are more commonly seen.

Ependymoma

Ependymoma is much less common, accounting for about 10 percent of the posterior fossa tumors in children. These lesions are intimately attached to the floor of the fourth ventricle, making complete removal impossible. They are malignant and classified as grade III or IV. In the posterior fossa they have a peak incidence at 3 to 7 years of age but may be encountered at any age.

The tumor grows to fill the fourth ventricle, causing hydrocephalus. Growth through the foramina into the cisterns is a characteristic feature. The tumor may "entrap" CSF around the periphery, creating a "halo" effect. Metastasis to the meninges of the brain and spinal column occurs, particularly after surgical resection.

On MRI the tumor is seen as an irregular, inhomogeneous fourth ventricular mass, hypointense on T_1- and hyperintense on T_2-weighted images (Fig. 6-6). Cystic change is relatively uncommon. The widespread growth is well defined with MRI. Calcification may be

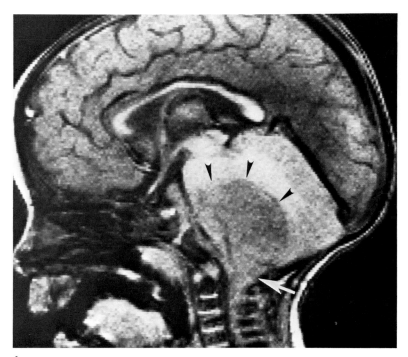

A

Fig. 6-6 Ependymoma. (A) T$_1$-weighted GRE image shows the hypointense large mass in the central portion of the posterior fossa occupying the fourth ventricle (arrowheads). Note the inferior extension into the foramen magnum and upper cervical canal (arrow). **(B)** T$_2$-weighted image showing the tumor as slightly hyperintense (arrowheads). *(Figure continues.)*

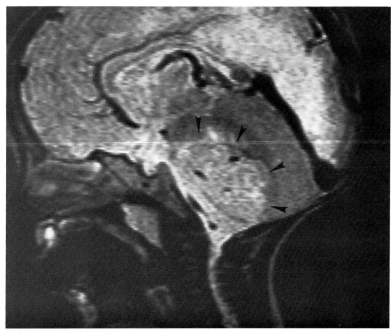

B

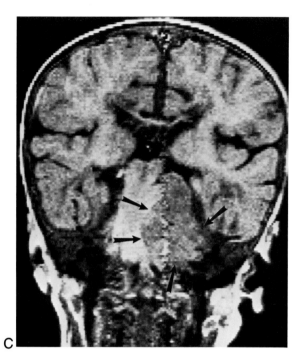

C

Fig. 6-6 *(Continued).* **(C)** Coronal T_1-weighted image shows the hypointense tumor with exophytic growth to the left into the peripontine and basal cisterns (arrows).

seen as signal void, especially on gradient echo imaging. Gd-DTPA enhancement occurs.

On the precontrast CT scan, ependymomas are usually isodense or slightly hyperdense. Calcification is especially common and may be fine or coarse. A densely calcified midline posterior fossa tumor is almost always an ependymoma. Accompanying hydrocephalus is the rule. The outline of the tumor is commonly irregular.

Contrast enhancement, almost always present, is usually inhomogeneous because of necrotic change (Fig. 6-7). Angiography shows an avascular intraventricular posterior fossa mass.

Brain Stem Glioma

Brain stem gliomas mostly occur in children and adolescents, with the peak incidence at 3 to 7 years. The histology of the astrocytoma is variable, although most of these tumors are of low grade malignancy. Almost all occur in the pons but may spread in any direction into the mesencephalon or medulla or show exophytic growth that may encase and elevate the basilar artery.

Cysts are common within the tumor. The usual presentation is gradually progressive cranial nerve dysfunction, often asymmetric. Hydrocephalus is uncommon, even with large tumors.

Although other lesions, such as lymphoma, granuloma, or angioma, can produce brain stem enlargement in children, they are rare. Therefore almost all solid or cystic masses in the pons are considered gliomas, and many are treated with irradiation without a definitive tissue diagnosis. Cysts are important to recognize, as decompression can be performed. Postirradiation calcification of the tumor is common.

The most effective imaging method for diagnosing pontine glioma is MRI. The tumor appears hypointense on T_1- and hyperintense on T_2-weighted images (Fig. 6-8). The pons is enlarged and distorted. Cysts are identified by round regions of CSF density. Hemorrhage may be seen within the tumor.

The precontrast CT scan may show some degree of pontine enlargement and obliteration of the peripontine cisterns, but the tumor is much more difficult to recognize with CT scanning than with MRI. The fourth ventricle is characteristically displaced posteriorly, so it becomes slit-like. About 50 percent of gliomas are hypodense, the remainder being isodense or of mixed density. About 50 percent show some degree of contrast enhancement in the solid portions of the tumor (Fig. 6-9). The enhancement may be uniform, patchy, or ring-like. Calcification does not occur, except after radiation therapy.

Acoustic Neurinoma

Acoustic neurinomas are benign tumors that are rarely seen in children. When they do occur, they are often bilateral and almost always in children with neurofibromatosis (NF-2). When discovered, the tumors are usually large with associated enlargement of the internal auditory canals. Hearing loss is the first symptom. (See Chapter 5.)

SUPRATENTORIAL TUMORS

Astrocytoma

The astrocytoma is the most common cerebral hemispheric tumor in children. The tumors are usually grade I and II, but almost all are locally invasive to some

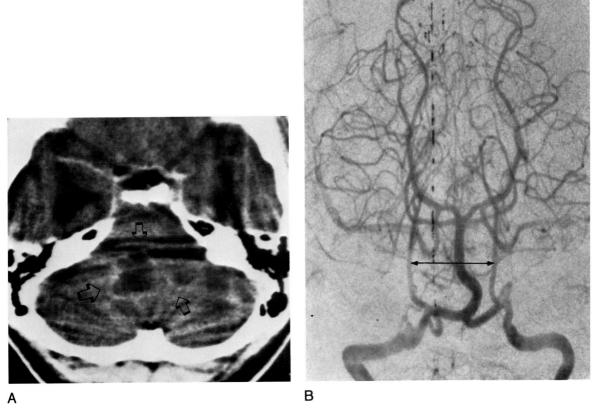

A   B

Fig. 6-7 Ependymoma (intraventricular tumor). (A) Contrast-enhanced CT study shows irregular ring-like enhancement surrounding regions of necrosis (arrows). The tumor lies within the fourth ventricle. **(B)** AP vertebral angiography showing wide separation of the PICAs by the intraventricular ependymoma (opposed arrows). *(Figure continues.)*

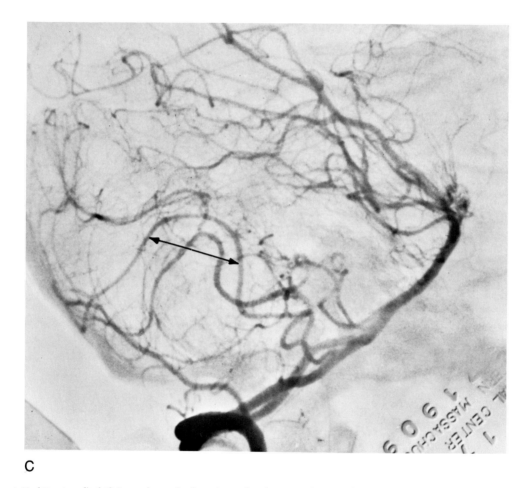

C

Fig. 6-7 *(Continued).* **(C)** Lateral vertebral angiography shows widening of the choroidal loop of the PICA by the intraventricular tumor (opposed arrows).

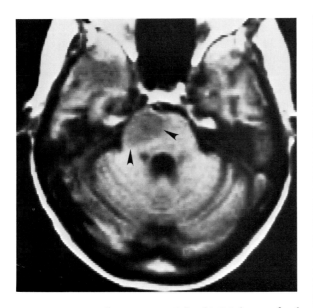

Fig. 6-8 Pontine glioma. T_1-weighted MRI shows a focal low intensity mass within the right anterolateral aspect of the pons (arrowheads). The contour of the pons is locally expanded. On T_2-weighted imaging the tumor would be hyperintense.

SUPRATENTORIAL TUMORS IN CHILDREN

Common tumors
    Astrocytoma (50%)
        Hemispheric
        Hypothalamic and optic chiasm
    Ependymoma
    Craniopharyngioma
    Pineal region tumors
    Choroid plexus papilloma
    Leukemia
Uncommon tumors
    Meningioma
    Hamartoma
    Histiocytosis X
    Cavernous hemangioma
    Neuroblastoma
    Primitive Neuroectodermal tumor
Other mass lesions
    Dermoid
    Epidermoid
    Arachnoid cyst

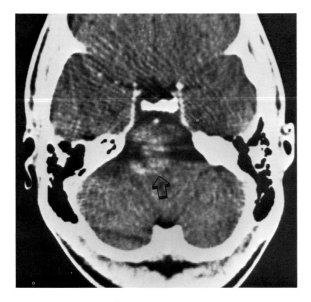

Fig. 6-9 Pontine glioma, CT scan. Contrast CT scan shows diffuse enhancement of a pontine astrocytoma (arrow).

extent. Most occur within the parietal or temporal lobes. Headache and seizures are the most common presenting symptoms.

The tumors may be solid or cystic and exhibit MRI and CT patterns similar to those seen with low grade astrocytomas in adults (see Ch. 5). When a small cystic tumor is first seen, it is impossible to differentiate it from the rare benign cyst of the brain (Fig. 6-10). All cystic lesions within the brain parenchyma must be considered a tumor until proved otherwise. Follow-up scans must be obtained.

Some tumors show varying amounts of calcification. Sometimes the only evidence of the tumor is a small "dot" of calcium on the CT scan. In this situation, follow-up scanning or MRI is necessary to finally diagnose the lesion as a tumor that may take many years to show any growth. Contrast enhancement indicates a higher grade of histologic malignancy.

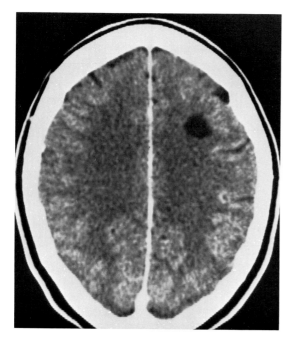

Fig. 6-10 Hemispheric cyst. Contrast CT scan shows a nonenhancing hypodense cyst-like lesion in the left posterior frontal subcortical white matter. It did not change over many years and presumably is a benign idiopathic cyst. A low grade astrocytoma might also have this appearance.

Hypothalamic and Optic Chiasm Astrocytoma

The hypothalamic and optic chiasm astrocytomas are almost always benign, grade I, pilocytic tumors. In the optic chiasm they most commonly occur with neurofibromatosis (NF-1). In the hypothalamus they produce the diencephalic syndrome, with signs of cachexia, particularly in infants. Diabetes insipidus and narcolepsy may occur.

On MRI the tumors show slight hypointensity on T_1- and slight hyperintensity on T2-weighted images (Fig. 6-11). On CT scans the tumors are either isodense or hyperdense and are occasionally calcified. Most of the tumors are solid, although sometimes those within the hypothalamus have a few cysts. There is strong homogeneous contrast enhancement of the solid portions of the tumor with MRI and CT scanning. The tumors cause partial obliteration of the suprasellar cistern. It is impossible to differentiate a hypothalamic astrocytoma from mixed glioma, histiocytosis X, "ec-

topic pinealoma" (midline germinoma), and hamartoma, which also occur in this region.

Ependymoma

Ependymomas arise from ependymal cells lining the walls of the ventricles or from ependymal "rests" that occur in the paraventricular white matter. Therefore the tumors may be found entirely within the ventricle or entirely within the white matter adjacent to the ventricle. Frequently, both ventricle and white matter are involved. The most common location is adjacent to the atrium of the lateral ventricle. The peak incidence is during adolescence and young adulthood. All carry a poor prognosis. An especially malignant form of the tumor, called *ependymoblastoma,* may grow rapidly and attain large size. It has a strong tendency to spread within the ventricular system and may form a tumor cast of the ventricular cavity.

The tumors appear similar to a posterior fossa ependymoma on both MRI (Fig. 6-12) and CT scanning. Calcification and cysts are common. About 50 percent are homogeneous and solid. Contrast enhancement is usually present.

Craniopharyngioma

Craniopharyngioma is a tumor with a peak incidence in children and adolescents and a second peak incidence in adults about 40 to 50 years old. There is a male predominance. The tumor usually arises in the suprasellar cistern within the pituitary stalk at the level of the tuber cinereum, although in 20 percent it is within the sella turcica (Fig. 6-13). It is the second most common tumor within the sella turcica. The most accepted theory states that the tumor develops from a remnant of Rathke's pouch, an invagination of epidermal tissue of the buccal mucosa. The suprasellar location of the tumor produces visual field deficits, diabetes insipidus, or hydrocephalus. The tumors have both solid and cystic components and may become large enough to occupy more than one-half of the brain. The epidermal tissue secretes keratin (protein) or cholesterol (fat) in varying amounts.

Enlargement of the sella occurs only with an intrasellar location of the tumor. With downward growth of the suprasellar mass, there may be truncation of the dorsum sellae without change in its normal forward-directed axis. Calcification is common in children (70

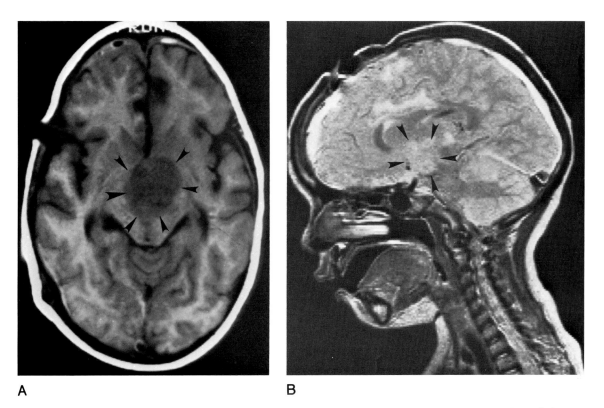

A   B

Fig. 6-11 Hypothalamic astrocytoma. (A) T_1-weighted MRI shows a hypointense mass in the hypothalamus extending upward to fill the third ventricle (arrowheads). **(B)** Parasagittal lightly T_2-weighted MRI shows a round, slightly hyperintense, midline mass in the region of the hypothalamus and third ventricle (arrowheads).

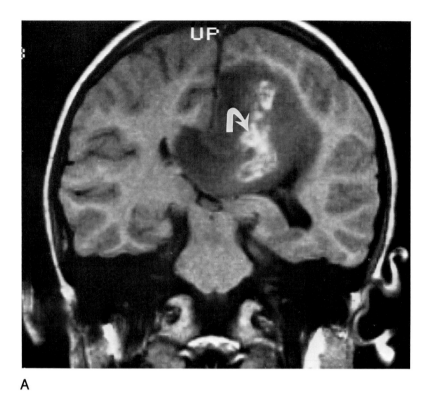

A

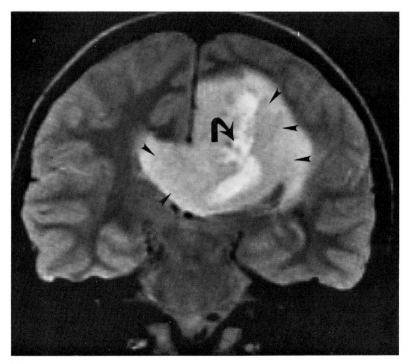

B

Fig. 6-12 Ependymoma. (A) T_1-weighted MRI shows a hypointense mass in the medial left posterior parietal lobe adjacent to and extending into the atrium of the left lateral ventricle. The tumor crosses the midline through the splenium of the corpus callosum. The high intensity region (arrow) represents hemorrhage. **(B)** Lightly T_2-weighted MRI shows the mildly hyperintense tumor mass (arrowheads) surrounded by a thin rim of edema with greater hyperintensity. The high intensity in the central portion of the tumor (curved arrow) represents hemorrhage.

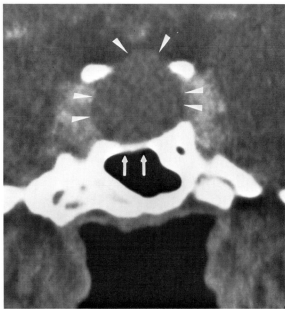

Fig. 6-13 Craniopharyngioma. (A) Coronal contrast-enhanced CT scan shows homogeneous nonenhancing mildly hypodense mass within the sella turcica, with just slight suprasellar extension (arrowheads). There is minimal erosion of the floor of the sella (arrows). In an adult, pituitary adenoma is the most common tumor with this appearance. **(B)** Intrasellar and suprasellar craniopharyngioma. The sella is grossly enlarged with undercutting of the anterior clinoid processes (arrowheads). The dorsum is truncated (arrow). Faint suprasellar calcification is seen within the tumor (open arrows).

A

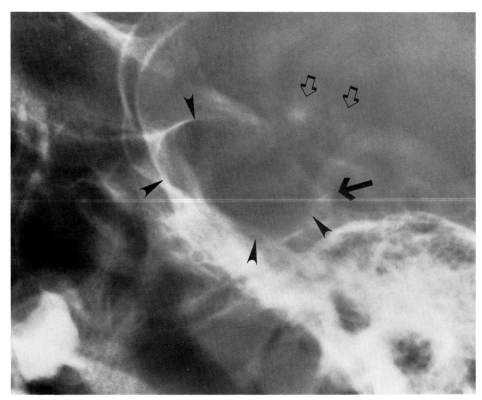

B

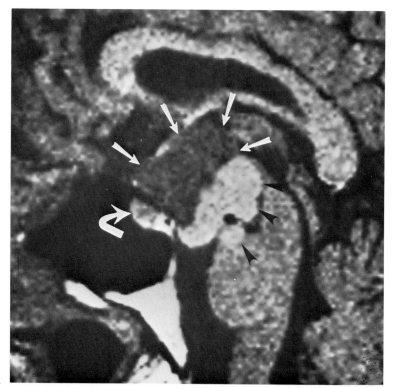

A

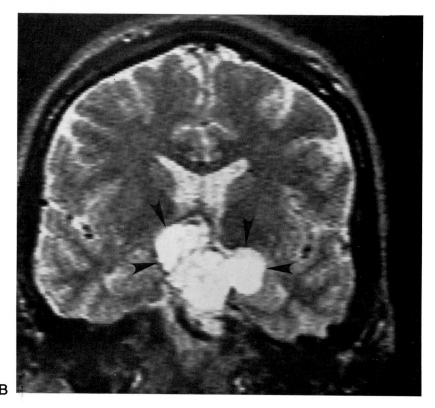

B

Fig. 6-14 Craniopharyngioma. (A) Parasagittal T_1-weighted MRI shows the large tumor within the suprasellar cistern and extending posteriorly into the interpeduncular and prepontine cisterns. The anterior portion is solid and is slightly hypointense (arrows), whereas the posterior portion is cystic and hyperintense (arrowheads). Note the normal pituitary gland and sella turcica (curved arrow). **(B)** Coronal T_2-weighted MRI shows the very high signal intensity of the cystic component of the tumor (arrowheads). The solid portion is moderately hyperintense. The tumor has extended superiorly to occupy the third ventricle and displace the basal ganglia.

percent) but less common in adults (30 percent). The calcification is variable in appearance and may be densely globular, diffusely speckled, or thin and rim-like.

The tumors are histologically benign; when large, however, they may become impossible to remove, and recurrence is common. Spillage of contents into the subarachnoid space may cause arachnoiditis.

Variable signal intensity is seen on MRI with this tumor (Fig. 6-14). The cystic components may have either high or low signal on T_1-weighted images depending on the amount of fat within the cyst contents. Focal calcifications may be difficult to detect. T_2-weighted images show variable intensity as well. Gd-DTPA enhancement may occur within solid portions of the tumor but is not necessary for diagnosis.

The CT appearance is also variable, as there are solid, cystic, and calcified portions (Fig. 6-15). The cystic regions usually are of a density approximately equal to that of the CSF, but they be hypodense owing to cho-

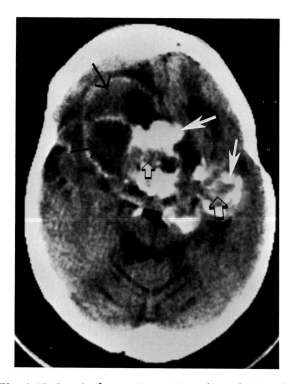

Fig. 6-15 Craniopharyngioma. Nonenhanced CT study shows a large tumor mass with cysts containing variable-density material (black arrows), solid tissue (open arrows), and dense calcification (white arrows). (Courtesy of Dr. Sam Mayerfield, UMDNJ.)

lesterol or hyperdense owing to increased protein content. About 66 percent show some contrast enhancement within the solid portions of the tumor.

Pineal Region Tumors

Most tumors in the region of the pineal gland occur in persons 10 to 20 years old. The presentation is usually that of hydrocephalus (headache, nausea, vomiting, confusion), often with Parinaud's syndrome (supranuclear impairment of upward gaze, defective convergence, and slow pupillary reaction to light). Tumors in this region are classified as being either of germ cell origin or neuroectodermal origin from the pineal parenchyma.

Germ cell tumors are the most common, accounting for more than 50 percent. They are similar to germ cell tumors occurring elsewhere in the body. Germinomas and teratomas are the most common type, although rarely an endodermal sinus tumor or choriocarcinoma appears.

Germinoma occurs almost exclusively in males, with a peak frequency at 15 years. If a germinoma occurs in a female, it almost always is located in the region of the anterior third ventricle. These tumors are slow-growing and well circumscribed. On CT scans the tumor is seen as a homogeneous, slightly hyperdense mass, usually without calcification and showing intense uniform contrast enhancement (Fig. 6-16). On MRI they tend to be isointense with the brain on both T_1- and T2-weighted images. Gd-DTPA enhancement occurs.

Teratoma is usually inhomogeneous with cystic, lipomatous, and calcific change, which can be seen with CT scanning and MRI. It shows irregular contrast enhancement. Endodermal sinus tumor has a nonspecific appearance but tends to be somewhat more aggressive with poorly defined margins.

Ectodermal pineal tumors are either pinealoma (pineocytoma) or pineoblastoma. Both of these tumors are either isodense or slightly hyperdense on CT scans, with intense contrast enhancement indistinguishable from that of germinoma. They occur with equal frequency in males and females. The pinealoma can be found at any age and is slow-growing. In contrast, the pineoblastoma behaves similar to a medulloblastoma, with rapid growth and the propensity for seeding in the subarachnoid space. Initially, the two tumors appear similar on all imaging studies and may be diagnosed only by the clinical findings, CSF cytology, or biopsy.

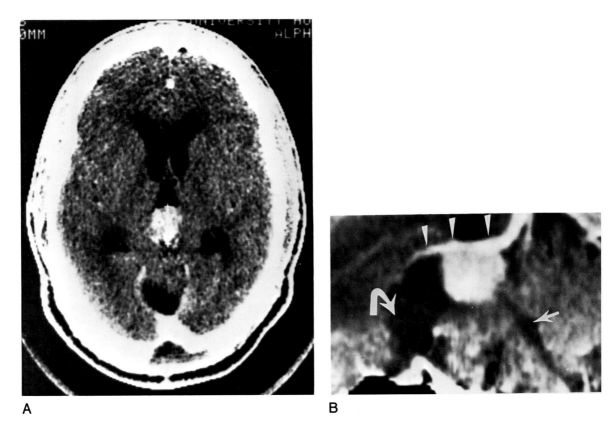

Fig. 6-16 Pineal dysgerminoma. (A) Transaxial contrast-enhanced CT scan shows an intensely enhancing mass in the posterior third ventricle in the region of the pineal gland. It is causing hydrocephalus. **(B)** Sagittal reconstruction shows the enhancing mass in the posterior third ventricle occluding the aqueduct. It lies underneath the internal cerebral veins and the vein of Galen (arrowheads). Note the dilated third ventricle extending into the sella turcica (curved arrow). The fourth ventricle is small (arrow). (Courtesy of Dr. Sam Mayerfield, UMDNJ.)

LESIONS IN THE PINEAL REGION

Germ cell tumor

    Germinoma

    Teratoma

    Endodermal sinus tumor

    Choriocarcinoma

Neuroectodermal tumor

    Pinealoma

    Pineoblastoma

Glioma

Metastasis

Arachnoid cyst

Vein of Galen aneurysm

Cavernous hemangioma

Lipoma

Other tumors or masses (Fig. 6-17; see also Fig. 6-21) that can occur in this region are listed in the box.

Choroid Plexus Papilloma

Choroid plexus papillomas are rare intraventricular tumors that arise from the ependymal layer of the choroid plexus. They occur most frequently in infants at the site of the glomus within the atrium of the lateral ventricle. Rarely, they are seen in the roof of the third or fourth ventricle. The tumors cause hydrocephalus from overproduction of CSF, which may be asymmetric. Hemorrhage sometimes occurs. Complete surgical removal is curative.

On precontrast CT scans the tumor is homogeneously isodense or hyperdense, with sharp undulating margins lying within a dilated ventricle. Calcification is common. There is intense homogeneous contrast enhancement. Malignant change is suggested when there is edema in the adjacent brain parenchyma.

Angiography is important for defining the vascular pedicle prior to attempting surgical removal. The tumor itself shows an angiographic "blush," similar to the common pattern of meningioma. The anterior choroidal artery enlarges to significantly contribute to a tumor of the glomus.

Leukemia

Central nervous system leukemia is occurring with increasing frequency, mainly because of the increased survival of children with leukemia. Therefore 25 to 50 percent with leukemia at some time develop CNS involvement, which can occur during peripheral remission. CNS leukemia always carries a poor prognosis.

The meninges are the usual sites of involvement, with sheets of tumor cells spreading diffusely throughout the subarachnoid space. This situation blocks the flow of cerebrospinal fluid, resulting in mild hydrocephalus. Rarely, there is focal peripheral infiltration of the brain with the formation of a tumor mass (chloroma).

On CT scanning there is almost always some degree of hydrocephalus when meningeal leukemic infiltration is present. The hydrocephalus may be minimal, indicated only by a slight increase in the size of the temporal horns. When there is extensive infiltrate, the meninges and sometimes the ependyma of the ventricles show diffuse contrast enhancement. Focal chloroma or infiltration in the brain is identified by a region of homogeneous enhancement (Fig. 6-18). The lesions tend to be isodense or slightly hyperdense on the nonenhanced scan. Hemorrhage may occur in the brain in the absence of leukemic infiltration, usually as a result of thrombocytopenia. Cerebral infections may occur secondary to pansinusitis and retrograde contamination through the veins into the cavernous sinus, the brain and the subdural space.

Subacute Necrotizing Leukoencephalopathy

Subacute necrotizing leukoencephalopathy is a significant disorder characterized by demyelination, axonal destruction, and coagulation necrosis, often with fibrinoid vascular change. It is the undesirable result of the combination of cranial radiotherapy and intrathecal methotrexate given to treat CNS leukemia. The greater the dose of each, the more likely is the development of destruction. Total cranial irradiation of more than 2000 R and total intrathecal methotrexate of more than 50 mg results in about 45 percent of patients developing the leukoencephalopathy. The changes are irreversible. The damage can be minimized if therapy is modified at the time of the early development of the lesions.

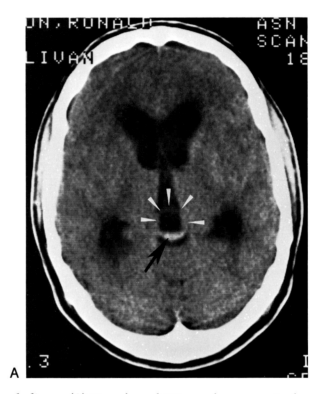

Fig. 6-17 Pineal cyst and glioma. (A) Nonenhanced CT scan shows a cyst in the region of the pineal with contents of just slightly higher density than CSF (arrowheads). Small uncomplicated cysts generally do not cause any problem. This cyst appears to have hemorrhage within it (arrow) and is causing hydrocephalus. *(Figure continues.)*

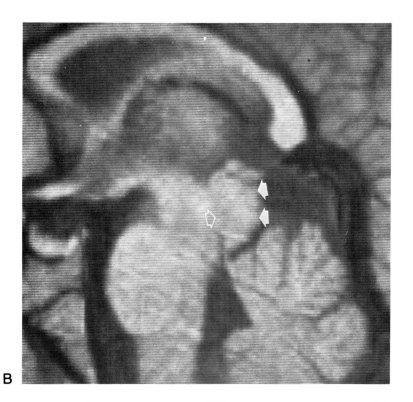

B

Fig. 6-17 *(Continued)*. **(B–C)** glioma of the quadrigeminal plate. **(B)** Midline parasagittal T$_1$-weighted MRI shows enlargement of the quadrigeminal plate expanding posteriorly into the cistern (arrows). The aqueduct is obliterated (open arrow). **(C)** Transaxial T$_1$-weighted MRI shows the enlargement of the right side of the quadrigeminal plate (arrows). Subtle hypointensity represents the glioma (arrowheads). Hydrocephalus is present from obstruction of the aqueduct.

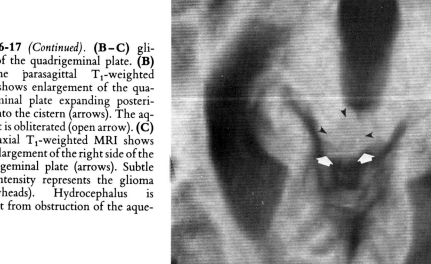

C

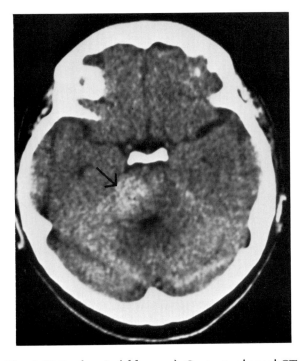

Fig. 6-18 Leukemia (chloroma). Contrast-enhanced CT study shows diffuse homogeneous enhancement in the right side of the pons and cerebellar peduncle. It was thought to represent leukemic infiltration of the brain and disappeared after treatment.

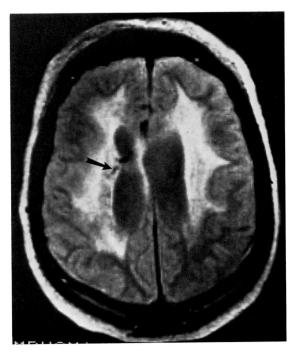

Fig. 6-19 Subacute necrotizing leukoencephalopathy. T_2-weighted MRI shows high signal intensity in the periventricular white matter throughout both hemispheres. There is dilatation of the lateral ventricular system due to atrophy; the low signal region (arrow) probably represents calcium.

The initial CT finding is a diffuse homogeneous decrease in the density of the paraventricular white matter, which is difficult to recognize in the early phase of the disease. MRI is much more sensitive for detecting early disease and shows paraventricular high signal intensity on T_2-weighted images (Fig. 6-19). Calcification may occur in the blood vessels and is seen as clumps within the white matter. Later, ventricular dilatation results from atrophy.

RARE TUMORS

Meningioma

Meningioma and meningeal sarcoma occur in children; 80 percent are supratentorial and 20 percent intraventricular. En plaque growth is common and often causes skull sclerosis. The most common sites are along the sphenoid ridge or the frontoparietal convexity, although the lesions may be found at any of the characteristic locations. Bone destruction may occur. The CT and angiographic characteristics are the same as those described in adults. (Chapter 5.)

Neuroblastoma

Intracranial neuroblastoma may be metastatic or primary. Metastatic neuroblastoma involves the calvarium as destructive lesions invading the orbit and intracranial epidural space; it almost never involves the brain parenchyma.

Primary neuroblastoma usually arises within the cerebral hemispheres, most often the medial posterior temporal lobe. On CT scan it appears hypodense, isodense, or of mixed density, sometimes with dense calcification and cysts. Contrast enhancement is present (Fig. 6-20). Hemorrhage occurs relatively frequently, a

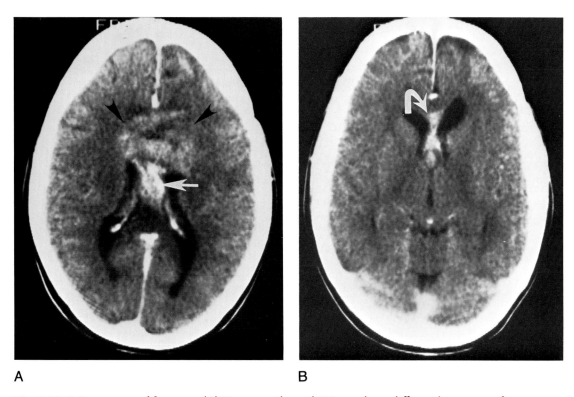

A   B

Fig. 6-20 Primary neuroblastoma. (A) Contrast-enhanced CT scan shows diffuse enhancement of a tumor mass within the corpus callosum and hemispheric white matter bilaterally (arrowheads). Calcification is present in the posterior portion (arrow). **(B)** Tumor has extended into the septum pellucidum (arrow).

finding that helps to differentiate the tumor from an astrocytoma, which it otherwise closely resembles. Peritumoral edema is common.

Aesthesioneuroblastoma is the term given to neuroblastomas originating from the olfactory nerve. These rare tumors penetrate the anterior frontal fossa and the superior nasal cavity. They are slow-growing but infiltrate and are locally destructive. Their great vascularity is well demonstrated on angiography. The CT findings are nonspecific, resembling those of other invasive tumors.

Hamartoma

Hamartomas are slowly growing gliomatous lesions. They are most common in the temporal lobe, where they may cause psychomotor seizures. Another common location is the hypothalamus near the tuber cinereum.

On CT scan they are seen as calcified, cystic, slightly contrast enhancing lesions. They cannot be accurately differentiated from other low grade gliomas. They are hyperintense on T_2-weighted MRI.

Cavernous Hemangioma

Cavernous hemangiomas are rare malformations of the brain. They can occur anywhere but most often are hemispheric. The lesions appear hyperdense on the precontrast CT scan and show a varying degree of contrast enhancement (Fig. 6-21). Most commonly they cause seizures, but they may cause intracerebral or subarachnoid hemorrhage. The peak incidence of presentation is during adolescence or young adulthood. Angiography does not demonstrate these lesions because of the slow blood flow through the malformation. (Also see Chapter 4.)

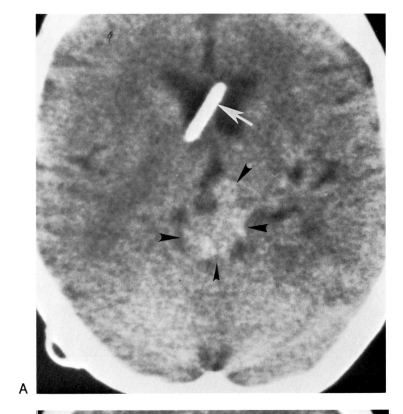

A

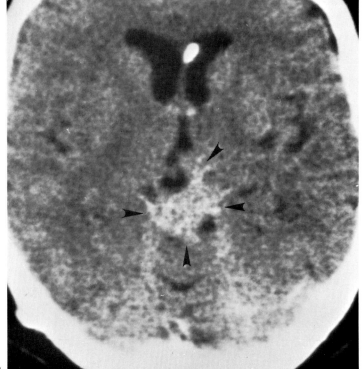

B

Fig. 6-21 Cavernous hemangioma. (A) Nonenhanced CT scan shows an irregular, slightly hyperdense lesion in the region of the pineal gland (arrowheads). The lesion had hemorrhaged and caused hydrocephalus. There is a shunt catheter in the right frontal horn (arrow). (B) Lesion shows diffuse homogeneous contrast enhancement (arrowheads).

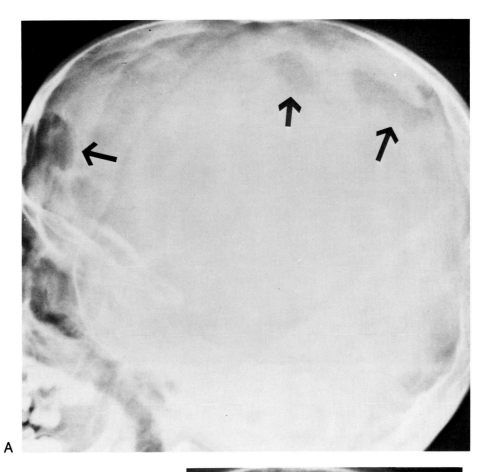

A

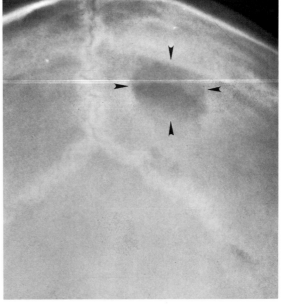

B

Fig. 6-22 Histiocytosis X and eosinophilic granuloma.
(A) Histiocytosis X. Plain skull radiograph shows multiple
lytic lesions of the calvarium (arrows). **(B)** Eosinophilic
granuloma. Skull radiograph shows a well circumscribed solitary lytic lesion of the calvarium (arrowheads). On tangential view the margins may appear beveled. Compare it with
the epidermoid shown in Figure 5-38A.

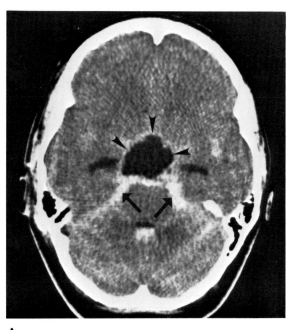

A

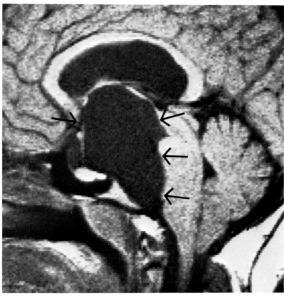

B

C

Fig. 6-23 Arachnoid cyst. (A) Transaxial CT positive-contrast cisternogram shows a noncommunicating cyst with CSF-density fluid (arrowheads). Aqueous contrast is seen in the cisterns (arrows). **(B)** Parasagittal T_1-weighted MRI shows a large cyst in the suprasellar prepontine cistern causing displacement of the brain (arrows). **(C)** Arachnoid cyst of the temporal region. CT scan shows the typical trapezoidal configuration with straight margins (arrows). Slight mass effect is present with contralateral shift of the frontal horns. The density of the contained fluid is equivalent to that of CSF. Arachnoidal cysts may be discovered in any age group.

Primitive Neuroectodermal Tumors

Primitive neuroectodermal tumors are highly aggressive, rapidly growing lesions that occur during the first decade of life. The tumors are poorly marginated and often infiltrate but cause little mass effect. Cystic change is frequently present. The tumors are hypodense or isodense on the precontrast CT scan and show moderate enhancement on the postcontrast scan.

Histiocytosis X

Histiocytosis X comprises a group of disorders characterized by abnormal proliferation of histiocytes in multiple organs including the skull and brain. The disease may occur at any age but is seen primarily in children and young adults. The brain is only rarely involved; but when it is, there is usually only a single lesion in the hypothalamus or sella turcica. Rarely, a lesion occurs in the cerebrum, cerebellum, optic chiasm, or spinal cord. It is associated with diabetes insipidus in about 50 percent of cases. Typical, purely lytic bone lesions are present in the skull (Fig. 6-22) and mandible.

On CT scans the lesions show as a homogeneously enhancing mass, surrounded by edema. On MRI, the lesion shows nonspecific prolongation of the T_1 and T_2 values.

Dermoid

Dermoids and epidermoids occur as a result of embryonic rests resulting from the infolding of the neural tube. Dermoids are most commonly seen in children, and epidermoids are discovered more often during adulthood. Both lesions tend to be in or near the midline.

Dermoid tumors are most often found in the posterior fossa. They assume a variety of configurations, from a small cyst in the occipital subcutaneous tissue to a large cyst that occupies the fourth ventricle, associated with a sinus tract connected to a skin pit. About 50 percent are associated with a sclerotic tract within the calvarium. In infants or children with an occipital skin pit or cyst, a CT scan of the posterior fossa is obtained to look for an intracranial component of the lesion. The dermoid causes problems by its mass effect, infection, or rupture into the subarachnoid space. When rupture occurs, fat density material is seen scattered in the cisterns and causes a chemical meningitis.

Dermoids contain partially saponified fatty tissues and are therefore seen as very low density, 0 to -150 H.U., on the CT scan. Rarely a tooth or calcification is present. There is usually no contrast enhancement. Dermoids have variable intensity on MRI images. (Also see section on epidermoid in Chapter 5).

Arachnoid Cyst

Arachnoid cysts are thought to result from separation of the arachnoid membrane with accumulation of CSF between the layers. Most are congenital. Some cysts result from adhesions that occur following meningitis, subarachnoid hemorrhage, or trauma. Suprasellar cysts are thought to be unique, occurring as a result of upward expansion of an imperforate membrane of Lilliquist into the hypothalamus. Frequently, there is atrophy of the underlying adjacent brain.

The cysts occur most commonly in the temporal fossa or sylvian fissure, posterior fossa, and suprasellar cistern. On CT scans they are homogeneous and of CSF density. Calcification or contrast enhancement does not occur. Large cysts in the suprasellar region expand into the third ventricle and obstruct the foramina of Monro, causing hydrocephalus. It may be difficult to detect these cysts on the initial CT scan, as they may mimic a dilated third ventricle. However, there is almost always widening of the prepontine cistern associated with the cyst. Lateral cysts may locally expand the calvarium. Because of the adjacent atrophy, there is less distortion of the brain than would be expected for the size of the cystic mass. MRI shows the cysts as CSF-intensity masses within the subarachnoid space (Fig. 6-23).

SUGGESTED READINGS

Barnes PD, Lester PD, Yamanshi WS, et al: Magnetic resonance imaging in childhood intracranial masses. Magn Res Imaging 4:41, 1986

Batnitzky S, Segall HD, Cohen ME: Radiologic guidelines in assessing children with intracranial tumors. Cancer 56:1756, 1985

Brandt-Zawadzki M, Kelly W: Brain tumors. In Brandt-Zawadzki M, Norman D (eds): Magnetic Resonance Imaging of the Central Nervous System. Raven Press, New York, 1987

Bydder GM: Magnetic Resonance Imaging of the Posterior Fossa. Magnetic Resonance Annual. Raven Press, New York, 1985

Curtin HD: CT of acoustic neuroma and other tumors of the ear. Radiol Clin North Am 22:77, 1984

Gentry LR, Smoker WRK, Turski PA, et al: Suprasellar arachnoid cysts. I. CT recognition. AJNR 7:79, 1986

Hasso AN, Fahmy JL, Hinshaw DB Jr: Tumors of the posterior fossa. p. 425. In Stark DD, Bradley WG Jr (eds): Magnetic Resonance Imaging. CV Mosby, St. Louis, 1988

Haughton VM, Daniels DL: The posterior fossa. In Williams AL, Haughton VM (eds): Cranial Computed Tomography. CV Mosby, St. Louis, 1985

Lee Y-Y, VanTassel P, Bruner J: Juvenile pilocytic astrocytomas: CT and MR characteristics. AJNR 10:363, 1989

Pusey E, Kortman KE, Flannigan BD: MR of craniopharyngiomas. AJNR 8:439, 1987

Segall HD, Batnitzky S, Zee C-S, et al: Computed tomography in the diagnosis of intracranial neoplasms in children. Cancer 56:1748, 1985

Yock DH Jr: Techniques in imaging of the brain. Part 1. The skull. p. 1. In Heinz ER (ed): Neuroradiology. Churchill Livingstone, New York, 1984

7

Head Trauma

Accidental injury is the most common cause of death and disability among adolescents and young adults. Fifty percent of the injuries are the result of vehicular accidents, and at least 40 percent of the deaths result from head injury, a percentage that is increasing. Many of the deaths inevitably result from severe impact injury; with lesser injuries, however, rapid resuscitation, diagnosis, and treatment of intracranial pathology can lead to a better outcome.

Post-traumatic events in the brain can occur with surprising rapidity. The gravity of the intracranial pathology does not necessarily correlate with the severity of the initial trauma or the condition of the patient immediately after the accident.

The changes demonstrated with CT scans or MRI may presage clinical events while there is still opportunity for effective therapy, especially generalized brain swelling and impending herniation. It is not enough for the radiologist simply to diagnose the presence of a hematoma or swelling. Rather, it is necessary also to assign some value regarding its severity and importance. Recommendations for the timing of follow-up scans must be given.

Skull radiographs are performed if a depressed or basal skull fracture is suspected because of the nature of the injury and the physical findings. A depressed fracture almost always occurs secondary to a blow with a relatively small-faced object such as a hammer. The clinical signs of a basal skull fracture are (1) hemotympanum, (2) hearing loss, (3) vestibular dysfunction, (4) peripheral type of facial nerve palsy, (5) Battle's sign (ecchymosis over the mastoid), (6) anosmia, or (7) otorrhea or rhinorrhea.

Life-threatening injury to organs outside the CNS take precedence, and in these cases CT scans of the head are deferred. Otherwise, CT scanning or MRI is done for persons with head injury that results in any neurologic symptoms or signs, including minor changes in mental status. Persons with minor head injury without neurologic dysfunction, loss of consciousness, or decrease in sensorium do not need a scan of the brain.

The CT scan remains the preferred initial examination, as all immediately important post-traumatic lesions can be detected. CT scanning is easier, faster, and less expensive than MRI, particularly if the patient requires life support systems. A nonenhanced CT scan of the whole head is obtained using 10-mm scan slice intervals. Intravenous contrast is of little use for acute head trauma and may be dangerous. Bone window images are routine.

The MRI technique is capable of diagnosing most important lesions as well, including acute hematomas. T_1- and T_2-weighted transaxial images are used. Axonal shear injury is better seen with MRI. Small extracerebral hematomas may be seen with MRI and not with CT scans, but the hematomas are not immediately important and do not require surgical removal. However, MRI does not reliably demonstrate subarachnoid hemorrhage. Coronal plane images may better demonstrate hematomas in the subfrontal and subtemporal regions.

Traumatic lesions can be characterized as primary or secondary, intracerebral or extracerebral. Primary lesions are those that occur at the instant of injury. They include axonal (shear) injuries, contusions, hematomas, lacerations, and extracerebral hematomas. Except for the removal of hematomas, there is little that can be done to alter the severity of the primary damage. The

241

TRAUMATIC LESIONS OF THE HEAD

Primary lesions
    Intracerebral lesions
        Contusion
        Axonal injury (shear)
        Hematoma
    Extracerebral lesions
        Subdural hematoma
        Epidural hematoma
        Subdural hygroma
        Subarachnoid hemorrhage
    Skull fracture
        Calvarium
        Basal
        Sinuses
    Vascular lesions
        Laceration
        Pseudoaneurysm
Secondary lesions
    Brain swelling
        Edema
        Hyperemia
        Increased intracranial pressure
    Delayed hemorrhage
    Herniation
    Infarction
    CSF fistula
    Infection
        Intracranial
        Sinus
        Mastoid
    Atrophy

severity and type of primary injury is the major determinant of the final outcome.

Secondary responses may occur within minutes of the injury or may not become apparent for days or weeks. Intracranially, these responses include brain swelling, delayed hemorrhage, herniation, infarction, infection, and atrophy. Sometimes, particularly in children, the severity of subsequent swelling is greater than would be expected for relatively minor injuries. Hydrocephalus after trauma is rare.

PRIMARY INJURY

Cerebral Contusion

Cerebral contusion is a common post-traumatic intracranial lesion. It consists in varying amounts of necrosis, hemorrhage, and edema. It is primarily a cortical lesion and may be just a small, superficial bruise. In its more severe forms, the necrosis and hemorrhage are extensive and not only involve a large portion of the cortex but extend deep into the subjacent white matter. Almost all of the damage is done at the time of the impact.

Most contusions occur at sites distant from the point of impact and represent the classic *contrecoup lesion.* Here the contusion is produced by acceleration and sudden deceleration of the head. With the sudden halt of the calvarial motion, the nonrigid brain continues its forward motion, riding over internal skull protuberances, particularly the orbital roof, sphenoid ridge, and petrous pyramid. Therefore the inferior surface of the frontal lobe and the anterior and inferior portions of the temporal lobes are the most commonly contused portions of the brain. Oblique motions can cause contusions of the medial surfaces of the cerebral hemispheres as they are momentarily displaced underneath the falx. Occipital, parietal, and cerebellar contusions are unusual, presumably because of the smoothness of these regions of the calvarium. A depressed skull fracture may penetrate the brain, causing cortical laceration.

Multiple lesions occur in more than 50 percent of persons with contusions, with subdural hematoma being the most common associated lesion. Skull fractures are frequently associated with contusions, and the prognosis is generally worse if a fracture is present.

The CT appearance of a cerebral contusion depends on its size, the amount of hemorrhage present, and the interval between the injury and the scanning. Some small contusions do not hemorrhage and show only edematous changes. A small peripheral bruise may not be detected on the initial CT scan, and only a small amount of focal atrophy may be detected after about 1 month. However, MRI can show the edema and hemorrhage of these small contusions (Fig. 7-1).

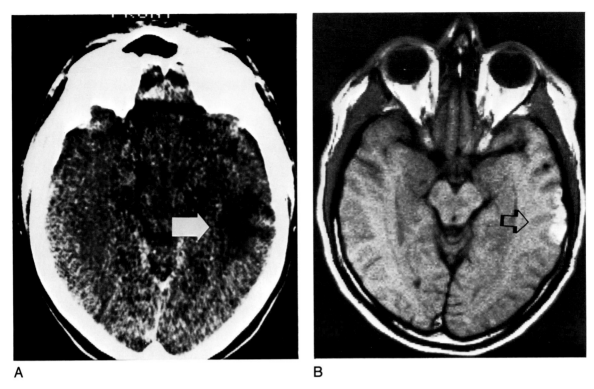

A   B

Fig. 7-1 Cerebral contusion. (A) Cortical contusion is present in the lateral left temporal lobe (arrow). The findings are subtle on the CT scan, with just minimal cortical hemorrhage and edema seen. **(B)** On T_1-weighted MRI, the high intensity change of subacute cortical hemorrhage is easily seen (arrow).

With more severe contusions, CT scanning shows a heterogeneous abnormality composed of (1) low density tissue due to necrosis and edema, and (2) regions of multifocal increased density, representing hemorrhage (Fig. 7-2). The mass effect is usually small during the initial phases of the lesion and is proportional to the size of the contusion. It becomes maximum at 4 to 7 days. If the hemorrhages are severe, the cortex may be completely replaced by homogeneous blood density. Hematomas may occur within deep structures (Fig. 7-2C).

The MRI scan shows contusions well. The regions of hemorrhage are seen as very low intensity signal on the T_2-weighted SE and GRE images. The hemorrhage is surrounded by high signal intensity edema (Fig. 7-3). During the acute phase, the hemorrhage is isointense on T_1-weighted images. Over a 3- to 10-day period, the hemorrhages begin the resorption process, losing density and sharpness on the CT scan. On MRI, the hemorrhages first become bright on T_1-weighted images and then later on T_2-weighted images.

Delayed hemorrhage may occur into the regions of contusion, usually within 48 hours of the injury. It may occur spontaneously or after surgical removal of an extracerebral hematoma. (Presumably the latter event results in removal of a tamponade effect.) Delayed hemorrhage can result in a significant increase in the intracranial pressure and deterioration of the patient. The prognosis thus becomes worse.

The CT examinations 2 weeks to 6 months after the injury demonstrate the gradual development of gliosis and encephalomalacia, which may become cystic. The density of any hemorrhage disappears, and there is a gradual decrease in the CT tissue density of necrotic tissue until it approximates that of CSF. On MRI, the late appearance of the contused tissue depends on the amount of hemorrhage that was present initially. For nonhemorrhagic contusions, as gliosis occurs there is a gradual decrease in the signal intensity of the tissue on T_1-weighted images and an increase in the signal intensity on T_2-weighted images. Hemorrhage within

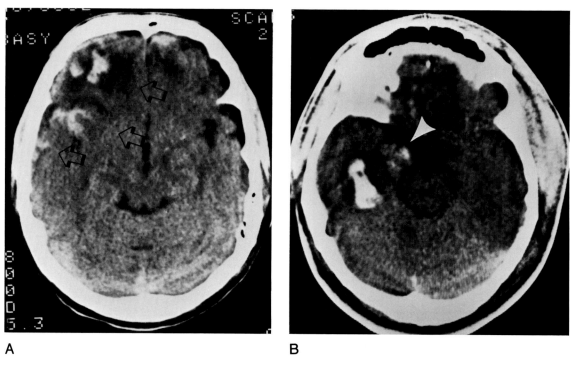

A

B

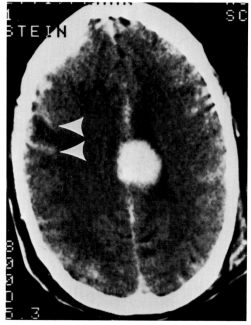

C

Fig. 7-2 Cerebral contusion. (A) Cortical and subcortical regions of hemorrhage and edema are present in the right frontal and right temporal lobes (arrows). **(B)** Right inferior temporal contusion adjacent to petrous ridge and a small contusion of the hippocampal gyrus (arrowhead) are seen. **(C)** Hematoma within the corpus callosum and subarachnoid hemorrhage (arrowheads).

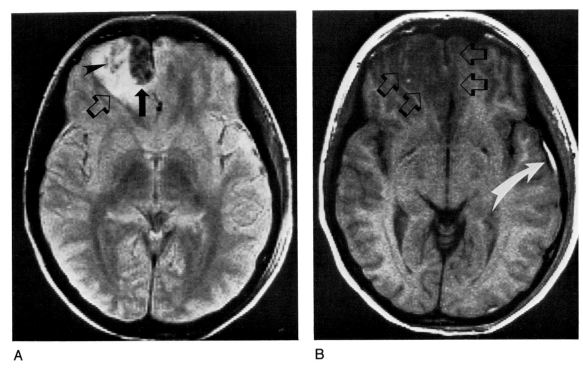

A   B

Fig. 7-3 Frontal contusion, MRI. (A) Proton density MRI shows the hemorrhage as low signal intensity in the medial frontal pole (solid black arrow). Petechial-type hemorrhages are seen laterally (black arrowhead). The edema is shown as high signal intensity (open arrow). **(B)** T_1-weighted MRI shows the hemorrhage to be isointense as it is imaged acutely (open black arrows). A small left temporal extracerebral blood collection has higher intensity than the intracerebral hemorrhage (white arrow).

the contusions is high intensity on T_1-weighted images, and this picture persists for months or even years after the injury. On T_2-weighted images the hemorrhage also becomes bright and persists indefinitely. Very low intensity hemosiderin rings surround the high intensity hemorrhages. Focal atrophy is present, and at this stage the contusion may mimic old infarction. Depending on the depth of the contusion injury, there may be associated focal dilatation of the adjacent lateral ventricle (Fig. 7-4).

As with infarctions, after about 5 days there is proliferation of peripherally located granulation tissue. These new vessels do not possess a blood-brain barrier, so there is ring-like or gyral enhancement on contrast CT scans that persists many months, although gradually decreasing in area and intensity. If a contrast CT examination is performed and the history of recent trauma is not known, it is possible to misdiagnose the lesion as a tumor, infarction, or infection.

The signs and symptoms of cerebral contusion are related to the size and location of the contusion. Small contusions may resolve without causing any deficit. Lesions in the motor or speech regions generally result in focal neurologic deficit.

Axonal Injury (Shear)

Axonal injury, or shear, is a diffuse type of brain damage. It occurs as an immediate consequence of the rotational forces associated with impact. Because the gray and white matter have different mass densities, with rapid rotation these two tissues deform at different rates, causing shearing of axons at gray–white matter interfaces. The lesions are characteristically found within the white matter at the corticomedullary junction or in the corpus callosum. They may also occur deep within the brain or in the brain stem when especially severe forces have occurred. Small intraventricu-

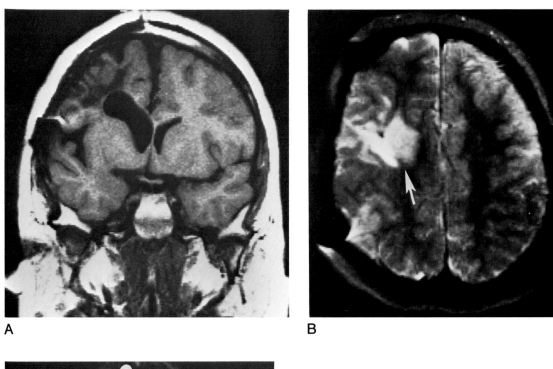

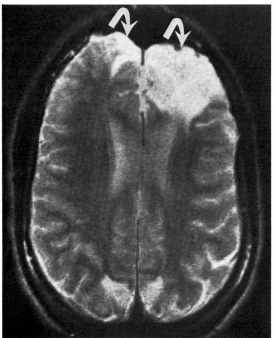

Fig. 7-4 Post-traumatic encephalomalacia. (A) T$_1$-weighted MRI shows right posterior frontal cortical atrophy, subcortical gliosis, and porencephalic dilatation of the adjacent lateral ventricle. **(B)** The gliosis is seen as high signal intensity on the T$_2$-weighted images (arrow). **(C)** Bifrontal contusion in another patient. T$_2$-weighted MRI shows gliosis and demyelination as regions of high signal intensity extending to the cortical surface (arrows).

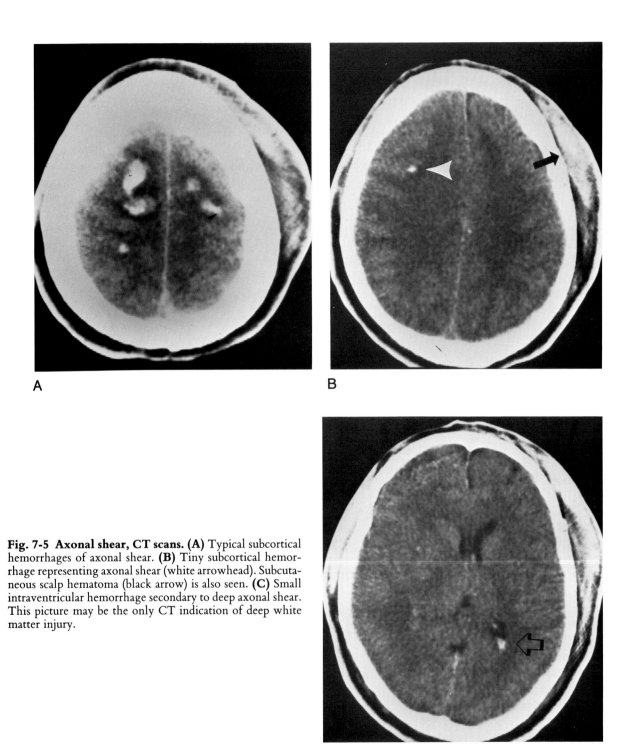

Fig. 7-5 Axonal shear, CT scans. (A) Typical subcortical hemorrhages of axonal shear. **(B)** Tiny subcortical hemorrhage representing axonal shear (white arrowhead). Subcutaneous scalp hematoma (black arrow) is also seen. **(C)** Small intraventricular hemorrhage secondary to deep axonal shear. This picture may be the only CT indication of deep white matter injury.

lar hemorrhages may be seen as an indirect sign of deep axonal injury (Fig. 7-5C).

Most axonal injuries are small, widely distributed, and nonhemorrhagic, producing only a small amount of local edema. About 20 percent have a small associated hemorrhage. There is a general correlation of the amount of axonal injury and neurologic dysfunction. This correlation is greatest with more severe injury. With lesser degrees of axonal injury, the effect on neurologic function is unpredictable. When severe, the summation of multiple lesions may produce significant diffuse brain swelling with compression of ventricles and sulci. Axonal injury produces significant white matter loss, which after 1 month results in ventricular enlargement.

T_2-weighted MRI is superior to CT scanning for detecting axonal injury. The injury is best seen during the acute phase. The lesions are seen as small, less than 1 cm, foci of high signal intensity within the white matter, representing the focal edema. Small hemorrhages are seen on T_2-weighted images as low intensity regions within the high intensity edema. In the subacute and chronic phase, hemorrhages are best detected as high signal on the T_1-weighted images. CT scans demonstrate only the hemorrhagic lesions (Fig. 7-5), as the small nonhemorrhagic regions of subcortical edema are usually too small for routine CT scan detection. The MRI findings of axonal injury must be differentiated from other multifocal white matter diseases, particularly multiple sclerosis, diffuse infection (fungus infection, AIDS), metastasis, and small subcortical infarctions which might pre-exist in the trauma patient.

Intracerebral Hematoma

Intracerebral hematomas are well defined homogeneous hemorrhages in the brain parenchyma, usually the white matter. They are formed when there is rupture of a major perforating artery from an acceleration-deceleration injury or when there is profuse hemorrhage in a region of contusion so that the hemorrhages coalesce. The differentiation of hemorrhagic contusion from hematoma can be difficult and somewhat arbitrary. Like contusions, 80 to 90 percent of hematomas occur most commonly in the frontal and temporal lobes. Hematomas may also occur underneath depressed skull fractures or be associated with penetrating wounds. They are rare in the cerebellum. The CT and MRI examinations show the findings of intracerebral hematoma (Fig. 7-2C) (also see Chapter 2).

Extracerebral Subdural Hematoma

A subdural hematoma (SDH) is a collection of blood within the subdural space. It almost always occurs as a result of trauma. These lesions have been arbitrarily classified according to their age relative to the trauma. An acute SDH is one that clinically manifests within the first 72 hours after the injury. Subacute refers to one that is 3 to 20 days old. Chronic SDH is one that is more than 20 days old. The CT and MRI appearances, their pathogenesis, and their epidemiology differ among the three groups, so they are discussed separately.

ACUTE SDH

Acute SDH almost always occurs as a result of significant head trauma, but it may occur spontaneously from dural AVM, mycotic aneurysm, or after the most minimal injury in those with coagulopathies. Rarely, it occurs after rupture of a berry type aneurysm. Mostly, it occurs over the cerebral convexity but may extend beneath the brain or into the interhemispheric fissure. A posterior fossa SDH is unusual. Post-traumatic SDH is thought to result from rupture of surface cortical veins or arteries at sites of brain contusion or from tearing of the bridging veins that drain into the dural venous sinuses.

Most patients with acute post-traumatic SDH have an underlying brain contusion that is often severe. The mass effect and elevation of the intracranial pressure may be predominantly due to the changes associated with the contused brain. The severity of the associated brain injury is the primary determining cause of the outcome of patients with SDH, even after its timely surgical evacuation.

In the hyperacute phase, MRI shows the SDH as a high protein solution, with isointensity on T_1- and high intensity on T2-weighted images. During the first day the SDH becomes of low intensity on T_2-weighted images.

On CT scan an acute SDH appears as a high density (50 to 90 H.U.) crescent-shaped extracerebral mass most commonly over the frontal or parietal convexity

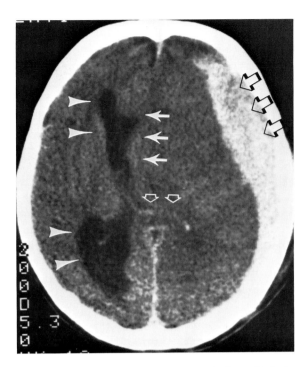

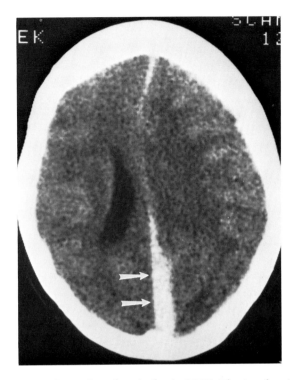

Fig. 7-6 Acute subdural hematoma. The large high density extracerebral fluid collection over the left frontal and parietal convexities represents an acute subdural hematoma (large open arrows). There is subfalcial herniation (white arrows) and transtentorial herniation as represented by enlargement of the right lateral ventricle (white arrowheads) and obliteration of the quadrigeminal plate cistern (small open arrows).

Fig. 7-7 Acute interhemispheric SDH. The interhemispheric SDH is seen with a flat medial border (arrows) and a convex lateral border. The shift of the brain is due to contusion.

(Fig. 7-6). Its medial border may be slightly angulated into the region of the sylvian fissure. SDH may also be found in the subtemporal, suboccipital, and interhemispheric regions (Figs. 7-7 and 7-8). The clot density may be uniform or may have low density regions within it, representing either unclotted blood or continued bleeding at the time of the CT scan. With unclotted blood a density level may be seen from red blood cells settling in the dependent region. It is possible for the SDH to have a relatively low density (30 to 40 H.U.) in patients with severe anemia (hemoglobin usually less than 9 mg/dl). The hematoma decreases in density with time, so that some time between 1 and 3 weeks the SDH is isodense with the adjacent brain. After 3 weeks, the SDH becomes hypodense.

Cerebral angiography demonstrates the SDH a high percentage of the time. It is seen as an avascular crescent-shaped mass over the frontal and parietal convexity, causing compression of the brain and displacement of the cortical arteries and veins away from the inner table of the skull (Fig. 7-9D).

SUBACUTE SDH

An SDH that is seen 3 to 20 days after injury is called a subacute SDH. During this period MRI easily detects a SDH. With the development of methemoglobin, the T_1-weighted images show the extracerebral blood collection as hyperintense, first at the periphery and then filling in centrally. The same change occurs with the T_2-weighted imaging, although at a slightly differing time, depending on the field strength used (Fig. 7-9).

During this time, the hematoma is more difficult to detect with CT scanning. An SDH decreases in CT radioabsorption properties with time, so that at some point, it appears isodense with the adjacent brain. Nev-

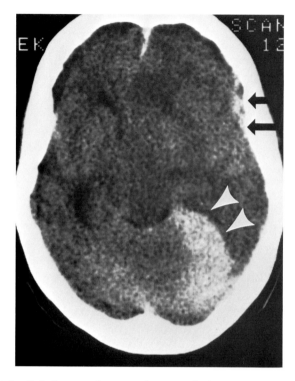

Fig. 7-8 Acute suboccipital SDH. The high density over the left tentorium represents a suboccipital SDH (white arrowheads). A small left convexity SDH also is seen (black arrows), and there is subfalcial herniation.

ertheless, it is possible to detect nearly all collections without resorting to the use of intravenous contrast. The extracerebral collection causes a mass effect that compresses the brain, which can be detected by recognizing (1) obliteration of the cerebral sulci; (2) inward displacement of the cortex, seen as "buckling" of the ipsilateral gray–white matter junction (Fig. 7-10A); (3) ipsilateral compression of the ventricles; and (4) subtle, mottled extracerebral density adjacent to the inner table of the skull, where normal brain sulci are usually seen. Bilateral subacute SDHs are more difficult to recognize because of symmetry.

In difficult situations, CT scanning with intravenous contrast helps to detect the subacute SDH. The contrast enhances the hypervascular inner membrane that forms around the SDH after 1 week. It defines the border between the SDH and the cortex of the brain (Fig. 7-10B).

Additionally, the contrast may outline cortical veins and the brain cortex itself, further defining the margin of the SDH.

CHRONIC SDH

Be definition, chronic SDHs are those that are more than 20 days old. In the elderly, an SDH is frequently not recognized until it has reached the chronic stage. Up to 50 percent of these patients cannot even recall a specific head injury; and those who can recall a mild injury. Fifty percent of persons who present with a chronic SDH are chronic alcoholics.

Most SDHs that present in the chronic stage produce few symptoms. They enlarge slowly and are not associated with underlying brain injury. They may be asymptomatic for weeks, probably at least partly a consequence of the greater compliance of an atrophic brain to accommodate an intracranial mass lesion. Bilateral chronic SDH is common, with an incidence of up to 50 percent in some series.

There are multiple clinical patterns of presentation: (1) dementia or inappropriate behavior; (2) acute motor or sensory loss mimicking a stroke; (3) transient neurologic deficit, mimicking a transient ischemic attack (TIA); (4) seizure; (5) increased intracranial pressure with headache and vomiting; and (6) gradual progression of neurologic signs, mimicking a tumor. Headache is a cardinal symptom and may be present without associated neurologic abnormality. Therefore in the elderly, headache is a definate indication for the performance of CT scanning or MRI.

In the elderly, the SDH is thought to result from rupture of the fragile bridging veins that connect the cortical veins with a dural sinus. These veins are under greater stretch in persons with cerebral atrophy. The hemorrhage begins as a small, silent, acute SDH. There is ingrowth of fibroblasts into the hematoma from the inner surface of the dura, forming a thick lateral membrane over the subdural blood collection. A thin membrane also forms along the medial margin of the hematoma. This formation occurs within the first 3 weeks after the injury, and the membrane can be imaged by either contrast-enhanced CT scans or radionuclide brain scanning because of its lack of a blood-brain barrier. The hematoma increases in size, usually because of repeated hemorrhages. It may take any shape; the most common is concave medially, similar to an acute SDH (Fig. 7-11). A biconvex shape is less common and usually indicates multiple bleeding episodes (Fig. 7-12A).

With MRI, the chronic SDH appears as an extracerebral high intensity collection on both T_1- and T_2-weighted images. Inhomogeneity may be present from

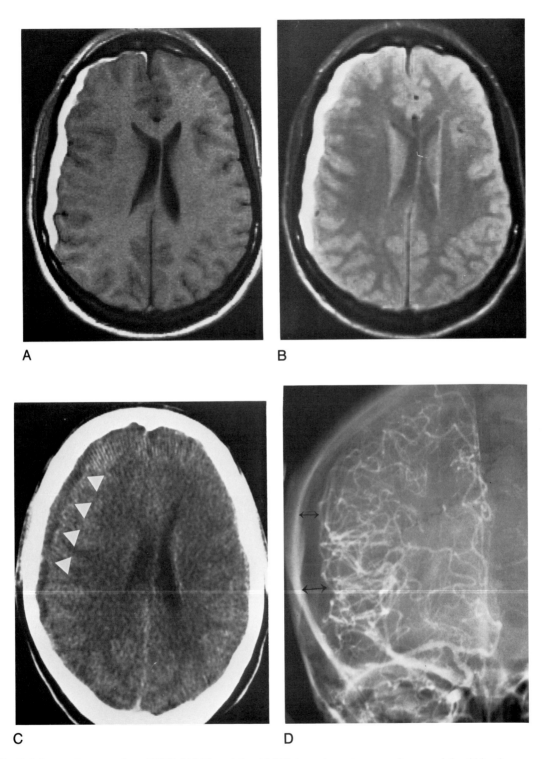

Fig. 7-9 Late subacute phase SDH. (A) T$_1$-weighted MRI shows hyperintense subacute subdural blood accumulation over the right convexity. **(B)** Proton density MRI shows high intensity fluid accumulation over the convexity. **(C)** CT scan shows slightly hypodense fluid accumulation over the right convexity. **(D)** Angiography shows cortical arteries displaced away from the inner table (opposed arrows).

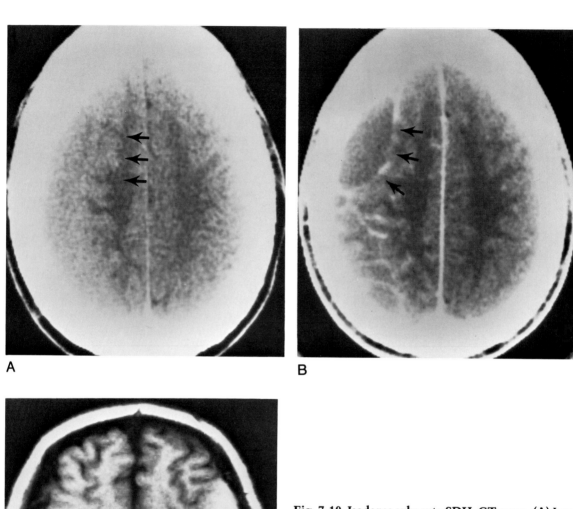

A

B

C

Fig. 7-10 Isodense subacute SDH, CT scans. (A) Inward displacement (buckling) of the gray–white matter junction on the right (arrows) secondary to the invisible SDH. **(B)** Contrast enhancement outlines the dural membrane (black arrows) and compressed cerebral cortex by the now visible SDH. **(C)** A subacute SDH is easily seen with T_1-weighted MRI.

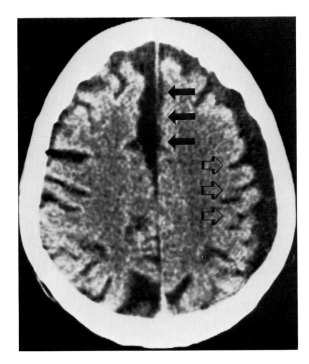

Fig. 7-11 Chronic SDH. CT scan shows a very low density extracerebral fluid collection on the left causing compression of the cerebral sulci (open black arrows) and narrowing of the ipsilateral interhemispheric fissure (solid black arrows).

loculated hemorrhages of differing ages. Because of contained protein, the chronic SDH is very hyperintense on the T_2-weighted images. After a few months the hematoma may become hypointense on T_1-weighted images, although it remains of high intensity indefinitely on T_2-weighted images. Peripheral hemosiderin deposits are much less common with extracerebral hemorrhages than with parenchymal hemorrhages.

With CT scanning the collection is primarily hypodense (Fig. 7-11). Multiple loculations of differing densities may be present, sometimes with a compartmentalized acute hemorrhagic density (Fig. 7-12A). Fresh blood elements may gravitate to the dependent portion of the collection. If rebleeding has not occurred for some time, the CT density of the SDH is very low, just slightly above that of the CSF, and may appear as enlargement of the subarachnoid space due to severe atrophy. However, mass effect is usually present with an SDH (Fig. 7-11). T_2-weighted MRI always shows a chronic SDH as high signal intensity and so easily dif-

ferentiates SDH from the enlarged subarachnoid space of severe atrophy.

It is generally not possible to completely evacuate a chronic SDH at the time of surgery in elderly patients because of underlying brain atrophy and the inability of the brain to reexpand to fill the extracerebral void. Serous fluid usually fills the remaining space. However, over weeks this fluid gradually resorbs (Fig. 7-12).

Subdural Hygroma

Subdural hygromas, collections of CSF in the subdural space, may occur following trauma or rapid decompression of the ventricular system after shunting. There may also be a small amount of blood within the fluid with acute head injury.

These peculiar collections probably result from a tear in the arachnoid, with escape of CSF into the subdural space. Because the fluid may not be able to escape from the subdural pocket, it can act as a mass effect. Small hygromas resorb on their own, but those associated with deteriorating neurologic signs may benefit from surgical drainage. However, hygromas that develop after ventricular over-shunting are treated by placement of a higher-pressure shunt valve rather than removal of the extracerebral fluid. On CT a hygroma may appear as a chronic SDH but is seen in a different clinical context (Fig. 7-13).

Subarachnoid Hemorrhage

Subarachnoid hemorrhage (SAH) is common after head injury. It is caused by rupture of small perforating vessels. It can be seen on CT scans as increased density within the cisterns and sulci (Fig. 7-2C). SAH is usually not detected with MRI. Although it does not cause any mass effect, SAH may cause a mild communicating hydrocephalus and contribute to increased intracranial pressure.

Epidural (Extradural) Hematoma

Acute epidural hematoma refers to a blood collection that occurs between the dura and the inner table of the skull. It is relatively infrequent—about one-tenth as common as SDH. Epidural hematoma is rare in individuals under the age of 2 or over age 60 because in these

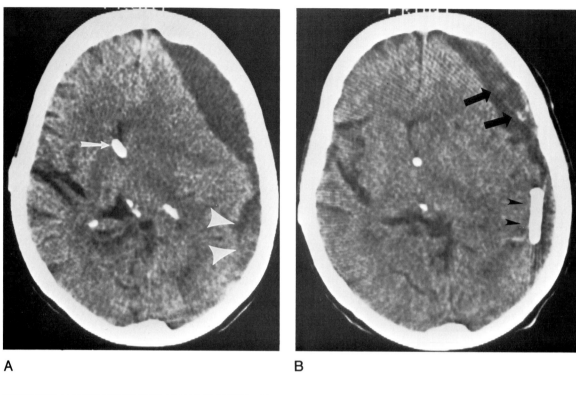

A

B

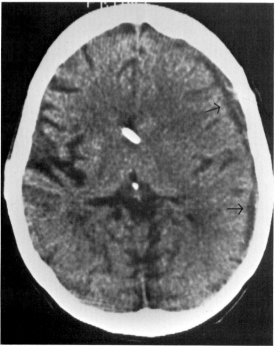

Fig. 7-12 Chronic SDH, surgical evacuation. (A) CT scan shows a moderately hypodense multiloculated chronic SDH on the left with a convex inner margin. Slight increased density is seen in the posterior loculation from recent hemorrhage (arrowheads). The brain is compressed and shifted. A shunt tube is present in the right frontal horn (arrow). (B) Subtotal removal of the SDH on the left. A small amount of rebleeding has occurred (black arrows). A drain is in place posteriorly (arrowheads). (C) One month later near-complete resorption of the extracerebral fluid collection has occurred (arrows).

C

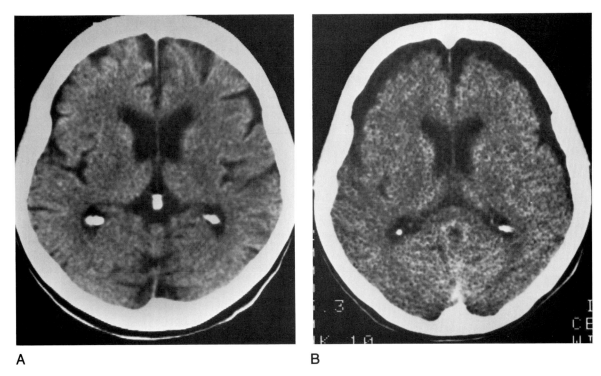

A   B

Fig. 7-13 Acute subdural hygroma. (A) CT scan of the brain obtained for other reasons just prior to a head injury. **(B)** Acute bilateral subdural low density fluid collections found at surgery to be CSF. Note the compression of the ventricles and cerebral sulci.

two groups the dura is firmly adherent to the undersurface of the skull. It occurs most commonly in the supratentorial region and only rarely in the posterior fossa.

Epidural hematoma is due to laceration of the meningeal arteries and veins that are on the calvarial surface of the dural membrane. Less commonly it is caused by laceration of a dural sinus. Eighty-five percent are associated with a local skull fracture that usually crosses a vascular groove or dural sinus. The force of the trauma produces inward bending of the calvarium, which in turn strips the dura from the inner table. This action creates an epidural pocket into which bleeding may occur. Venous bleeding remains localized to the original pocket. Arterial bleeding may exert enough force to enlarge the pocket. If the associated fracture is large, the hemorrhage may decompress outward into the subgaleal space instead of into the epidural space.

An epidural hematoma may enlarge rapidly, and so most must be evacuated immediately. Because there is usually relatively little underlying brain injury, the results of surgical removal are much better than with

acute SDH. Small epidural hematomas (less than 1 cm thick) tend not to enlarge and may be followed with serial CT scans. They resorb without surgical evacuation.

With CT scanning the acute epidural hematoma appears as a homogeneous high density (40 to 90 H.U.) biconvex mass underneath the inner table (Fig. 7-14). It causes local displacement of the brain, with compression of the sulci and the ventricles, and midline shift; but underlying brain injury is uncommon. A skull fracture can often be demonstrated with the use of bone window images. Hematomas that are due to a tear of the sagittal sinus are seen high on the convexity and often cross the midline. Small epidural hematomas that are not removed gradually decrease in density and size, eventually becoming hypodense lesions and disappearing. There may be slight thickening of the inner table of the skull with healing.

Epidural hematomas appear on MRI with the intensity characteristics of any hematoma. The shape is the same as that described with CT scans (Fig. 7-15).

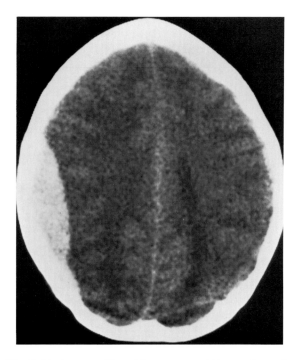

Fig. 7-14 Acute epidural hematoma. CT scan shows the typical high density extracerebral collection on the right with a convex medial border. The right lateral ventricle is compressed, and there is a slight shift of the falx.

SECONDARY INJURY

Intracranial Pressure

The intracranial pressure is normally below a mean of 15 mmHg. This steady state is maintained by a balance of the formation of CSF, resorption of CSF, resistance to the flow of CSF through the ventricles and cisterns, and compliance of the intracranial fluid volume to accommodate increased cerebral mass. After cranial trauma, the normal mechanisms controlling intracranial pressure may be disturbed or overwhelmed so there is a devastating increase in intracranial pressure.

It is important to understand the concept of intracranial compliance and the nature of the CSF pressure–volume curve. Because of the buffer of the vascular system, an increase in CSF volume or the formation of brain edema is compensated for by a decrease in the intracerebral vascular volume. Similarly, the CSF spaces surrounding the brain and the ventricular cavities can accommodate changes in brain size by displacement of fluid. Clearly, these mechanisms can work

only to a point. If the brain volume (e.g., from edema) becomes so great that all of the blood is displaced from the vascular system and the CSF is displaced from the ventricles and cisterns, the intracranial pressure rises rapidly to the level of the blood pressure. The intracranial blood flow ceases, and brain death ensues.

At conditions close to normal, small changes in the cerebral volume (brain swelling) can be accommodated with little increase in the intracranial pressure. However, when the capacity of the cisterns and the vascular system is approached, an equally small incremental increase in the intracranial volume results in a large, possibly detrimental increase in the intracranial pressure. At this point the intracranial compliance has become markedly reduced. The converse is also true, and a small decrease in cerebral volume due to therapeutic maneuvers results in a significant decrease in the intracranial pressure. The brain volume–intracranial pressure curve is shown in Figure 7-16.

The nature of the pressure–brain volume curve has important imaging implications. From the curve alone, one can predict that there can be a considerable amount of brain swelling present with little increase in the intracranial pressure. It is also true that it is impossible to determine where the patient is on the curve simply by measuring the intracranial pressure. Therefore serial CT or MRI scans become important for management of the trauma victim, as the findings of cerebral swelling may be seen on the CT examination before there is a significant rise in the intracranial pressure or a change in the patient's clinical state. The scans can also predict the amount of compliance present by determining the size of the cisterns. If the cisterns are small or obliterated, the intracranial compliance for an increase in brain volume is low.

Other factors reduce the compliance of the brain to absorb changes in intracranial volume. Compliance is reduced by any intracranial hematoma, hydrocephalus, subarachnoid hemorrhage, transtentorial or tonsillar herniation (increased resistance to flow of CSF in the cisterns), systemic hypertension, or fluid overload. These factors must be considered when evaluating the CT or MRI scan.

Brain Swelling

Brain swelling is a poorly understood phenomenon that may accompany any type of head injury. It may be severe after either major and surprisingly minor inju-

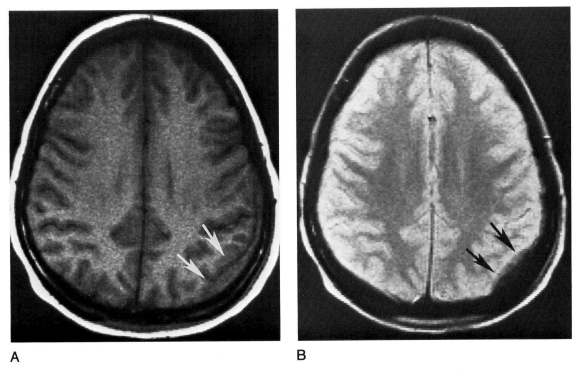

A   B

Fig. 7-15 Acute epidural hematoma. (A) Small epidural left posterior parietal blood collection is isointense on the T_1-weighted image (arrows). **(B)** T_2-weighted image shows the acute small collection as extreme low signal intensity (arrows).

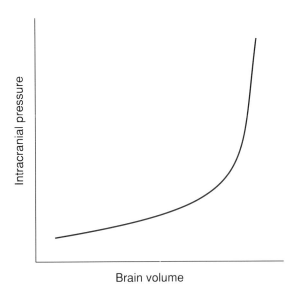

Fig. 7-16 Relation of cerebral volume to intracranial pressure. The intracranial pressure rises only slightly until a critical brain volume is reached. The pressure then increases greatly with slight increases in brain volume.

ries. The effects of the swelling are additive to the effects of the primary injury itself and may become the most significant factor determining outcome.

Acute brain swelling is usually the result of increased intracerebral blood volume brought about by changes in the autoregulation of the cerebral vessels. Delayed swelling is usually due to brain edema. The mechanism of the swelling has important therapeutic ramifications. Hyperventilation therapy through vasoconstriction is aimed at decreasing intracranial vascular volume. Mannitol therapy is aimed at decreasing actual cerebral edema. Severe post-traumatic brain swelling is difficult to control by any means.

Brain swelling is identified on the CT scan by a decrease in the size of the ventricles, cortical sulci, and basal cisterns. Special attention is given to observing the size of the cisterns. If the supratentorial and incisural cisterns are totally obliterated, cranial-caudad transtentorial herniation is either imminent or has already occurred (Fig. 7-6). This sign indicates extreme danger and may be recognized on the CT scan before clinical

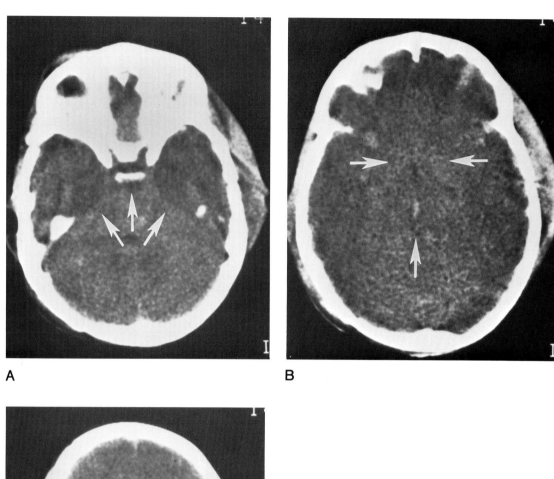

A

B

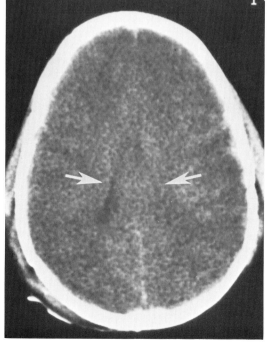

C

Fig. 7-17 Severe acute brain swelling. (A) Obliteration of the prepontine and cerebellopontine angle cisterns (arrows). **(B)** Obliteration of the suprasellar and quadrigeminal plate cisterns (arrows). **(C)** Compression of the lateral ventricular system (arrows). All the scans show loss of gray–white matter differentiation, obliteration of cerebral sulci, and small contusions at typical sites. The findings on this scan indicate increased intracranial pressure and low compliance.

signs of herniation have occurred. When this degree of swelling is present, even small changes in intracranial volume due to edema or bleeding result in a rapid increase in the intracranial pressure. In severe situations, the posterior fossa cisterns are also obliterated (Fig. 7-17).

The CT density of the swollen brain following trauma is variable, and depends on a complex relation between blood volume, edema, and microhemorrhages. The brain may be any density, from slightly hypodense to slightly hyperdense; it is unpredictable.

Herniation

Internal herniations are common with severe head injuries. There are many types. Subfalcian herniation occurs when the brain shifts across the midline underneath the relatively rigid falx (Fig. 7-6). Such a shift results from unilateral hemispheric or extracerebral lesions. The frontal horns of the ventricles are distorted. Infarctions may result in the distribution of the compressed pericallosal arteries. Cranial-caudad transtentorial herniation is due to a large unilateral or bilateral supratentorial mass lesion. Here the base of the brain is forced downward into the tentorial hiatus, which obliterates the perimesencephalic and quadrigeminal plate cisterns. Acute hydrocephalus results from compression of the aqueduct. The ventricular dilatation may be asymmetric depending on the side of the maximal lesions (Fig. 7-6). There may be unilateral or bilateral third cranial nerve (CN III) compression.

Uncal herniation is the result of lesions within or adjacent to the temporal lobe. Here the medial portion of the temporal lobe (uncus) is forced medially and downward into the ipsilateral tentorial hiatus, and the brain stem is displaced contralaterally. There is ipsilateral compression of CN III (see Fig. 5-10A).

Infarction

Focal cerebral infarctions may result from injured or compressed vessels. Most commonly they occur in the: (1) pericallosal region, due to compression by subfalcial herniation; (2) occipital lobes, due to compression of the posterior cerebral arteries against the tentorium with transtentorial herniation (Fig. 7-18); (3) posterior parietal "watershed" region; (4) middle cerebral territory, due to compression of the supraclinoid internal carotid artery against the anterior clinoid processes; and

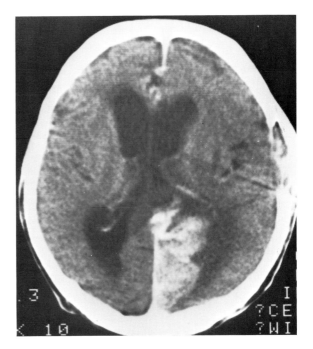

Fig. 7-18 Occipital infarction after transtentorial herniation. This contrast-enhanced CT study shows diffuse enhancement in a left occipital infarct. It is the postoperative CT scan of the acute SDH shown in Figure 7-6.

(5) global infarction, due to a substantial increase in the intracranial pressure.

Atrophy

Atrophy is common after head injury. It may be mild or severe and focal or diffuse. After the subsidence of swelling, it progresses in a linear fashion to become maximal about 2 months after the injury. The white matter is usually most affected, resulting in dilatation of the ventricles that may be considerable (Fig. 7-4A). The cerebral sulci show less enlargement. Ventricular enlargement from atrophy must not be misdiagnosed as hydrocephalus, which is uncommon after head injury.

Pneumocephalus (Pneumocranium)

A careful search is made for air within the calvarium. It most frequently collects in the anterior portion of the frontal fossa and can be seen best on the transaxial CT scan but also on a cross-table lateral skull radiograph

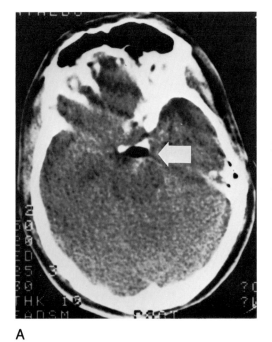

Fig. 7-19 Pneumocranium. (A) Air behind dorsum sellae (arrow). **(B)** Plain film showing air within frontal cortical sulci (arrow). A compound depressed fracture is seen posteriorly (arrowheads).

A

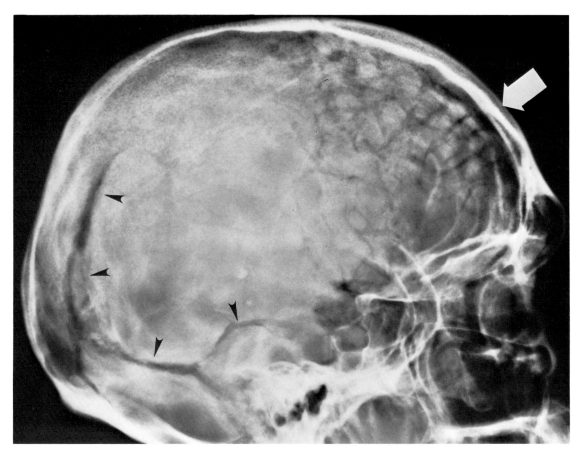

B

(Fig. 7-19). It implies rupture of the dura, most commonly due to fracture through the posterior wall of the frontal sinus or the ethmoidal plate. Parasellar air suggests a fracture through the sphenoid sinus. Fracture of the petrous bone only rarely produces pneumocranium. Air may collect anywhere after a compound depressed fracture. The presence of intracranial air indicates risk of subsequent meningitis.

Infections

Intracranial infections are surprisingly rare after head injury. Most occur as a postoperative complication or with dural tears. Paranasal sinus infection is a problem in the immobilized head-injured patient and may cause sepsis. It can be identified as fluid in the paranasal sinuses on head scans (Fig. 7-20). However, not all fluid collections within a sinus represent infection. Fluid is common within the sphenoid sinus with nasotracheal intubation.

SKULL RADIOGRAPHY AND SKULL FRACTURES

The important observations to make from the skull radiograph of the person with head trauma are pineal shift, fracture, pneumocranium, and facial fracture.

Pineal Shift

A shift of the pineal gland of more than 3 mm is considered significant. The presence of a shift denotes an emergency, and the shift is considered to be caused by either brain swelling or hematoma. A CT scan or MRI must be done immediately to determine the nature of the problem.

Because the pineal is positioned directly above the odontoid process and therefore is at the center of rotation of the skull, rotation of up to 20 degrees has little effect on the measured position of the gland. Calcific densities in the tentorium and choroid must not be

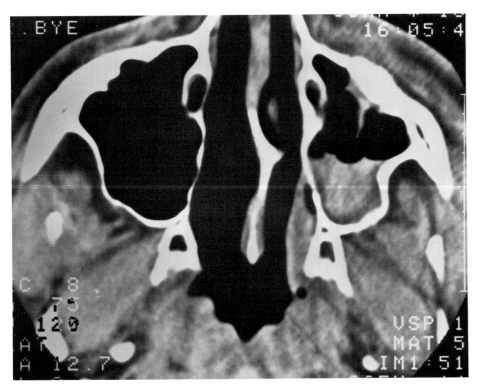

Fig. 7-20 Acute sinusitis. A fluid level is seen in the left maxillary sinus. This infection was the source of a troublesome fever after severe head injury.

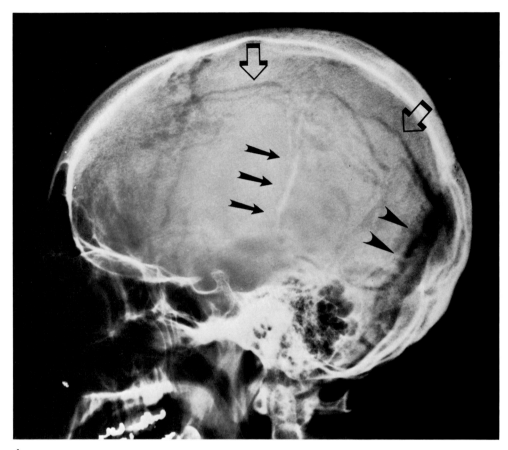

A

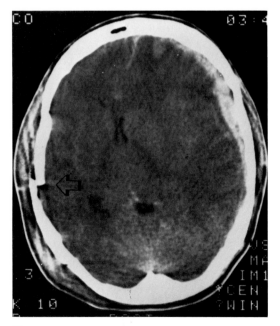

B

Fig. 7-21 Depressed skull fracture. (A) Lateral skull radiograph shows a linear region of increased density over the right parietal bone representing the overlapping bone margins of the depressed skull fracture (arrows). A diastatic linear parietal fracture is seen (open arrows). There is diastasis of the lambdoid suture (arrowheads). **(B)** CT scan shows overlapped edges of the right parietal depressed skull fracture. There is also an acute left SDH and subfalcial herniation.

misinterpreted as representing the pineal gland. To be visible on the frontal projections, the pineal must also be visible on the lateral projection. Atrophy of the brain and posterior fossa masses usually do not cause pineal shift.

Depressed Fracture

A depressed fracture is considered significant if the fragment is displaced inward a distance equal to, or greater than, the width of the calvarium. There is a high incidence of an associated dural tear with communication of the subarachnoid space with the outside air (compound fracture) and cortical laceration. Pneumocranium (air within the cranial cavity) indicates a compound fracture (Fig. 7-19). It is estimated that 85 percent of depressed fractures are compound. The development of post-traumatic seizures is thought to occur with greater frequency if a completely displaced fragment is not elevated.

A depressed fracture may be recognized by observing the inward displacement of bone fragments at the tangential portions of the calvarium or the increased density of overlapping bone margins when the fracture is viewed en face (Fig. 7-21). Special note is made of a depressed fracture that overlies a dural sinus. Angiography may be necessary to determine precisely the relation of a fracture to a sinus. CT scanning with bone windows is also an excellent means of evaluating depressed fractures. Unconventional scan planes may be needed to optimally view the fracture.

Linear Fracture

Linear fractures are the most common type of fracture and require the least amount of kinetic energy. They are of little consequence unless they are diastatic or cross meningeal vessels or dural sinuses. When this situation is present, they may be associated with a dural tear or epidural hematoma. A normal suture line or vascular groove must be differentiated from a fracture. A fracture line appears more radiolucent than a vascular groove and does not have sclerotic margins. Fractures also tend to be straight or to make angular changes in direction. Occasionally, sutures are mistaken for fractures. The common suture lines are shown in Figure 7-22. Linear fractures heal within 1 to 2 years in adults.

Diastatic Fractures

A diastatic fracture is a widened linear fracture or a separated sutural fracture. These fractures may be associated with dural tears. In young children, less than 2 years old, the separated fracture may fail to heal because of interposition of meninges into the fracture site. This problem may cause progressive expansion of the fracture, the "growing fracture" (post-traumatic leptomeningeal cyst) (Fig. 7-23). All diastatic fractures of the calvarium in young children require follow-up radiographs to ensure proper healing of the fracture.

Basal Fractures and CSF Fistula

Basal skull fractures are those that involve one of the five bones that make up the base of the skull: cribriform plate of the ethmoid bone, orbital plate of the frontal bone, sphenoid bone, petrous and squamous portions of the temporal bone, and occipital bone. Basal fractures are of considerable significance because the regional dura may be disrupted, allowing communication of the subarachnoid space with an underlying paranasal or mastoid sinus. A dural disruption here places the person at increased risk for the development of meningitis or a CSF fistula.

Fractures through the petrous bone are either horizontal or vertical. Horizontal (longitudinal) fractures are caused by blows to the temporal or parietal region. The fracture may be in any plane. It is best viewed with coronal or transaxial high resolution CT scanning. More than one plane of scanning may be required for detection of these fractures. There may be tearing of the membranes of the external auditory canal and tympanic cavity or ossicular dislocation. Patients may have bleeding from the external canal, otorrhea, or conductive hearing loss (Fig. 7-24).

Vertical fractures of the petrous bone result from an occipital blow. The fracture is orthogonal to the petrous pyramid and is usually in the sagittal plane. It can be identified with tomography or CT scans in either the frontal or transaxial plane. The tympanic membrane is usually intact, and therefore otorrhea does not occur. If the fracture passes through the cochlea and vestibular structures, there is sensorineural hearing loss. CN VII and CN VIII may be damaged.

A severe complication of a basal fracture is a CSF fistula into the sinuses. It is recognized clinically by the

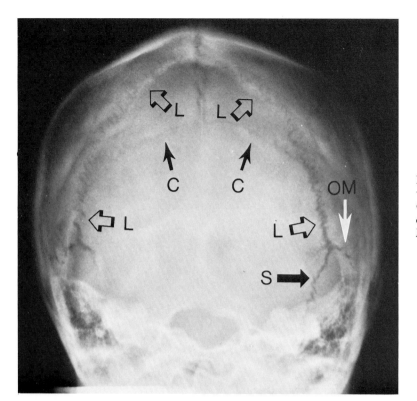

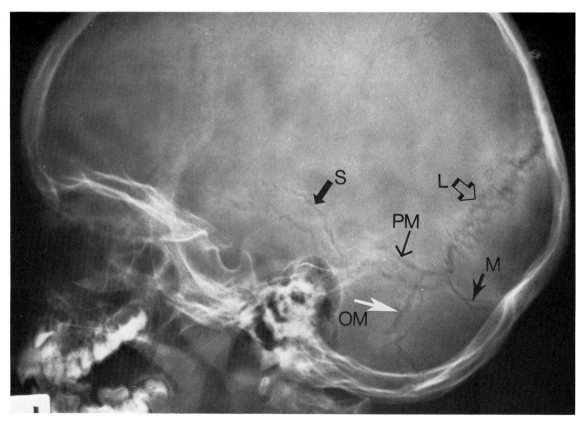

Fig. 7-22 Cranial sutures. (A) Towne view. **(B)** Lateral view. L = lambdoid; C = coronal; S = squamosal; OM = occipitomastoid; PM = parietomastoid; M = mendosal.

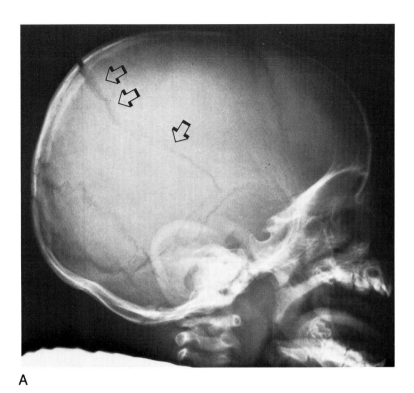

A

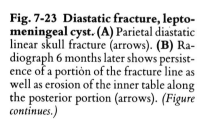

Fig. 7-23 Diastatic fracture, lepto-meningeal cyst. (A) Parietal diastatic linear skull fracture (arrows). **(B)** Radiograph 6 months later shows persistence of a portion of the fracture line as well as erosion of the inner table along the posterior portion (arrows). *(Figure continues.)*

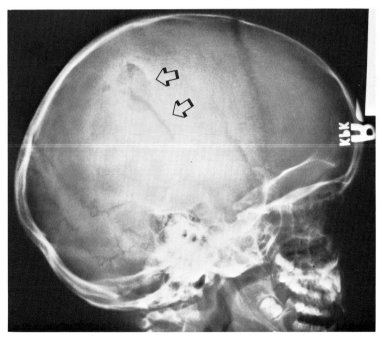

B

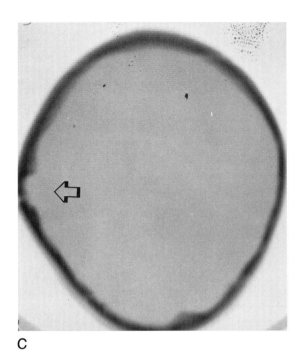

C

Fig. 7-23 *(Continued)*. **(C)** CT scan shows persistence of the fracture line with erosion of the inner table and some local thickening of the calvarium (arrow).

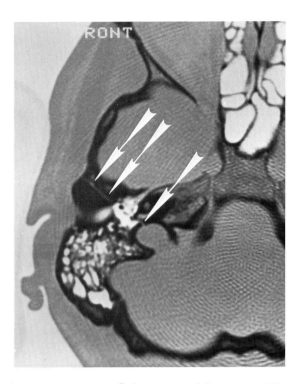

Fig. 7-24 Fracture of the temporal bone. An oblique fracture line is seen in the temporal bone passing through the middle ear cavity and into the lateral margin of the jugular foramen. High-resolution CT scanning with bone windows is the best method for demonstrating basal skull fractures.

presence of rhinorrhea or otorrhea. The site of the fistula must be determined for successful surgical repair. A basal fracture may cross several sinus cells, and the actual site of the fistula may be indeterminate. Fluid within a sinus is an indirect sign (Fig. 7-25) but may be present owing to other causes (hemorrhage, a prolonged recumbent position, or a nasotracheal tube). Special studies may be necessary.

Positive-contrast CT cisternography, done with the patient in the position that produces a leak, most frequently demonstrates the fistula. Contrast accumulating within a sinus cell is diagnostic. Sometimes repeated studies are necessary, occasionally with the use of positive pressure in the subarachnoid space. Demonstration of herniation of brain into the sinus is rare but diagnostic. Radionuclide cisternography with nasal pledgets can be used to lateralize the fistula if other studies are not informative.

Frontal Sinus Fractures

Fractures through the anterior wall of the frontal sinus, if depressed, may need surgical cosmetic repair but do not affect the intracranial structures. However, it is

important to recognize a fracture of the posterior wall of the frontal sinus as these fractures present a risk for development of meningitis or CSF fistula (Fig. 7-26).

VASCULAR INJURIES OF THE HEAD AND NECK

Intracranial and extracranial vascular injuries are relatively rare but important. Because angiography is no longer routinely performed in the acute trauma situation, vessel injuries may go undiagnosed. They are important because of their associated high mortality rate and the potential for repair. Vascular injury is suspected and angiography considered when there is (1) a history of a blunt or penetrating injury to the neck; (2) a hematoma in the neck; (3) a focal neurologic deficit suggesting a stroke or TIA; or (4) a local bruit.

Extracranial vascular injury may be the result of direct laceration of the vessel against a bone, especially

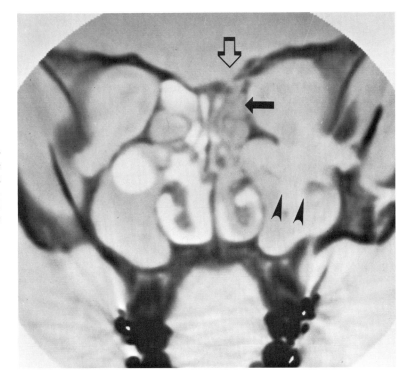

Fig. 7-25 Fracture through ethmoid plate. The diastatic fracture through the ethmoid plate can be seen on the coronal CT scan (open arrow). Fluid is present in an ethmoid air cell (arrow). A blow-out fracture of the orbit is also seen (arrowheads).

Fig. 7-26 Fracture of the posterior wall of the frontal sinus. An oblique fracture line courses through the posterior wall of the right frontal sinus and orbital roof (arrow).

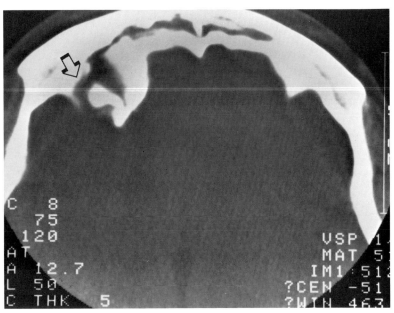

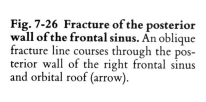

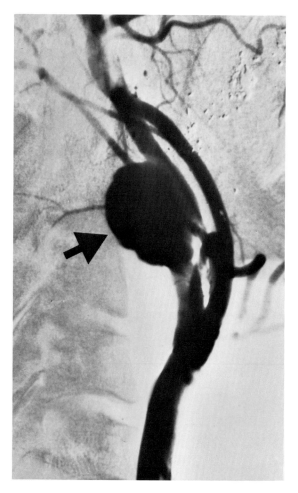

Fig. 7-27 Pseudoaneurysm of the internal carotid artery. Vascular injury (arrow) may follow blunt trauma, gunshot wounds, or knife wounds.

the transverse process of C2. Dissection of the ICA may result from stretching. Intimal injury may lead to thrombosis, which can embolize or progress to vessel occlusion. Adventitial injury results in pseudoaneurysm formation. The apparent trauma that causes the vascular injury may be minimal.

Selective angiography of the extracranial vessels is generally necessary for the diagnosis. The usual findings are pseudoaneurysm at the injury site (Fig. 7-27), mural hematoma with vessel constriction, or total occlusion from intimal injury or thrombosis. Two orthogonal views are needed to exclude injury of a vessel.

Intracranial vascular injury may result from a basal or depressed fracture, internal herniation of the brain, or a direct penetrating injury (bullet or knife wound). Dissection may occur, particularly of the middle cerebral artery. Traumatic aneurysms may be found in the cortical vessels over the convexities or at the base of the skull. Depressed fractures in the region of the posterior portion of the sagittal sinus or the transverse sinuses often cause excessive hemorrhage from dural sinus laceration or occlusion of the sinus with resultant hemorrhagic brain infarction, frequently accompanied by intractable seizures. Dural arteriovenous fistula may be seen. Intracranial angiography is performed when there are infarctions not directly explained by the trauma.

Injury to the cavernous portion of the internal carotid artery is particularly apt to result from severe head trauma. Often there is a fracture of the sphenoid bone, but not necessarily. A carotid-cavernous fistula occurs when laceration of the internal carotid artery or one of its small cavernous dural branches allows communication between the carotid artery and the venous channels of the cavernous sinus. If the rupture is contained by a noncommunicating compartment of the cavernous sinus, a pseudoaneurysm results (Fig. 7-28).

The clinical diagnosis of a carotid-cavernous fistula is usually straightforward. The rush of blood to the cavernous sinus generally drains anteriorly to the ophthalmic veins, causing proptosis, chemosis, bruit, ophthalmoplegia, loss of vision, and headache. Despite the large amount of blood flow that may occur through the fistula, focal cerebral neurologic deficit is rare. Angiography in patients with a carotid-cavernous fistula is done with rapid serial filming so the size and location of the fistula can be determined. The fistula may be successfully treated by catheter placement of detachable balloons.

Gunshot Wounds

Gunshot wounds of the head are becoming more common in civilians, especially in the United States. Military and civilian wounds usually differ, mainly because of the slower bullet velocity of the common civilian weapons. The higher velocity missiles used by the military are much more lethal, and a direct hit in the head almost always produces death. Unfortunately, military weapons are becoming much more available for civilian use.

The amount of injury produced in the brain follow-

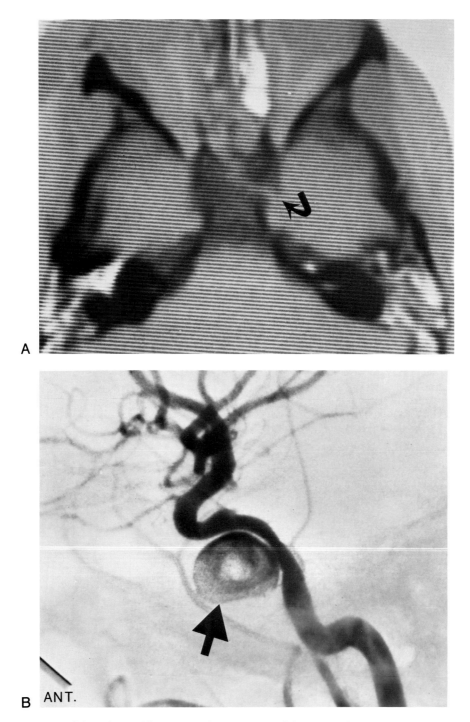

Fig. 7-28 Fracture of the sphenoid bone, pseudoaneurysm of the internal carotid artery. (A) CT scan with bone windowing shows a fracture through the sphenoid bone displaced into the left cavernous sinus (arrow). **(B)** ICA angiography demonstrates a pseudoaneurysm of the cavernous segment (arrow). If the ICA rupture had been into a different compartment of the cavernous sinus, a carotid-cavernous fistula might have resulted.

ing penetration by a bullet is directly proportional to the amount of kinetic energy deposited from the bullet into the tissues. The amount of kinetic energy of a moving bullet is proportional to the mass of the bullet and the square of its velocity. The impact and penetration of the bullet causes a shock wave that produces an instantaneous rise in tissue pressure. Although the shock wave lasts only several microseconds, the pressure is high and is transmitted to the central axis of the brain, often causing deep irreversible pontine damage or even herniation of brain tissue through the tentorium. Thus a relatively peripheral bullet tracking can produce immediate death if enough energy is deposited.

There is cavitation of the tissue along the missile path. A permanent cavity is produced that nearly corresponds with the width of the bullet fragment. Also, a transient cavitation is produced more peripheral to the permanent tract, the width of which is proportional to

the velocity of the bullet; it may be up to 30 times the width of the central cavity. Because the missile slows as it traverses tissue, the path of destruction is more or less conical in shape, being widest at the site of entry. Deformation of the bullet or bullet yaw may alter the shape of the path of damage in an unpredictable way.

When the bullet enters the skull, bone fragments are driven inward but always to a lesser distance than the final resting place of the bullet. Therefore the bone fragments are embedded in the part of the brain that is closest to the site of entry. If the bullet exits the opposite side of the skull, the path of the bullet is nearly a straight line from the entry to the exit site. If the bullet does not possess enough kinetic energy to penetrate the opposite skull table, the bullet may ricochet backward and come to rest away from the expected path. In this situation, the path of the bullet cannot be determined with certainty. Normally, in the civilian situation, only large-caliber bullets fired at close range exit the skull.

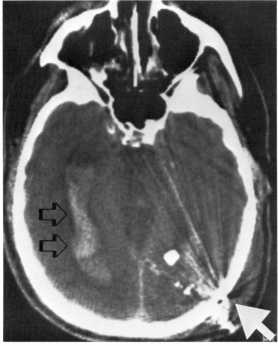
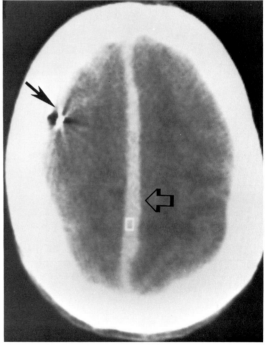

A B

Fig. 7-29 Low velocity gunshot wound. (A) The bullet has entered the left occipital region (white arrow). Intraventricular blood is seen in the right temporal and occipital horn (open black arrow). **(B)** The bullet fragment has come to rest against the inner table of the right posterior frontal bone (black arrow). Interhemispheric blood is also present (open arrow), and there is diffuse brain edema.

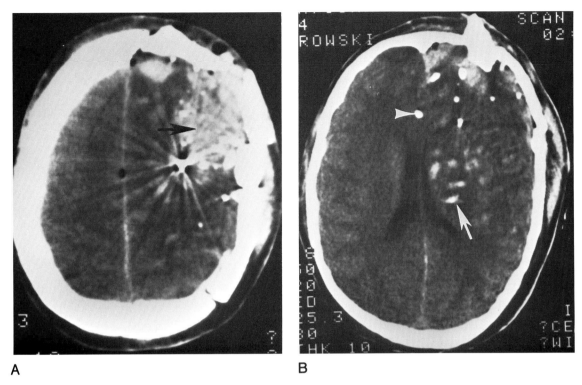

Fig. 7-30 High velocity gunshot wound. (A) CT scan superiorly near the tract of the bullet demonstrates the explosive force produced by a high velocity missile. The comminuted fracture fragments are displaced outward, and there is a large hemorrhage (arrow) in severely contused brain. **(B)** CT scan at a lower level, some distance from the bullet tract, demonstrates the punctate hemorrhages of multiple axonal injuries (arrow) and severe acute brain swelling. Small bullet fragments are scattered widely (arrowhead).

The site of the bullet fragments must be reported with accuracy, as they must be removed if possible (Figs. 7-29 and 7-30).

Hemorrhage occurs along the track of the bullet because of laceration of the large and small vessels. Large vessels at the base of the skull may be lacerated completely, resulting in massive hemorrhage and infarction. Incomplete lacerations of major arteries may result in aneurysms or pseudoaneurysms. Special note is made of bullet wounds in the region of the sagittal or transverse sinuses, as there may be life-threatening hemorrhage or thrombosis. Subdural or epidural hematoma may result from rupture of bridging veins or laceration of cortical or dural arteries.

It is important to identify the site of entry so the surgeon may be directed to the site of dural tear. This point is especially true for a bullet that has passed through a paranasal sinus, as the risk for subsequent infection is increased.

Plain skull radiographs and CT scanning of the brain are the basic neuroradiologic examinations. The prognosis of intracranial gunshot wounds is poor and for the most part depends on the neurologic conditions and the state of consciousness at the time of evaluation.

CHILD ABUSE

In the United States there are more than one million cases of reported child abuse annually, and about 50 percent of them involve inflicted trauma. It is the group with bodily injury that comes to attention of the radiologist. Most of the children with head injuries are under 2 years of age. Cerebral damage can result from many factors, including direct impact, shaking, whiplash, asphyxia, and vascular occlusion due to strangulation. Clinically visible signs of injury and a history of injury are often lacking, so the responsibility may fall to the

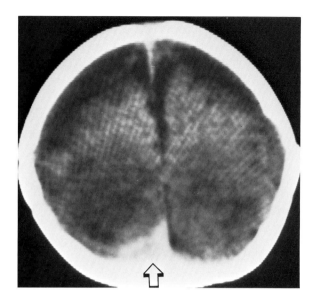

Fig. 7-31 Child abuse; interhemispheric subdural blood collection. CT scan shows a high density blood collection in the posterior interhemispheric fissure extending over the right convexity (arrow). This finding has a high association with inflicted injury.

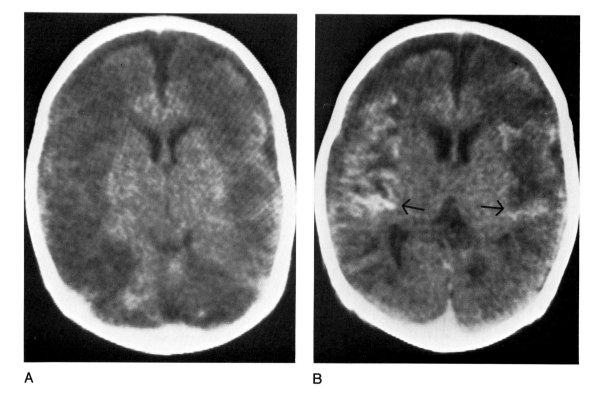

A   B

Fig. 7-32 Child abuse; anoxic/ischemic encephalopathy. (A) There is peripheral low density with general preservation of normal density of the deep basal ganglionic and posterior fossa structures. Extracerebral fluid collections are also present. **(B)** A few days later there is hemorrhage into the ischemic tissue (arrows).

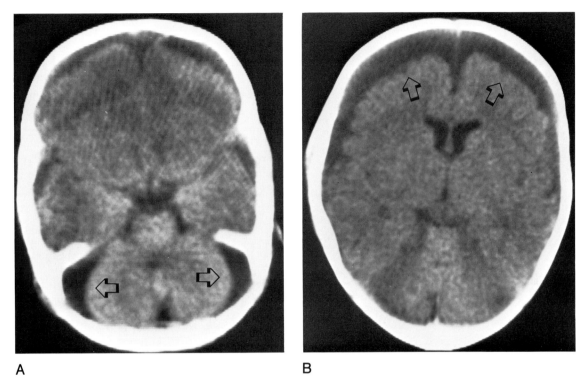

A   B

Fig. 7-33 Child abuse; low density extracerebral collections.

radiologist to suggest child abuse. A key component to diagnosis is the "discrepant history," i.e., the description of an injury that does not match the clinical or radiographic findings.

The main imaging modalities used to evaluate possible child abuse include plain film radiography, CT scanning, and MRI. Ultrasonography and radionuclide scanning are sometimes of additional value.

The primary imaging technique here is the CT scan, as it is sensitive for detecting intracranial hemorrhage and skull fracture. The most common finding is subarachnoid hemorrhage (SAH), seen in about 75 percent of abused children with intracranial head injury. It may be subtle, seen only as a slight increase in the density of the subarachnoid space. SAH in the interhemispheric fissure is common, but blood may also be seen in the basal cisterns, sylvian fissures, and cerebral sulci. CT scanning is superior to MRI for detecting SAH. In infants, SAH is far more common in the child abuse situation than with trauma due to other causes, such as falls or car accidents. Whenever SAH is seen in a child under 2 years old, child abuse must be considered.

Interhemispheric subdural hematoma (SDH) is also a common finding with child abuse (Fig. 7-31). It is seldom found with other causes of head injury. It appears as a unilateral interhemispheric region of high attenuation, usually posteriorly. It has a flat medial border but a slightly convex lateral border. It may extend over the posterior convexity of the brain, or the tentorium. In the chronic phase, there is usually a small residual low density region, confirming the diagnosis. It may be impossible to differentiate an interhemispheric SDH from SAH. However, this point is not a particularly important distinction, as both blood collections have the same diagnostic implication.

It is important to differentiate interhemispheric blood from a normally dense falx. The normal falx may appear especially dense if there is adjacent brain edema. The falx is generally much thinner than blood collections, but repeat scans may be necessary to make this important distinction. It is equally important to avoid overdiagnosis of child abuse.

Cerebral anoxic or ischemic encephalopathy may occur as a result of child abuse. Resulting from coma, seizures, aspiration, or strangulation, it is reflected in the brain as diffuse cerebral edema, similar to global

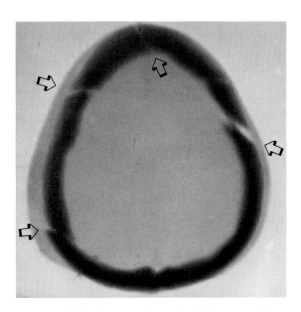

Fig. 7-34 Child abuse; multiple skull fractures. Multiple skull fractures (arrows) have a high association with abuse in infants.

ischemic encephalopathy due to any cause. Most commonly, the cerebral hemispheres have uniform low density with loss of gray–white matter distinction. The thalami, cerebellum, and brain stem are usually spared and remain of relatively normal density (Fig. 7-32). Sometimes the pattern is that of near-drowning or carbon monoxide poisoning, with low density seen in the basal ganglia (see Ch. 2).

Focal infarction may result from strangulation, due to occlusion of the carotid artery in the neck. The infarction usually involves multiple vessel territories supplied by the internal carotid artery. Spontaneous hemiplegia of childhood due to cerebrovascular disease usually involves only the internal capsule or a single cerebral vessel distribution.

Focal cerebral parenchymal hemorrhages occur, most of which represent contusion. A well circumscribed triangular hemorrhage pointing toward the ventricle indicates laceration of the brain. Low density extracerebral fluid collections represent hygromas, which are common following child abuse (Fig. 7-33).

Skull fractures result from direct impact trauma. The more severe or comminuted a fracture in a child, the more likely it is the result of inflicted injury (Fig. 7-34). Radiography of other regions is worthwhile and may reveal additional fractures of different ages. This exam-

ination includes the ribs, clavicles, spine, and long bones. Radionuclide bone scanning can identify otherwise occult regions of injury but cannot give the age of the lesion. Organ injury also may occur. MRI is used in cases of suspected child abuse when the CT scan is nondiagnostic. Small subdural blood collections or regions of infarction, axonal injury, or contusion may be seen with MRI that cannot be seen with the CT scan.

Atrophy is often seen after head injury caused by abuse. It is particularly severe after anoxia or infarction. The ventricles may become large. The brain damage of inflicted injury is often irreparable, and post-traumatic neurologic dysfunction is common and often devastating.

SUGGESTED READINGS

Allen WE III, Kier EL, Rothman SLG: Pitfalls in the evaluation of skull trauma: a review. Radiol Clin North Am 11:479, 1973

Cooper PR (ed): Head Injury. Williams & Wilkins, Baltimore, 1982

Eskridge JM: Interventional neuroradiology: state of the art. Radiology 172:991, 1989

Fobben ES, Grossman RI, Atlas SW, et al: MR characteristics of subdural hematomas and hygromas at 1.5 T. AJNR 10:687, 1989

Gentry LR, Godersky JC, Thompson B: MR imaging of head trauma: review of the distribution and radiopathologic features of traumatic lesions. AJNR 9:101, 1988

Gentry LR, Godersky JC, Thompson BH: Traumatic brain stem injury: MR imaging. Radiology 171:177, 1989

Gentry LR, Godersky JC, Thompson B, et al: Prospective comparative study of intermediate-field MR and CT in the evaluation of closed head trauma. AJNR 9:91, 1988

Genieser NB, Becker MH: Head trauma in children. Radiol Clin North Am 12:333, 1974

Kelly AB, Zimmerman RD, et al: Head trauma: comparison of MR and CT experience. AJNR 9:699, 1988

North CM, Ahmadi J, Segall HD, Zec C-S: Penetrating vascular injuries of the face and neck: clinical and angiographic correlation. AJNR 7:855, 1986

Williams A: Trauma. In Williams A, Haughton VM (eds): Cranial Computed Tomography. CV Mosby, St. Louis, 1985

Wright JW Jr: Trauma of the ear. Radiol Clin North Am 12:527, 1974

Zimmerman RD, Balaniuk LT: Head trauma. In Heinz RE (ed): The Clinical Neurosciences: Neuroradiology. Churchill Livingstone, New York, 1984

Zimmerman RD, Danziger A: Extracerebral trauma. Radiol Clin North Am 20:105, 1982

8

Infections

PYOGENIC INFECTIONS

Pyogenic (pus-forming) bacterial infections of the CNS occur by direct spread from contiguous structures, hematogenous seeding, or trauma. The infection may be seen in many forms, such as meningitis, ventriculitis, cerebritis, brain abscess, and subdural and epidural empyema. Although the incidence of pyogenic infections of the CNS has decreased, the disease is still important and causes significant morbidity.

Meningitis

Meningitis is an inflammation of the arachnoid, pia, and CSF. It is the most common form of pyogenic infection of the CNS. Most often it is a result of hematogenous seeding, but it may result from trauma, direct extension from a sinus infection or pre-existing brain abscess, or a congenital fistula. The etiologic agent of the infection depends on the age of the victim and the clinical setting in which the infection occurs. Neonates are most commonly infected with *Escherichia coli* or a group B streptococcus. Infants up to age 5 are most often infected with *Hemophilus influenzae*. If infection occurs with these agents later in life, it suggests a congenital neurologic defect that allows direct infection of the CSF. In those over age 5 and throughout adulthood, *Neisseria meningitidis* and *Streptococcus pneumoniae* are the predominant agents. After trauma and surgery, *Staphylococcus aureus* and gram-negative organisms are most commonly found.

The purulent material is widely distributed throughout the subarachnoid space and ventricles (ventriculitis). Ventricular empyema (pus-filled ventricle) is

rare. Brain abscess does not result from meningitis, as the pia is an effective barrier to the spread of infection. However, underlying brain edema may be present and can become severe enough to cause increased intracranial pressure and herniation. A cortical thrombophlebitis, or secondary arteritis may result in brain infarction. This problem is particularly likely with *H. influenzae* and may progress to gross devastation of the cerebral hemispheres despite appropriate treatment of the infection. Hydrocephalus may result from obstruction by pus, but it tends to be mild and occurs almost exclusively in children. Sterile subdural effusions may occur, most frequently in infants and most often after *H. influenzae* infection. Subdural empyema as a result of meningitis is rare.

The diagnosis of meningitis is best accomplished by lumbar puncture and CSF analysis. Imaging during the acute phase of the infection is of little use, as the results are usually normal or demonstrate only a subtle hydrocephalus. If contrast enhancement is used with MRI or CI scanning, there may be enhancement of the meningeal surface, particularly at the base of the brain. This picture is indistinguishable from the enhancement that may be seen with acute subarachnoid hemorrhage or meningeal carcinomatosis (Fig. 8-1). With severe infections, the cerebral sulci may appear widened owing to gross pus.

Imaging is used primarily to define complications and the underlying etiologic process. Studies are performed on patients who develop seizures, focal neurologic signs, persistent fever, an enlarging head, or signs of increased intracranial pressure. A nonenhanced MRI or CT scan is preferred and should include the paranasal and mastoid sinuses. Hydrocephalus is detected by the

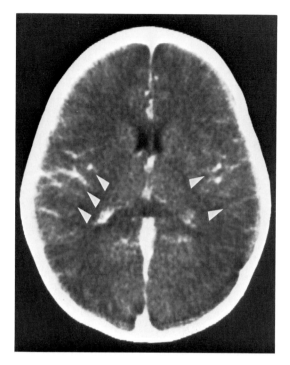

Fig. 8-1 Meningitis, meningeal contrast enhancement, CT scan. There is enhancement of the meningeal surface of the sulci (arrowheads). This pattern of enhancement can also be seen with SAH and meningeal carcinomatosis.

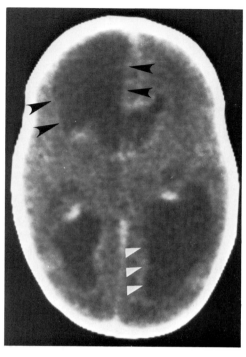

Fig. 8-2 Meningitis, infarction, and hydrocephalus. A large right frontal region of hypodensity represents infarction (black arrowheads). The large ventricles represent hydrocephalus and developing porencephaly (white arrowheads).

enlargement of the ventricles. Special attention is directed to observing any septations within the ventricles, as they may loculate fluid and cause persistent infection. An entire ventricle may become isolated by adhesions and remain enlarged after routine lateral ventricular shunting. Focal brain abnormalities almost always represent ischemia or infarction and may be global and severe (Fig. 8-2). Contrast is used to define etiology if the diagnosis is uncertain. Enhancement may occur in the gyri, representing loss of the blood-brain barrier, but it does not necessarily represent infarction or infection (Fig. 8-3). Ependymal enhancement, however, does represent significant ventriculitis (Fig. 8-4).

Subdural effusions are seen as crescent-shaped fluid collections nearly equivalent to CSF density over the frontal and parietal lobes (Fig. 8-5). They occur almost exclusively in children. Those which are infected (rare empyema) show contrast enhancement along the inner thickened membrane. Severe edema with herniation is recognized by the compression of the lateral ventricles and the obliteration of the basal cisterns. MRI shows simple effusions as CSF-equivalent intensity and empyema as a high protein solution with very high T_2 signal.

Computed tomography and MRI are both useful for defining a possible cause of the meningitis. Multiplanar scanning through the paranasal sinuses, inner ear, or mastoids may detect sinusitis, CSF fistula, encephalocele, otitis media, or cholesteatoma. Bone windows are essential. MRI may better show small effusions and ischemia. Skull radiography is useful in post-traumatic situations. Angiography may show the changes of vasculitis but has little practical usefulness. Mycotic aneurysm following meningitis is rare. CT scans and radionuclide cisternography may help with the diagnosis of CSF fistula (see CSF rhinorrhea, Ch. 7).

Cerebritis and Brain Abscess

Brain abscess is encapsulated or free pus within the brain parenchyma. The abscess may vary in size from a microscopic focus to a large region of suppurative ne-

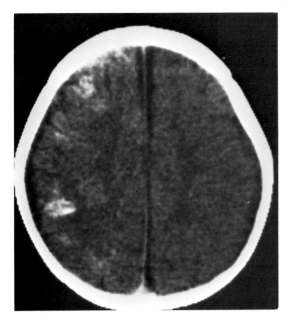

Fig. 8-3 Meningitis, gyral enhancement. This picture indicates damage to the blood-brain barrier but not necessarily infarction. It must not be interpreted as cerebritis.

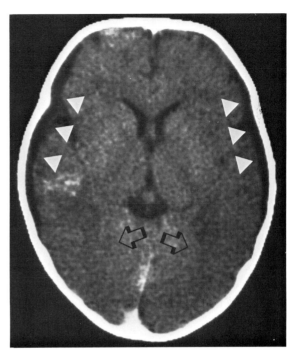

Fig. 8-5 Subdural effusion. Bilateral low density fluid accumulations of CSF-equivalent density are present. They represent effusions (arrowheads). Additionally, note the low density abnormalities present bilaterally in the posterior temporal and occipital lobes, representing ischemia (open arrows).

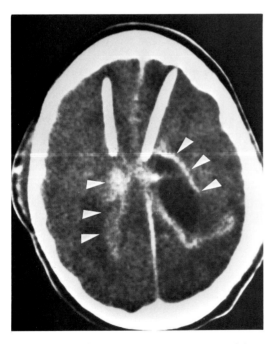

Fig. 8-4 Ventriculitis. Contrast enhancement of the ependyma is seen in a patient with ventriculitis (arrowheads). Bilateral shunt catheters are present, but the left shunt is malfunctioning.

crosis. *Cerebritis* refers to a region of infection and inflammatory response but without associated necrosis. The abscess may be single or multiple and always occurs within the white matter, sparing completely the gray matter. It is most common in the cerebral hemispheres, thought it may also occur in the cerebellum (almost always a direct extension from otologic infection), thalamus, pons, and pituitary gland. MRI and CT scans are the primary imaging modalities used.

The infection begins with local inflammation (cerebritis) limited to the white matter. This area is surrounded by vasogenic edema. CT scanning and MRI with contrast show enhancement in the region of infection, (Fig. 8-6). MRI, without or with contrast, is more sensitive for detection of this phase. The edema of inflammation is seen as high signal intensity on T_2-weighted images. Small hemorrhages may be detected on the T_1-weighted images.

With progression, central necrosis develops in regions of cerebritis. After about 10 days, the abscess becomes walled off by a reticular-collagen capsule that

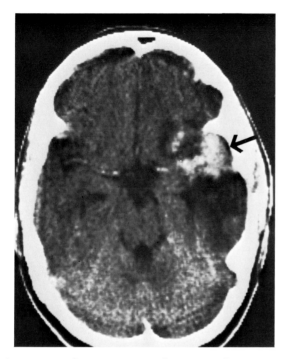

Fig. 8-6 Cerebritis. A region of contrast enhancement is present in the left anterior temporal and posterior frontal lobe (arrow). There is considerable surrounding edema, particularly in the left temporal lobe.

is formed by fibroblasts migrating into the region. With virulent infection or immunocompromise, the encapsulation takes longer and is less complete or absent. The capsule is always thinner on the ventricular side of the abscess, and infection may escape medially to form daughter abscesses or reach the ventricle to cause ependymitis. Ventriculitis results if pus spills into the ventricular cavity.

On CT scan, the capsule is represented by a ring of contrast enhancement (Fig. 8-7). It is impossible to determine the maturity of the encapsulation solely by the nature of the contrast-enhanced ring, but it is presumed to develop sometime during the 14- to 21-day stage of the abscess. The central low density accurately represents the abscess cavity. Ependymitis is indicated by contrast enhancement of the ventricular surface. Ventriculitis from actual spillage of inflammatory cells and bacteria into the ventricular CSF is indicated by ventricular enlargement and intense enhancement of the choroid plexus. The ventricular fluid may become more dense owing to accumulation of pus.

T_1-weighted MRI shows the capsule as an isointense ring separating the central low intensity abscess cavity and surrounding edema (Fig. 8-7). On the T_2-weighted images the pus of the central abscess cavity is seen as very high intensity separated from the surrounding edema by the hypointense capsule. Gd-DTPA results in very high signal intensity of the capsule on T_1-weighted images following the principles of contrast enhancement in CT scanning.

The peripheral edema is maximum at the beginning of the abscess stage but subsides with the formation of the capsule. A decrease in the diameter of the ring and the size of the central cavity indicates a favorable response to treatment. An abscess may recur after complete CT scan disappearance, so follow-up scans are necessary for up to 2 years.

Cerebral angiography shows an abscess as a well circumscribed ring-like "blush," without tumor neovascularity (Fig. 8-8). The primary use of angiography was for differentiating abscess from tumor, but this task is better done with needle biopsy. Radionuclide brain scanning has no inherent advantage over the other modalities, although gadolinium- or indium-labeled white blood cell studies may differentiate abscess from tumor.

An abscess may occur by direct extension from cranial sinuses (Fig. 8-9), trauma, or metastatic seeding (Fig. 8-10), particularly from infection in the lungs. For a few, no source of infection is found. Brain abscess occurs relatively infrequently with bacterial endocarditis. The most common organisms isolated are aerobic and anaerobic streptococci. Staphylococcal infection occurs most often after trauma but may be seen in intravenous drug users as well. Mixed infections are common.

Percutaneous needle aspiration of the abscess may be done with CT or MRI guidance. Material can be obtained for culture through a needle as small as 22 gauge. Anaerobic organisms must be handled efficiently so they grow in vitro. Ideally, the microbiologist is present to transfer the aspirate, so all significant organisms will be later identified. Complete aspiration of the abscess cavity may be curative, obviating surgical excision (Fig. 8-11).

Differentiation between abscess, glioblastoma, and metastasis is at best difficult if not impossible with either CT scans or MRI. The shape of the lesion, the thinness of the ring enhancement and its regularity, and the density of the central fluid may suggest an

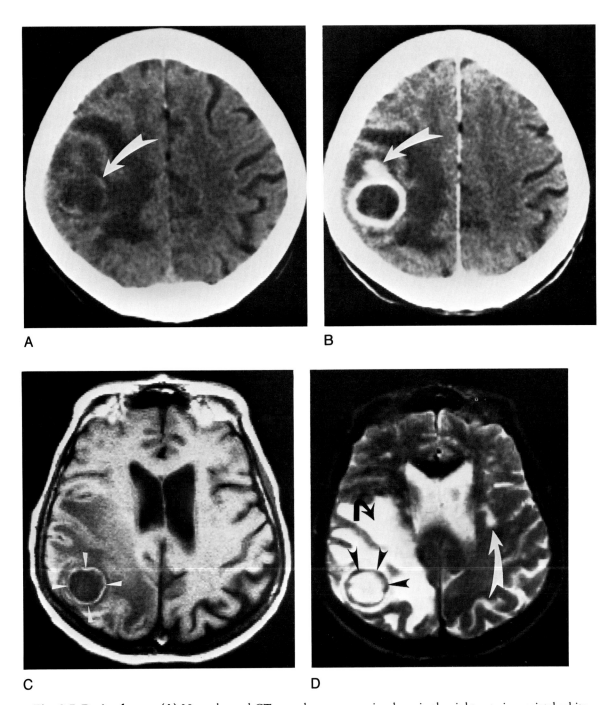

A

B

C

D

Fig. 8-7 Brain abscess. (A) Nonenhanced CT scan shows vasogenic edema in the right anterior parietal white matter. The isointense ring of the abscess capsule can be seen (white arrow). **(B)** Contrast-enhanced study shows a thick but uniformly enhancing capsule with the beginnings of a daughter abscess anteriorly (arrow). The enhancement of abscess is typically circular and nearly uniform except along the medial surface. **(C)** T_1-weighted MRI shows the abscess cavity as hypointense surrounded by an isointense capsule (arrowheads). **(D)** T_2-weighted MRI shows the high intensity white matter edema (black arrow) and a high intensity central pus collection. The capsule is hypointense (arrowheads). A small region of cerebritis is present in the left hemispheric white matter (white arrow).

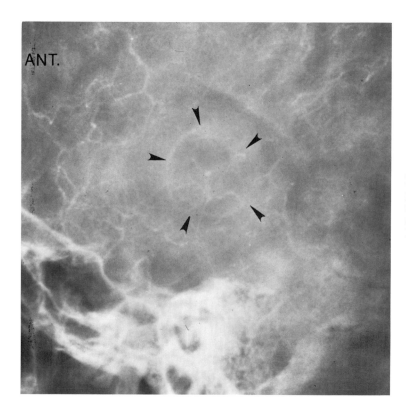

Fig. 8-8 Brain abscess, angiography. The capillary phase of the carotid angiography shows the abscess capsule as a faint ring-like "blush" (arrowheads) with surrounding edema.

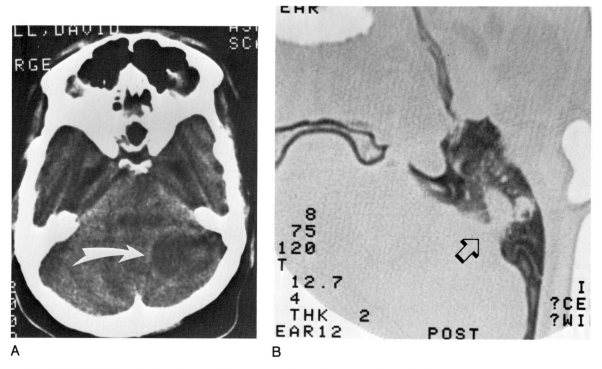

A

B

Fig. 8-9 "Otitic" cerebellar abscess. (A) Contrast-enhanced CT scan shows faintly enhancing ring of a large left cerebellar abscess (arrow). **(B)** Destruction of the temporal bone from purulent mastoiditis (arrow).

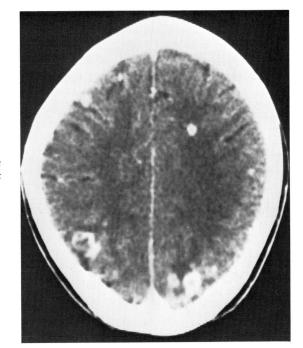

Fig. 8-10 Multiple metastatic brain abscesses. Multiple brain abscesses are seen in various stages. Multiple metastatic tumors could also produce this same picture.

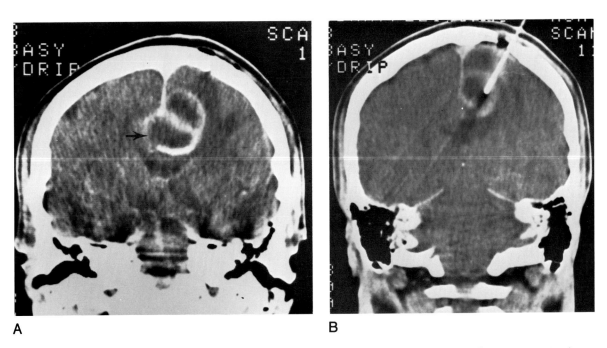

A   B

Fig. 8-11 Percutaneous needle aspiration of brain abscess. (A) Irregular contrast-enhancing mass in the medial parietal lobe extending into the corpus callosum. Note the deficient capsule (arrow). It is impossible to differentiate between an abscess and glioma in this case. **(B)** Needle aspiration of the central cavity.

abscess; but the diagnosis cannot be made with certainty. Gas within the central cavity is the only pathognomonic finding of abscess. The diagnosis of brain abscess must be considered whenever ring-like enhancing lesions are seen (see block, page 154).

Septic Embolization

Septic thromboembolization to the brain commonly occurs in association with subacute bacterial endocarditis (SBE). About 15 percent of those with SBE are affected. The embolus causes infarction that is sometimes hemorrhagic, but abscess rarely occurs. About 5 percent of those with septic embolization develop a mycotic aneurysm, most commonly in a peripheral branch of the middle cerebral artery. Hemorrhage in the brain, or subarachnoid or subdural space suggests its presence (Fig. 8-12). To identify the aneurysm prior to rupture, angiography is recommended in all those who have diagnosed septic emboli.

Subdural Empyema

Subdural empyema is a rare but grave form of intracranial infection, with pus collecting within the subdural space. The infection is rapidly progressive, and emergency surgical drainage is usually required. Most commonly it results from infection within the frontal sinuses or middle ear. Other causes include trauma, surgery, septicemia, and osteomyelitis of the calvarium.

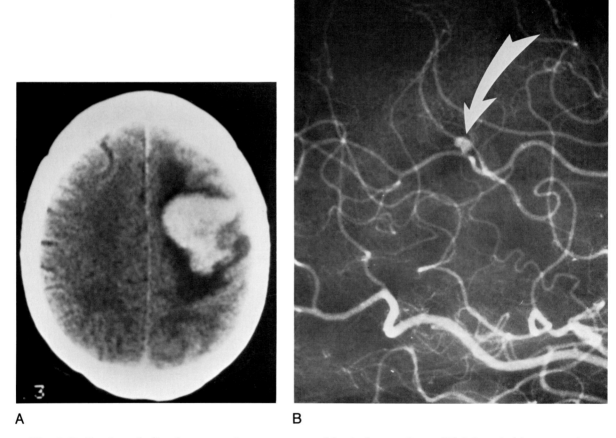

A   B

Fig. 8-12 Septic embolization, mycotic aneurysm, and brain hemorrhage. (A) Subcortical hematoma is present in the left anterior parietal lobe. **(B)** Small mycotic aneurysm in a peripheral left middle cerebral artery branch (arrow).

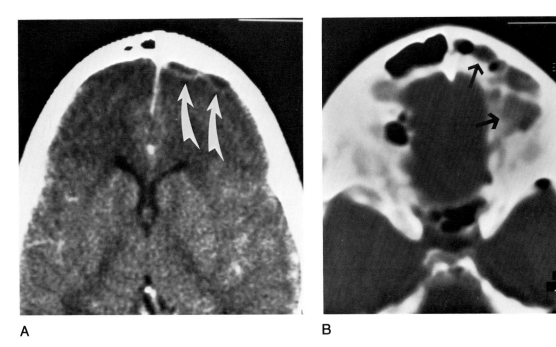

A   B

Fig. 8-13 Subdural empyema. (A) Small extracerebral fluid collection is seen over the left frontal lobe with membrane enhancement (arrows). The findings are subtle but important. **(B)** Left frontal sinusitis (arrows), which was the cause of the subdural empyema.

On CT scan the empyema appears as an extracerebral hypodense collection of fluid over the convexity or within the interhemispheric fissure of slightly greater density than CSF. Rarely, it is along the tentorium. Contrast enhances the inner membrane (Fig. 8-13). Over the convexity, large collections may have the same appearance as a chronic subdural hematoma or epidural abscess. Bone windows may show osteomyelitis. On MRI the collection is seen as low intensity on T_1- and as very high intensity on T_2-weighted images. The signal characteristics are those of a proteinaceous fluid.

Epidural Empyema

The findings for epidural empyema by CT scan are similar to those for subdural empyema except that there is usually a convex margin medially (Fig. 8-14). The epidural collections do not extend into the interhemispheric fissure. The etiologic factors are the same as for subdural empyema, although the epidural infection most commonly occurs following craniotomy (Fig. 8-15). Angiography may define the epidural location of

extracerebral fluid if the dural sinuses are elevated away from the inner table of the calvarium. Epidural infections do not advance nearly as rapidly as those within the subdural space.

Major Dural Sinus Thrombosis

The dural sinuses may become thrombosed because of infection. This situation occurs when the sinuses are adjacent to epidural or subdural empyema. The venous sinus thrombosis produces local brain infarction usually hemorrhagic. On CT scan the sinus is seen not to fill normally with contrast, and on MRI there is signal intensity within the thrombosed vein. Care must be taken with MRI diagnosis of thrombosis, as flow-related enhancement effects can produce the same appearance. Angiography shows sinus occlusion and collateral venous flow (see Chapter 2).

Cavenous sinus thrombosis may be caused by facial, orbital, or paranasal sinus suppuration. Usually, the afflicted person is severely ill with high fever, edema, and cyanosis of the upper face and eyelid. There may be ophthalmoplegia. MRI shows signal intensity within

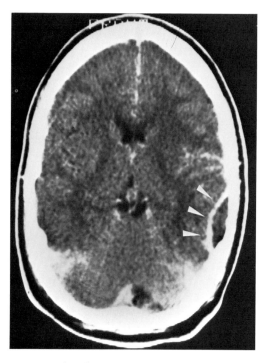

Fig. 8-14 Epidural empyema. Low density extracerebral fluid collection is seen over the left posterior temporal lobe. There is a convex medial border with membrane enhancement (arrowheads). This collection was secondary to mastoiditis.

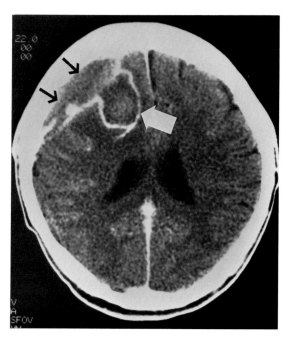

Fig. 8-15 Epidural abscess, postcraniotomy. Relatively high density extracerebral fluid collection is present over the right frontal lobe with an enhancing medial margin (black arrows). Abscess was also found within the tumor bed (white arrow). This same appearance can be found with sterile hemorrhagic postoperative collections.

the cavernous sinus instead of the low signal of "flow-void." The cavernous sinus does not become hyperintense after Gd-DTPA enhancement. Dynamic contrast CT scanning also shows an absence of contrast within the cavernous sinus.

VIRUS INFECTIONS

Acquired Immunodeficiency Syndrome

The acquired immunodeficiency syndrome (AIDS) was first described in 1981. Since that time the disease has exploded to epidemic proportion and is now considered one of the major health problems of the world. At the time of this writing, most persons with AIDS in the United States are homosexual or bisexual men, but heterosexual intravenous drug abusers of either sex are accounting for an increasing percentage. The remaining (10 percent) are infants of infected mothers, sexual partners of bisexual or drug-addicted men, persons who have received contaminated transfusions, or health workers accidentally infected by needle puncture or splashes of contaminated blood or body fluid. A few individuals with AIDS have no identifiable risk factor. AIDS is pandemic in much of Africa.

AIDS is caused by a retrovirus — human T-cell leukemia virus (HTLV III) — now called human immunodeficiency virus (HIV-I). Almost certainly, there are other subtypes of retrovirus that are responsible for the disease, and HIV-II has now been found associated with AIDS. These specific RNA retroviruses primarily infect the T-lymphocyte. Containing reverse transcriptase, the virus is capable of replicating its code into DNA and then inserting the DNA into the genetic code of the host cell. The end result is destruction of the T-cell-mediated defense functions within the body. Being immunocompromised, the host then develops unusual infections and tumors, some of which are far more common than others.

There are variations in the severity of the immuno-deficiency among patients with AIDS. Those with the greatest deficiency present with opportunistic infections, most commonly intrapulmonary *Pneumocystis carinii*. Those with less severe deficiency present with Kaposi's sarcoma and have a more favorable prognosis.

Neurologic involvement is common, found clinically in about 50 percent of patients and at autopsy in 80 percent. Neurologic complications occur earlier in those with more severe immunodeficiency. Neurologic involvement of any kind portends a severe clinical course and poor prognosis. About 10 percent of individuals with AIDS present with a neurologic complaint. Neurologic complication is seen less commonly with the AIDS-related complex (lymphadenopathy syndrome).

The neurologic complications of AIDS are protean. They are best studied with either CT scans or MRI. The more common afflictions are discussed separately below, and detailed accounts for some of the infections or tumors may be obtained in their respective sections elsewhere in this book. Multiple processes within the same patient are common, and in many instances it is impossible to diagnose an etiology from the imaging, serologic study, or clinical symptoms. Therefore biopsy of the CNS lesions becomes important for accurate diagnosis and timely treatment of the complications.

The AIDS–dementia complex, or subacute encephalitis, is the most common neurologic complication of those with AIDS, occurring in more than 30 percent. Minimal dementia (depression, social withdrawal) is the usual presenting symptom. The dementia relentlessly advances to a state of global mental impairment with behavioral and motor dysfunction, often leaving the patient with rudimentary intellect as death draws near. Rarely, a myelitis may occur.

Although a precise etiology cannot be given at this time, the syndrome correlates positively with the finding of HIV and to a lesser degree with cytomegalovirus (CMV) within monocytes in the cerebral parenchyma. The vacuolar lesions are primarily in the subcortical white matter and are variably associated with an inflammatory reaction. The subcortical gray matter (basal ganglia) may be involved.

The most common finding with both MRI and CT scans in the AIDS—dementia complex is generalized atrophy. There is a progressive enlargement of both the cerebral sulci and the ventricles. Additionally, MRI often demonstrates multifocal patchy or punctate re-

---

NEUROLOGIC COMPLICATIONS WITH AIDS (AUTOPSY DATA, COMBINED SERIES)

Infections
  Virus infections
    Common
      HIV subacute encephalitis (30%)
      Cytomegalovirus encephalitis (25%)
      HIV atypical meningitis (8%)
      ? HIV vacuolar myelopathy, etiology unknown to date (30%)
    Uncommon
      Herpes simplex encephalitis (3%)
      Progressive multifocal leukoencephalopathy (2%)
      Varicella-zoster encephalitis (2%)
  Nonvirus infections
    Common
      Toxoplasma gondii encephalitis (25%)
      Cryptococcus neoformans meningitis (12%)
    Uncommon
      Other fungi, mycobacteria, bacteria (2%)
Neoplasia
  Lymphoma
    Primary CNS (5%)
    Secondary CNS (4%)
  Kaposi's sarcoma, metastatic (1%)
Other complications
  Infarction, hemorrhage, and unknown lesions (2%)

---

gions of increased signal intensity on T_2-weighted images (Fig. 8-16). These regions are bilateral and often become large and confluent in the subcortical white matter (Fig. 8-17). This picture is thought to be representative of the HIV encephalitis. CT scanning

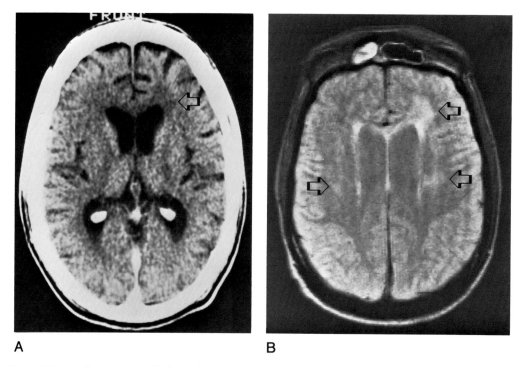

Fig. 8-16 AIDS, subacute encephalitis. (A) CT scan shows generalized cerebral atrophy. There is subtle low density in the white matter adjacent to the left frontal horn (arrow). **(B)** Lightly T_2-weighted MRI shows patchy paraventricular high signal intensity in the white matter (arrows).

has not been able to consistently demonstrate these lesions. High T_2 signal abnormality may also be seen in the basal ganglia and spinal cord with MRI (Fig. 8-17). Rarely, CT scans show these lesions as regions of abnormal enhancement. The lesions in the basal ganglia are thought to represent CMV infection.

Herpes simplex infection occurs uncommonly. It may assume its characteristic appearance on CT scans with slightly hemorrhagic, contrast-enhancing, low density mass lesions bilaterally within the temporal or frontal lobes. However, because the immune response of the brain is diminished there is often little necrosis associated with the infection, and the CT scan may show only atrophy. MRI also shows edema and hemorrhage. Varicella-zoster has been isolated in autopsy series, but there are no reports of its detection by imaging.

Progressive multifocal leukoencephalopathy, with its characteristic findings (discussed in a section to follow) occurs in about 2 percent of those with AIDS. The high T_2 signal intensity lesions on MRI tend to be large and focal, but may have widespread distribution.

Toxoplasma gondii causes, by far, the most common secondary nonviral infection of the brain. Depending on the series cited, this infection occurs in 10 to 40 percent of patients with AIDS. The trophozoites invade the brain, producing regions of necrosis that are often large. The lack of immune response allows the infection to persist, even with appropriate antimicrobial therapy, so recurrence is common even after apparent clearance.

The contrast-enhanced CT examination detects all but a few of the cases of cerebral toxoplasmosis. A diffuse *Toxoplasma* encephalitis without necrosis may occur and not be detected with CT scans. A high dose drip/delayed examination may detect some lesions when the routinely enhanced study is negative. The imaging test is important, as the diagnosis from serologic data is unreliable and is frequently negative when infection is raging.

The most common CT pattern is a large low density region, with mass effect, showing ring-like contrast enhancement within and often involving the basal ganglia (75 percent of cases). Mild hydrocephalus may re-

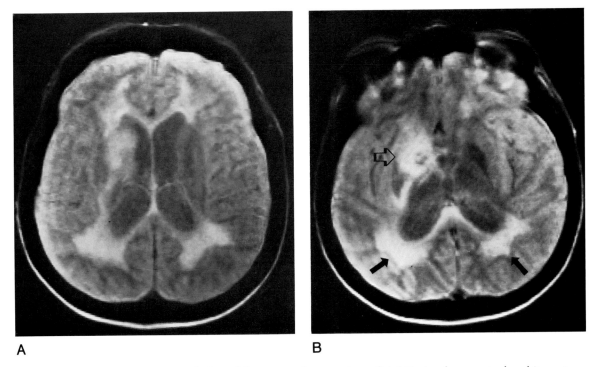

A   B

Fig. 8-17 AIDS, subacute encephalitis. (A) Large confluent regions of high T_2 signal are seen in the white matter with MRI. **(B)** High T_2 signal may also be seen in the basal ganglia (open arrow). Confluent high T_2 signal is seen about the ventricular atria (black arrows). Toxoplasma can produce identical basal ganglionic lesions.

sult from third ventricular compression. The lesions are often multiple (66 percent). Small hemorrhages may occur. About 33 percent of the lesions do not show enhancement or else show nonspecific enhancement of the cortical surface near more peripheral lesions. Occasionally, the enhancement is uniform (homogeneous) throughout the lesion. *Toxoplasma* encephalitis and lymphoma commonly coexist in the same region. The lesions may regress but frequently remain visible even with adequate antimicrobial therapy (Fig. 8-28).

All the lesions seen with CT scanning are also seen on MRI, and more. The lesions of *Toxoplasma* infection are seen as either single or multiple discrete high intensity regions on T_2-weighted images (Fig. 8-18). MRI may show abnormality when the CT scan is entirely negative except for atrophy. Gd-DTPA enhancement increases the sensitivity on MRI with the principles similar to CT scanning. If the CT scan or MRI does not show focal disease, it is unlikely that there is infection present in the brain.

Cryptococcus meningitis, sometimes associated with *Cryptococcus* encephalitis, is common, occurring in about 10 percent of those with AIDS. Meningitis is suggested when contrast enhancement is seen in the meninges. Other opportunistic infections that have been reported are *Candida albicans* infection, *Mycobacterium* infection, *coccidioidomycosis,* and pyogenic abscess. These lesions are indistinguishable from those of toxoplasmosis. (See the specific headings for these infections in this chapter.)

Non-Hodgkins lymphoma is the most common CNS neoplasm, occurring in 9 percent of those with AIDS. Primary and secondary involvement occurs with equal frequency. On CT scans lymphoma lesions may be hypodense and demonstrate ring-like enhancement —and so be indistinguishable from the lesions of *T. gondii* infection or they may be hyperdense and show homogeneous enhancement. In about 25 percent of cases the enhanced CT scan does not show the lesions. MRI shows greater sensitivity for detecting the process but with nonspecific high density signal abnormality on the T_2-weighted images.

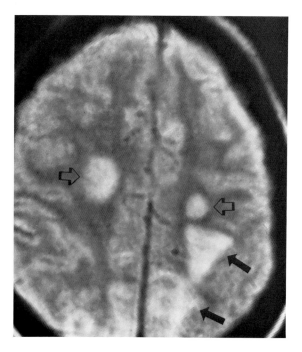

Fig. 8-18 AIDS, toxoplasmosis. The rounded regions of high T_2 signal in the white matter represent toxoplasmosis (open arrows). The more confluent regions of high T_2 signal posteriorly (black arrows) are undiagnosed. These findings could just as well represent lymphoma or Kaposi's sarcoma.

Table 8-1 MRI Patterns in AIDS

Pattern	Pathologic Correlation
Generalized atrophy	Subacute encephalitis
	AIDS – dementia complex
	Effects of chronic illness
Multiple discrete high intensity foci on T^2-weighted images	Opportunistic infection: *Toxoplasma gondii* by far the most common (see text)
	Lymphoma, metastatic Kaposi's sarcoma
Large, bilateral patchy white matter high signal lesions on T^2-weighted images	Subacute encephalitis
	Progressive multifocal leukoencephalopathy
Solitary high signal lesion on T_2-weighted images	Opportunistic infection: *Toxoplasma gondii*, most common
	Lymphoma, Kaposi's sarcoma

Kaposi's sarcoma infrequently metastasizes to the brain. It has been shown on CT scans as a homogeneously enhancing mass. However, CT scanning has failed to diagnose some lesions found at autopsy. No data on MRI scanning are available at this time.

In summary the lesions seen with CT scanning and MRI are nonspecific in character. Therefore no etiologic diagnosis can ever be given with certainty from the scan alone. The lesions of HIV, *Toxoplasma gondii,* CMV, lymphoma, and other infections may appear alike; and in fact they frequently coexist, even in the same biopsy specimen. Before specific treatment is given, biopsy of one or more of the lesions is recommended. Biopsy may be done efficiently by the percutaneous needle aspiration technique using CT or MRI guidance or stereotaxis (Table 8-1).

Herpes Simplex Encephalitis

Herpes simplex encephalitis is the most common type of sporadic viral encephalitis. In adults, type 1 herpes simplex virus (HSV-1) is the infective agent. Most cases of encephalitis seem to result from primary infection, although some patients have had recurrent oral or cutaneous herpes. In neonates, HSV-2 is the agent, transferred from a maternal genital infection.

Most cases are severe, and the disease carries a 70 percent mortality rate with great morbidity in those who survive. In the brain there are necrotic lesions with microscopic hemorrhages that are characteristically bilateral but often asymmetric. The limbic system is most often involved, especially the anterior medial temporal lobes, the insula, and the orbital surface of the frontal lobes. In those who survive, there is severe remaining regional atrophy.

In neonates the infection may cause global devastation of the brain with cystic encephalomalacia. Intense diffuse gyral enhancement may be seen with contrast CT scanning. Gross low density abnormality in the white matter represents the encephalomalacia. The ventricles are enlarged because of brain atrophy, and there may be paraventricular calcification. Congenital intrauterine infection rarely occurs.

In adults, CT scans may be normal in mild cases. In severe cases, low density abnormality is seen in the characteristically involved regions about 5 days after the onset, and blotchy contrast enhancement occurs after 7 to 10 days. The hemorrhages are usually not demonstrable. Late atrophy is seen with gross dilation of the temporal horns of the lateral ventricles. Radionuclide scanning may show abnormal accumulation of radionuclide in the temporal lobes a day or two sooner than with CT scans.

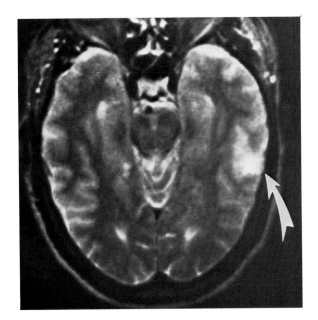

Fig. 8-19 Herpes encephalitis. T$_2$-weighted MRI shows high signal intensity in the left middle temporal gyrus (arrow). This abnormality is nonspecific, and the diagnosis must be made by biopsy. This lateral temporal location is unusual for herpes encephalitis.

The most sensitive method for detecting infection seems to be MRI. High signal abnormality representing edema is seen on T$_2$-weighted images in the inferior frontal and medial temporal lobes and extending to the insula. Atypical distribution may occur (Fig. 8-19), and small hemorrhages may be seen. The coronal image is helpful for defining the characteristic distribution. The lesions are seen at least as early as with radionuclide scanning. Biopsy has been recommended for accurate diagnosis prior to antiviral treatment, although because of morbidity from the biopsy in herpes-involved tissue many patients are treated on the basis of the MRI results and the clinical diagnosis.

Subacute Sclerosing Panencephalitis

Subacute sclerosing panencephalitis is a post-measles viral encephalitis of obscure etiology. It usually occurs in persons 4 to 20 years of age. The onset is insidious and may not be until years after the measles infection. The disorder gradually produces relentless mental deterioration and eventual death. CT scanning and MRI show multifocal regions of edema in the subcortical

and paraventricular white matter associated with atrophy. Contrast enhancement does not occur. Both MRI and CT scans may show only progressive atrophy.

Progressive Multifocal Leukoencephalopathy

Progressive multifocal leukoencephalopathy is caused by a papova virus infection, occurring only in immunodeficient persons. It is most commonly associated with Hodgkin's disease, chronic lymphocytic leukemia, and AIDS. The infection causes demyelination primarily of the posterior parietal and occipital white matter; it may be bilateral but asymmetric. This state is seen on CT scans as ill-defined, low density regions in the posterior white matter, characteristically without contrast enhancement or mass effect. T$_2$-weighted MRI shows high signal abnormality in the characteristic locations. The disease can be successfully treated with cytosine arabinoside, so making the diagnosis is important. Biopsy is necessary for accurate diagnosis.

Chronic Mononucleosis-like Syndrome, Epstein-Barr Virus Infection

A syndrome of chronic fatigue, recurrent infections, headache, memory disturbance, and cognitive malfunction is becoming recognized. It is thought to be caused by infection with the Epstein-Barr virus or possibly the human B-cell lymphotrophic virus (HBLV). It most commonly affects late adolescents and young adults. MRI of the brain has shown small punctate regions of high signal intensity in the immediate subcortical frontal and parietal lobes. Occasionally, the lesions were larger and sightly deeper, but they were not distributed in the paraventricular region. This pattern is different from the usual distribution of lesions in multiple sclerosis. No pathologic correlation is available at this time.

OTHER INFLAMMATORY DISEASES

Fungus Infections

Fungus infections of the CNS occur as part of disseminated systemic infection. The infection may affect normal individuals in endemic regions (coccidiomycosis,

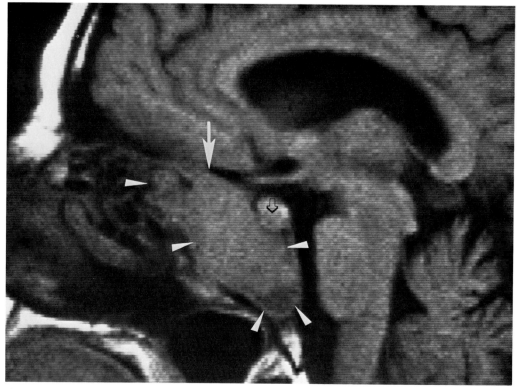

A

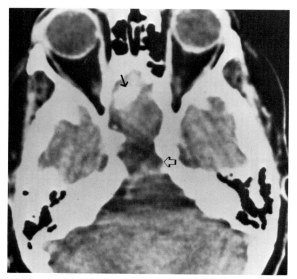

B

Fig. 8-20 Fungus infection of the sphenoid sinus. (A)
Parasagittal T_1-weighted MRI shows an isointense, nearly
homogeneous mass within the sphenoid sinus (arrowheads).
It has destroyed the upper clivus and eroded through the
planum sphenoidale into the inferior frontal fossa (arrow).
The pituitary is preserved (open arrow). A carcinoma could
have this appearance. **(B)** Transaxial CT scan shows an isodense mass within the sphenoid sinus causing destruction of
the upper clivus (open arrow). Calcification is present within
the lesion (arrow), a relatively common finding with fungus
infections but not with tumor.

histoplasmosis, blastomycosis, chromomycosis) or immunodeficient persons without geographic limitation (candidiasis, aspergillosis, cryptococcosis, nocardiosis, mucormycosis, and actinomycosis).

Basal meningitis is common and is seen as contrast enhancement of the leptomeninges on both CT scans and MRI. The basal cisterns may show increased intensity on T_1-weighted MRI. Hydrocephalus is common, and there may be focal ventricular entrapments from ependymitis. Focal fungal abscesses occur within the brain and may be single or multiple. On contrast-enhanced CT scans and MRI they appear as round, homogeneous enhancing lesions when small, but when large they are usually ring-like with central necrosis. MRI shows the cerebral infections as nonspecific regions of high signal intensity on T_2-weighted imaging. More mature granulomatous lesions have lower central intensity. The lesions are indistinguishable from metastatic tumor, multiple pyogenic abscesses, or tuberculosis.

Most fungus infections appear similar on imaging, with a few exceptions. Large fungi (hyphal fungi), particularly *Aspergillus,* tend to cause occlusion of major cerebral arteries with secondary brain infarction. *Mucormycosis* (phycomycosis) occurs primarily in diabetic patients with ketocidosis. It involves the nasal cavity and paranasal sinuses. The infection is highly invasive, entering the base of the frontal fossa through the cribriform plate *(rhinocerebral phycomycosis)* and extending into the orbits. Here a fungal inflammatory mass may mimic tumor (Fig. 8-20). *Cryptococcus* primarily causes a meningitis with occasional secondary involvement of the brain parenchyma.

Syphilis

Neurosyphilis may occur anytime after the primary stage of the infection. Most commonly, it is an asymptomatic aseptic meningitis. However, if it is more severe, meningovascular syphilis causes endarteritis and vascular thrombosis of major arteries at the base of the brain, which may result in cerebral infarction indistinguishable from that due to other causes. The pattern of basal meningitis is similar to that found with tuberculosis and fungal infections; however, the CSF VDRL is positive with meningovascular syphilis. CT scanning and MRI may show infarction and contrast enhancement at the base of the brain, and angiography may show narrowing of the lumen or thrombosis of major

vessels at the base of the brain. In the chronic stage, gummas may occur within the brain parenchyma and appear as nonspecific, focal, round, contrast-enhancing lesions. Severe atrophy is also present with tertiary syphilis.

Granulomatous Meningitis and Pachymeningitis

Granulomatous meningitis results primarily from fungal or tuberculous infections but may occur in association with other systemic inflammatory granulomatous processes such as sarcoidosis. The meninges may become thick, particularly at the base of the brain. This change causes cisternal block to the flow of CSF, resulting in hydrocephalus, the primary cause of morbidity in this group of patients. Cranial nerve palsies may also occur.

The MRI or CT scans demonstrate the hydrocephalus. The meninges show varying degrees of contrast enhancement, from none at all to pronounced enhancement, confined primarily to the basal cisterns. Dense calcification of the basal meninges may occur in chronic inflammations, particularly tuberculosis. The fungus and tuberculous infections may be associated with cerebral granulomas, usually appearing as ring enhancing focal lesions. The pattern may be indistinguishable from that of metastatic disease to the brain and meninges. The diagnosis usually is made by biopsy at the time of ventricular shunting.

Sarcoidosis

Sarcoidosis is a relatively common granulomatous process of unknown etiology. The CNS is involved 5 percent of the time. There may be meningitis, meningoencephalitis, or granulomas within the brain, spinal cord, or lytic round lesions in the skull.

Hydrocephalus is the most common finding on MRI and CT scans, usually occurring as a result of obstruction to the outlet of the fourth ventricle or basal CSF pathways by granulomatous meningitis, as described in the preceding section. The dural surfaces, including the falx and tentorium, may show lesions that are indistinguishable from meningioma. These lesions may become thick and extensive (Fig. 8-21). Encephalitis may appear as diffuse patchy enhancement of the brain.

Parenchymal sarcoid granulomas are slightly hyperdense on the nonenhanced CT scan and show homoge-

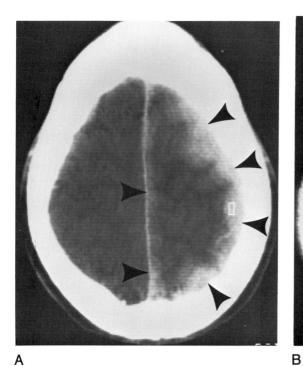

A

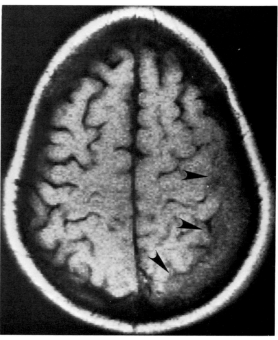

B

C

Fig. 8-21 Sarcoidosis, pachymeningitis. (A) Contrast-enhanced CT scan shows homogeneous enhancement of the grossly thickened meninges over the left hemisphere and in the left interhemispheric fissure (arrowheads). (B) T_1-weighted MRI shows the thickened dura as being slightly hypointense to the brain (arrowheads). (C) Slightly T_2-weighted image shows the extracerebral inflammatory tissue as very hypointense (arrowheads). (MRI courtesy of Dr. Paul Markarian, Springfield, MA.)

neous enhancement with contrast. Calcification some-times occurs. The lesions are most common in the hypothalamus, pituitary stalk, or pons, but they may occur anywhere, including the spinal cord. The clinical presentation may suggest tumor.

MRI demonstrates the CNS granulomas as regions of nonspecific high signal intensity on T_2-weighted images sometimes with slightly less intensity centrally. MRI may show lesions not seen with CT scans, but calcified lesions are poorly seen. It is important to recognize neurosarcoid, as the outcome is much improved with steroid therapy. The hydrocephalus is treated with shunting. Biopsy is usually necessary for diagnosis.

Tuberculosis

Tuberculosis remains a common and important intracranial infectious disease worldwide. The intracranial infection results from hematogenous spread of *Myco-bacterium tuberculosis,* usually from a pulmonary site. Untreated miliary tuberculosis increases the likelihood of intracranial infection.

The intracranial infection may be focal in the brain parenchyma (tuberculoma) or cause meningitis, when the infection spreads from a tuberculoma into the subarachnoid space. Both processes may occur simultaneously. It is usually a subacute illness that develops insidiously over 3 to 6 weeks.

The tuberculoma is equivalent to the pulmonary granuloma and forms a discrete mass within the brain parenchyma. On CT scans it appears as a contrast-enhancing, round, nonspecific mass that is variable in size and may be multiple. Like all metastatic processes to the brain, it tends to occur at the corticomedullary junction (Fig. 8-22). Larger lesions appear ring-like (Fig. 8-23). On MRI, the lesions have high signal on T_2-weighted images and may have a ring-like appearance. Because of frequent hemorrhage within the lesions, they have high signal intensity on T_1-weighted images and regions of low signal on T_2-weighted SE and GRE images. Edema around the lesion is variable and may be minimal.

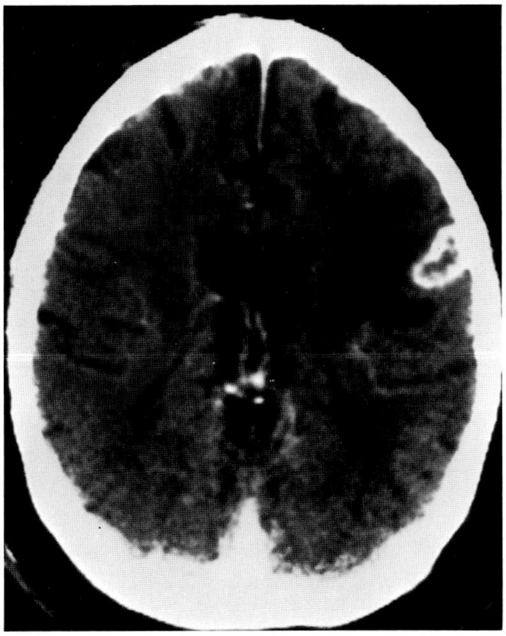

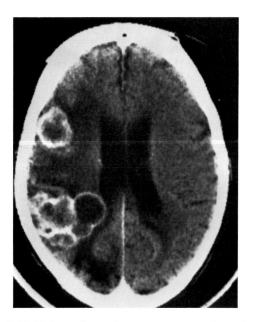

Fig. 8-22 Tuberculoma. Contrast-enhanced CT scan shows a ring-like enhancing lesion at the corticomedullary junction extending to the cortical surface of the left posterior frontal lobe. There is moderate surrounding edema. This lesion is indistinguishable from a metastasis or early phase glioma. (Courtesy of Dr. Sam Mayerfield, UMDNJ.)

Fig. 8-23 Tuberculous abscess. Contrast-enhanced CT scan shows multiple large tuberculomas in the right frontal and posterior temporal lobes. This picture is indistinguishable from that of multicentric glioma.

If the infection spills over into the subarachnoid space, meningitis occurs. Characteristically, a thick exudate is present at the base of the brain, which frequently produces hydrocephalus from either blockade of the cisternal flow of CSF or the outlet of the fourth ventricle. CT scans and MRI show the process as intensely contrast-enhancing and thickened meninges frequently with associated hydrocephalus and demonstrable tuberculoma. This constellation of findings suggests the diagnosis of tuberculosis. Heavy calcification of the meninges may be seen during the chronic phase, and cranial nerve compression and vascular occlusion of major arteries may occur (Fig. 2-51).

PARASITIC INFESTATIONS

Parasites that infest the lungs, intestines, liver, and muscle may also infest the brain. These organisms include cestodes (tapeworms: cysticercosis, hydatidosis), protozoans (unicellular organisms: toxoplasmosis), nematodes (roundworms: trichinosis), and trematodes (flukes: schistosomiasis, paragonimiasis). The cestodes and protozoans involve the CNS relatively commonly, but involvement by nematodes and trematodes is rare. Only the first two categories are discussed here.

Cysticercosis (Cestode Infestation)

Cysticercosis is caused by infection with the larval form of the pork tapeworm, *Taenia solium.* This infection is becoming more prevalent not only in non-industrialized regions of the world but also in industrialized countries without endemic disease, principally because of the migration of infected persons. The disease is particularly common in Mexico, Central America, South America, Africa, India, China, eastern Europe, and Indonesia.

Knowledge of the life cycle of *T. solium* is essential for understanding the disease cysticercosis. The pig is the primary source of the infection. Humans acquire the adult tapeworm by ingesting undercooked pork. The tapeworm then attaches to the human intestine, producing a large number of eggs, which are discharged in the feces. This stage can result in the contamination of food or in autoinfection if the person harboring the tapeworm contaminates his or her hands and so ingests the eggs. The ingested eggs hatch in the small intestine, burrow into venules, and are carried in the blood to distant sites, most commonly muscle and brain. Here they develop into mature larvae, or cysticerci, within about 2 months.

The larvae remain for years, as the viable cysts do not cause any significant inflammatory reaction. After about 4 to 5 years the larvae die, the cysts degenerate, and the inflammatory reaction begins, resulting in enlargement of the lesions and surrounding inflammatory edema. It is only at this time that the patient becomes symptomatic.

The cysticerci (5- to 10-mm spheres) are found in the brain parenchyma, the ventricular system, or the subarachnoid space. The location of the cysts determines the nature of the clinical presentation. The symptoms are produced by the mass effect, the surrounding inflammatory reaction, and the obstruction of the flow of CSF in the ventricles or the subarachnoid cisterns. Any combination of findings may occur, as multiple cysts usually exist in various locations. Seizures, focal deficits, and headache from hydrocephalus with increased intracranial pressure are the most common symptoms, mimicking tumor.

The diagnosis is based on clinical or CT findings. Subcutaneous nodules are present in 50 percent of those afflicted, and biopsy of the nodules is diagnostic. Serologic antibody test is usually positive. CSF examination shows the nonspecific findings of chronic meningitis, with a lymphocyte-predominant pleocytosis and elevated protein and pressure. Eosinophilia occurs in only 20 percent of patients. Plain film findings are helpful only when there is calcification of the cysts in the brain or muscle.

The CT scan is overall the most useful test for diagnosis of cysticercosis. During the earlier stages the cysts within the brain parenchyma appear as spherical or nodular lesions of poorly defined low density (slightly greater than that of CSF) of varying size. They are usually located at the gray-white matter junction. The cysts may become large, measuring 5 cm or more (Fig. 8-24). The scolex may be seen as density in the cyst. MRI will show these viable lesions as cysts with CSF equivalent fluid, and may also demonstrate the scolex within the cyst.

Degenerated lesions can best be seen with contrast enhancement. Small lesions homogeneously enhance, appearing as solid nodules, whereas large lesions tend to show central low density. Thin, ring-like enhancements may occur (Fig. 8-25), although some lesions do

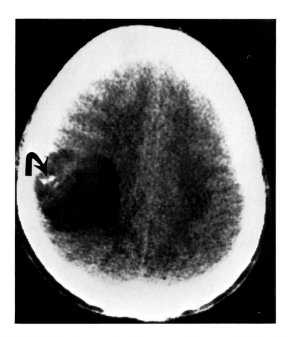

Fig. 8-24 Cysticercosis. A large cyst is present in the right parietal lobe containing fluid of near-CSF density. The calcification represents the dead larva (arrow).

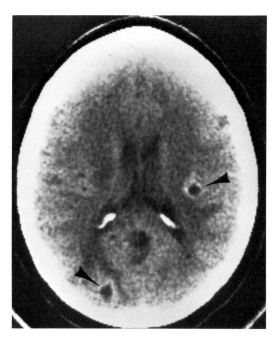

Fig. 8-25 Cysticercosis. Contrast-enhanced CT scan shows multiple ring enhancing lesions with central low density (arrowheads). (Courtesy of Dr. Sam Mayerfield, UMDNJ.)

not enhance at all. The picture may mimic that of metastatic neoplastic disease. Edema frequently surrounds the lesion. At this stage MRI shows the lesions as moderately high T_2 signal with higher intensity perifocal edema that mimics a tumor. Infarctions may result from the intense perivascular inflammatory reaction, arteritis, and vascular occlusion. Angiography may show the typical changes of arteritis with narrowing, "beading," or occlusion. With the death of the cysticercus, either naturally or after treatment, the scolex partially or totally calcifies (Fig. 8-24). The calcified lesions are easy to detect with CT scanning, but are difficult to detect with MRI.

Within the ventricular system or the subarachnoid space, the cysts have about the same CT absorption spectrum as the CSF and are therefore difficult or nearly impossible to detect. The cysts are attached to the ependyma or are free-floating. Ring-like abnormal contrast enhancement or the scolex may be seen allowing one to discern the lesions, but it occurs less frequently than with cysts in the brain parenchyma. The cysts assume the shape of the ventricular cavity and so may appear to be the ventricle itself, particularly within the fourth ventricle. Positive contrast cisternography

or ventriculography may be necessary to define the cyst which is seen as a negative defect within the contrast filled ventricle. MRI may be helpful here as sometimes the rim of the cyst and adjacent ependyma may have very high T_2 signal intensity or the cyst may contain proteinaceous fluid with higher signal intensity than CSF allowing for its identification within the ventricle. The intraventricular cysts may cause obstruction of the foramina, with the development of hydrocephalus. Surgical excision of critical lesions can be helpful in relieving the patient of symptoms.

Calcifications does not occur in cysts within the ventricles or the subarachnoid space. Rarely, a cyst within the CSF shows homogeneous contrast enhancement and mimics a solid tumor. Rupture of a cyst may lead to diffuse meningitis. The infection may occur along the spinal cord in the subarachnoid space and is seen with myelography as intradural, extramedullary masses. Intramedullary spinal cord lesions are rare.

Treatment consists in shunting of the hydrocephalus, removal of the critical lesions in the ventricular system, steroids, antiseizure medication, ^{131}I-tagged specific immunoglobulins, and praziquantel, a broad-spectrum antitrematodal agent.

Hydatidosis (Cestode Infestation)

Hydatidosis is caused by the larval form of the tapeworms *Echinococcus granulosa* or *Echinococcus multilocularis.* It is endemic in South America, northern and eastern Africa, central Europe (particularly the Mediterranean countries), and the Middle East. The dog is the primary host; and humans, sheep, cattle, and horses are the intermediate hosts. The life cycle is similar to that described in the above section on cysticercosis. The human becomes infected when he or she comes into contact with soil or dogs contaminated with eggs.

The CT appearance is characteristic. The hydatid cysts in the brain is usually large and unilocular, containing fluid of nearly CSF density. There is little surrounding edema and only occasional calcification. The cyst is round (Fig. 8-26). This feature may help to differentiate hydatid disease from a congenital arach-

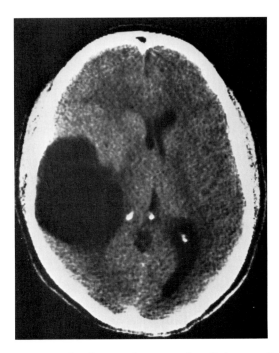

Fig. 8-26 Hydatid cyst. A large, round, well circumscribed cyst of near-CSF density is present in the right temporal lobe. There is little surrounding edema but considerable mass effect from the cyst itself.

noidal cyst, which tends to have at least one straight border. The cyst itself causes a mass effect, leading to increased intracranial pressure; and it may rupture, causing dissemination of the scolices throughout the subarachnoid space.

Toxoplasmosis

Toxoplasmosis is a protozoan infection occurring as either a severe congenital form manifested by destructive lesions of the CNS, the eyes, and viscera or as an acquired form with acute lymphadenopathy, ocular lesions, and an illness resembling infectious mononucleosis. The disease is caused by *Toxoplasma gondii,* which multiplies intracellularly and persists in the CNS and the eye. Elsewhere it subsides in response to the development of antibodies. The infectious agent resides in cattle, swine, sheep, dogs, and rabbits as well as in several domestic birds. The disease prevalence is increasing, primarily because of the relatively high incidence in immunodeficient individuals, particularly those with AIDS.

With congenital toxoplasmosis, maternal infection is transferred to the infant. The maternal infection may be chronic and occult. The brain and eyes are the primary target organs. A severe encephalitis causes extensive tissue destruction resulting in microcephaly, severe psychomotor retardation, and chorioretinitis. Calcifications are deposited in granulomas in the ependymal walls of the lateral ventricles, basal ganglia, peripheral frontal and parietal lobes, and choroid plexi. The calcifications may take any form and be curvilinear, nodular, or plaque-like, or they may be in clumps. The ventricular enlargement is most commonly the result of the severe brain destruction, although rarely a granuloma will obstructs the aqueduct of Sylvius causing hydrocephalus (Fig. 8-27). Congenital toxoplasmosis and cytomegalic inclusion disease are the two most common causes of intracranial calcifications in infants. Cortical and basal ganglionic calcifications are more common in congenital toxoplasmosis, although the two processes cannot be reliably differentiated by imaging alone.

Acquired adult toxoplasmosis is now occurring with increasing frequency in immunosuppressed patients. It is seen in those with tumors of the hematopoietic system, those with AIDS, and those receiving chemotherapy for malignant disease. Because of the impaired immune reaction in these patients, the serologic test for

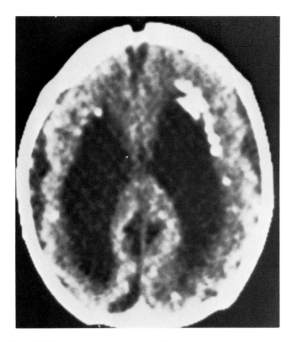

Fig. 8-27 Congenital toxoplasmosis. CT scan shows gross ventricular dilatation and periventricular calcifications. Small extracerebral fluid collections are also present.

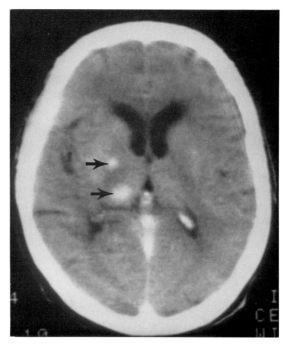

Fig. 8-28 Toxoplasmosis. Contrast-enhanced CT scan shows two densely enhancing, solid-appearing lesions in the thalamus and lenticular nuclei (arrows). This appearance is characteristic of acquired toxoplasmosis.

toxoplasmosis may be negative. Most commonly, a multifocal encephalitis causes densely enhancing lesions seen on CT scans (Fig. 8-28). They may be up to 4 cm in diameter and are distributed throughout the brain but preferentially in the paraventricular white matter or at the level of the corticomedullary junction. The appearance of the lesions on CT scans are nonspecific, being ring-like with central low density due to necrosis and surrounded by a rim of edema. MRI shows the lesions as nonspecific round regions of high T_2 signal intensity (Fig. 8-18). The lesions themselves have the same appearance as metastatic tumor or pyogenic abscesses. Because the disease is relatively acute in onset, the lesions tend to be of the same size within an individual. Metastatic tumors to the brain, when multiple, are frequently varied in size, a result of blood-borne embolization occurring over an extended period. In most cases, biopsy of a lesion is required for definitive diagnosis. Many clinicians believe that these multiple lesions, when seen in the appropriate clinical setting, are sufficiently diagnostic of toxoplasmosis that treatment should be initiated immediately.

Lyme Disease

Lyme disease is the result of infection with the spiochete Borrelia burgdorferi. The disease is widespread occurring in the United States, Europe, the Soviet Union and Asia. The infection is transmitted to humans through the bite of an infected tick of the ixodid group (I. ricinus complex). The ticks may be found on a wide variety of animals, deer being the most common. Humans pick up the tick when in infected regions.

The infection begins locally around the site of the tick bite usually producing a characteristic skin lesion, erythema migrans. Within days to weeks the infection becomes disseminated to a wide variety of organs including the meninges and brain. Afflicted persons may suffer severe headache from meningitis, and Bell's palsy and other cranial or peripheral neuropathies from radiculoneuritis. Imaging of the brain is usually normal during this phase. Malaise, migratory muscle and joint pains, lymphadenopathy and symptoms of myopericarditis may be present.

Late neurologic abnormality may occur from six months to as long as six years after infection. Most commonly, this is from a progressive encephalomyelitis which may produce paraparesis, bladder dysfunction, ataxia, cranial nerve palsies and dementia. At times the symptoms may mimic a demyelinating disease (multiple sclerosis), and oligoclonal bands may be found in the CSF. During this stage MRI has shown focal high intensity lesions within the white matter in some patients suggesting demyelination. The correct diagnosis is made by serologic testing with specific enzyme-linked immunosorbent assay (ELISA).

SUGGESTED READINGS

Dalakas M, Wichman A, Sever J: AIDS and the nervous system. JAMA 261:2396, 1989

Enzmann DR, Britt RR, Obaua WG, et al: Experimental Staphylococcus aureus brain abscess. AJNR 7:395, 1986

Enzmann DR, Britt RR, Placone RC Jr: Staging of human brain abscess by computed tomography. Radiology 146:703, 1983

Haimes AB, Zimmerman RD, Morgello S: MR imaging of brain abscesses. AJNR 10:279, 1989

Hayes WS, Sherman JL, Stern BJ, et al: MR and CT evaluation of intracranial sarcoidosis. AJNR 8:841, 1987

Heck AW, Phillips LH II: Sarcoidosis and the nervous system. Neurol Clin 7:641, 1989

Kieburtz K, Schiffer RB: Neurologic manifestations of human immunodeficiency virus infections. Neurol Clin 7:447, 1989

Post MJD, Tate LG, Quencer RM, et al: CT, MR, and pathology in HIV encephalitis and meningitis. AJNR 9:469, 1988

Sze G, Zimmerman RD: The magnetic resonance imaging of infectious and inflammatory diseases. Radiol Clin North Am 26:839, 1988

Teitelbaum GP, Otto RJ, Lin M, et al: MR imaging of neurocysticercosis. AJNR 10:709, 1989

Weingarten K, Zimmerman RD, Becker RD, et al: Subdural and epidural empyemas: MR imaging. AJNR 10:81,1989

Zimmerman RD, Leeds NE, Danziger A: Subdural empyema: CT findings. Radiology 150:417, 1984

9

White Matter Disease

Most diseases of the white matter affect myelination. If myelin has formed normally, it may be broken down by the disease process (demyelination, myelinoclastic process). Alternatively, the myelin may not have formed properly in the first place (dysmyelination). The dysmyelinating diseases are discussed in Chapter 12.

Myelin is hydrophobic. Therefore myelinated white matter normally has a low water content. If myelin is deficient, broken down, or abnormally formed, the water content of the tissue is much greater than that of normally myelinated tissue. Regions of abnormal or absent myelin are seen on CT scans as regions of hypodensity. On MRI they are of low signal intensity on T_1-weighted images and high signal intensity on T_2-weighted images. MRI is more sensitive than CT scanning for detection of a demyelinating process.

A myelinoclastic process (prime example multiple sclerosis) may have an associated inflammatory component that sometimes produces a mass effect or abnormal breakdown in the blood-brain barrier, which results in enhancement after contrast infusion. Dysmyelination does not produce these changes. Demyelination has many causes, including multiple sclerosis, ischemia, trauma, infection, radiation damage, and metabolic factors.

NORMAL MYELINATION PATTERN

The CT and MRI appearance of the central white matter varies with age. There are infantile, transitional, adult, and aging patterns. Myelination is a dynamic process that progresses in an orderly fashion over the first 3 years of life. The most ancient phylogenetic tracts are myelinated first and the telencephalon last. This development proceeds in a more or less caudal to rostral direction (see Ch. 12). Prior to myelination, the white matter has relatively high water content, which shows as relative hypodensity with CT scanning and relative high signal with T_2-weighted MRI. Transition in the cerebrum occurs at about 10 to 12 months, when the white matter of the centrum semiovale first becomes isointense and then hypointense on the T_2-weighted images. The white matter assumes the adult level of hypointensity at about 36 months. Delays in myelination can be determined if the infantile pattern persists longer than normal. After 3 years, the pattern of the white matter remains the same until late adulthood.

In normal persons of all ages there is frequently a

DEMYELINATING DISEASES OF THE WHITE MATTER

Multiple sclerosis

Radiation damage (see also Ch. 2)

Progressive multifocal leukoencephalopathy (see Ch. 8)

Subacute sclerosing panencephalitis (see Ch. 8)

Acute disseminated encephalomyelitis

Central pontine myelinolysis

Subcortical arteriosclerotic encephalopathy (Binswanger's disease) (see Ch. 10)

Marchiafava-Bignami disease

---

small focal region of high T_2 signal intensity within the white matter adjacent to the frontal and occipital horns of the lateral ventricles. It is thought to represent a concentration of water about to be absorbed into the lateral ventricles. The flow of CSF here is centripedal; it is opposite that seen with transependymal absorption associated with hydrocephalus. There may also be a thin "pencil line" of high intensity outlining the whole ventricular system. These regions must not be mistaken for pathologic change. However, at times it is impossible to determine if the amount of high signal in the paraventricular white matter is physiologic or pathologic.

UNIDENTIFIED BRIGHT OBJECTS

Increasingly frequent with increasing age, small focal or punctate regions of high T_2 signal intensity, or unidentified bright objects (UBOs), are seen within the white matter on MRI. They occur predominantly in the paraventricular white matter but may be in the subcortical region and brain stem as well. These high signal foci have been found to represent a variety of lesions. Most commonly they represent small infarctions, either cystic or noncystic. Other causes include gliosis, focal demyelination (possible subclinical multiple sclerosis), brain cyst, or ventricular diverticulum. In some cases no lesion is found within the brain at autopsy.

The significance of these lesions is not known, although there is a positive correlation with atherosclerosis of the perforating arteries, dementia, hypertension, and diabetes. On MRI scans, they cause confusion, as they sometimes cannot be differentiated from small metastases or regions of multiple sclerosis. Clinical correlation, contrast enhancement and follow-up scanning can usually determine if they are of relevance.

MULTIPLE SCLEROSIS

Multiple sclerosis (MS) is by far the most common primary demyelinating disease. It typically occurs in persons 20 to 50 years old who live in the northern parts of the United States, Europe, and Asia and in southern Australia. It causes dissolution of the myelin sheaths of the brain and spinal cord with preservation of the nerves. Proliferating astrocytes form the firm "plaques" characteristic of the lesions. Inflammatory changes are present with edema and eventual scar formation. The cause is unknown.

Multiple sclerosis produces variable neurologic signs and symptoms that are characterized by exacerbations and remissions. The diagnosis is made clinically by history, physical findings, CSF analysis, and evoked potential tests. Imaging is used for confirmation of the clinical diagnosis. The diagnosis of MS cannot be made on the basis of imaging alone.

The lesions, which vary from a few millimeters to centimeters in diameter, are characteristically located adjacent to the ventricles of the cerebral hemispheres. Lesions may also be found in the peripheral subcortical white matter, but there they tend to be smaller and less numerous. Less commonly, they occur within the cerebellum, pons, and spinal cord. Multiple lesions may become confluent. Occasionally, a single large lesion has the appearance usually associated with a glioblastoma. Edema may accompany the larger lesions. Cerebral atrophy is seen after the disease has been present for some time causing both the ventricles and the sulci become enlarged.

The most sensitive imaging modality for the detection of MS is MRI. Lesions are seen in 95 percent of those who have the clinical diagnosis of MS. However, many more lesions are seen pathologically than are seen with MRI. The lesions are of high signal intensity on the T_2-weighted images. Those in the immediate paraventricular region are best seen with proton density images (long TR with relatively short TE; e.g., SE 2500/30), so the ventricular CSF is made to appear isointense with the normal white matter allowing the paraventricular lesions to stand out. Most commonly, the lesions are discrete or confluent adjacent to the frontal and posterior horns. Those in the more peripheral white matter are best demonstrated with long echo T_2-weighted images (e.g., SE 2500/120) (Fig. 9-1).

The lesions seen with MRI may be acute (inflammatory change) or chronic (scar). The activity of the lesions cannot be determined with routine MRI, although the older lesions tend to have lower intensity on the T_1-weighted images. Once established, most of the lesions on MRI remain indefinitely, although they sometimes change slightly in size. The size and number of the lesions imaged do not necessarily correlate with the clinical activity or severity of the disease. The lesions generally do not change with steroid therapy, so

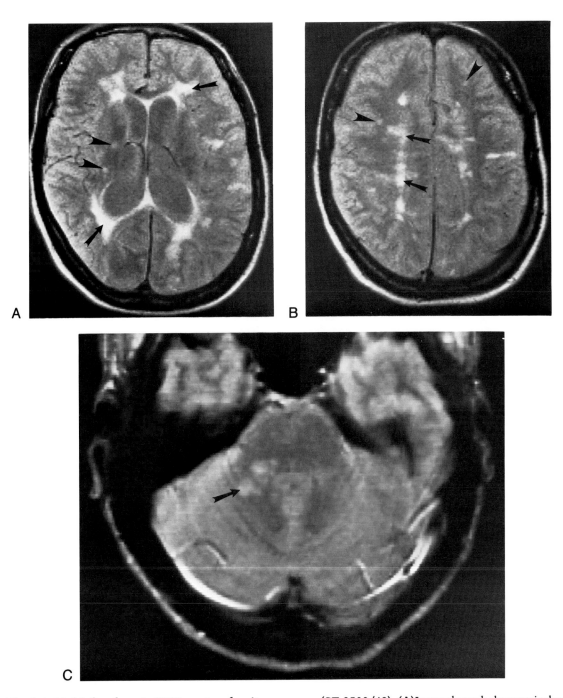

Fig. 9-1 Multiple sclerosis, MRI, proton density sequence (SE 2500/40). (A) Image through the ventricular system shows the CSF isointense with the white matter. This image is optimal for visualization of paraventricular white matter abnormality. Confluent high T_2 signal abnormality is seen in the paraventricular white matter (arrows). Smaller, discrete lesions can be seen in the internal capsule on the right (arrowheads). **(B)** Scan through a higher level shows the confluent paraventricular high T_2 signal abnormality (arrows). The more peripheral subcortical lesions are smaller and less intense (arrowheads). This distribution is typical of MS lesions. **(C)** High T_2 signal abnormality is seen in the cerebellar peduncle (arrow).

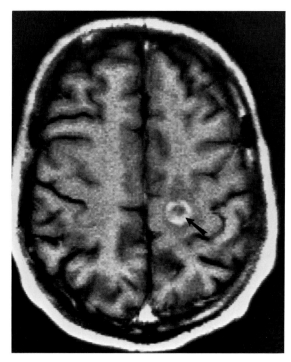

Fig. 9-2 Multiple sclerosis, MRI with Gd-DTPA enhancement. T_1-weighted MRI demonstrates a ring-like enhancing lesion of multiple sclerosis in the left hemispheric white matter (arrow). Such lesions are indistinguishable from some other lesions, e.g., metastasis or infection, except for their association with typical MS changes in the brain and the appropriate clinical history.

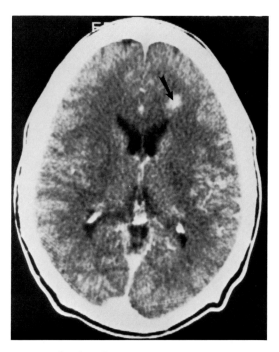

Fig. 9-3 Multiple sclerosis, CT scan with contrast enhancement. High dose drip/delay contrast-enhanced CT scan shows a homogeneously enhancing lesion adjacent to the left frontal horn (arrow). The lesion is nonspecific in appearance and can be diagnosed as MS only in the appropriate clinical setting.

routine MRI cannot be used to follow treatment effectiveness.

Gd-DTPA enhancement seems to occur only with inflammatory activity and may be used to define the progression or response to therapy (Fig. 9-2). However, unlike CT scanning, Gd-DTPA generally does not demonstrate more lesions than were seen on the nonenhanced T_2-weighted scan.

The lesions of MS must be differentiated from "normal" paraventricular high signal intensity, paraventricular high intensity associated with hydrocephalus, UBOs, multiple subcortical infarctions (Binswanger's disease), arteritis (e.g., lupus), axonal (shear) injury, migraine, Lyme disease, and postirradiation change.

The nonenhanced CT scan is relatively insensitive to the detection of MS lesions. High dose contrast infusion (80 g of iodine) and 1-hour delayed scanning increases the sensitivity, so that about 50 percent of patients with clinical MS show focal lesions (Fig. 9-3).

Only the active lesions are detected with the enhancement. Low density white matter lesions may be seen with the nonenhanced scan but far fewer than are actually present (Fig. 9-4). The contrast-enhanced lesions have a positive correlation with the activity of the lesions and their response to treatment.

RADIATION DAMAGE

Radiation causes white matter damage with nonspecific changes of demyelination, vacuolation, edema, and gliosis. It is thought to be a result of small vessel hyalinization, with the most severe changes in the deep paraventricular region. The damage occurs only within irradiated tissue.

The CT scans most commonly show only atrophy with dilatation of the ventricles and the sulci. Hypodensity of the white matter may occur. More severe focal regions of necrosis may have intense contrast enhancement, with surrounding edema appearing indis-

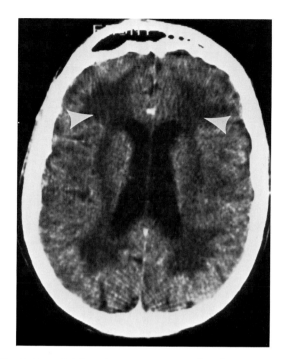

Fig. 9-4 Multiple sclerosis: severe and end-stage. Nonenhanced CT scan shows generalized hypodensity of the hemispheric white matter. The ventricles are enlarged because of deep white matter atrophy.

tinguishable from recurrent tumor. MRI shows regions of radiation effect as high signal intensity in the white matter on T_2 images (see Fig. 2-54 and 2-55). It represents edema, demyelination, and gliosis (see Ch. 2).

ACUTE DISSEMINATED ENCEPHALOMYELITIS

Acute disseminated encephalomyelitis includes the syndromes of postinfectious encephalomyelitis, postvaccinal encephalomyelitis, and acute hemorrhagic leukoencephalitis. It consists in demyelination that follows 1 to 2 weeks after vaccination or a viral illness that usually does not directly infect the nervous system, particularly varicella or influenza. The lesions may be widespread or limited and discrete, e.g., optic neuritis or transverse myelitis (spinal cord involvement at a single level).

The CT scans and MRI show the typical pattern of demyelination with low density of the white matter on CT scans and high signal intensity of the white matter on T_2-weighted MRI. Contrast enhancement has not been reported. Brain swelling may occur. The lesions can regress if the patient survives.

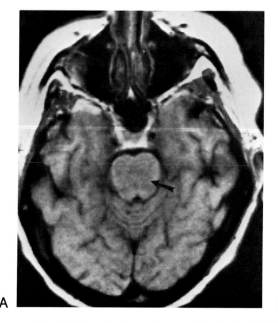

A

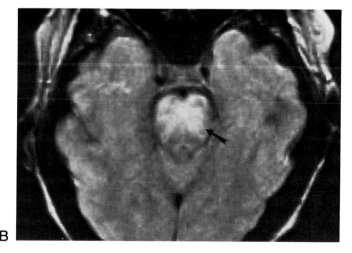

B

Fig. 9-5 Central pontine myelinolysis, MRI. (A) T_1-weighted MRI through the upper pons shows slight enlargement of the pons and central hypointensity (arrow). **(B)** Lightly T_2-weighted MRI shows high signal intensity through most of the pons with minimal peripheral sparing (arrow).

CENTRAL PONTINE MYELINOLYSIS

Central pontine myelinolysis is a relatively rare form of demyelination that occurs primarily within the pons but may extend upward into the mesencephalon and thalamus. It was first described in alcoholics but occurs also with such other metabolic disorders as hyponatremia or poorly controlled diabetes. The course of the disease is variable and may be mild or severe. The demyelination can best be seen with MRI as diffuse high T_2 signal intensity within the brain stem and mesencephalon (Fig. 9-5). Peripheral sparing may be present. The MRI findings do not always correlate with the clinical severity.

MARCHIAFAVA-BIGNAMI SYNDROME

The Marchiafava-Bignami syndrome is a rare disorder occurring in patients with severe malnutrition, often alcoholics. Middle-aged men are most often affected. The course is variable, but recovery is rare. The neurologic disturbance suggests bilateral frontal lobe disease. The lesion is demyelination of the corpus callosum beginning anteriorly and extending contiguously posteriorly. The lesion can be seen as high intensity signal in the corpus callosum with T_2-weighted MRI and sometimes as low density with CT scans.

SUGGESTED READINGS

Braffman BH, Zimmerman RA, Trojanowski JQ, et al: Brain MR: pathologic correlation with gross and histopathology. 2. Hyperintense white matter foci in the elderly. AJNR 9:629, 1988

Grossman RI, Braffman BH, Brorson JR, et al: Multiple sclerosis: serial study of gadolinium-enhanced MR imaging. Radiology 169:117, 1988

Maravilla K: Multiple sclerosis. p. 344. In Stark DD, Bradley WG Jr (eds): Magnetic Resonance Imaging. CV Mosby, St. Louis, 1988

Uhlenbrock D, Seidel D, Gehlen W, et al: MR imaging in multiple sclerosis: comparison with clinical, CSF and visual evoked potential findings. AJNR 9:59, 1988

10

Atrophy, Aging, and Dementia

Dementia is the deterioration of intellectual capacity. It is a clinical entity defined by behavior. Memory loss is a major feature. In addition, there is the inability to learn new material, calculate, reason, and speak. Emotional disturbance, particularly depression, is common. Any pathologic process affecting the cerebral hemispheres may result in dementia. Although Alzheimer's disease is the most common specific cause of dementia, a small percentage of patients have other, correctable causes for their dementia. The major reason for neuroradiologic examination of persons with dementia is to define the degree of atrophy and to identify any correctable pathologic process. The causes of dementia are given below.

Physiologic changes naturally occur with *aging*. These changes must be taken into account when evaluating the brains of patients with dementia and other degenerative syndromes.

ATROPHY AND AGING

Atrophy refers to the decrease in brain volume that occurs with the loss of brain tissue. It is irreversible, except perhaps in young infants, in whom there appears to be some regenerative capability. With CT scanning and MRI, atrophy is evidenced by enlargement of the CSF spaces within and surrounding the brain.

Atrophy is categorized as deep when it involves the white matter and basal ganglia and as cortical when it involves the gyral gray matter. Most commonly, both types are found together, and the atrophy is then said to be generalized or mixed (Fig. 10-1).

With deep atrophy the frontal horns, bodies of the lateral ventricles, and the third ventricle are enlarged. The temporal horns enlarge relatively little, a finding that helps to differentiate atrophy from hydrocephalus. A useful guide when determining the "normal" size of the lateral ventricles is to calculate the bicaudate or bifrontal indices. The *bicaudate index* (Fig. 10-1B) is the width of the ventricles at the most medial margins of the caudate nuclei, expressed as a percentage of the internal diameter of the skull at that level. The mean adult index is 0.15. The *bifrontal index* is the maximum width of both frontal horns expressed as the percentage of the internal diameter of the skull at the level of measurement. The mean bifrontal index is 0.30. The mean width of the third ventricle is 3.5 mm; greater values indicate ventricular enlargement. With deep atrophy the callosal angle of the frontal horns is obtuse (more than 110 degrees). There is no periventricular edema with atrophy.

With cortical atrophy the cerebral sulci enlarge as the gyri shrink. Fortunately, simple visual inspection and intuitive grading of the degree of atrophy into four categories (none, mild, moderate, severe) is, for practical purposes, adequate for defining the presence of atrophy.

A gradually accelerating loss of brain substance occurs with aging, so that the average adult brain diminishes from about 1,400 g at age 25, to 1,375 g by age 45, and to 1,200 g by age 80. Presently, brain atrophy is considered an inevitable part of the aging process. Normally, there is little or no cortical atrophy present up to age 50. From age 50 to 75 there is mild

CAUSES OF DEMENTIA IMPORTANT FOR IMAGING

Alzheimer's disease
Angiopathic dementia
    Subcortical atherosclerotic encephalopathy (of Binswanger)
    Multi-infarction dementia
    Amyloid (congophilic) angiopathy
Low-pressure hydrocephalus
Creutzfeldt-Jakob disease
Pick's disease
Huntington's chorea
Wilson's disease
Parkinson's disease
Multisystem atrophy
Brain trauma
Mass lesions
    Tumor
    Abscess
    Large infarction
    Chronic subdural hematoma
Pugilistic encephalopathy
AIDS
Toxic/metabolic causes
    Alcohol
    Lead

BRAIN CHANGES WITH AGING

Gradual cerebral volume loss (atrophy)
Multifocal high T_2 signal intensity lesions in white matter
Increased brain iron in the globus pallidus, substantia nigra, red nucleus, and dentate nucleus

high T_2 signal intensity foci with MRI in 90 percent of this population. The changes are not seen in normal persons under 45 years of age. They represent small regions of demyelination, necrosis, and gliosis, most likely from microinfarctions. When the changes are

CAUSES OF DIFFUSE CEREBRAL ATROPHY

Degenerative disease of the brain
    Alzheimer's disease
    Binswanger's disease
    Creutzfeldt-Jakob disease
    Huntington's disease
    Pick's disease
    Parkinson's disease
    Multiple sclerosis
    Leukodystrophies
Trauma
    Shear injuries, contusion
Vascular disease
    Migraine
    Vasculitis
    Anoxia/global ischemia
    Postmeningitis
Toxic causes
    Alcohol
    Marijuana and other substances
    Cancer chemotherapy
    Radiation therapy to brain
    Chronic illness

atrophy; and over age 75 moderate atrophy is present. Severe atrophy or atrophy occurring prematurely suggests a degenerative process, possibly associated with dementia. There is about a 75 percent correlation of the degree of atrophy with the degree of mental impairment.

Additionally, there is the gradual development of paraventricular leukomalacia (softening of the white matter), which is positively correlated with the blood pressure level and the degree of hyalinization of the small, deep arterioles. This change has a slight positive correlation with intellectual function and gait disturbance. These changes are seen as hypodensity on CT scans in about 30 percent of those over 75 years and as

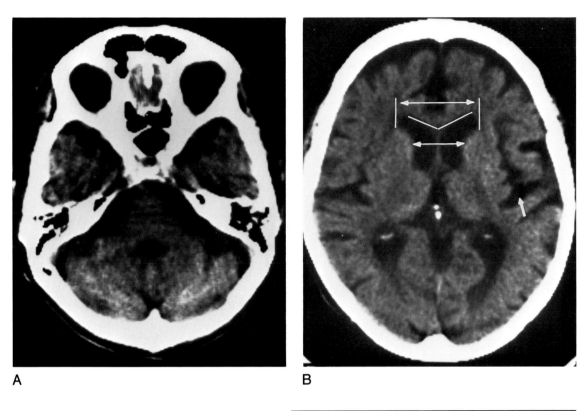

A

B

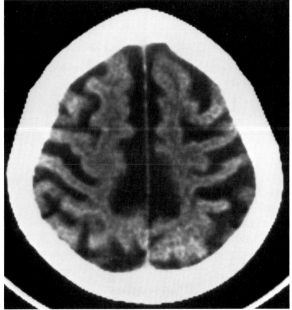

Fig. 10-1 Generalized atrophy, CT scans. (A) Scan through the posterior fossa shows enlargement of the pericerebellar and peripontine cisterns. **(B)** There is enlargement of the lateral ventricles, third ventricle, sylvian fissure (arrow), and subarachnoid spaces over the frontal lobes. The long opposed arrows represent the bifrontal dimension. The short opposed arrows indicate the bicaudate dimension. The white lines outline an obtuse frontal horn (callosal) angle. **(C)** Gross widening of both the interhemispheric fissure and the cerebral sulci is seen.

C

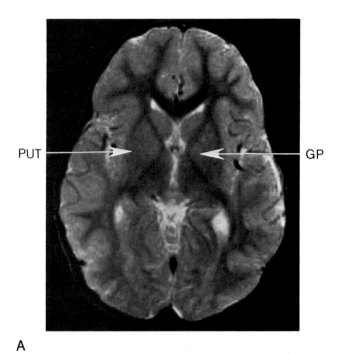

A

B

Fig. 10-2 Brain iron, MRI. (A) Normal 2-year-old brain. The globus pallidus (GP) is isointense with the putamen (PUT). The globus pallidus (medial) and putamen together constitute the lenticular nuclei (lentiform nucleus). **(B)** Normal 40-year-old brain. Iron has deposited within the globus pallidus, which is now hypointense to the putamen on this T_2-weighted image. *(Figure continues.)*

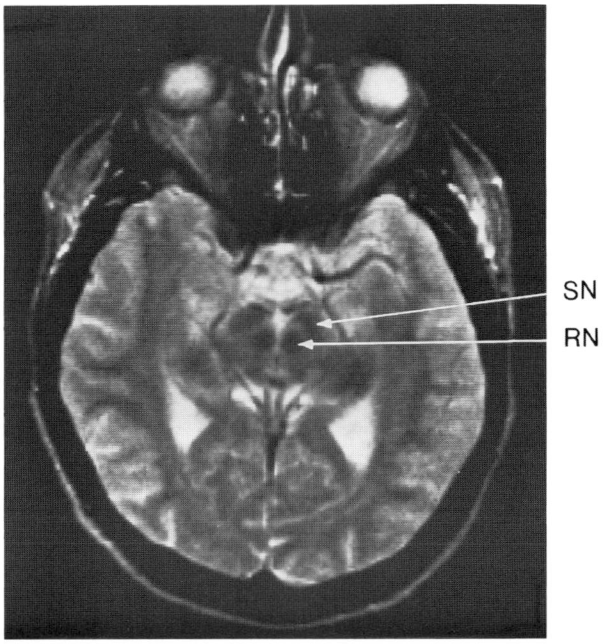

Fig. 10-2 *(Continued)* **(C)** Scan through the upper mesencephalon shows the hypointense T_2 signal from iron deposition in the red nucleus (RN) and the substantia nigra (SN). These regions become more hypointense with aging.

C

mild, they are considered part of the aging process. When more severe, they may be associated with Alzheimer's disease or Binswanger's subcortical arteriosclerotic encephalopathy (SAE). The line is indistinct between normal aging and pathologic change.

Focal atrophy results from a focal destructive process. It is identified by local enlargement of the CSF spaces surrounding the abnormality. Therefore with CT scans or MRI, the lesion is indicated by focal enlargement of the cerebral sulci or adjacent ventricular cavity. There may be density changes seen within the brain on CT scans and MRI representing encephalomalacia or

---

CAUSES OF FOCAL ATROPHY

Infarction
Contusion
Hemorrhage
Surgical removal of tissue
Arteriovenous malformation
Abscess

---

gliosis. It is most commonly seen following head trauma (see Fig. 7-4) or infarction (see Figs. 2-8 and 2-13). Rarely, dystrophic calcification occurs within focal atrophic regions, particularly around arteriovenous malformations. Focal cerebellar atrophy may result from prolonged phenytoin (Dilantin) therapy. The causes of focal atrophy are given below.

BRAIN IRON

At birth there is no ferric iron within the brain. At about 6 months, beginning traces of iron deposits can be found within the globus pallidus. Soon thereafter, iron also can be found in the zona reticulata (lateral portion) of the substantia nigra within the mesencephalon and then later in the red nucleus and the dentate nucleus of the cerebellum (Fig. 10-2). Ferric iron is paramagnetic and on MRI causes reduced signal intensity on the T_2-weighted SE and GRE images. It cannot be imaged with CT scanning.

The amount of iron deposition increases with age, so the loss of signal intensity becomes prominent after age 60. Brain iron may deposit in unusual regions with some degenerative diseases and may be of some diagnostic use (see Multisystem Atrophy, below).

ALZHEIMER'S DISEASE

Alzheimer's disease is a devastating, progressive, terminal disease resulting from a degenerative process in the brain. It occurs in about 5 percent of the population over age 65. The onset is insidious, with memory loss for recent events the most common early manifestation. After a few years, this stage is followed by disturbance of other cognitive functions, such as judgment, comprehension, and abstract reasoning. Anxiety and depression are prominent features. Because of cortical involvement in the degenerative process, aphasia, apraxia (inability to perform tasks), and agnosia become evident. Focal or generalized seizures occur late in about 15 percent of persons affected. There may be myoclonus and extrapyramidal signs in severe cases. Death usually occurs 6 to 10 years after the onset. The diagnosis can be made with certainty only after autopsy.

Pathologically, the disease is characterized by generalized brain atrophy, with frontal and temporal lobe predominance. Atrophy is particularly striking in the region of the hippocampus, amygdala, and the inferior and middle temporal gyri. Microscopically, there are specific changes consisting in neurofibrillary tangles, "senile" plaques, and decreased numbers of neurons. In addition, there is a high incidence of paraventricular leukomalacia in brains of those with the clinical diagnosis of Alzheimer dementia. There is no essential pathologic difference between presenile dementia (classic Alzheimer's disease), occurring before age 60, and senile dementia of the Alzheimer's type (SDAT), occurring after age 60. The cause is unknown.

With CT scanning and MRI, atrophy is the major finding. It is both deep and superficial. The scans show generalized enlargement of the cerebral sulci, which may be more prominent in the parasylvian region resulting in enlargement of the sylvian fissure. The lateral and third ventricles dilate owing to deep atrophy, which may be pronounced. The degree of ventricular enlargement generally correlates with the deterioration of mental impairment. The moderate enlargement of the temporal horns, the choroidal-hippocampal fissure, and suprasellar cistern reflects the atrophy in the hippocampus and basal ganglia. Scans 2 years apart show progression of atrophy in those with Alzheimer's disease but little appreciable change in normal individuals. A clinical diagnosis of Alzheimer's disease must be questioned if the ventricles are not enlarged and especially if the temporal horns are normal. The major difficulty in differential diagnosis is Alzheimer's disease and normal-pressure hydrocephalus, which may also cause ventricular enlargement. The two processes may also coexist.

Paraventricular abnormalities of the white matter are demonstrated with both CT scans and MRI. On CT scans they appear as low density regions, predominantly adjacent to the frontal horns but also extending more posteriorly with severe involvement. These lesions do not enhance with contrast. The MRI shows the lesions best as high signal intensity with T_2-weighted images. CT scans demonstrate these lesions in about 30 percent of those with SDAT, whereas MRI shows them to be present in about 90 percent.

Positron emission tomography (PET) has shown changes in the brains of demented persons that appear specific for Alzheimer's disease. Using ^{18}F-2-fluoro-2-deoxy-D-glucose ([18]FDG), PET demonstrates that the rate of metabolism in the parietal cortex is exceedingly low. Also, those who have specific cognitive defects (aphasia, apraxia, or spatial difficulties) have a corresponding regional decrease in measured cortical metabolism. These changes do not occur with other dementing diseases, such as Parkinson's or Huntington's dementia.

NORMAL-PRESSURE HYDROCEPHALUS

The normal-pressure hydrocephalus syndrome (synonyms: NPH, low-pressure hydrocephalus, Hakim-Adams syndrome) consists of the triad of gait apraxia, dementia, and urinary incontinence associated with ventriculomegaly. The ventricular enlargement is from a communicating obstructive hydrocephalus that has minimal or intermittent increase in intraventricular pressure. The gait disturbance manifests as unsteadiness, ataxia, shuffling, and rigidity sometimes described as "magnetic." It precedes the onset of dementia and is initially more disabling. Typically, the dementia consists in memory impairment, with little disturbance in language function. Its onset is insidious over many years. Urinary incontinence occurs late in the course of the illness.

The disease must be considered in the differential diagnosis of dementia. It can occur without any known antecedent event, or it may result from meningitis,

SAH, meningeal carcinomatosis or, rarely, head trauma.

The CT or MRI scans show the usual findings of hydrocephalus (detailed in Chapter 11). However, many of the persons afflicted also show atrophic changes, making interpretation of the scan difficult. In general, hydrocephalus is considered a possibility when there is considerable enlargement of the temporal horns, narrowing of the callosal angle of the ventricles (less than 100 degrees), periventricular edema, and relatively small cerebral sulci for the person's age. When the bifrontal span is more than 50 mm, hydrocephalus is almost always present. Extensive paraventricular high T_2 signal abnormality on MRI also suggests hydrocephalus rather than simple atrophy.

Radionuclide cisternography may help with the diagnosis. It is performed by injecting ^{111}In-DTPA (or an equivalent tracer) into the lumbar subarachnoid space and imaging the migration of the tracer substance through the intracranial subarachnoid space and ventricles. Iodinated intrathecal contrast and CT scanning may also be used. Normally, the tracer reaches the basal cisterns within 1 hour. Over the next 24 hours, it migrates over the cerebral convexities to concentrate in the region of the sagittal sinus within the interhemispheric fissure. The tracer does not normally enter the ventricular system. In persons with large ventricles due to atrophy, some tracer may reflux into the ventricular system, but the amount is generally small and clears completely by 48 hours.

In persons with normal-pressure hydrocephalus or any type of communicating hydrocephalus, there is continuous reflux of the tracer into the ventricular system, where it remains for at least 72 hours (Fig. 10-3).

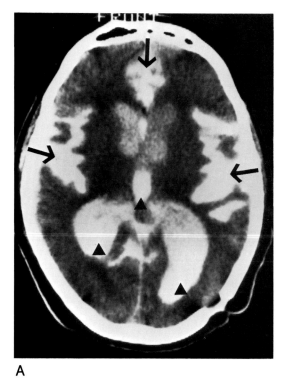

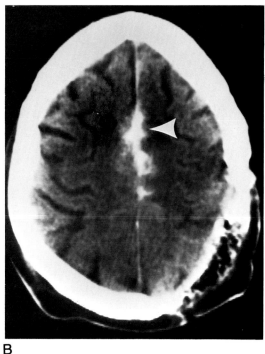

A   B

Fig. 10-3 Normal-pressure hydrocephalus, CT cisternography. Aqueous contrast is injected into the lumbar subarachnoid space. Serial CT scans are then obtained to follow the intracranial distribution of the contrast. **(A)** View through the ventricular system at 24 hours shows dense contrast within the sylvian and interhemispheric fissures (arrows). Dense contrast is also seen within the visualized ventricular system (arrowheads). **(B)** Scan through the vertex shows only a small amount of contrast collecting in the region of the sagittal sinus (arrowhead). There is no contrast at other regions of the interhemispheric fissure or within the cerebral sulci.

Additionally, the tracer does not reach the region of the sagittal sinus but is held up at some point, usually within the basal cisterns, at the incisura, or at the sylvian fissures. This pattern, thought to represent the "block" to the flow of CSF through the subarachnoid space, is diagnostic of communicating hydrocephalus. A "mixed" pattern may be seen that shows delay of the migration of tracer over the convexities (eventually concentrating in the parasagittal region) and transient reflux into the ventricular system that mostly clears by 48 hours. The positive predictive value of the mixed pattern for the diagnosis of hydrocephalus is low.

The treatment of normal-pressure hydrocephalus is shunting of CSF, usually by intraventricular catheter. In about 50 percent of those shunted, there is improvement in gait and mental functioning. Selection of the appropriate persons for shunting remains inaccurate. There are no absolute criteria. In general, the closer the patient's symptoms are to the typical syndrome, including the order of onset of the symptoms, and the more firm the findings of hydrocephalus on the CT,

MRI, and radionuclide scans, the more likely there is to be a favorable result from the shunting.

ANGIOPATHIC DEMENTIA

Multiple Infarction Dementia

Whenever 100 cc or more of brain volume has been destroyed by infarction, there is almost always some deficit in cognitive function. Smaller regions of infarction can produce cognitive dysfunction if they occur in the hippocampal gyri, the thalamic nuclei, or other regions of the limbic system. The mental decline may occur in a stepwise fashion. MRI and CT scans show the multifocal ischemic infarctions. However, it is often difficult to determine if the infarcts seen on CT and MRI are sufficient cause for the mental impairment, and the diagnosis of multiple infarction dementia is most often a judgmental decision. Carotid or vertebral artery stenosis alone is not thought to produce

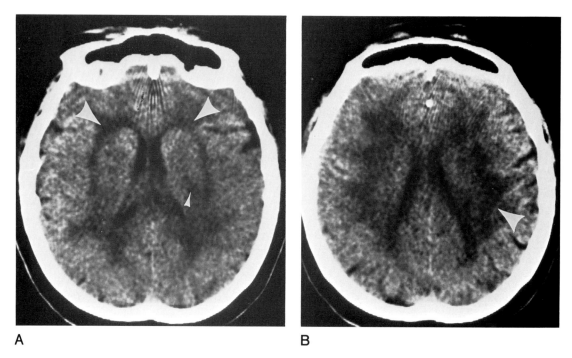

A   B

Fig. 10-4 Binswanger's SAE, CT scans. (A) Scan through the ventricular system shows hypodensity in the paraventricular white matter (large arrowheads). A lacunar infarction is seen in the left posterior internal capsule (small arrowhead). The ventricular system is dilated but less than average for a patient with this disease. **(B)** White matter changes are severe, extending into the subcortical regions (arrowhead). The cerebral sulci are not dilated.

dementia, even when the decrease in blood flow is significant.

Subcortical Arteriosclerotic Encephalopathy of Binswanger

Although somewhat controversial, subcortical arteriosclerotic encephalopathy (SAE), or Binswanger's disease, is now thought to be a discrete disease entity. Most persons with the disease have had long-standing hypertension and a history of infarctions, particularly of the lacunar type. Most neuropathologists consider Binswanger's disease a form of multiple infarction dementia that results from diffuse small vessel arteriosclerotic disease found deep within the brain. The deep ischemic lesions are thought to be the cause for the dementia, gait apraxia, motor deficits, and urinary incontinence seen in affected patients. However, the disease is not associated with language disturbance, which is a distinguishing feature from Alzheimer's disease. SAE may be the cause of up to 55 percent of those with dementia over the age of 70.

The CT scan shows nonenhancing multifocal low density lesions within the paraventricular white matter (Fig. 10-4). The lesion extends more peripherally within the centrum semiovale when the involvement is severe. Ischemic infarctions, mostly lacunar, are usually present, and there is ventricular enlargement due to diffuse deep cerebral atrophy. Cortical atrophy is less severe. The temporal horns are usually near normal in size, helping to distinguish these patients from those with the clinically similar normal-pressure hydrocephalus syndrome.

The most sensitive modality for the detection of SAE is MRI. It shows the bilateral symmetric multifocal lesions as hypointense on T_1- and hyperintense on T_2-weighted images (Figs. 10-5 and 10-6). Confluence of the lesions into a diffuse region of high T_2 signal intensity usually occurs adjacent to the ventricles and when severe also involves the external and internal capsules. Smaller, focal, round lesions are generally seen in the more peripheral white matter and may reach the subcortical zones. In any given patient, the lesions appear more severe and widespread on MRI than on CT scans.

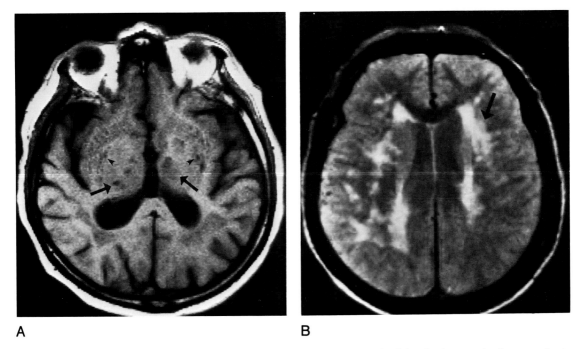

A

B

Fig. 10-5 Binswanger's SAE, MRI. (A) T_1-weighted MRI at the level of the third ventricle shows multiple lacunar-type infarctions in the thalamic nuclei bilaterally (arrows). The Virchow-Robin spaces are enlarged (arrowheads). **(B)** Proton density image through the ventricular system shows multifocal and confluent high T_2 signal intensity in the paraventricular white matter (arrow). The ventricles are moderately enlarged.

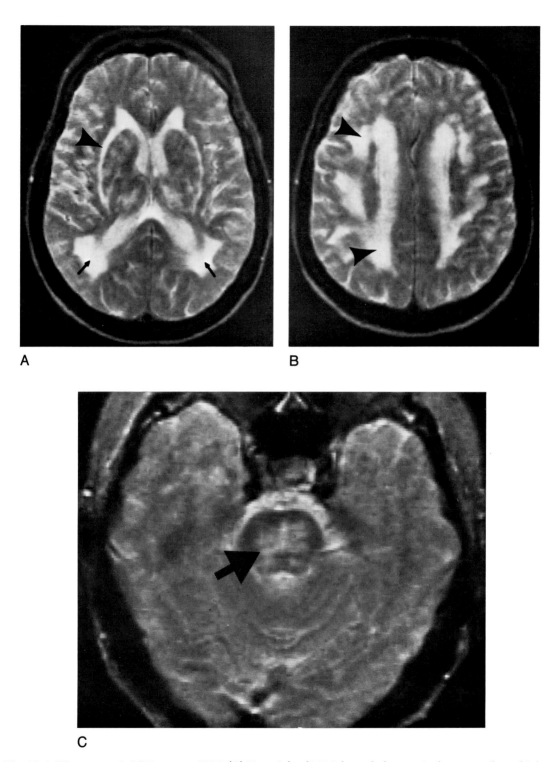

A

B

C

Fig. 10-6 Binswanger's SAE, severe, MRI. (A) T_2-weighted MRI through the ventricular system shows high T_2 signal in the white matter adjacent to the atria (arrows) and in the external capsule (arrowhead). **(B)** Scan at a higher level shows an extreme confluent high T_2 signal white matter abnormality (arrowheads). **(C)** Scan through the pons shows symmetric high T_2 signals throughout the white matter of the brain stem (arrow). Brain stem involvement is present only in the most severe cases.

Binswanger's disease can probably be considered an advanced form of the lacunar state.

Amyloid (Congophilic) Angiopathy)

Amyloid (congophilic) angiopathy is a relatively rare form of angiopathy characterized by amyloid deposition in the walls of small intracranial vessels. It usually occurs only within the brain, although in some there is evidence of amyloid deposits in the vessels of other organs, particularly the gastrointestinal tract. Most often patients present with cortical or subcortical hemispheric hemorrhages that tend to be recurrent. The hemorrhages may be indistinguishable from the subcortical hemorrhages that occur secondary to hypertension and atherosclerosis. The diagnosis is made by biopsy of the meninges at the time of surgical removal of the cerebral blood clot. Sometimes patients present with a slowly progressing dementia that is clinically indistinguishable from SDAT. Amyloid angiopathy may be suggested if the CT or MR scans show evidence of old hemorrhage or infarction in the posterior regions of the brain.

OTHER CAUSES OF DEMENTIA

Creutzfeldt-Jakob Spongiform Encephalopathy

Creutzfeldt-Jakob encephalopathy is a rare, severe, rapidly progressive, infectious degenerative disease of the brain resulting in presenile dementia. It is believed to be caused by a "slow virus" infection that is transmitted by contact with the diseased tissue, including organ transplants of all types. The cerebral cortex is the region most involved, but there may be atrophy of the basal ganglia, thalamus and cerebellum as well.

The onset usually consists in focal neurologic deficits, particularly visual, followed shortly thereafter by dementia, myoclonus, and gait disturbance. The dementia is severe, coming on much more rapidly than the dementia of Alzheimer's disease. Changes may even be observable on a day-to-day basis. Death usually occurs within 1 year from the onset of symptoms. The electroencephalogram shows characteristic periodic spike–wave complexes, often associated with virus infections of the brain. The usual onset is between the ages of 40 and 60, but the disease can be seen at any age, even rarely in teenagers.

The CT scans and MRI show nonspecific changes of cerebral atrophy that are rapidly progressive when compared with other dementing illnesses. There is demonstrable change from month to month. Sometimes there is evidence of demyelination.

Pick's Disease

Pick's disease is a relatively rare cause of dementia. Neuropathologically, there is degeneration of neurons with cytoplasmic swelling, called Pick's bodies. The dementia tends to involve language and behavior more than memory. The atrophy is usually more focal than with Alzheimer's disease and may be limited to the anterior temporal and frontal lobes. The basal ganglia may be involved as well.

The CT scans and MRI reflect these gross anatomic changes (Fig. 10-7). There is severe widening of the frontal horns of the lateral ventricles, third ventricle and temporal horns, sylvian fissures, and frontal and temporal gyri. The remainder of the brain shows much less atrophic change.

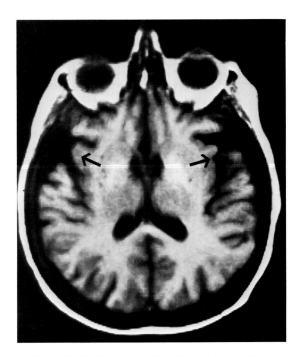

Fig. 10-7 Pick's disease, MRI. T_1-weighted MRI shows severe enlargement of the sylvian fissures (arrows). The posterior sulci show only slight enlargement.

Huntington's Chorea

Huntington's chorea is a rare hereditary dementing disease that usually manifests during middle adulthood. Generalized atrophy is present, but the characteristic anatomic finding is shrinking of the caudate nuclei, which produces widening of the intercaudate region of the frontal horns of the lateral ventricles. The lateral walls of the frontal horns may become convex outward at the level of the caudate head. When the ratio of the maximum width of the frontal horns to the intercaudate distance is less than 1.6, the diagnosis of Huntington's disease can be made.

However, there is relatively poor anatomic correlation with the clinical symptomatology, and patients with severe chorea may have a nearly normal-appearing brain. No distinctive changes are present during the preclinical phase of the disease. The diagnosis is usually made on a clinical basis by the presence of a family history for the disease, decreased levels of γ-aminobutyric acid in the CSF, and abnormality in the fourth chromosome.

Wilson's Disease

Hepatolenticular degeneration, or Wilson's disease, is an autosomal recessive inherited disease resulting from an abnormally low concentration of serum ceruloplasmin. This condition allows accumulation of abnormal amounts of copper within the lentiform nuclei (putamen and globus pallidus), caudate nucleus, thalamus, brain stem, dentate nuclei, and subcortical cerebral white matter, which leads to gliosis and cavitation.

The amount of copper is usually too low for detection with CT scanning. Atrophy is the major finding and is most prominent in the basal ganglia and brain stem. Sometimes focal, low density, nonenhancing lesions are seen involving the regions of copper deposition listed above. There is general correlation between the degree of atrophy and the severity of the dementia. The atrophy may progress even after treatment with penicillamine, a chelating agent. The CT scan of the liver is normal in persons with Wilson's disease.

Increased T_2 signal representing gliosis in the regions of copper deposition listed above but most commonly within the lenticular nuclei and the brain stem are seen on MRI. The lesions are most often symmetric and show little change with therapy. There is general correlation with the severity of the clinical disease and the amount of MRI signal abnormality found.

Parkinson's Disease

Parkinson's disease is the most common disorder of the extrapyramidal system, affecting about 1 percent of the population of the United States over the age of 50. There are four cardinal signs of the disease: tremor at rest, bradykinesia (general slowing of movement, masked face, decreased frequency of blinking), rigidity, and the loss of postural reflexes. It is classified into three etiologic groups: the idiopathic primary form, referred to as Parkinson's disease; secondary, or acquired, parkinsonism; and parkinsonism-plus syndromes, in which nonparkinsonian neurologic findings are present in addition to those of parkinsonism. The final underlying pathologic process is loss of dopamine activity in the striatum (caudate nucleus and putamen).

With primary Parkinson's disease, there is depigmentation and loss of neurons in the substantia nigra and the locus ceruleus of the brain stem, the site of production of the neurotransmitters dopamine and norepinephrine. Focal gliosis may occur. Because of the striatonigral connections, this condition leads to a secondary loss of these transmitters in the striatum.

The etiology is unknown. Clinical improvement can occur after replacement therapy with levodopa or dopamine agonist drugs. About 20 percent of individuals with Parkinson's disease eventually become demented.

The CT scans show moderate, nonspecific generalized atrophy with no recognizable specific changes in the brain stem or basal ganglia. MRI may show changes not seen with CT scanning. Commonly, there is a decrease in the width of the pars compacta of the substantia nigra to about 2 mm (normal 2.5 mm). In practice, this change is difficult to detect. On heavily T_2-weighted images, some observers have described hypointensity of the putamen and slight increased intensity of the lateral substantia nigra (reticulata) so it becomes isointense with the pars compacta, but these findings have not been consistently confirmed. There is moderate nonspecific atrophy and occasional focal high T_2 signal in the brain stem most likely due to gliosis.

With secondary parkinsonism, the findings on the MRI or CT examination depend on the etiology of the process. Postinfarction parkinsonism often shows lucunar-type infarctions in the basal ganglia or thalamic nuclei. Carbon monoxide poisoning, trauma, and Wilson's disease result in bilateral basal ganglionic atrophy. Hypoparathyroidism may cause parkinsonism associated with calcium deposits in the basal ganglia, although idiopathic basal ganglionic calcification does not cause symptoms. Rarely, deep tumors cause parkinsonism.

Parkinson-plus refers to parkinsonism that occurs along with other degenerative diseases of the CNS. It is considered below.

Multisystem Atrophy (Degeneration)

The multisystem atrophy syndrome refers to a group of similar idiopathic brain degenerations that have varied anatomic distributions and clinical manifestations. These disorders are rare. Some studies have shown increased iron deposition within the putamen associated with the multisystem degenerations, which may be demonstrated as low signal intensity on heavily T_2-weighted SE and GRE images. Atrophy in the distribution of the degeneration is also seen.

Alcoholism

The effects of chronic excessive alcohol intake on the CNS are complex and serious. There may be direct toxicity or indirect effects from nutritional deficiencies or trauma.

Alcohol withdrawal may produce various CNS symptoms from mild tremors to life-threatening delerium tremens. Withdrawal seizures are relatively com-

---

SUBCATEGORIES OF MULTISYSTEM ATROPHY

Olivopontocerebellar degeneration

Striatonigral degeneration

Progressive supranuclear palsy

Shy-Drager syndrome

Friedrich's ataxia

Cerebellar degeneration

Hallervorden-Spatz disease

---

mon. These usually consist of one to six convulsions occurring within a six hour period and consisting of tonic-clonic movements. When there is no associated focal deficit or evidence of head trauma, CT or MR scanning is unecessary.

Wernicke's encephalopathy is a relatively common disorder that is caused by associated thiamine deficiency. It is probably more common than is usually recognized. Oculomotor abnormalities (nystagmus, palsy, gaze paresis), gait ataxia and encephalopathy (indifference, disorientation, agitation, depressed consciousness or coma) are present to varying degrees. Treatment is prompt parenteral administration of thiamine. The lesions in the brain are characteristic and consist of demyelination about the third and fourth ventricles and the intervening aqueduct. This may be imaged as hypodensity on CT, and hyperintensity on T2-weighted MRI. In addition, the mamillary bodies are small which can be diagnosed on the parasagittal T_1-weighted MR study.

True dementia may occur in alcoholics and is usually associated with one of two syndromes: 1) Marchiafava-Bignami disease, a rare disorder consisting of necrosis of the corpus callosum and adjacent white matter, or 2) Korsakoff's syndrome which is associated with necrosis in the dorsal medial thalamus. These syndromes may be sometimes diagnosed by finding the necrotic lesions in their characteristic locations on either CT or MRI.

Central pontine myelinolysis is a rare demyelinating disorder of the pons that is seen most commonly in alcoholics. It may be quite extensive, involving the thalami and corpera striatum as well. It has a variable association with clinical symptoms. It is best diagnosed with MRI as high T2 signal abnormality in the characteristic distribution. The disease is most often found in those with severe hyponatremia sometimes occuring only after rapid "over correction" of the electrolyte abnormality (See Chapter 9).

Cerebral volume loss is common in alcoholics, but it is controversial as to whether true atrophy is present. Most alcoholics will show enlarged ventricles and sulci, but this will usually revert to normal about one month after the cessation of drinking. The degree of cerebral volume loss does not correlate with either the duration of alcohol abuse or any associated mental impairment. Cerebellar loss is common, particularly of the anterior superior vermis, but it does not correlate with the degree of ataxia. Post-traumatic intracranial hemorrhage is common, particularly acute or chronic subdural hematomas.

SUGGESTED READINGS

Aisen AM, Martel W, Gabrielsen TO, et al: Wilson disease of the brain: MR imaging. Radiology 157:137, 1985

Braffman BH, Grossman RI, Goldberg HI, et al: MR imaging of Parkinson disease with spin echo and gradient echo sequences. AJNR 9:1093, 1988

Braffman BH, Zimmerman RA, Trojanowski JQ, et al: Brain MR: pathologic correlation with gross and histopathology. 2. Hyperintense white matter foci in the elderly. AJNR 9:629, 1988

Drayer BP: Imaging of the aging brain. I. Normal findings. Radiology 166:785, 1988

Drayer BP: Imaging of the aging brain. II. Pathologic conditions. Radiology 166:797, 1988

Drayer B, Burger P, Darwin R, et al: Magnetic resonance imaging of brain iron. AJNR 7:373, 1986

Hendrie HC, Farlow MR, Austrom MG, et al: Foci of increased T_2 signal intensity on brain MR scans of healthy elderly subjects. AJNR 10:703, 1989

Jack CR Jr, Mokri B, Laws ER Jr: MR findings in normal-pressure hydrocephalus: significance and comparison with other forms of dementia. J Comput Assist Tomogr 11:923, 1987

Lemay M: CT changes in dementing diseases: a review. AJNR 7:841, 1986

Lotz PR, Ballinger WE Jr, Quisling RG: Subcortical arteriosclerotic encephalopathy: CT spectrum and pathologic correlation. AJNR 7:817, 1986

Pastakis B, Polinsky R, DiChiro G, et al: Multiple system atrophy (Shy-Drager syndrome): MRI imaging. Radiology 159:499, 1986

Rutledge JN, Hilal SK, Silver AJ: Study of movement disorders and brain iron by MR. AJNR 8:397, 1987

Simmons JT, Pastakia B, Chase TN: Magnetic resonance imaging in Huntington disease. AJNR 7:25, 1987

11
Hydrocephalus

Hydrocephalus is pathologic enlargement of the cerebral ventricles, accompanied by an increase in CSF volume. The term implies obstruction to the flow, or a decrease in absorption, of the CSF. About 70 percent of the CSF is produced by the choroid plexi within the cerebral ventricles at the average rate of 0.5 ml/min (600 ml/day), although there is considerable individual variation.

The CSF must flow through the ventricular system to reach the exit foramina of the fourth ventricle. From this point most of the CSF flows over the cerebral convexities to be absorbed through the arachnoid villi into the sagittal venous sinus. A much smaller amount is absorbed through the spinal villi at exiting root sleeves. If production of CSF is greater than absorption, there is an increase in the intracranial volume and pressure of CSF with secondary dilatation of the ventricular system.

The usual cause of hydrocephalus is obstruction to the flow of CSF. Hydrocephalus from overproduction of CSF is rare, becoming a factor only with choroid plexus papilloma. Hydrocephalus is said to be "active" when there is increased intraventricular pressure causing progressive enlargement of the ventricles. It is "arrested" when compensatory mechanisms have caused the intraventricular pressure to return to normal with no further tendency for enlargement of the ventricular system. In infants and young children with open cranial sutures, hydrocephalus causes enlargement of the head. In older children and adults with closed cranial sutures, hydrocephalus causes increased intracranial pressure. The clinical signs and causes of hydrocephalus are given below. Obstructive hydrocephalus is further classified as being noncommunicating or communicating. Ventriculomegaly from atrophy is not considered to be hydrocephalus.

CLINICAL SIGNS OF
HYDROCEPHALUS AND INCREASED
INTRACRANIAL PRESSURE

Infants
    Enlarging head and anterior fontanelle
    Distended scalp veins
Children/adults
    Headache
    Diplopia (CN VI compression)
    Vomiting
    Papilledema and visual blurring
    Gait apraxia

CAUSES OF HYDROCEPHALUS

Noncommunicating type
    Infants
        Aqueduct obstruction
        "Congenital tumor," particularly of
          the fourth ventricle
        Hemorrhage, with adhesions within
          the ventricles or aqueduct
        Arachnoidal cyst
        Vein of Galen aneurysm
        Chiari II malformation
        Dandy-Walker malformation
(continued)

Children

    Posterior fossa tumor (medulloblastoma, astrocytoma, ependymoma, epidermoid

    Craniopharyngioma

    Germ cell tumors of the pineal region

    Arachnoidal cyst of the quadrigeminal cistern

    Hypothalamic or thalamic glioma

    Tuberous sclerosis

    Pontine glioma (rarely)

Adults

    Tumors, particularly metastatic tumors, within the posterior fossa or near the aqueduct

    Cerebellar hemorrhage

    Cerebellar infarction

    Tentorial meningioma

    Large glioma

    Pituitary marcroadenoma

    Colloid cyst of the third ventricle

    Giant aneurysm, particularly of the basilar artery

    Transtentorial herniation

    Pachymeningitis of the basal cisterns

    Cysticercosis

Communicating type

  Infants/children

    Congenital "external" hydrocephalus

    Posthemorrhage

    Postmeningitis

    Meningeal tumor (leukemia, medulloblastoma)

  Adults

    Subarachnoid hemorrhage

    Meningitis, especially fungal or tuberculous

    Idiopathic low-pressure hydrocephalus syndrome

    Meningeal carcinomatosis (breast, small cell of lung)

    Very high CSF protein

NONCOMMUNICATING HYDROCEPHALUS

Noncommunicating hydrocephalus results from an obstruction to the flow of CSF that occurs within the ventricular system or at the level of the outlet foramina of the fourth ventricle. The obstruction isolates the intraventricular CSF that is proximal to the obstruction. Noncommunicating hydrocephalus most commonly results from an intracerebral mass lesion or congenital narrowing of the aqueduct of Sylvius. Rarely, pachymeningitis due to a chronic inflammatory process obstructs the outlets of the fourth ventricle.

The ventricles enlarge proximal to the obstruction, and the cisterns and sulci are compressed by the expanded brain. There may be unilateral enlargement or enlargement of only a portion of the lateral ventricle by a mass within the ventricle. Occasionally, multiple lesions produce entrapment of portions of a ventricular cavity. Multiple shunts may be required for decompression.

Obstruction at the level of the foramina of Monro is most commonly due to a colloid cyst of the third ventricle (see Fig. 5-18). Other causes include a large pituitary macroadenoma, craniopharyngioma, meningioma (from the floor of the frontal fossa or rarely within the third ventricle), septal and hypothalamic gliomas, and tubers (tuberous sclerosis). The lateral ventricles enlarge, and the third and fourth ventricles are small. Bilateral intraventricular shunting may be necessary to relieve the hydrocephalus.

Obstruction at the level of the aqueduct of Sylvius or posterior third ventricle causes enlargement of both lateral ventricles and the third ventricle associated with a normal or small fourth ventricle. Congenital aqueduct stenosis is by far the most common cause during the first 15 years of life (Figs. 11-1 and 11-2). In young adults, pineal region tumors are most common (see Figs. 6-16 and 6-17). In later life, periaqueductal tumors, metastasis, and subependymoma are the most common. Other causes include compressive nearby lesions, such as arachnoid cyst of the quadrigeminal cistern, vein of Galen aneurysm, giant aneurysm of the basilar artery, and meningioma about the tentorial hiatus. It is possible for small tumors in this region to cause obstruction. Therefore a thorough investigation of the region is mandatory preferably with MRI in the parasagittal and transaxial projections with contrast enhancement. The characteristics of the various lesions

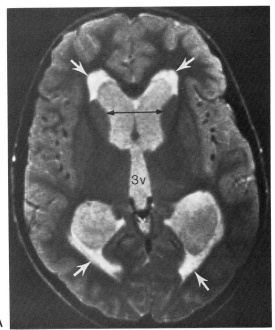

Fig. 11-1 Hydrocephalus, aqueduct stenosis. (A) Transaxial T$_2$-weighted MRI shows enlargement of the lateral (opposed arrows) and third ventricle (3V). High paraventricular signal intensity represents increased fluid content in the white matter from reversal of transependymal flow (white arrows). **(B)** Parasagittal T$_1$-weighted MRI shows enlargement of the third ventricle (3V) and a normal-size fourth ventricle (4V). The problem was caused by a short obstruction within the aqueduct (black arrow).

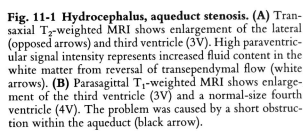

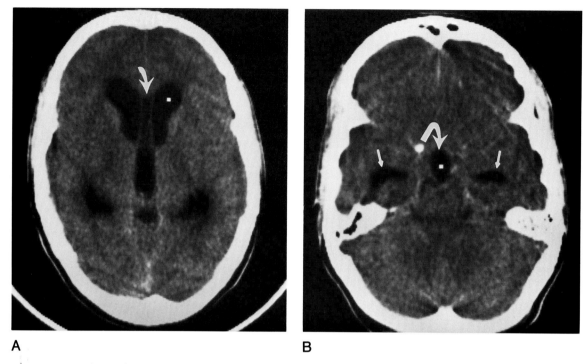

A   B

Fig. 11-2 Hydrocephalus, aqueduct stenosis. (A) Transaxial CT scan shows enlargement of the lateral and third ventricles and a cavum septum pellucidum (arrow). There is only minimal paraventricular edema, as reflected by "smudginess" of the borders of the ventricles. **(B)** Transaxial CT scan at a lower level shows a dilated anterior third ventricle (curved arrow) and temporal horns (small arrows). The fourth ventricle is not dilated and cannot be seen at this scan level. The basal cisterns are compressed from the hydrocephalus.

are described under their specific headings elsewhere in the text. It may be only after a follow-up examination that a benign nonprogressive process can be diagnosed.

Tumor masses within the ventricular cavity or adjacent to the ventricle may cause obstruction to the fourth ventricle. The aqueduct and the third and lateral ventricles are dilated. The fourth ventricle may also be dilated, especially when the obstruction is at the foramina of Luschka (lateral) and Magendie (medial) from tumor or adhesive meningitis.

The diagnosis of basilar adhesions as the cause of fourth ventricular outlet obstruction is often difficult. The adhesions may occur particularly after meningitis from tuberculosis, fungus infection, or sarcoidosis. The diagnosis may be suspected only by the generalized ventriculomegaly including a large fourth ventricle and without a visible mass. Occasionally, there is contrast enhancement of the basal meninges on CT scan or MRI. Nevertheless, the exact etiology may be apparent only at surgery. An intraventricular cyst of cysticercosis

may exactly mimic the ventricular cavity itself and may require CT ventriculography for diagnosis. The clinical history of residence within an endemic region is suggestive of this diagnosis.

COMMUNICATING HYDROCEPHALUS

Communicating hydrocephalus is the most common type of hydrocephalus in adults. It is common with subarachnoid hemorrhage (see Fig. 3-1) meningeal carcinomatosis or meningitis. It is rare after trauma. With these conditions the hydrocephalus is usually mild and self-limited, the ventricles returning to near normal with time and appropriate treatment. Sometimes the hydrocephalus is progressive and symptomatic, and it may be severe. Shunting is required in these instances. (see also Normal-pressure hydrocephalus, Ch. 10) Communicating hydrocephalus implies obstruction to the flow of CSF outside the brain, within the cisterns or at the level of the arachnoid villi. Sometimes, no antecedent cause can be determined for communicating hydrocephalus.

The ventricles enlarge, although the fourth ventricle may remain relatively small; and the cisterns show variable enlargement. There is free flow of CSF between the ventricular system and the subarachnoid space. Radionuclide or positive contrast CT cisternography demonstrates "reflux" of the contrast agent into the ventricular system and block to the flow of radionuclide or contrast over the cerebral convexities.

Diagnosis of Hydrocephalus

The hallmark for the diagnosis of hydrocephalus is enlargement of the ventricular system, best demonstrated with MRI or CT scanning. However, there is no precise measurement for distinguishing normal from abnormal size. Some have defined ventricles as being abnormally enlarged when the frontal horn span measured at the widest point is more than 30 mm or the

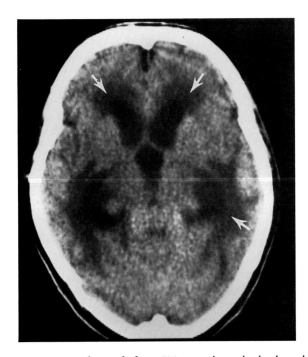

Fig. 11-3 Hydrocephalus. CT scan through the lateral ventricles shows striking periventricular edema (arrows) most commonly associated with acute hydrocephalus. It will disappear after adequate shunting of the hydrocephalus.

ventricular-intracranial index is more than 0.30. However, change from a baseline size is most helpful for defining ventricular enlargement.

With hydrocephalus, alternative pathways of CSF resorption are found. The most prominent is the transependymal absorption from the lateral ventricles. Through breaks in the ependyma, fluid is forced into the paraventricular white matter; and from there it is resorbed into the venous system, producing paraventricular edema, which can be imaged with MRI and CT scanning (Figs. 11-1 and 11-3).

The pattern of the ventricular enlargement is important for differentiating the ventricular enlargement of hydrocephalus from the ventricular enlargement of atrophy. The major anatomic features of hydrocephalus are the following. (See also Chap. 10.)

1. Enlarged lateral ventricles
2. Commensurate enlargement of the temporal horns, usually more than 7 mm in width (Fig. 11-2B)
3. An acute callosal angle, formed by the frontal horns (less than 95 degrees)
4. Bulbous enlargement of the frontal horns so there is a relatively wide frontal horn radius for the size of the ventricles
5. Periventricular white matter edema from compensatory transependymal absorption of CSF (Figs. 11-1 and 11-3)
6. Decreased size and number of visible cortical sulci
7. Decreased size of the subarachnoid cisterns

Hydrocephalus may also be diagnosed with angiography. The enlarged frontal horns can be outlined on the AP projection by the spread subependymal veins, particularly the thalamostriate vein, which is stretched and bowed laterally (Fig. 11-4A). Similarly, the lenticulostriate and the sylvian vessels are stretched and bowed laterally. The pericallosal artery is stretched in a smooth, curving arc around the stretched corpus callosum (Fig. 11-4B). On the lateral vertebral study, the posterior pericallosal arteries are displaced and stretched posteriorly, and the posterior lateral choroidal arteries are pushed forward and downward by the enlarged atria of the lateral ventricles (see Fig. 1-28).

Nonspecific changes of the calvarium result from the increased intracranial pressure associated with hydrocephalus. They can be seen on plain film skull radiography (Fig. 11-5). Most of the skull changes to be listed

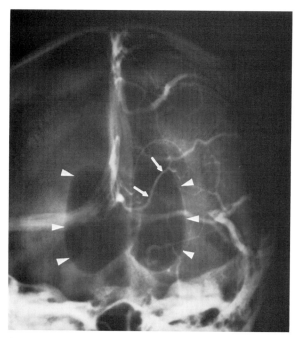

A

Fig. 11-4 Hydrocephalus, angiography. (A) AP venous view shows the thalamostriate vein (arrows) being stretched laterally by the hydrocephalus. The enlarged ventricles are outlined by air from prior pneumoencephalography (arrowheads). (B) Lateral arterial angiography shows stretching of the pericallosal arteries around the enlarged frontal horns (arrows). The sylvian vessels are also displaced upward by the enlarged temporal horn (arrowheads).

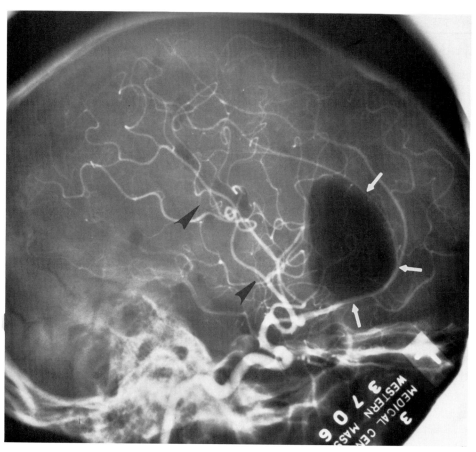

B

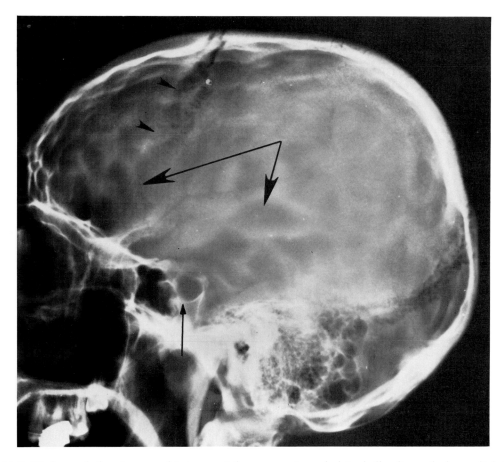

Fig. 11-5 Hydrocephalus, increased intracranial pressure. Lateral plain skull radiograph shows slightly enlarged sella turcica with loss of the cortical margin along the floor (small arrow) and at the chiasmatic sulcus. There are prominent convolutional markings (large arrows) and widening of the cranial sutures with elongation of the interdigitations (arrowheads).

occur after hydrocephalus has been present for some time.

1. Separation of the cranial sutures in infants and children.

2. Elongated sutural interdigitations.

3. Persistence or excessive prominence of the convolutional marking of the inner table of the calvarium. This sign is most useful in the 8- to 12-year age group. Before this age, prominent convolutional margins are normal. This sign infrequently occurs in adults.

4. Thinning and bone resorption of the floor of the sella, beginning at the posterior inferior portion. Thinning may also occur along the planum sphenoidale.

5. Enlargement of the sella and truncation of the dorsum by downward expansion of an enlarged third ventricle.

6. Enlargement of the emissary vein channels, particularly in the occipital region.

7. Enlargement of the internal auditory canals.

When severe hydrocephalus occurs acutely, transtentorial cranial-caudal herniation of the brain may occur, sometimes quickly, causing death. It is especially true when shunt occlusion occurs in "shunt-dependent" individuals. This potential may be recognized by the obliteration of the basal cisterns caused by the compressed brain. Immediate action must be taken when this situation is observed. Severe hydrocephalus may also cause occlusion of the posterior cerebral arteries

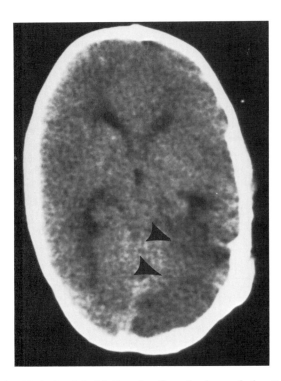

Fig. 11-6 Occipital infarction from hydrocephalus. Severe hydrocephalus has caused compression of the left posterior cerebral artery as it crosses over the tentorium. It has caused infarction in the left occipital and subtemporal regions (arrowheads). Hydrocephalus has been shunted.

(Fig. 11-6). If the hydrocephalus is acute, there is usually complete recovery of the compressed brain after decompression. Prolonged hydrocephalus causes atrophy of brain tissue.

Whereas the diagnosis of hydrocephalus is easy in most circumstances, the differentiation from atrophy may be difficult if not impossible. In these situations it is best to describe the ventricles as enlarged but indicate that an accurate etiology cannot be given at the time. Follow-up scans showing progression may be the only way to diagnose hydrocephalus if the clinical features are not obvious.

AQUEDUCT STENOSIS

The aqueduct of Sylvius is normally a small channel connecting the posterior third ventricle with the superior fourth ventricle. Congenital aqueductal stenosis

refers to the maldevelopment of the aqueduct such that the normal single channel is subdivided, or "forked," into two or more small channels that have inadequate capacity to drain the CSF adequately. Atresia or focal stenosis is rare. The abnormality may occur as an isolated event or in association with the Arnold-Chiari (type II) deformity.

Aqueduct stenosis usually produces severe hydrocephalus, which shortly after birth manifests as a rapidly enlarging head. The diagnosis is generally made with ultrasonography or CT scans. The scans show enlarged lateral and third ventricular cavities with no demonstrable mass in the periaqueductal region. The occipital horns are usually larger than the frontal horns. The left occipital horn is often asymmetrically enlarged. The fourth ventricle is small or normal in size (Figs. 11-1 and 11-2). If left untreated, the head becomes grotesquely enlarged.

The condition responds to ventricular shunting. It is remarkable how a thin cortical mantle reconstitutes so that the brain returns to a relatively normal appearance. These infants are normally "shunt-dependent," meaning that the relief of hydrocephalus depends entirely on adequate shunt function.

If the condition is mild and goes undetected, a few infants reach a state of compensation of CSF production and drainage. This state, often called "arrested hydrocephalus," usually occurs after a moderate degree of ventricular dilatation has developed. A few of these persons function normally and go undetected into adulthood and then are discovered only by chance.

Occasionally, aqueductal stenosis develops during adulthood. Many are new cases that result from periaqueductal gliosis, which may be a response to some unknown inflammatory process. Rarely, prior intraventricular hemorrhage produces adhesions within the aqueduct. A careful search for small periaqueductal tumor must be made, with Gd-DTPA enhanced MRI the single best examination.

NORMAL-PRESSURE HYDROCEPHALUS

Normal-pressure hydrocephalus is also known as low-pressure hydrocephalus, occult hydrocephalus, normal-pressure hydrocephalus, and the Hakin-Adams syndrome. It is discussed in Chapter 10.

EXTERNAL HYDROCEPHALUS

External hydrocephalus is a condition in infants consisting in an enlarging head with widened subarachnoid spaces and normal, or only slightly enlarged, ventricles. The subarachnoid spaces show disproportionate widening over the frontal lobes and in the frontal interhemispheric fissure. The cerebral sulci are prominent over the frontal lobes but are normal elsewhere (Fig. 11-7). The condition is thought to be a communicating hydrocephalus resulting from decreased absorption of CSF at the arachnoid villi in the presence of open cranial sutures.

External hydrocephalus may occur spontaneously or following subdural hematoma, meningitis, and prematurity with associated intracranial hemorrhage. The process is almost always self-limited and resolves without treatment in 2 to 3 years. Atrophy may be a delayed finding in those with the other associated conditions, and the clinical course is determined more by the underlying damage than the external hydrocephalus.

External hydrocephalus must be differentiated from atrophy, which may have a similar CT appearance. With atrophy, the head size is normal or small, the subarachnoid space is more uniformly enlarged, there is little widening of the interhemispheric fissure, and both the ventricles and the sulci are diffusely large. The differential diagnosis is important as the prognosis with external hydrocephalus is good, whereas atrophy implies brain damage. The conditions that may cause macrocranium in infants and children are given in a box.

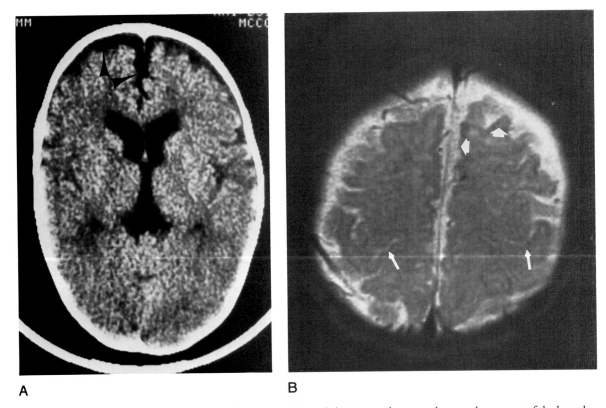

A   B

Fig. 11-7 "External" communicating hydrocephalus. (A) CT scan shows moderate enlargement of the lateral ventricles from hydrocephalus. There is disproportionate enlargement of the cerebral space over the frontal lobes and in the interhemispheric fissure (arrowheads). **(B)** T$_2$-weighted MRI through the vertex shows the widened subarachnoid space over the frontal lobes and in the interhemispheric fissure (fat arrows). The sulci and extracerebral spaces posteriorly are much smaller (thin arrows).

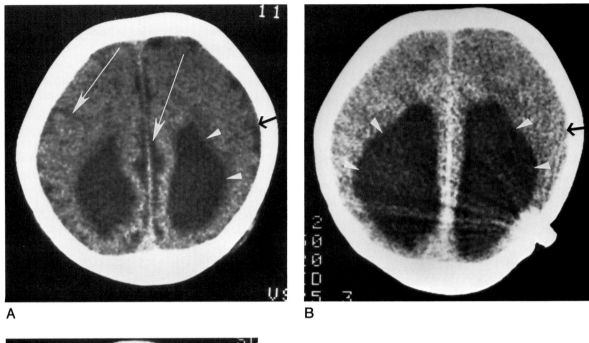

A

B

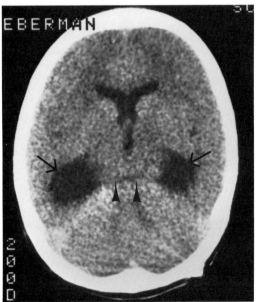

C

Fig. 11-8 Shunt malfunction. (A) Scan superiorly shows enlarged lateral ventricles (arrowheads) but visible subarachnoid space in the interhemispheric fissure and cerebral sulci (white arrows). A small hygroma is present on the left (black arrow). The presence of these spaces indicates adequate shunt function of the preexisting hydrocephalus. **(B)** Shunt malfunction. A scan sometime later shows greater enlargement of the lateral ventricles (arrowheads). The cerebral sulci, interhemispheric fissure, and extracerebral fluid collection on the left have been obliterated. **(C)** Scan at a lower level shows considerable enlargement of the temporal horns (arrows), but the frontal horns are relatively small. The quadrigeminal plate cistern is compressed (arrowheads).

VENTRICULAR DECOMPRESSION: SHUNTS

The usual treatment for hydrocephalus is the surgical establishment of any one or more of a variety of shunts (see below). The object is to divert the intracranial CSF into the peritoneum, pleural space, or bloodstream, thereby reducing the intracranial volume and pressure of the CSF. The shunt may be temporary or permanent. Even when the hydrocephalus is severe, the brain may return to a normal appearance, especially in infants and young children. Acute hydrocephalus responds better to shunting than chronic hydrocephalus. Long-standing hydrocephalus causes irreversible atrophic changes.

The ventriculoperitoneal shunt is the one most commonly employed. The intracranial portion of the tube is preferably passed through the nondominant hemispheric tissue into the ipsilateral ventricle, entering the skull in the posterior parietal region or through the coronal suture. Optimally, the tip of the catheter is within the frontal horn. It may cross through the sep-

TYPES OF SHUNT

Ventricular-peritoneal
Ventricular-pleural
Ventricular-right atrial
Ventricular-cisternal (Torkildsen)
Lumbar-peritoneal

tum pellucidum to the opposite side with no adverse consequence. A shunt that resides within the temporal horn or the atrium of the lateral ventricle can easily become plugged with the surrounding choroid. Care must be taken before diagnosing a catheter as being outside the ventricular cavity, as collapse of a decompressed ventricle or partial volume averaging may spuriously suggest a catheter within brain tissue.

The shunt function is usually evaluated by observing the change in the size of the ventricular system with CT. MRI may be used, but it has no particular advantage. If the ventricles become smaller, the shunt is considered to be working. With successful decompression, the ventricles begin to decrease in size within 24 to 48 hours. The lower the functioning pressure setting of the shunt, the faster do the ventricles decompress. After acute hydrocephalus, the ventricles usually return to normal with fully functioning shunts. If atrophy is

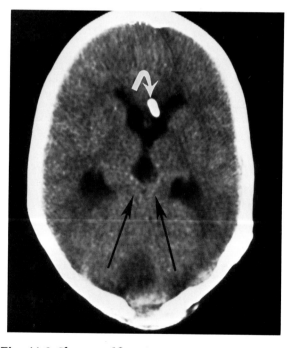

Fig. 11-9 Shunt malfunction, imminent herniation. The ventricles are mildly enlarged, and the shunt catheter is present in the left frontal horn (curved arrow). The basal cisterns are totally obliterated (arrows), indicating increased intracranial pressure in this child who is shunt-dependent. This finding indicates risk of imminent cranial caudal herniation, and the function of the shunt must be reestablished immediately.

present, the ventricles become stabilized at some larger size. Higher-pressure shunts leave slightly larger ventricles.

Shunt malfunction can usually be diagnosed with CT scanning by observing enlargement of previously decompressed ventricles. Initially, the dilatation may be subtle, but it can be recognized by careful comparison with prior examinations. The sulci and interhemispheric fissure become compressed (Fig. 11-8). The condition of the cisterns must be consciously noted so that any potential for herniation can be predicted (Fig. 11-9). Particularly in children, fibrosis of the ventricular ependyma may prevent appreciable enlargement of the ventricles when the shunt has failed. This situation is especially prone to occur with the "slit ventricle syndrome," a condition where the ventricles become extremely small because of shunting. With this condition it is difficult to determine shunt malfunction by scanning, and the clinical symptoms alone must be used to make the correct diagnosis. Scans are repeated at frequent intervals (hours to days) in questionable cases to detect subtle changes.

Ventricular shunts may create extracerebral fluid collections, either subdural hygromas or hematomas (Fig. 11-10). This problem is especially likely to occur when the ventricles are rapidly decompressed, especially in older individuals and those with underlying brain atrophy. In this situation, the brain parenchyma is relatively noncompliant and cannot regain its original volume. The relative negative pressure within the collapsed ventricles causes the cerebral hemispheres to fall away from the inner table of the calvarium. The extracerebral space created is then filled with near-water-density fluid. The extracerebral collections are a sign of "overshunting." Subsequent hemorrhage into the hygroma occurs frequently, causing a mass effect. If the shunt is blocked, or a higher pressure valve is placed, the ventricles reexpand and the extracerebral fluid decreases or disappears. This complication can be prevented by initially using higher-pressure valves and anti-siphon devices in the shunt. Other complications of shunts (Figs. 11-11 and 11-12) are given below.

With noncommunicating hydrocephalus, there can be herniation of the brain after shunting. In the presence of a large posterior fossa tumor, the decompression

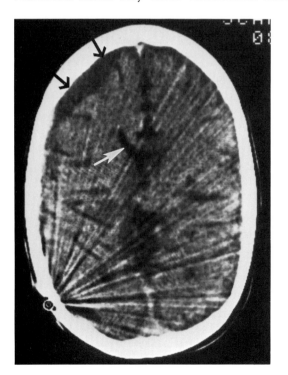

Fig. 11-10 Subdural hygroma, overshunting. CT examination shows small, nearly slit-like ventricles (white arrow). A low density extracerebral collection has developed on the right (black arrows), agenesis of corpus callosum.

COMPLICATIONS OF SHUNTS

Shunt malfunction (poor drainage)
> Poor placement
>> Not within ventricle
>> Plugged by choroid within temporal horn, atrium, or third ventricle
> Disconnection or kinking
> Loculated CSF fluid collection within peritoneum or pleural space (Fig. 11-11)
> Plugged by blood clot

Extracerebral fluid collection (overshunting) (Fig. 11-10)

Hemorrhage around shunt catheter (Fig. 11-12)

Local cerebral infarction

Infection with ventriculitis

Thrombosis and septic emboli from right atrial shunt

Intraperitoneal spread of primary CNS tumor or infection

Brain herniation from asymmetric decompression

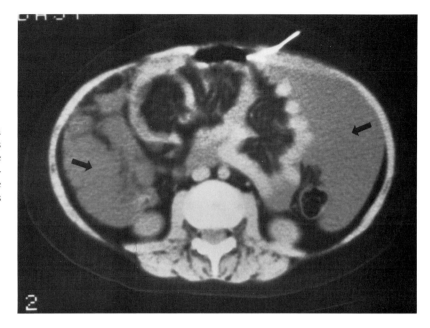

Fig. 11-11 CSF accumulation in the abdomen. CT scan shows a large amount of fluid within the peritonial cavity (arrows), indicating failure of resorption of the shunted fluid. The collections may be focal or diffuse.

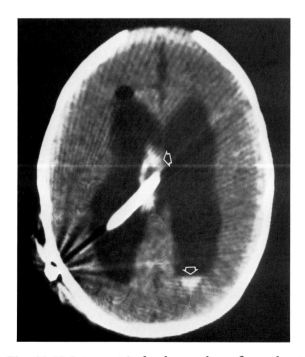

Fig. 11-12 Intraventricular hemorrhage from shunt placement. A small hemorrhage has occurred in the region of the choroid plexus from placement of the shunt. Blood is present in the dependent ventricle (arrows).

of the hydrocephalic lateral ventricles may allow upward transtentorial herniation of the cerebellum, resulting in severe hemorrhage or death. Similarly, when the obstruction is at the level of the foramina of Monro, decompression of only the lateral ventricle may cause subfalcial herniation of the opposite "trapped" ventricle. The trapped ventricle requires shunting with an additional catheter. These potential disasters must be anticipated from the findings on the preshunt CT or MRI scans.

SUGGESTED READINGS

Atlas SW, Mark AS, Fram EK: Aqueductal stenosis: evaluation with gradient-echo rapid MR imaging. Radiology 169:449, 1988

Bradley WG Jr: Hydrocephalus. p. 451. In Stark DD, Bradley WG Jr (eds): Magnetic Resonance Imaging. CV Mosby, St. Louis, 1988

Gammal TE, Allen MB Jr, Brooks BS, Mark EK: MR evaluation of hydrocephalus. AJNR 8:591, 1987

Maytal J, Alvarez LA, Elkin CM, Shinnar S: External hydrocephalus: radiologic spectrum and differentiation from cerebral atrophy. AJNR 8:271, 1987

Naidich TP, Schott LH, Baron RL: Computed tomography in evaluation of hydrocephalus. Radiol Clin North Am 20:143, 1982

12

Congenital Abnormalities of the Brain

Structural congenital abnormalities are thought to result from insults to the developing brain. The timing of the insult is considered the most important factor. Most insults affect the entire brain, so frequently several anomalies are seen. Malformations are classified on the basis of anatomic features.

Other congenital abnormalities include destructive disorders, dysmyelination and the neurocutaneous syndromes. These conditions tend to exhibit inheritance and some have a known metabolic basis.

The preferred imaging technique for identifying these structural malformations is MRI. T_1 imaging is usually better for anatomic definition, and the sagittal and coronal planes are often helpful. T_2-weighted MRI is better for dysmyelinating diseases. CT scanning may be used but is generally less precise.

EMBRYOLOGIC REVIEW

The development of the nervous system begins with the thickening of the dorsal neural ectodermal plate. At about the T12-L1 level and progressing rostrally, the ectodermal plate infolds to produce the neural tube, which then forms the brain and spinal cord. Below this level there is a regressive type of differentiation process that forms the lower spine and dural tube. Failures of the normal tube closure and differentiation process results in abnormalities such as anencephaly, cephalocele,

myeloschisis, myelomeningocele, and the Chiari malformation. This process occurs during the fourth to seventh weeks of gestation.

Once the neural tube is formed, ventral induction occurs in the rostral end, which forms the face and the brain. The prosencephalon, mesencephalon, and rhombencephalon are created. There is division into two hemispheres, which then roll over to form lobes and the major fissures. The connecting corpus callosum and the vermis of the cerebellum are formed in a rostral-caudal direction. Disorders during this phase result in various anomalies, including agenesis of the corpus callosum, holoprosencephaly, septo-optic dysplasia, cerebellar aplasia, and the Dandy-Walker syndrome. These events occur during the fifth to tenth weeks of gestation.

After formation of the gross structure of the brain, cellular migration and differentiation occur. Neurons are formed in the germinal matrix of the paraventricular region and then migrate outward to the cortex. Failure of this migration results in deformation of the gyral pattern—either too few and too thick (agyria, pachygyria) or too thin and too many (polymicrogyria). Abnormal differentiation or inclusion of foreign cells results in vascular malformations, teratomas, hamartomas, and other tumors from embryonal rests. These processes occur during the second to fifth months of gestation.

Myelination begins later, after 5 months of gestation.

333

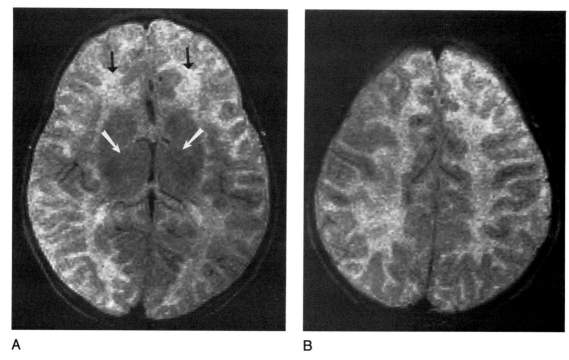

A   B

Fig. 12-1 Normal 3-month-old brain, immature white matter; T_2-weighted MRI SE2500/80. (A) Transaxial slice through the basal ganglia shows relatively high intensity of the hemishperic white matter, particularly the frontal lobes (black arrows). This pattern is opposite that of normal adult myelin. Myelination has occurred within the posterior limbs of the internal capsules and the thalamic nuclei (white arrows). These areas are the more "primitive" portions of the brain. The white matter of the cerebellum and pons also have low intensity by this age. **(B)** Slice through the centrum semiovale shows the typical high intensity signal of immature nonmyelinated white matter. It must not be interpreted as dysmyelination.

Myelin first appears in the cerebellum and brain stem and then in the thalamus and posterior limb of the internal capsule (Fig. 12-1). The myelination process continues to include the entire cerebellum, the posterior optic radiations, and finally the centrum semiovale of the cerebral hemispheres. This process is complete at about 15 months of age with final maturation of the myelin at 3 years. Various disorders of myelin formation result in a multiplicity of syndromes, discussed below.

The congenital disorders discussed below are grouped according to their most likely etiology. When placed into this somewhat arbitrary framework, the disorders make some sense and are easier to remember.

DISORDERS OF CLOSURE OF THE NEURAL TUBE

Anencephaly

Anencephaly is the most severe of anomalies and causes death of the fetus or infant. It may be diagnosed with ultrasonography as early as 20 weeks' gestation. The brain and calvarium may be totally deficient, or there may be rudimentary brain at the base and severe microcephaly. Polyhydramnios and increased levels of α-fetoprotein in the amniotic fluid are usually associated with these defects of closure of the neural tube.

Cephalocele

Cephalocele is a congenital defect resulting in herniation of intracranial contents outside the calvarium. Most occur in the midline. In Europe and the United States the defect is most commonly occipital. In Asia it is most commonly nasofrontal. It may also occur in parietal, frontal, and nasopharyngeal sites.

Meningocele refers to herniation of only the meninges. *Encephalomeningocele* indicates herniation of brain tissue along with the meninges. *Encephalocystomeningocele* includes the ventricle within the herniation (Fig. 12-2A). Microcephaly is present with large encephaloceles. The herniated brain may be normal or dysgenetic. It is impossible to predict this condition accurately with imaging or angiography. Sphenoethmoidal encephaloceles are frequently associated with facial midline defects and always hypertelorism, but these sacs usually do not contain herniated brain (Fig. 12-2B). Low occipital encephaloceles containing the cerebellum are called Chiari III malformations. Low cephaloceles may include posterior dysraphism of the upper cervical spine. A midline dermoid may mimic the skull defect of cephalocele.

Chiari Malformations

The Chiari malformations are considered under a separate heading, as they are a diverse group with poorly understood pathogenesis. There is notorious confusion about them. There were four entities described by Chiari, which he labeled types I to IV. The four are not related pathologically.

CHIARI I

Chiari I refers to a malformation of both the cerebellum and cervicomedullary junction of the spinal cord usually associated with malformation of the cervical spine and craniovertebral junction. The cerebellar tonsils are small, pointed inferiorly, and situated through the foramen magnum into the posterior upper cervical spinal

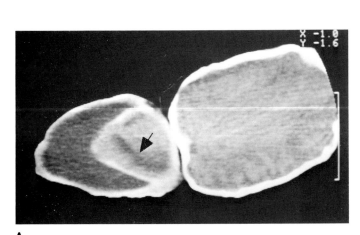

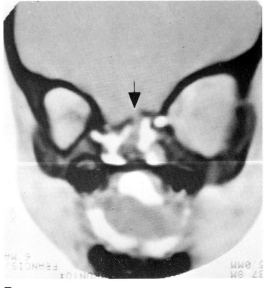

A   B

Fig. 12-2 Occipital encephalocystomeningocele. (A) CT scan shows a large hernia sac posteriorly. It contains CSF, brain, and what appears to be a rudimentary ventricular cavity (arrow). **(B)** Frontoethmoidal encephalocele. Coronal view (reverse gray scale) of the brain of a 7-month-old infant. There is hypertelorism and hypoplasia of the right orbit. The encephalocele extends through the frontal bone and into the nasal ethmoid region through a small ethmoid defect (arrow). (From Fitz, 1984, with permission.)

canal. The fourth ventricle is usually small and slightly low in position. The cisterna magna is small. Associated bone abnormalities include basilar impression, occipitalization of the atlas, incomplete ossification of the atlas, and Klippel-Feil anomaly. Hydromyelia is common. Chiari I is discussed further in Chapter 13.

CHIARI II

The Chiari II malformation is a complex abnormality almost always associated with a myelomeningocele. The malformation affects many diverse structures (Fig. 12-3). The tentorium is low, creating a small posterior fossa. The brain stem is inferiorly positioned within a large foramen magnum and the upper cervical spinal canal. There may be actual buckling of the medulla behind the upper cervical cord, forming a characteristic kink. The fourth ventricle is elongated inferiorly. The cerebellum is poorly differentiated, herniates inferiorly, and expands anteriorly around the pons. There is a posteroinferior vermian peg behind the medulla. Hydrocephalus is common (usually a result of aqueduct stenosis) and often requires shunting. There may also be a "beaked" collicular plate, agenesis of the corpus callosum, a large massa intermedia, inferior frontal horn beaking, anatomic polymicrogyria (stenogyria), anomalous cisterns, syringohydromyelia, clival scalloping, and craniolacunia (Fig. 12-4). Craniolacunia is a dysplastic scalloping of the calvarium that resolves after 6 months.

CHIARI III

The Chiari III malformation is a cervico-occipital encephalocele with the sac containing nearly all of the cerebellum.

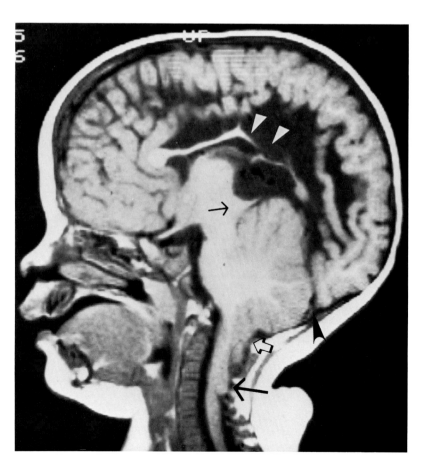

Fig. 12-3 Chiari II malformation. Sagittal T$_1$-weighted MRI shows the characteristic findings. Elongation and buckling of the medulla (large arrow), a vermian peg (open arrow), beaking of the tectum (small arrow), agenesis of the posterior corpus callosum (white arrowheads), and stenogyria (polymicrogyria). The foramen magnum is large, and there is a low position of the tentorium, allowing inferior extension of the occipital lobes (black arrowhead). The fourth ventricle, not seen on this image, is small, elongated, and inferiorly positioned.

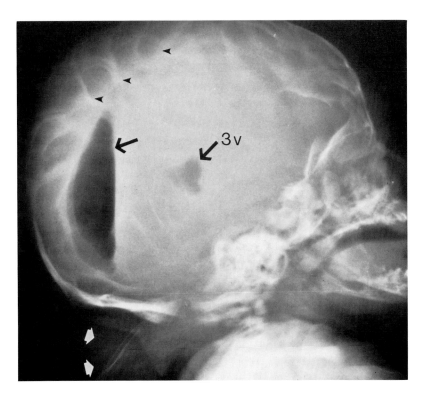

Fig. 12-4 Craniolacunia, Chiari III. Plain skull radiograph shows a scalloped appearance of the calvarium (arrowheads). This infant has undergone ventriculography, and air is seen in the dilated occipital horns in the posterior third ventricle (3V, black arrows). The posterior fossa is small, and there is a cervico-occipital encephalocele (white arrows). This picture represents a Chiari III malformation.

CHIARI IV

The Chiari IV malformation is severe cerebellar hypoplasia.

DISORDERS OF ORGANOGENESIS

Dysgenesis of the Corpus Callosum

The corpus callosum may be partially or completely absent. The corpus callosum begins development from the region of the anterior commissure, and the growth proceeds posteriorly. Therefore with partial absence, the anterior genu is formed but there is aplasia of the body or posterior splenium (Figs. 12-3 and 12-5B&C). The anomaly occurs most commonly in association with other defects of brain formation, particularly Chiari II, Dandy-Walker cyst, Aicardi's syndrome (chorioretinopathy and mental retardation), and holoprosencephaly. Callosal dysgenesis may occur as an isolated defect causing minor mental impairment.

Callosal dysgenesis is best diagnosed with sagittal MRI (Fig. 12-5) but may also be diagnosed with CT scanning (Fig. 12-6). The corpus callosum is absent or partially absent. Large longitudinal parasagittal white matter bundles of Probst indent and splay the frontal horns, causing a "bull's horns" appearance on the coronal scan (Fig. 12-6). The frontal horns are small with sharp lateral angles. The third ventricle is usually large and superiorly positioned. Owing to the absence of the splenium and the forceps major, the atria and occipital horns are large and extend medially to nearly the cortical interhemispheric surface of the occipital lobe (Figs. 12-5C and 12-7). The interhemispheric sulci are radially oriented and reach the ventricular surface (Fig. 12-5B). There may be an associated interhemispheric arachnoid cyst or lipoma (Fig. 12-7).

Lipoma

Intracranial lipomas almost always occur near the midline, usually in or along the corpus callosum, at the collicular plate, or the tuber cinereum. They are thought to represent a form of dysraphism. Large inter-

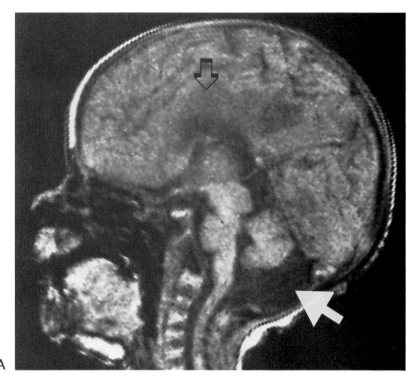

A

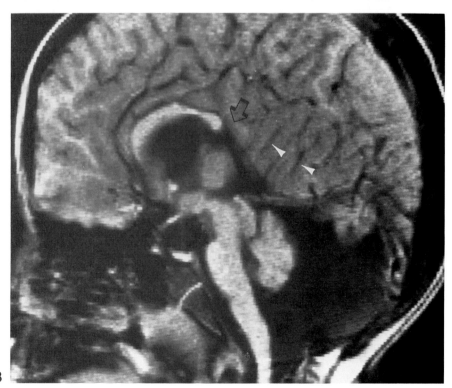

B

Fig. 12-5 Agenesis of the corpus callosum. (A) Parasagittal T_1-weighted MRI shows complete agenesis of the corpus callosum (open arrow). There is also cerebellar hypoplasia and an arachnoid cyst within the posterior fossa (white arrow). **(B)** Agenesis of the corpus callosum, cerebellar hypoplasia, and posterior fossa arachnoid cyst. Parasagittal T_1-weighted MRI shows agenesis of the posterior portion of the corpus callosum (open arrow). The medial sulci are oriented in a radial fashion (arrowheads). There is a large collection of CSF-intensity fluid in the posterior fossa representing an arachnoid cyst. The cerebellum and vermis are hypoplastic. (*Figure continues.*)

Fig. 12-5 (*Continued*) **(C)** Partial agenesis of the corpus callosum. Transaxial T_1-weighted MRI shows normal anterior corpus callosum and frontal lobe white matter (black arrows). The posterior corpus callosum and splenium are absent (open arrow). The occipital horns are dilated and extend more medially than normal because of the absence of the forceps major (white arrows). **(D)** Total agenesis of the corpus calosum, as seen by angiography. The pericallosal artery has a meandering posterior and superior course instead of its normal curving sweep around the genu of the corpus calosum (arrows).

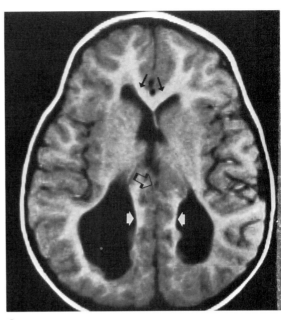

C

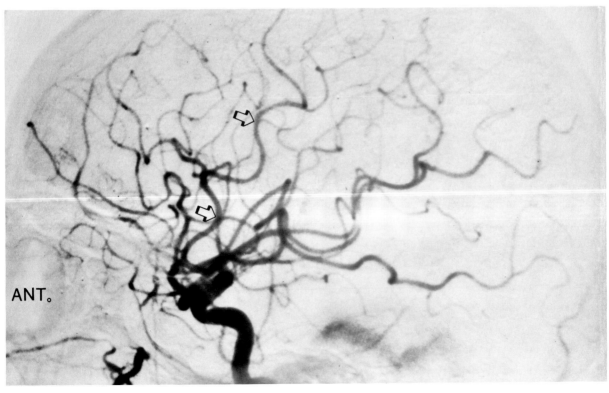

ANT.

D

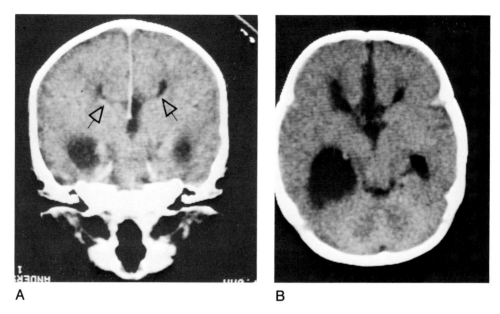

A   B

Fig. 12-6 Agenesis of the corpus callosum. (A) Coronal CT scan shows the typical "bull's horns" separation of the frontal horns (arrows). The third ventricle rides high between the lateral ventricles. **(B)** Transaxial CT scan shows widening of the frontal horns and posterior extension of the interhemispheric fissure. (From Fitz, 1984, with permission.)

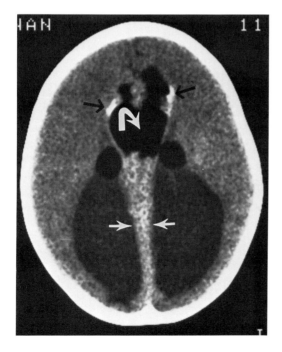

Fig. 12-7 Lipoma with agenesis of the corpus callosum. A large multilobulated interhemispheric lipoma is present (white curved arrow) associated with agenesis of the corpus callosum. There is calcification associated with the lipoma (black arrows). Note the medial enlargement of the atria of the lateral ventricles due to the absence of posterior white matter fibers (white arrows).

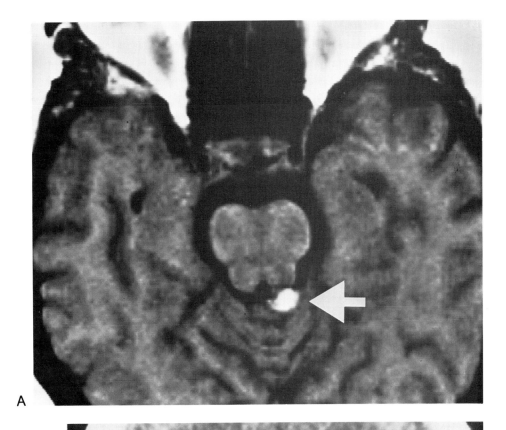

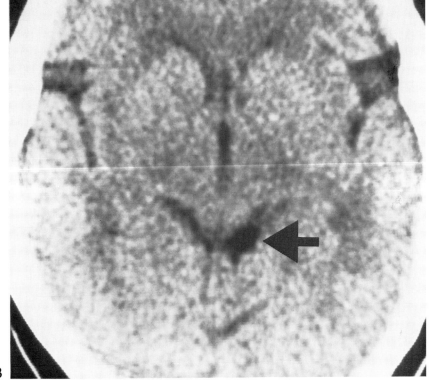

Fig. 12-8 Lipoma. (A) T$_1$-weighted MRI shows a small lipoma in the quadrigeminal plate cistern as being very hyperintense (arrow). **(B)** CT scan shows the lipoma as a region of hypodensity (arrow). This location is common.

hemispheric lipomas are found in association with seizures and callosal dysgenesis (Fig. 12-7). Small lipomas are usually incidental findings (Fig. 12-8).

Holoprosencephaly

Holoprosencephaly refers to failure of the brain to separate into hemispheres. There is a spectrum of abnormality classified into three forms.

Alobar holoprosencephaly. There is complete failure to form separate hemispheres and lobes. The mass of the brain is fused, and there is a central monoventricle. A large posterior cyst is usually present, thought to arise from the roof of the third ventricle. It fills the posterior calvarium, compressing the brain anteriorly (Fig. 12-9). There is no falx. The thalami are completely fused.

Semilobar holoprosencephaly. This form is less severe. The posterior occipital and temporal lobes partially separate with partial differentiation of the ventricles into occipital and temporal horns. The frontal half of the brain is fused, but there is only partial fusion of the thalami (Fig. 12-10).

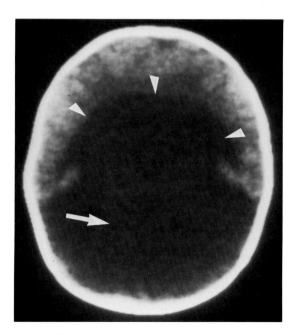

Fig. 12-9 Alobar holoprosencephaly. CT scan shows the anterior monoventricle (arrowheads). The characteristic large cyst is seen posteriorly (arrow).

Lobar holoprosencephaly. This form is least severe. Only the antero-inferior part of the frontal lobes are fused. The frontal horns of the lateral ventricles are "squared off," and there is absence of the septum pellucidum. The interhemispheric fissure and falx are nearly complete. The occipital and temporal horns are well formed, and there is a third ventricle separating the thalami (Fig. 12-11).

Facial anomalies are common. There is always hypotelorism. The other common facial abnormality is absence of the intermaxillary segment (the middle third of the upper lip, the palate, and the incisors). A spectrum of more severe abnormalities also occurs, including cyclopia.

Septo-optic Dysplasia (DeMosier Syndrome)

Septo-optic dysplasia is a rare syndrome consisting of hypoplasia of the optic nerves and chiasm, absence of the septum pellucidum, and dilatation of the anterior third ventricle and lateral ventricles. Occasionally, callosal dysgenesis is present. Clinically, there is short stature, visual loss, and nystagmus.

Dandy-Walker Syndrome and Cysts of the Posterior Fossa

The Dandy-Walker malformation is thought to be caused by defective development of the roof of the fourth ventricle and failure of the foramen of Magendie (median aperture) to open. This deformity causes variable expansion of the fourth ventricle, resulting in the more common Dandy-Walker variant, or the "full-blown" Dandy-Walker cyst;. Large cystic dilatation of the fourth ventricle causes inferior vermian aplasia, cerebellar hemispheric hypoplasia, and expansion of the posterior fossa.

With the classic Dandy-Walker cyst, the entire posterior fossa is filled with a cyst that balloons upward, often through the incisura. The torcula is high, and the falx cerebelli is absent. The foramen of Magendie is closed (Fig. 12-12).

The Dandy-Walker variant is seen as a less severe form of the malformation with a somewhat formed but enlarged fourth ventricle that communicates with a retrocerebellar cyst. There is less severe vermian and

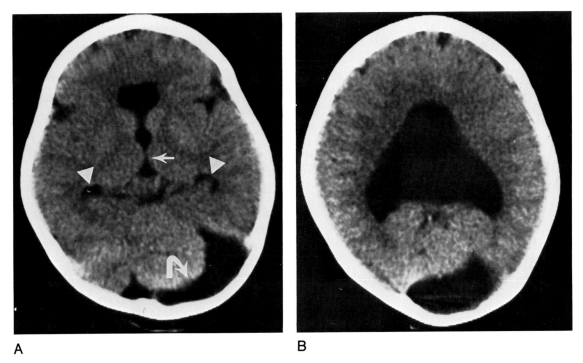

A   B

Fig. 12-10 Semilobar holoprosencephaly. (A) Transaxial CT scan shows anterior fusion of the frontal horns, partial fusion of the basal ganglia (arrow), and differentiation into well formed temporal horns (arrowheads). Note the arachnoid cyst of the posterior fossa (curved arrow). **(B)** Scan at a slightly higher level shows the fusion of the body of the lateral ventricles and separation into atria. The falx is absent anteriorly.

Fig. 12-11 Lobar holoprosencephaly. Transaxial CT scan shows enlargement of the fused frontal horns with a "squared off" anterior margin (arrowheads). The septum pellucidum is absent (arrow). There is a well formed third ventricle and separation of the basal ganglia (open arrow).

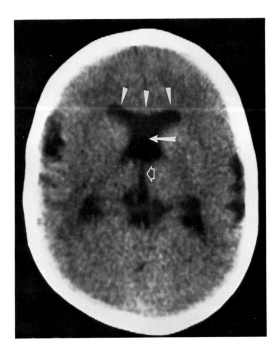

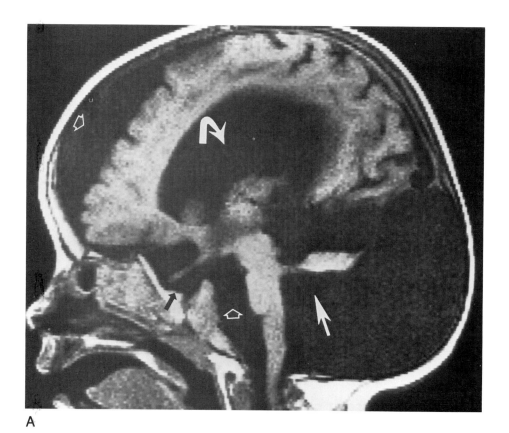

A

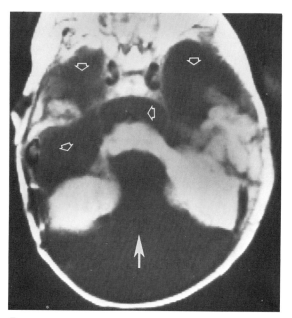

B

Fig. 12-12 Dandy-Walker cyst, MRI. (A) Parasagittal T₁-weighted MRI shows a large cyst within the posterior fossa in continuity with the fourth ventricle (arrow). There is hypoplasia of the cerebellum, and hydrocephalus is present (curved arrow). There are also arachnoid cysts over the frontal convexity and in the prepontine and suprasellar cisterns (open arrows). The sella turcica is grossly enlarged (black arrow). **(B)** Transaxial MRI shows the large cyst in the posterior fossa and its wide communication with the fourth ventricle (white arrow). Arachnoid cysts are seen in the temporal fossae and the prepontine cisterns (open arrows).

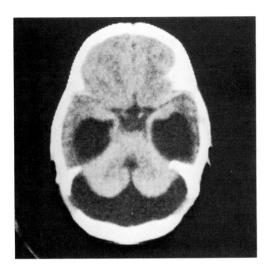

Fig. 12-13 Dandy-Walker variant. A moderately large posterior fossa cyst is connected to the relatively normal fourth ventricle by a small interhemispheric cleft. Hydrocephalus is present with large temporal horns. (From Fitz, 1984, with permission.)

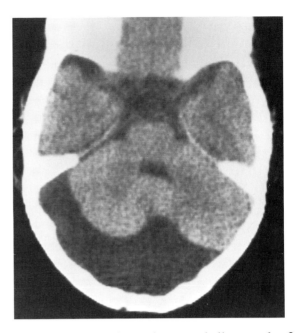

Fig. 12-14 Arachnoid cyst (retrocerebellar pouch of Blake). CT scan shows CSF-containing space behind normally formed cerebellar hemispheres and cerebellar vermis. There is no mass effect or hydrocephalus.

cerebellar hypoplasia and a relatively normal-size posterior fossa (Fig. 12-13).

Hydrocephalus is commonly present but, surprisingly, not always. Dysgenesis of the corpus callosum, holoprosencephaly, and cortical dysgenesis are often associated anomalies.

The retrocerebellar pouch (of Blake) is an arachnoidal cyst that evaginates from the choroid of the fourth ventricle behind normally formed cerebellar hemispheres and vermis (Fig. 12-14). It communicates with the fourth ventricle and subarachnoid space. Although it usually does not cause problems, it is probably responsible for what is often called the "mega cisterna magna." Differentiation between a cyst and a large cisterna magna is not necessary unless hydrocephalus or a posterior fossa mass effect is present.

Cerebellar Hypoplasia

There are varying degrees of cerebellar and vermian hypoplasia. The vermis forms in a rostrocaudal direction. Therefore there is either complete vermian agenesis or aplasia of the inferior portion (Fig. 12-15). It may form part of Down or Joubert syndrome. Severe cerebellar hypoplasia is the Chiari IV malformation.

Craniosynostosis

Craniosynostosis is considered to be a result of deformity of the base of the calvarium, which secondarily causes failure of proper formation of the cranial sutures. The abnormality is usually present at the time of birth. It is generally first recognized by skull deformity.

The abnormality consists of varying lengths of either fibrous or bone fusion of the cranial sutures. Part or all of one or more of the sutures may be involved. With time a bone ridge forms at the suture line. Usually only some of the cranial sutures are involved, resulting in asymmetric deformity of the calvarium (plagiocephaly).

The major problem of craniosynostosis is cosmetic deformity of the skull. Constriction of brain growth and increased intracranial pressure occur only with synostosis of all of the cranial sutures. The diagnosis of craniosynostosis is made by plain skull radiography or by CT scanning with bone images. Multiple tangential views may be required if there is partial stenosis of only one suture (Fig. 12-16).

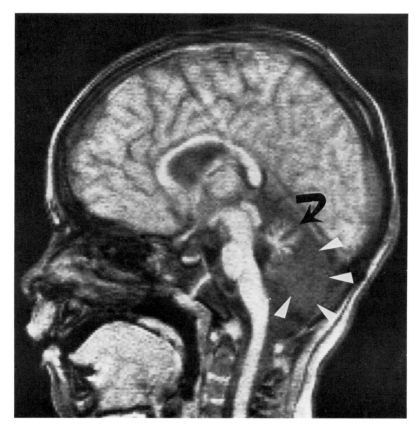

Fig. 12-15 Cerebellar hypoplasia. Severe hypoplasia of the vermis is present, although portions of the superior vermis remain (curved arrow). There is an arachnoid cyst (pouch of Blake) in the posterior fossa (arrowheads).

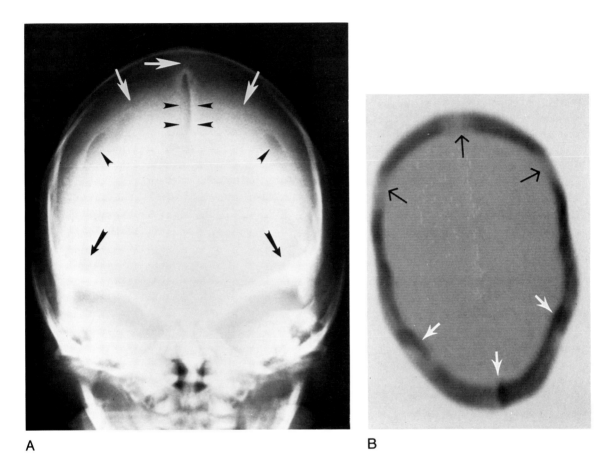

A   B

Fig. 12-16 Craniosynostosis. (A) Plain AP skull radiograph shows complete bone fusion of portions of the sagittal and coronal sutures (white arrows). Parts of the sutures show fibrous union with sclerotic margins (arrowheads). Note the deformity of the orbits from abnormal skull growth (black arrows). **(B)** Bone window CT images show the bone fusion and ridging of the posterior sagittal and lambdoid sutures (white arrows). The metopic and inferior coronal sutures appear open (black arrows).

MIGRATION ANOMALIES

The normal cerebral cortex is populated by a process of radial migration of neurons from the paraventricular germinal matrix. It occurs predominantly during the 8th through the 16th fetal weeks. When migration is interrupted, a thickened, disorganized cortical layer results. The underlying white matter is small, as there are correspondingly fewer axons present. The severity of the interruption determines the type of anomaly. There seems to be a strong genetic control of migration. There are multiple types of migration anomaly.

Lissencephaly (Agyria, Pachygyria)

Lissencephaly is a rare, severe malformation consisting of a total loss of the gyral and sulcal organization of the cerebrum so the brain appears smooth. The cortical gray matter is much thicker than normal and the white matter correspondingly smaller. The sylvian fissures have the appearance of shallow, open grooves, creating a "figure-of-eight" configuration of the brain as viewed in the transaxial plane. The ventricles are somewhat large and relatively formless (Fig. 12-17). It is sometimes familial. Agyria refers to absence of a gyral pattern and is the most severe form. Pachygyria refers to broadening of the gyri and is thought to be a milder form of the malformation. These conditions are associated with microcephaly and severe retardation.

Polymicrogyria

Polymicrogyria occurs relatively frequently and is less severe than the other malformations. It can be imaged only with MRI. It is characterized by a regional thickening of the cortex with excessive but shallow and poorly formed convolutions. The normal finger-like subcortical projections of the white matter are absent. The condition may be seen alone or associated with other anomalies, particularly schizencephaly. The opercular regions are characteristically involved. The condition of too many but normally formed gyri is called *stenogyria* and is seen with the Chiari II malformation (Fig. 12-3).

Schizencephaly

Although the exact etiology for schizencephaly is unknown, it probably results from an early injury or defect in the germinal matrix. This defect interrupts the neuronal migration process at its origin. The result is a full-thickness cleft in the cerebral cortex that may be unilateral or, more commonly, bilateral.

There is an infolding of the adjacent cortex along the margins of the cleft, with the intervening pia becoming fused with the ependyma of the subjacent ventricle. Gray matter is seen to extend along the cleft from the ventricle to the cerebral cortex. The septum pellucidum is usually absent. Callosal dysgenesis occurs at the cleft.

There are two types. Type I is mild with a small slit defect ("closed lips") and normal ventricles. Type II is move severe with larger, fan-like cortical defects ("open lips") and ventriculomegaly (Fig. 12-18).

Unilateral Megalencephaly

Unilateral megalencephaly may be mild or severe, causing seizures, hemiplegia, and retardation. The MRI is characteristic, showing unilateral ventricular

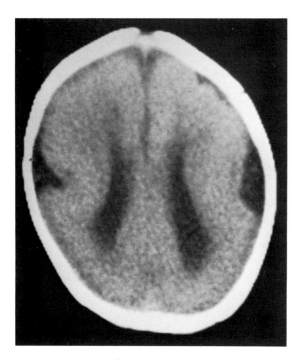

Fig. 12-17 Lissencephaly. CT scan shows a smooth cortical surface, thickened gray matter, wide sylvian fissures, and mild ventricular dilatation. (From Fitz, 1984, with permission.)

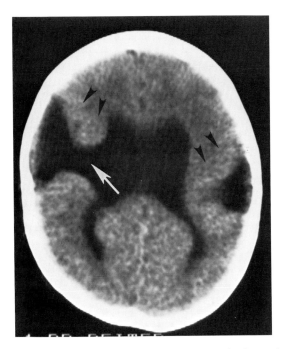

Fig. 12-18 Schizencephaly, type II. CT study shows the characteristic deep clefts extending to the ventricular system (white arrow). The margins of the clefts are lined with cortical gray matter (arrowheads).

dilatation and a thickened, distorted cortex of lissencephaly or polymicrogyria. The hemisphere is overgrown, and there is contralateral shift of the falx. The underlying white matter has high T_2 signal intensity due to demyelination. CT shows the anatomic abnormalities and low density in the white matter. Unilateral megalencephaly associated with somatic hemihypertrophy does not have the cortical abnormalities.

Heterotopic Gray Matter

Heterotopic gray matter may occur anywhere in the white matter. The abnormal nodules of neurons are thought to result from interruption of migration of neuroblasts. They are seen on MRI (and less obviously on CT scans) as foci of gray matter within the white matter. They may cause seizures. Heterotopia may occur as an isolated event or be found as part of other migrational or structural malformations such as dysgenesis of the corpus callosum or Chiari II.

DESTRUCTIVE LESIONS

Porencephaly and Atrophy

Porencephaly refers to a cyst in the brain parenchyma that usually communicates with the ventricular system but not the subarachnoid space. Most cysts are encephaloclastic; that is, they occur as a result of brain destruction, e.g., from infarction or severe hemorrhage. They are seen with CT or MRI as large CSF-containing structures within the brain (Fig. 12-19A). They normally do not cause any mass effect except when large and partially obstructed or when hydrocephalus is also present.

Hemiatrophy of the brain may result from events in utero or during early infancy. One hemisphere becomes smaller with dilatation of the ipsilateral ventricles and sulci. When it occurs early in life, the skull on the side of the atrophy becomes thicker and the sinuses enlarge to fill the void. This condition is called the Dyke-Davidoff-Mason syndrome (Fig. 12-19B–D).

Hydranencephaly

Hydranencephaly is severe destruction of the cerebral hemispheres thought to be a result of bilateral occlusions of the internal carotid arteries and massive infarction. It could possibly be a result of abnormal histogenesis. CT scans and MRI show a fluid-filled cranial cavity with preservation of the occipital lobes, cerebellum, and basal ganglia (Fig. 12-20). If a small amount of brain tissue is present, the entity cannot easily be differentiated from severe hydrocephalus (Fig. 12-21). Angiography shows an atretic carotid vascular system with hydranencephaly and stretched but normal vessels with hydrocephalus.

DYSMYELINATING DISEASES (LEUKODYSTROPHY)

Dysmyelination refers to the formation of abnormal myelin, most often a result of a deficient enzyme. Most are inherited as autosomal recessive. They share many features. MRI shows the regions of dysmyelination as high signal intensity on T_2-weighted imaging and low intensity on T_1-weighted images. CT scans demonstrate the abnormal myelin as regions of low density (Fig. 12-22). Some specific types of dysmyelination

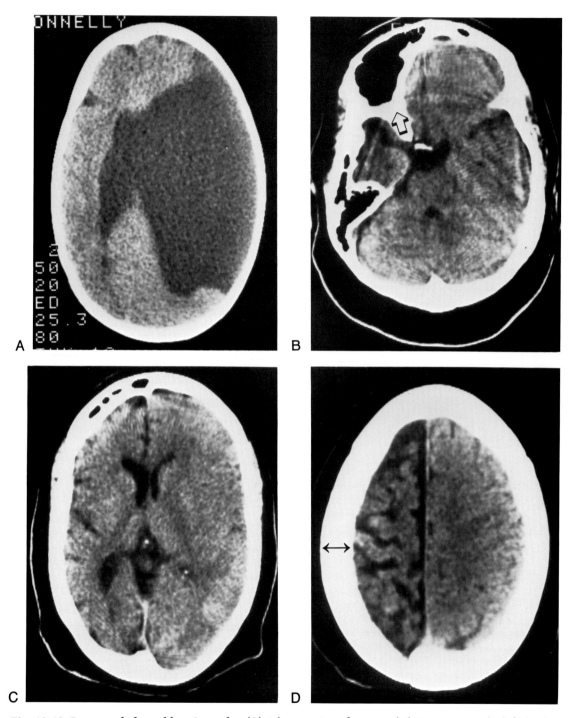

Fig. 12-19 Porencephaly and hemiatrophy. (A) A large region of porencephaly is present on the left that has caused enlargement of the left side of the calvarium. **(B–D)** Dyke-Davidoff-Mason syndrome. These three CT scans show the effects from hemiatrophy, which occurred in utero or during infancy. The right hemisphere is atrophic with dilatation of the ventricular system and cerebral sulci. There is gross enlargement of the frontal (open arrow) and mastoid sinuses and elevation of the ipsilateral sphenoid ridge, anterior clinoid process, and petrous pyramid. The right hemicalvarium is thickened (opposed arrows).

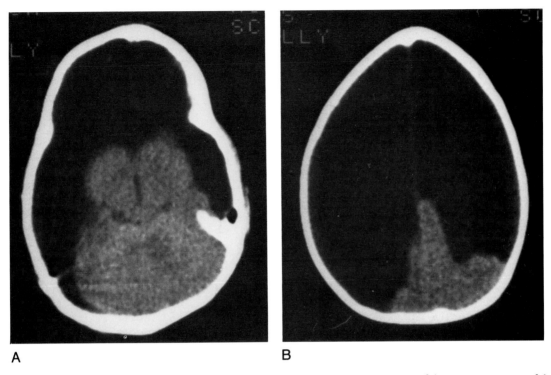

A   B

Fig. 12-20 Hydranencephaly. (A & B) Transaxial CT scan shows total destruction of the anterior portion of the cerebral hemispheres, with CSF filling the cranial cavity. The cerebellum, thalamic nuclei, and portions of the occipital lobes are preserved.

Table 12-1 Dysmyelinating Diseases

Disease	Age of Onset	Distribution	Laboratory Findings	Specific Finding
Metachromatic leukodystrophy	<2 mo	Diffuse	Arylsulfatase A in urine	
Canavan's spongy degeneration	2–9 mo	Bilateral, variable	0	Large head
Krabbe's disease (globoid cell leukodystrophy)	4–6 mo	Severe atrophy (with dysmyelination)	β-Galactocidase deficiency	High CT density in thalami and cerebellum
Alexander's disease	<1 yr	Frontal white matter	Rosenthal bodies	Large head
Cockayne's disease	<2 yr	Patchy white matter; calcium in basal ganglia and cerebellum	0	Absent subcutaneous fat
Adrenoleukodystrophy	4–6 yr males only	Occipital lobes		Primary adrenal failure
Pelizaeus-Merzbacher disease	Infancy, males	Diffuse	0	0
Aminoacidurias	Infancy	Diffuse	Specific deficit	0
Leigh's disease	Infancy childhood	Basal ganglia, white matter	0	0

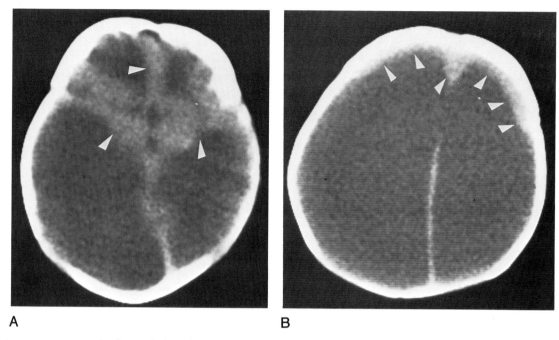

A   B

Fig. 12-21 Severe hydrocephalus. (A) CT slice through the base of the brain shows preservation of some hemispheric tissue (arrowheads). **(B)** More superiorly, a small amount of cortical mantle can be seen (arrowheads). Compare with Figure 12-20.

have distribution signatures, but in general the specific diagnosis cannot be made accurately with imaging. Histologic or chemical confirmation is necessary. Atrophy usually accompanies the process. The characteristics of the dysmyelination diseases are given in Table 12-1.

Metachromatic Leukodystrophy

Metachromatic leukodystrophy, with autosomal recessive inheritance, is the most common of the leukodystrophies. It produces a diffuse nonspecific pattern of dysmyelination on both MRI and CT scanning. Metachromatic material is found in the urine. Progressive mental deterioration that ends in death within 2 to 4 years is characteristic.

Spongy Degeneration (Canavan's Disease)

Many biochemical disorders cause spongy degeneration and dysmyelination, particularly the aminoacidurias. When no specific etiology can be determined, the process is referred to as Canavan's disease. It has autosomal inheritance and is particularly common in European Jews. Macrocephaly is common. Death usually occurs within 2 years.

Globoid Cell Leukodystrophy (Krabbe's Disease)

Globoid cell leukodystrophy is an autosomal recessive inherited disorder that usually presents during the first few months of life. The CT scan may be relatively normal at first but progressively demonstrates atrophy, periventricular and pontine dysmyelination, and sometimes high density of the caudate and cerebellar hemispheres. The disease progresses to death.

Adrenoleukodystrophy (Schilder's Disease)

Adrenoleukodystrophy is a sex-linked inherited disease in males associated with adrenal insufficiency. There is visual and intellectual impairment. Abnormal fatty acids accumulate in the lipids of the cerebral white

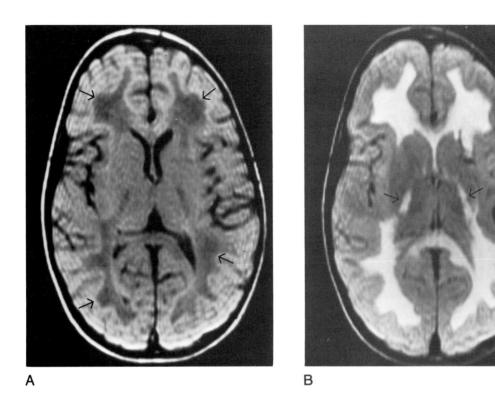

A

B

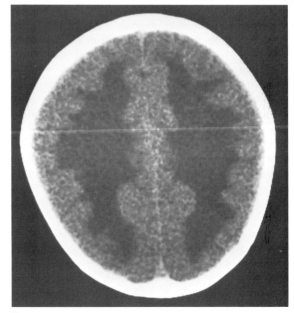

C

Fig. 12-22 Dysmyelinating disease. (A) T$_1$-weighted MRI shows the hypointense white matter in this 2-year-old with an undiagnosed leukodystrohy (arrows). There is mild atrophy. **(B)** T$_2$-weighted MRI shows the extreme hyperintensity of the white matter, including the posterior limbs of the internal capsules (arrows). **(C)** CT scan of the same patient shows the leukodystrophy as diffuse hypodensity of the centrum semiovale.

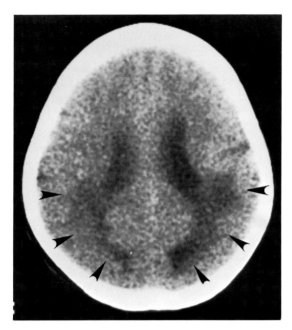

Fig. 12-23 Adrenoleukodystrophy. Transaxial CT scan shows bilateral symmetric hypodensity in the posterior temporal and occipital white matter (arrowheads).

matter and adrenal glands. The occipital lobes are predominantly involved. Clinical onset is usually at age 4 to 6 years.

The CT scan typically shows bilateral, symmetric, low density abnormality in the occipital lobe white matter (Fig. 12-23). There may be mass effect. Peripheral rim contrast enhancement indicates the active phase of the disease. The white matter changes extend anteriorly as the disease advances. Early in the disease the changes may be unilateral, mimicking a tumor. Occasionally, calcification is seen.

The white matter lesions are demonstrated on MRI as high intensity abnormality on T_2-weighted images. More extensive involvement can also be seen with MRI, including lesions in the brain stem and visual and auditory pathways.

An autosomal recessive form of the disease exists that presents during infancy and causes early death. Polymicrogyria may also be present.

Pelizaeus-Merzbacher Disease

Pelizaeus-Merzbacher disease is a rare diffuse leukodystrophy that affects males starting in early infancy. Its cause is unknown.

Leigh's Disease (Subacute Necrotizing Encephalomyelopathy)

Subacute necrotizing encephalomyelopathy affects both gray and white matter of infants and children. MRI is more sensitive than CT for defining the lesions, particularly in the white matter. The characteristic finding is high T_2 signal intensity or low CT density in the putamen and thalamus (Fig. 12-24). The disease progresses to severe global atrophy.

NEUROCUTANEOUS DISORDERS

Neurocutaneous disorders encompass a group of congenital disorders characterized by dysplasia or neoplasia of the skin, brain, peripheral nervous system, and eyes (ectodermal structures). However, abnormalities of bone, blood vessels, and gut may also be included in the syndromes. These diseases are genetically determined. Equivalent terms for this group of disorders are phakomatosis (from Greek, meaning birthmark) and congenital neuroectodermal dysplasia.

Neurofibromatosis

Neurofibromatosis is actually a group of disorders. The most common and well known types are neurofibromatosis 1 (von Recklinghausen's neurofibromatosis, peripheral NF, NF-1) and neurofibromatosis 2 (bilateral acoustic neurofibromatosis, central NF, NF-2). Other types are, for the most part, variants of NF-1 and NF-2; overlap among groups occurs. They are autosomal dominant genetic disorders.

NEUROFIBROMATOSIS 1

Neurofibromatosis 1 consists in multiple abnormalities of both ectoderm and mesoderm. The defining features of NF-1 are café au lait spots, peripheral neurofibromas, and iris hamartomas (Lisch nodules). All persons with NF-1 have these three features but only some of the other features listed below. Thus the syndrome is highly variable.

A far-ranging variety of abnormalities may be seen in the brain. Optic pathway glioma is the most common tumor (Fig. 12-25). This lesion may involve the optic

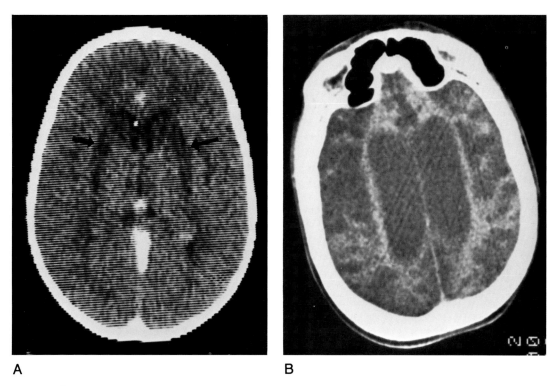

A   B

Fig. 12-24 Leigh's disease. (A) CT study shows hypodensity involving the basal ganglia and adjacent white matter. **(B)** Scan done many years later shows severe progression of the necrotizing process with development of global atrophy. The calvarium is thickened and the sinuses are enlarged because of the brain atrophy.

NEUROFIBROMATOSIS 1

Defining features

    Café au lait spots (>6)

    Peripheral neurofibromas (>2) or plexiform neurofibroma

    Lisch nodules

Other features

    Optic pathway glioma

    Astrocytoma

    Osseous dysplasia of the sphenoid ridge, tubular bones, spine

    Scoliosis

    Vascular dysplasia (brain, kidneys)

    Macrocephaly

    Cerebral heterotopia

    Intestinal plexiform neurofibromas

    Pheochromocytoma

    Axillary freckles

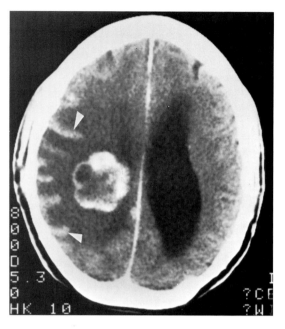

Fig. 12-26 NF-1, anaplastic astrocytoma. Contrast-enhanced CT scan shows an enhancing white matter tumor fund to represent a grade III astrocytoma. Note the pseudoenhancement of compressed gyri (arrowheads).

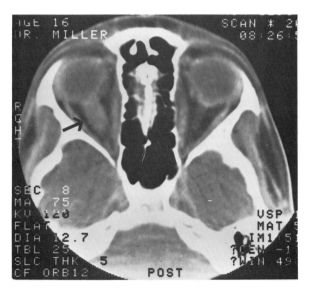

Fig. 12-25 NF-1, optic nerve glioma. CT scan of the orbits shows enlargement of the right optic nerve (arrow).

nerves, chiasm, or tracts. It is a slow-growing tumor and is often asymptomatic. Astrocytomas occasionally occur elsewhere in the brain (Fig. 12-26). Malignant tumors are rare.

Ventricular dilatation occurs most commonly because of central brain atrophy, but it may also indicate hydrocephalus due to aqueductal stenosis. Macrocephaly is also common. Vascular dysplasia, particularly stenosis of the arteries at the base of the brain, may lead to cerebral infarctions or even moyamoya (Fig. 12-27). Sphenoid wing dysplasia may allow herniation of temporal lobe tissue into the orbit, causing pulsating exophthalmos (Fig. 12-28). A round skull lucency near the lambdoid suture is characteristic. Large craniofacial plexiform neurofibromas may grow into the cranial cavity, particularly from the orbit (Fig. 12-28). Arachnoid cysts occur.

Regions of high T_2 signal intensity are seen with MRI anywhere in the white matter (Fig. 12-29) and basal ganglia, most commonly within the internal capsules and globus pallidus. Their etiology and significance are presently unknown, but most likely they represent glial dysplasia.

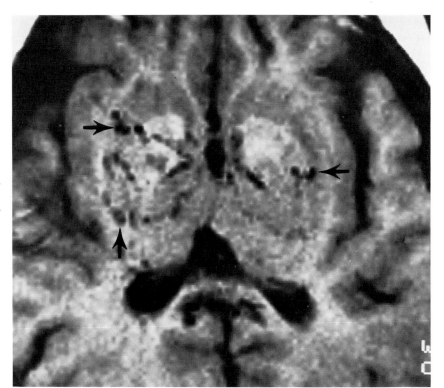

Fig. 12-27 NF-1, moyamoya.
T_1-weighted MRI through the base of the brain shows the prominent collateral vascular channels of moyamoya (arrows). The collateral vessels have developed as a result of severe vascular dysplasia of the major arteries of the base of the brain.

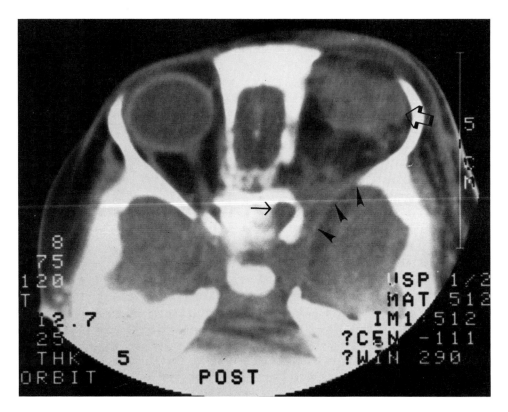

Fig. 12-28 NF-1, sphenoid dysplasia, plexiform neurofibroma. There is dysplasia of the left sphenoid bone, allowing expansion of the left temporal lobe into the posterior orbit (arrowheads). A plexiform neurofibroma is present in the anterior left orbit (open arrow). The left optic canal is enlarged because of an optic nerve glioma (arrow).

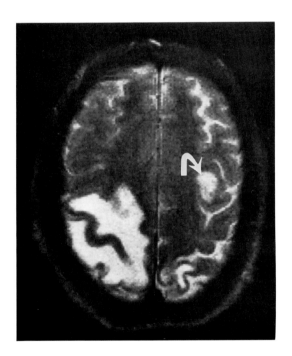

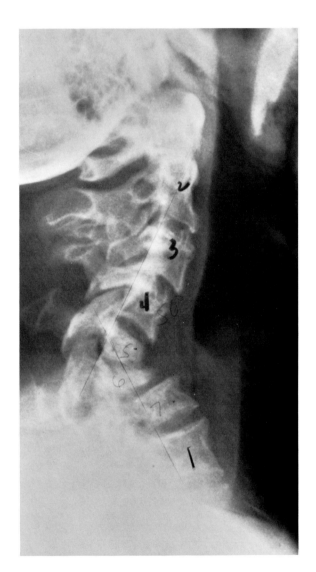

Fig. 12-29 NF-1. On this T$_2$-weighted MRI, a small subcortical region of high signal intensity is seen (arrow). It probably represents gliodysplasia. The white matter edema on the right is secondary to a glioma (see Fig. 12-26).

Fig. 12-30 NF-1, spinal dysplasia. Severe spinal dysplasias may occur, causing scoliosis and gibbus deformities.

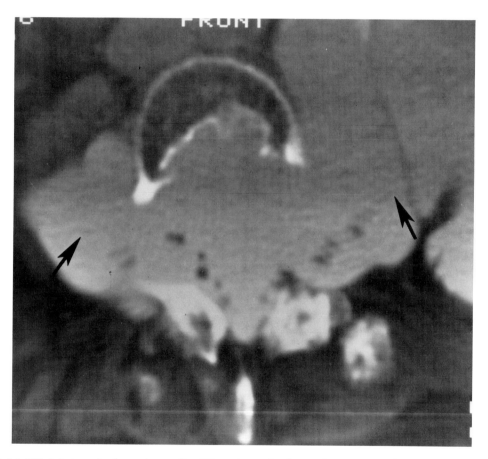

Fig. 12-31 NF-1, intraspinal meningocele. CT myelography shows a large contrast-filled intraspinal meningocele causing enlargement of the spinal canal, erosion of the posterior vertebral body, enlargement of the intervertebral foramina, and extension into the paraspinal space (arrows). Dural dysplasia is common with NF-1.

The cranial nerves are only rarely involved with tumor in NF-1. Only the extracranial portion of cranial nerve (CN) V is frequently involved with a large plexiform neurofibroma. Acoustic neurinoma is rare and occurs almost exclusively in NF-2.

The peripheral nerves, including the parasympathetic and visceral nerves, are extensively involved with neurofibromas. Significant gastrointestinal hemorrhage occurs from tumors involving the bowel wall. Angiography demonstrates the vascular tumors and often the bleeding site. There may be multiple small or large neurofibromas anywhere. Large major nerve plexes are frequently involved. Spine erosion is caused by paraspinal tumors. Occasionally, sarcomatous degeneration occurs, which may cause increased pain but no distinguishing imaging features. Pheochromocytoma occurs occasionally.

The spine and spinal cord are affected secondarily from adjacent neurofibromas and scoliosis. Severe spine dysplasia (Fig. 12-30) and intraspinal meningoceles (Fig. 12-31) can be found.

NEUROFIBROMATOSIS 2

Bilateral acoustic (vestibular nerve) neurinomas are characteristic of NF-2, occurring in 90 percent with this form of the disease. These tumors may be small or large, slow- or fast-growing. Changes in the rate of growth occurs so the tumors need to be followed at frequent intervals, at least annually. They tend to present during the second or third decade, earlier than sporadic unilateral acoustic neurinoma. Acoustic neurinoma presenting in a person under age 40 suggests NF-2.

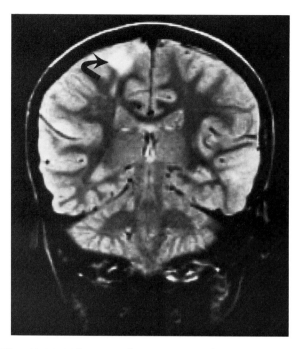

Fig. 12-32 Tuberous sclerosis. T_2-weighted MRI shows high intensity cortical and subcortical region (arrow), which represents a cortical tuber.

Other CNS tumors are common with NF-2. Schwann cell tumors may occur on the cranial and spinal nerves, and occasionally an intramedullary schwannoma is seen, indistinguishable from a spinal cord astrocytoma. Astrocytoma is seen within the cerebrum but almost never in the optic pathways. Meningiomas, often multiple, are common. A meningioma in a child suggests NF-2.

NF-2 characteristics are given below. Many of the features of NF-1 are absent, particularly the cutaneous manifestation. However, the division between NF-1 and NF-2 is not sharp. NF-2 is much less common than NF-1. Other types of neurofibromatosis have been defined, but they are mixed variants.

Tuberous Sclerosis

Tuberous sclerosis is a genetic disorder, about half of the cases being inherited as autosomal dominant. It is widely distributed with no sex predominance. The characteristic lesion is the hamartoma, which occurs in many organs. Reddish-brown papules (adenoma sebaceum) characteristically occur on the face, particularly

---

NEUROFIBROMATOSIS 2

Definite feature
    Bilateral acoustic neurinoma
Other features
    Cerebral astrocytoma
    Cranial nerve schwannoma
    Spinal nerve or cord schwannoma
    Meningioma

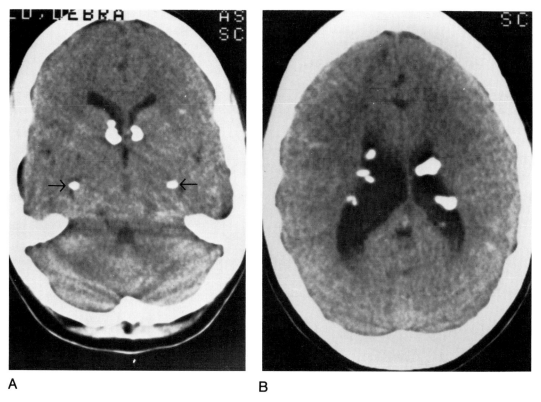

A

B

Fig. 12-33 Tuberous sclerosis. (A) CT scan through the lower portion of the brain shows the typical calcified tubers in the caudate nuclei adjacent to the foramina of Monro. Note also the tubers along the temporal horns (arrows). **(B)** Calcified subependymal nodules along the ventricular surfaces.

near the nose. Other skin lesions are shagreen patches, hypomelanotic spots, and subungual fibromas. The syndrome is associated with a high incidence of angiolipoma of the kidney, rhabdomyoma of the heart, and thickening of the calvarium. Periosteal reaction and bone cysts occur, especially in the digits. Rarely, there is lymphangiomatosis of the lung. The diagnosis may be made with MRI or CT scans; but MRI is more sensitive in younger patients before the lesions calcify.

The tuber, the characteristic lesion in the brain, consists of giant cells resembling astrocytes, focal gliosis, and abnormal myelination of regional axons. Tubers occur on the cortical surface causing a widened gyrus. They may occur anywhere but are seen most commonly in the frontal lobes; they infrequently calcify. The lesions may be seen with MRI as thickened gyri that have central high T_2 signal intensity (Fig. 12-32). Radially oriented high T_2 signal intensity is also seen in the white matter and correlates with regions of abnormal collections of giant cells and gliosis.

Subependymal nodules occur along the ventricular surface, most commonly at the caudate nucleus and in the thalamostriate sulcus. Although these lesions are similar to the cortical tuber, there are some differences with imaging. There is a high incidence of calcification easily seen on CT scans (Fig. 12-33). They tend to have low T_2 signal intensity with MRI. A subependymal nodule near the foramen of Monro, a characteristic location, may cause hydrocephalus.

Subependymal giant cell astrocytomas occur in about 10 percent of these patients. These lesions tend to be near the foramen of Monro and may become large; they are histologically benign and slow-growing. These tumors can be differentiated from subependymal nodules by their large size, high T_2 signal intensity on MRI, and contrast enhancement on CT scan (Fig. 12-34). Resection is done only for control of hydrocephalus. Other brain tumors are rare.

Von Hippel-Lindau Disease

Von Hippel-Lindau disease is an inherited autosomal dominant disorder that occurs equally in the sexes. The common abnormalities that may occur are retinal hemangioblastoma (50 percent), cerebellar or spinal hemangioblastoma (50 percent), renal cell carcinoma (30 percent), and pheochromocytoma (10 percent). Other findings are polycythemia, cutaneous nevi, and pancreatic cysts. Cerebellar hemangioblastoma is described in the section on brain tumors.

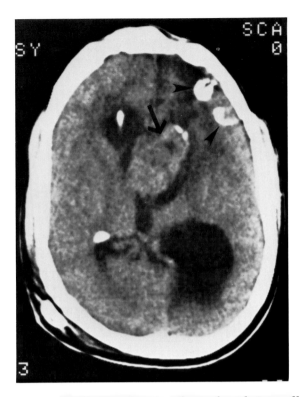

Fig. 12-34 Tuberous sclerosis, subependymal giant cell astrocytoma. Nonenhanced CT scan shows a large isodense tumor mass at the level of the foramen of Monro (arrow). It is causing hydrocephalus. Note the calcified cortical tubers (arrowheads).

Sturge-Weber Syndrome

Sturge-Weber syndrome is probably a noninherited genetic disorder consisting in a cutaneous vascular nevus of the face and a leptomeningeal angiomatous malformation on the ipsilateral occipital cortical surface. Serpiginous cortical calcification is characteristic. The malformation is described in more detail in Chapter 4.

MESIAL TEMPORAL SCLEROSIS

Mesial temporal lobe sclerosis (MTS) is an uncommon abnormality that consists in gliosis of the anterior hippocampus of one or both temporal lobes. Its importance is related to its presumed role in the causation of temporal lobe type seizures. The etiology is not definitely known, although the lesion is thought to be a result of ischemia.

The abnormality is best imaged with MRI. The re-

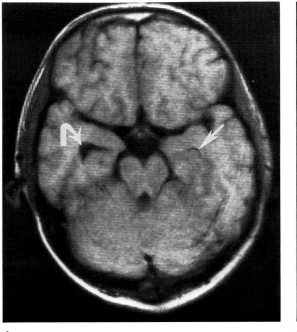 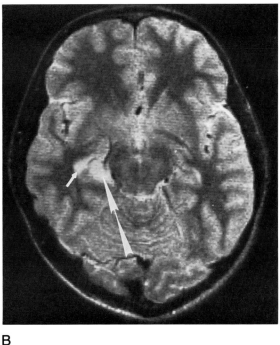

A   B

Fig. 12-35 Mesial temporal sclerosis. (A) T$_1$-weighted MRI shows focal enlargement of the right anterior temporal horn (curved arrow). The left temporal horn is normal (arrow). **(B)** T$_2$-weighted MRI shows high signal intensity in the right hippocampus (long arrow) medial to the temporal horn (small arrow).

gion of gliosis is seen as high signal on the T$_2$-weighted images. Local atrophic change causes slight regional enlargement of the temporal horn (Fig. 12-35). In some instances of intractable seizures, removal of the gliotic region has been curative. Only about 50 percent of those with MTS show abnormalities on MRI, and internally placed electroencephalography electrodes are generally a more sensitive means of defining abnormal seizure foci within the brain.

SUGGESTED READINGS

Aoki S, Barkovich AJ, Nishimura K, et al: Neurofibromatosis 1 and 2: cranial MR findings. Radiology 172:527, 1989

Barkovich AJ, Chuang SH, Norman D: MR of neuronal migration anomalies. AJNR 8:1009, 1987

Bird CR, Hedberg M, Dreyer BP, et al: MR assessment of myelination in infants and children: usefulness of marker sites. AJNR 10:731, 1989

Bognanno JR, Edwards MK, Lee TA, et al: Cranial MR imaging in neurofibromatosis. AJNR 9:461, 1988

Brassman BH, Bilaniuk LT, Zimmerman RD: The central nervous system manifestations of the phakomatoses on MR. Radiol Clin North Am 26:773, 1988

Byrd SE, Naidich T: Common congenital brain anomalies. Radiol Clin North Am 26:755, 1988

Curnes JT, Laster DW, Koubek TD, et al: MRI of corpus callosal syndromes. AJNR 7:617, 1986

Fitz CR: Developmental abnormalities of the brain. p. 215. In Heinz ER (ed): Neuroradiology. Churchill Livingstone, New York, 1984

Jacobson RI: Abnormalities of the skull in children. Neurol Clin 3:117, 1985

Lee BCP, Engel M: MR of lissencephaly. AJNR 9:804, 1988

Nixon JR, Houser OW, Gomez MR, et al: Cerebral tuberous sclerosis: MR imaging. Radiology 170:869, 1989

Nowell MA, Grossman RI, Hackney DB: MR imaging of white matter disease in children. AJNR 9:503, 1988

Osborn RE, Byrd SE, Naidich TP, et al: MR imaging of neuronal migrational disorders. AJNR 9:1101, 1988

Smith AS, Ross JS, Blaser SI, et al: Magnetic resonance imaging of disturbances in neuronal migration: illustration of an embryologic process. Radiographics 9:509, 1989

Van der Knapp MS, Valk J: Classification of congenital abnormalities of the CNS. AJNR 9:315, 1988

Wolpert SM, Anderson M, Scott RM, et al: Chiari II malformation: MR imaging evaluation. AJNR 8:783, 1987

13
Spine

Spine imaging has changed markedly with the introduction of CT scanning, MRI, and the water-soluble intrathecal contrast agents. Examination of the spine and its contents constitutes a major part of neurodiagnosis.

MYELOGRAPHY

New nonionic, hypo-osmolar, iodine-containing contrast agents are now in general use for myelography. Presently there are a number of similar compounds including iohexol, iopamidol, iotrol, and ioglunide. They have many advantages over Pantopaque, the previously used oily agent. Because the materials are less viscous and less radiodense, they produce much improved definition of nerve root sleeves and small structures within the subarachnoid space. Moreover, the compounds are completely resorbed from the subarachnoid space within hours.

The aqueous agents are absorbed unaltered from the CSF into the blood through the arachnoid villi located along the sagittal sinus and in the thecal sac at the nerve root sleeves. The normal flow of the CSF always carries some of the contrast over the convexities. Once in the bloodstream, the agent is handled like any ionic water-soluble contrast material. About 90 to 95 percent is excreted through the kidneys, with a small amount exiting in the bile and feces. The biologic half-life of the contrast in the blood is approximately 4 hours. Only 5 percent of the contrast remains in the CSF after 24 hours.

The toxicity of contrast agents is based primarily on the ionic properties, its osmolality, and the intrinsic chemotoxicity of the particular molecule. With the nonionic hypo-osmolar agents, the intrinsic toxicity of the compound becomes the most significant factor, and it is low. Seizures are rare with the newer agents but were relatively common with the earlier ionic material metrizamide. Electroencephalographic changes infrequently occur (10 percent) with the newer agents and are usually the less significant slow-wave type. The more ominous spike activity is uncommon. Nevertheless, use of the newer water-soluble agents is contraindicated in persons using drugs that lower the seizure threshold (monoamine inhibitors, tricyclic antidepressants, phenothiazines, and CNS stimulants). Myelography is safe if these medications are withheld for 48 hours prior to the examination and premedication with diazepam or phenobarbital is given. Alcoholics and epileptics are also given anticonvulsive prophylaxis.

The major risks from myelography are postmyelographic headache, nausea, muscular twitching, sciatica, seizures, mental dysfunction (psychic symptoms), and allergic reactions. These symptoms may be delayed, occurring as late as 24 hours after the injection, with the average delay of onset about 8 hours. The overall incidence of postmyelographic reaction is about 33 percent. The incidence of adverse reaction has a positive correlation with the total amount of contrast instilled and the amount reaching the brain.

Headache is the most common problem. It may be severe and last up to 10 days. Once it has occurred, there is little that can be given for treatment except analgesics. Hydration and a slightly upright position immediately after the myelography helps to decrease the incidence and severity of the headache. Postmyelographic arachnoiditis is not a problem with the water-soluble agents. A history of adverse allergic-type reaction to iodinated contrast agents is associated with an increased incidence of similar reaction from myelography.

Ordinarily, a lumbar puncture is performed with a 22- to 23-gauge spinal needle at L3-L4. The puncture is not done above L2-L3. For lumbar examinations, 170 to 200 mg I/ml is used. Contrast is carried superiorly to outline the conus medullaris. The cervical examination

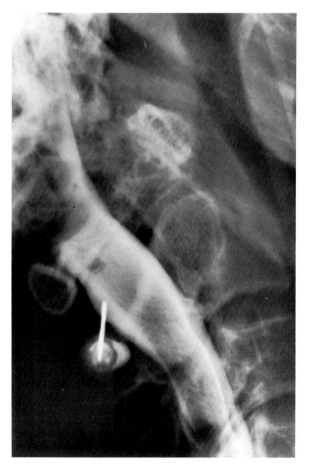

Fig. 13-1 C1-C2 needle puncture for cervical myelography. Excellent opacification of the cervical region can be obtained by administration of contrast at C1-C2. The needle is always placed in the posterior 20 percent of the C1-C2 space. The cervical examination is done promptly without lowering the head. Then, as soon as the fluoroscopic pictures are completed, the head is raised and the contrast medium is dumped into the lumbar space to decrease the cranial reabsorption. (From Sage, 1984, with permission.)

can usually be accomplished by lumbar instillation of the contrast, particularly if the contrast is initially pooled in the upper lumbar lordotic curve with the patient in the slightly head-down position. If the patient is large or difficult to position, the lateral C1-C2 puncture is used for instillation (Fig. 13-1), which allows better control of the contrast and less chance of having the contrast enter the head in high concentrations. It may be necessary to perform CT scanning (CT myelography) for adequate evaluation of regions difficult to examine. Contrast is carried only to the region of interest to keep the intracranial concentration to a minimum. Excessive hyperextension of the neck should be avoided. The indications for myelography are discussed under the various subsections of this chapter.

MAGNETIC RESONANCE IMAGING

The MRI technique has broad application for imaging the spine. The examination is done in multiple planes, depending on the problem to be studied. T_1- and T_2-weighted images are basic, and an interslice gap (25 percent) is usually necessary for "clean" images. Surface coils greatly improve the quality of the image and are necessary for detailed examinations.

Gradient echo (GRE) imaging is useful for examining the spine and has the advantage of short imaging times. T_1 and T_2^* weighting is accomplished by manipulating the flip angle. Flip angles of less than 20 degrees provide T_2 weighting, which is more useful. It produces the "myelographic appearance" of the image and good demonstration of the gray and white matter of the spinal cord. As with T_2-weighted spin-echo technique, edema in the cord is seen as high signal intensity. The bones and ligaments are especially well defined as very low signal. Short echo times (TE less than 15 msec) are used to reduce the error produced by the magnetic susceptibility effect of bone. With a longer TE, protuberances such as osteophytes appear spuriously large.

Gd-DTPA enhancement can be useful for examining the spine. The contrast defines abnormalities of the blood-brain barrier (BBB). As in the brain, the BBB is normally present within the spinal cord and the intradural segments of the spinal nerves. Lesions that destroy the BBB show enhancement, but the intensity of the enhancement is not as predictable as in the brain. Strong enhancement is most common with primary cord tumors and intradural-extramedullary metastasis. Other metastatic tumors, inflammatory lesions, and multiple sclerosis show less consistent enhancement. Osseous metastases within vertebral bodies enhance slightly so they may become isointense with surrounding fatty marrow and be obscured. Therefore Gd-DTPA is not used routinely if vertebral metastasis is sought. Epidural postoperative scar shows consistent enhancement.

The epidural venous plexus strongly enhances because of its slow blood flow. Being extradural, the dorsal root ganglion also shows marked enhancement. In confusing cases, Gd-DTPA can be used to define anatomy.

As a rule, Gd-DTPA enhancement is used for specific problems. It is best for evaluation of intramedullary tumors, intradural-extramedullary tumors (particularly meningeal metastasis), and differentiation of scar from disc herniation in the postoperative spine. The major uses are given below. Other potential uses include multiple sclerosis and transverse myelitis, although the value here is not as clear at this time.

Artifacts are a significant problem with MR imaging of the spine. Motion of the CSF and vascular system can cause periodic linear artifacts. Multiple strategies have been devised to control these degradations, the most useful of which are the presaturation and motion rephasing techniques. Truncation (Gibbs) artifact also produces linear alternating bands of high and low signal parallel with sharp borders of strongly differing signal intensity. It is a function of the Fourier transform that is inherent in the image reconstruction. Truncation artifact can be reduced with larger matrix size (256×256). Chemical shift artifact occurs along the frequency encoded direction and produces changes in the appearance of the cortical bone, which lies in the orthogonal plane. Patient motion must be kept to a minimum.

It is better to use MRI, rather than CT scanning, for the evaluation of intrinsic spinal cord pathology, spinal cord compression, intradural-extramedullary lesions, osteomyelitis, and vertebral metastasis. It is the preferred examination for the evaluation of myelopathy. Its accuracy is about equal to that of CT scans for the diagnosis of herniated disc disease. It is generally not as accurate for defining most other bone pathology or for small disc herniations, particularly in the cervical region.

COMPUTED TOMOGRAPHY

Computed tomography remains the benchmark examination for the spine, especially for evaluation of lumbar disc disease, spinal stenosis and fracture. It is fast, available, and relatively inexpensive. The examination is done in the high resolution mode using thin, contiguous slices. Disc spaces are usually examined parallel with the end-plates, unless reformatting the images into other planes is planned. Intravenous contrast is generally of little use except for the differentiation of postoperative scar from disc. Cord tumors show inconsistent enhancement, which is difficult to detect because of the artifact from surrounding bone.

In defined situations CT myelography is valuable. It can be performed up to a few hours after the injection of a small amount of contrast in the subarachnoid space. It is used to outline the cord and to define intradural-extramedullary lesions, arachnoiditis, perineural cysts, meningoceles, extradural lesions compressing the theca (metastasis), difficult disc herniations, spinal stenosis, and empyema.

USES FOR Gd-DTPA IN MRI OF THE SPINE

Common uses

  Differentiation of postoperative scar from disc herniation

  Intradural-extramedullary tumors, particularly meningeal metastasis

  Cord tumor

Other uses

  Distinguishing large extradural tumor from cord

  Defining viable tumor for biopsy

  Arachnoiditis

  Determination of the tumoricidal effect of radiation therapy

  Transverse myelitis

  Multiple sclerosis

The major disadvantages of CT scanning for examination of the spine are the relatively high radiation dose given and the inability to easily define the internal structure of the spinal cord and intrathecal contents. However, it is accurate for the diagnosis of degenerative disc disease and spinal stenosis, the most common problems involving the spine. It remains essential in cases of trauma.

DEGENERATIVE DISC DISEASE AND SPONDYLOSIS

The intervertebral disc is a fibrocartilaginous cushion occupying the interval between two vertebral bodies. It has three distinct anatomic units.

1. Cartilaginous plate of the adjacent vertebral body
2. Nucleus pulposus, the soft ovoid gelatinous core
3. Annulus fibrosis, a thick fibrous ring that is attached to the vertebral rim and the posterior longitudinal ligament

The water content of the nucleus decreases with age from 88 percent at birth to 66 percent at age 70, and accounts for much of the loss in height of the spine that occurs with aging. On MRI, a decreased T_2 signal intensity of the disc reflects this process (Fig. 13-2) and correlates with the degree of degenerative change demonstrated by discography or postmortem examination.

Biochemical explanation for the pathogenesis of disc degeneration is incomplete. It is known that the end result of the degeneration of the nucleus is loss of water, protein content, and turgor, which reduces the functional efficiency necessary for normal movement and stress resistance of the spine. The disc becomes brittle, fibrotic, and inelastic. Ultimately, the nucleus disappears. The degenerative process begins during the late teens or early twenties and probably starts with an initial increase in water content. This initial expansion is thought to contribute to the development of Schmorl's nodes, which are herniations of the nucleus through weak points in the degenerating cartilaginous plate. Following this stage there is dehydration and the progressive collapse and loss in height of the disc space.

Spondylosis is vertebral osteophytosis that occurs secondary to disc degeneration. Degeneration of the disc causes the disc space to narrow, which in turn causes the annulus to bulge in a circumferential man-

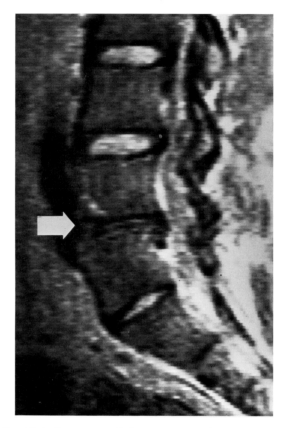

Fig. 13-2 Degenerated disc. Parasagittal proton density MRI (SE 2500/40) shows loss of T_2 signal within the L4-L5 disc interspace (arrow). The disc interspace is narrowed.

ner. The bulging lifts the periosteum at the sites of attachment to the rim of the vertebral body, causing the subperiosteal osteogenesis that forms the osteophytes. This change is most prominent in the anterior two-thirds of the vertebral body, where the annulus and ligament attachment is most easily elevated. Posterior osteophytes are unusual in the lumbar and thoracic regions. However, because uncinate joints are present in the cervical spine, posterior osteophytes are common here. Osteophytes always indicate degenerative disc disease. Those arising from the vertebral rim may cause nerve compression by narrowing the foramina and the lateral recesses.

Posteriorly in the spine there are zygoapophyseal joints between the opposing superior and inferior facets of the articular processes. They are the only true diarthrodial articulations in the spine. These joints are surrounded by a capsule and are lined by a synovium.

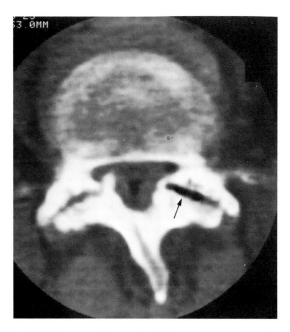

Fig. 13-3 Facet arthropathy. Transaxial CT scan shows severe bilateral degenerative arthropathy of the facet joints. The joint spaces are narrow, and the left space contains gas (arrow). Periarticular osteophytes may protrude into the spinal canal, a lateral foramen, or a lateral recess. A periarticular cyst may develop and protrude into the canal. The cyst sometimes contains gas. (From Haughton, 1984, with permission.)

With degeneration of the intervertebral disc, abnormal stress is transferred to these facet joints, producing painful degenerative arthritis with secondary hypertrophic changes (Fig. 13-3).

Disc Herniation

As a result of the degenerative process, the annulus develops fissures, first in a circumferential orientation but later becoming radial. The annulus becomes weak, so it may bulge or rupture allowing herniation of the nucleus pulposus to a position underneath the posterior longitudinal ligament. Most often, this change occurs in the posterior lateral portions of the annulus where the posterior longitudinal ligament is thinnest. Consequently, central disc herniation is less common.

The herniated disc material may perforate the posterior longitudinal ligament into the epidural space. Rarely, with chronic extrusion, the dura may also be perforated so that some of the disc material becomes intradural. The strength of the annulus determines whether there is simple bulging of the annulus or herniation of disc material. To herniate, the nucleus must be mobile and not completely fibrotic. Therefore, herniated disc disease is generally an affliction of young adults (under 45 years of age), although herniated disc material may be seen at any age.

The terminology used to describe degenerative disc disease and disc herniation is important but confusing. Different textbooks use different terms. What follows is a somewhat arbitrary compilation that I think describes the stages of disc herniation.

Bulging of the annulus. This phrase refers to a circumferential annular bulge so the annulus extends beyond the margins of the rim of the adjacent vertebral bodies. It usually does not cause nerve root compression except when associated with spinal stenosis.

Protrusion of the nucleus. Partial herniation of the nucleus pulposus occurs through some of the layers of the annulus, but the outer annular layers remain intact. For the most part, this specific type of partial herniation can be described accurately only by direct vision at the time of surgery. Sometimes the partial herniation can be diagnosed with MRI, but it cannot be differentiated from complete herniation on CT scans. It has the same clinical significance as complete herniation, the size of the focal bulge being the critical factor. This form is often called "prolapsed disc."

Herniation of the nucleus pulposus. Here there is complete herniation of the nucleus through all the layers of the annulus fibrosis. The herniated material is still contained by the posterior longitudinal ligament. The herniated material may migrate up or down behind a vertebral body but still be contained by the posterior longitudinal ligament. Some refer to it as "disc extrusion."

Extrusion of the nucleus. Complete herniation of the nucleus pulposus occurs through all layers of the annulus and the posterior longitudinal ligament. If a fragment separates from the disc level, it is called a free or sequestered fragment. This fragment may migrate up or down the epidural space or into a lateral neural canal or recess. Most large herniations are extrusions.

Herniated disc disease is most common in the lumbar and cervical segments of the spine. Thoracic disc herniation is uncommon. The diagnostic problems are different for each region.

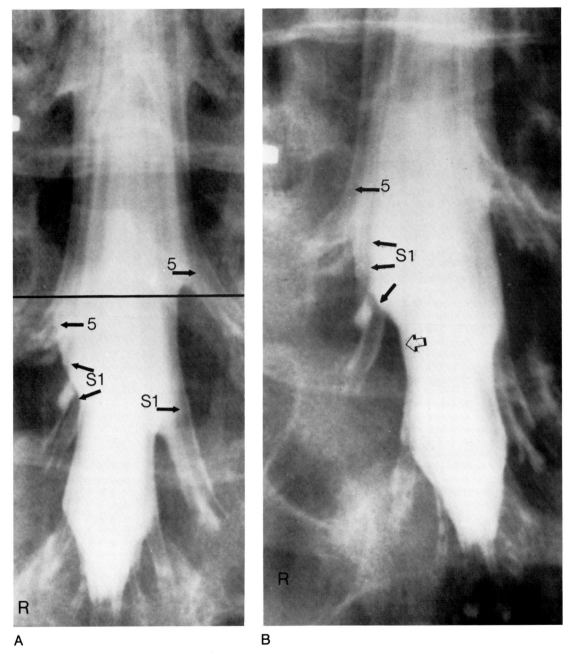

Fig. 13-4 Normal myelography, conjoined right L5-S1 root sleeves. (A) AP myelography shows the conjoined right L5 and S1 root sleeves. The normal arrangement of the root sleeves is seen on the left. Note the lower level of exit of the right L5 root compared with the left. Two preganglionic nerve roots can be seen within each sleeve. **(B)** Oblique view shows the conjoined roots on the right, which changes the contour of the dural tube. It may be misinterpreted as showing disc herniation (open arrow). (*Figure continues.*)

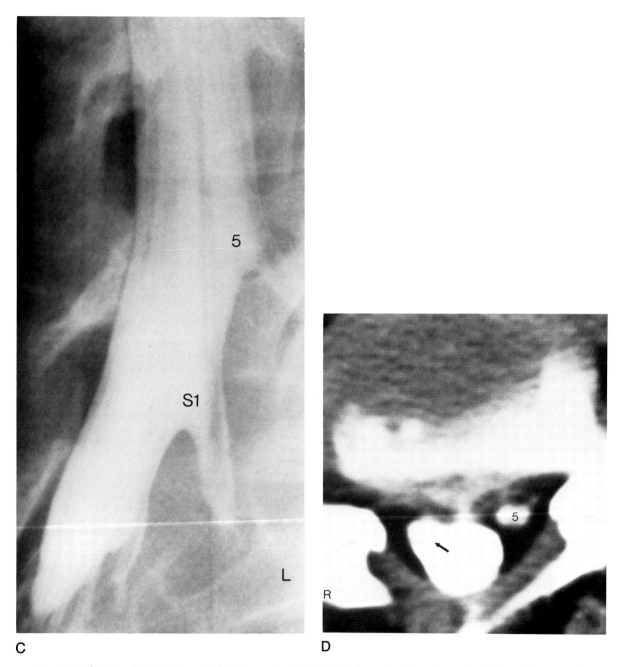

C

D

Fig. 13-4 (*Continued*) **(C).** Normal left oblique view. **(D)** CT Myelography shows the conjoined root sleeves on the right (arrow). The normal left L5 sleeve is separated from the dural tube (5). The horizontal line in Fig. A shows the level of the CT scan. Conjoined sleeves are reported, as they may cause difficulties during surgical exploration.

Lumbar Disc Disease

Most commonly, posterolateral disc herniation in the lumbar region causes nerve root compression resulting in radiculopathy (pain, sensory loss, muscular weakness, and hyporeflexia): The nerve root syndromes are listed in Table 13-1. Small central disc herniations most often cause deep, poorly localized, scleratogenous-type pain. Large central herniations, particularly in association with spinal stenosis, may cause the cauda equina syndrome, which if severe is a surgical emergency. Deep pain that is poorly localized may also be caused by annular bulge and facet disease.

Plain film examination of the lumbar spine is recommended as the initial examination. AP and lateral projections are all that are routinely required. Narrowing of the disc spaces and osteophytes indicate degenerative disc disease but not necessarily disc herniation. The lumbar disc spaces normally increase slightly in width through successively lower levels with the exception of L5-S1. If the L5 vertebral body is sacralized, it is referred to as a "transitional vertebra." Here the width of the L5-S1 disc space inversely correlates with the degree of sacralization of the L5 vertebral segment. The plain films can also be used to diagnose other processes, such as spondylolisthesis, osteomyelitis, discitis, and osseous tumors. Degenerative facet disease and narrowing of the neural foramina and spinal canal can be seen. The plain film examination provides the most accurate means of numbering the vertebral body levels and can be correlated with intraoperative films.

Lumbar myelography includes the AP, both obliques, and the upright lateral projections. The contrast is carried superiorly to outline the conus medullaris. Normal lumbar myelography shows the lumbar roots as they exit the dural sac in their sleeves. The root exits the spine underneath the pedicle corresponding at the root segment. For example, the L5 root courses inferolaterally underneath the pedicle of L5 in the su-

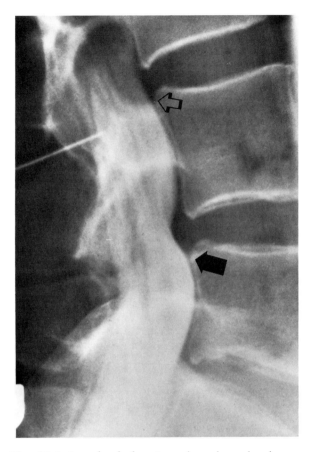

Fig. 13-5 Annular bulge. Lateral myelography shows a large annular bulge at the L4-L5 level. Note that the displacement of the dural tube does not extend significantly beyond the disc margins (black arrow). A small central disc herniation could have the same appearance. A normal posterior disc margin is present at the level above (open arrow).

perior portion of the intervertebral foramen. Conjoined root sleeves must be recognized so this anomaly is not misinterpreted as an extradural defect (Fig. 13-4).

In the upper lumbar region, the anterior margin of the subarachnoid space is closely applied to the poste-

Table 13-1 Synopsis of Lumbar Root Syndromes

Root	Usual HNP	Sensory	Muscle	Reflex
L4	L3–4	Posterolateral thigh, anteromedial leg	Quadriceps	Knee jerk
L5	L4–5	Anteromedial leg and foot	Anterior tibial, ext. hallicus long	None
S1	L5–S1	Posterolateral leg	Calf	Ankle jerk
Cauda equina L2-sacrum	Any level large	Buttocks, back of legs	Legs and feet, bladder, rectum	Ankle jerk Knee jerk

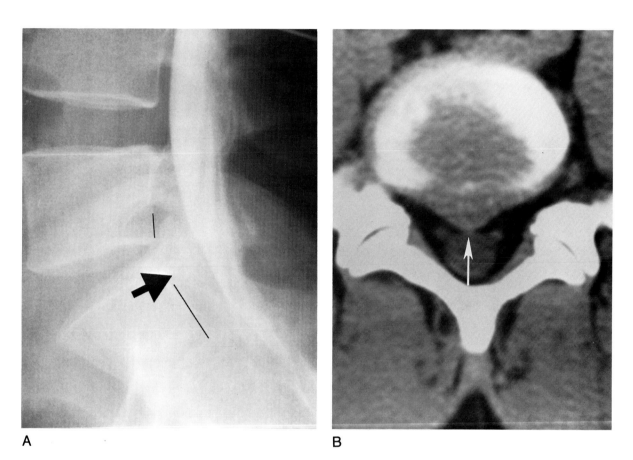

A   B

Fig. 13-6 Large lumbar epidural space, with herniated disc. (A) Lateral lumbar myelography shows a large
epidural space at L5 and S1 with a tapered dural tube. It is a normal variation. When this anatomy is present, lower
lumbar myelography has low sensitivity for detection of disc herniation. **(B)** CT scan at L5-S1 in the same patient.
The large central disc herniation was not seen with myelography. It just barely abuts the dural tube (arrow).

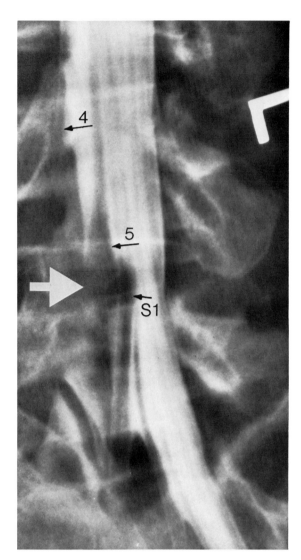

Fig. 13-7 Posterolateral L4-L5 disc herniation. An oblique myelographic view shows compression and flattening of the right L5 root as it crosses the disc interspace (arrow). The right S1 nerve root is also medially displaced.

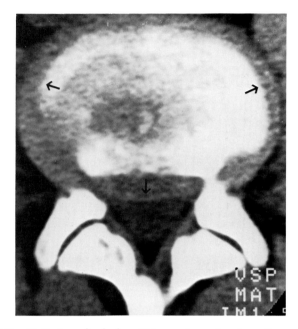

Fig. 13-8 Annular bulge. CT scan shows the circumferential bulging of the annulus about the entire disc margin (arrows). The bulge is generally uniform with slight posterior convexity. The dural tube is indented.

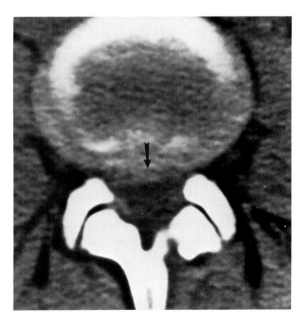

Fig. 13-9 Annular bulge. The disc annulus is bulged about the posterior two-thirds of the interspace. There is slightly greater bulge centrally along the posterior margin (arrow). In this instance it is impossible to differentiate between annular bulge and small broad-based central herniation.

rior margins of the vertebral bodies and disc spaces. Normally, there are slight indentations in the contrast column at the level of the disc spaces, representing the annulus and the thick posterior longitudinal ligament (Fig. 13-5). These indentations are accentuated with extension. The thickness of the anterior epidural space at the lower levels, especially L5-S1, is variable and may be large. The lower lumbar thecal sac may taper and be small. This pattern renders myelography less accurate for the detection of epidural lesions (Fig. 13-6).

The "extradural defect" is the hallmark sign of either bulging of the annulus (Fig. 13-5) or herniation of the nucleus pulposus (HNP). The most common defect caused by an HNP has some specific features. The dural sac is deviated away from the disc space by the herniation. The nerve root crossing the disc space is compressed and may appear widened (Fig. 13-7). For lateral herniations the displacement is best seen on the oblique projections. For central herniations the lateral projection is best.

The nerve root sleeve exiting the intervertebral foramen at the level of disc herniation is compressed only by lateral herniations, by superior migration or by herniations that have migrated into the lateral neural canal (see Fig. 13-13). Lateral disc herniations into the neural canal may show no abnormality on the myelogram.

Centrally occurring annular bulge or central disc herniation produces similar defects on the anterior portion of the dural sac, as seen on the lateral film (Fig. 13-5). Disc herniation tends to produce a larger, more "angulated" defect that extends beyond the margins of the disc space. It is difficult to reliably differentiate bulge from HNP with myelography alone. Myelography has a sensitivity of about 80 percent and specificity of about 90 percent for diagnosis of HNP.

On CT scans the diagnosis of both bulging of the annulus and herniation of the nucleus is based on detection of hyperdense disc material displacing the hypodense epidural fat of the spinal canal and the shape of the posterior disc margins. The normal disc margins conform to the rims of the vertebral bodies. Bulging of the annulus causes the entire margin of the disc to extend beyond the margins of the vertebral body (Fig. 13-8). The posterior margin of the bulged annulus usually becomes convex posteriorly, although sometimes it retains its normally central concavity, being held by the strong central portion of the posterior longitudinal ligament. The bulge may indent the anterior margin of the dural sac. In general, the bulged annulus does not cause nerve root compression, and surgery is not rec-

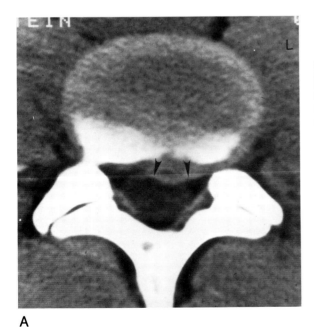

A

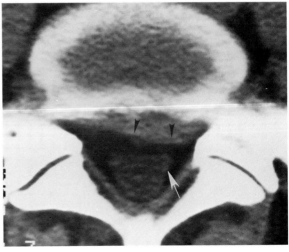

B

Fig. 13-10 Common posterolateral disc herniation. (A) CT scan shows the high density disc herniation extending posteriorly into the epidural space on the left (arrowheads). The dural sac is indented. **(B)** A more broad-based herniation extends into the epidural space on the left (arrowheads). There is just subtle posterior displacement of the left S1 nerve root (white arrow) because the epidural space is large and can accommodate the herniation.

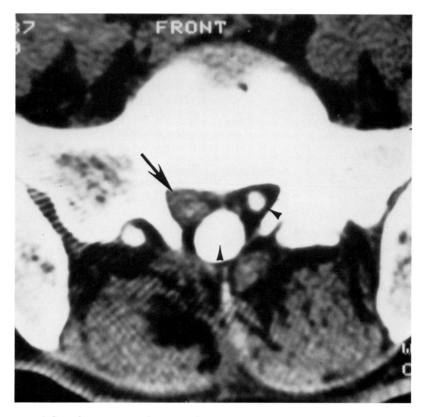

Fig. 13-11 Migrated free fragment. A fragment from disc herniation has migrated inferiorly behind the S1 vertebral body (arrow). It obliterates and displaces the right S1 root. A normal thecal sac and left S1 root are filled with contrast (arrowheads). The left S1 root is seen within a normal sized lateral recess.

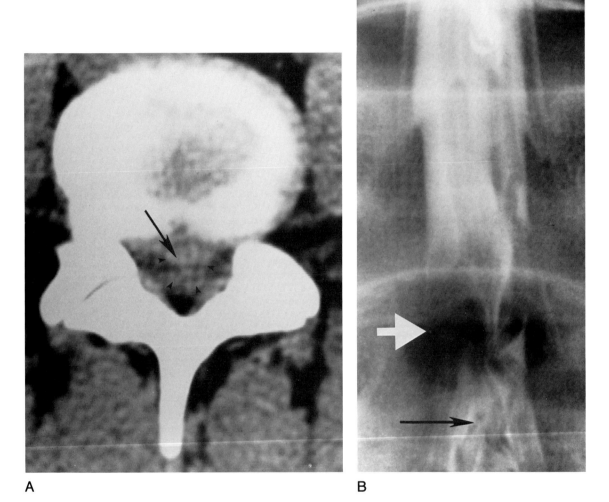

A **B**

Fig. 13-12 Huge central disc herniation. (A) CT examination shows huge disc herniation occupying the central spinal canal (arrow and arrowheads). The density of the herniated material is slightly greater than the density of the thecal sac, which would normally occupy this space. This type of herniation is difficult to recognize. **(B)** Myelography performed on the same patient shows the impression of the dural tube and high grade partial block from the large disc herniation (white arrow). MRI or myelography is performed when huge disc herniation is suspected. Note the buckled roots below the dural constriction (black arrow).

ommended. However, annular bulge may contribute to cauda equina compression when there is associated spinal stenosis. It is impossible to differentiate a small bulge of the annulus from a small, broad, central herniation of the nucleus (Fig. 13-9).

The CT findings for the diagnosis of a herniation of the nucleus pulposus are as follows (Figs. 13-5B and 13-10): (1) a focal hyperdensity in the epidural space arising from the posterior, posterolateral, or lateral portion of the disc margin; and (2) displacement of a nerve root or the thecal sac. Occasionally, there is calcification or gas in the herniated nuclear material. Most commonly, the abnormal epidural density of the herniated disc is at the level of the disc space, but sometimes it is separated and has migrated away from the disc margin, which may appear normal (Fig. 13-11). A large central herniation may have an appearance similar to the thecal sac and go unrecognized (Fig. 13-12). In this situation, the epidural fat is usually totally obliterated and the region of the thecal sac is of higher density than expected. If there is any doubt, myelography or MRI can make the diagnosis. The disc may herniate from the lateral portion of the disc into the intervertebral foramen (lateral neural canal) (Fig. 13-13). The rare neurofibroma may have a similar appearance but almost always enlarges the neural canal.

The herniated disc must be differentiated from dilated epidural veins (which appear round in the epidural space and may enhance with intravenous contrast infusion), conjoined spinal root sleeves, spondylolisthesis, metastatic or primary tumors, infection, and hemorrhage. Both the sensitivity and specificity of CT scanning for the evaluation of HNP is about 90 to 95 percent. Routine CT scans are relatively insensitive to intrathecal pathology.

MRI has replaced much of CT scanning for the lumbar spine. It is generally preferred, as it avoids irradiation of the pelvic region that is inherent with CT scanning. Its sensitivity and specificity are approximately the same, however. Sagittal and transaxial planes are routine. T_1-weighted SE and T_2-weighted GRE images are the most useful for disc disease. T_2-weighted spin-echo images show degenerative discs as having low signal intensity compared with the normal disc interspaces. GRE T_2-weighted imaging shows all disc interspaces as high signal intensity, so correlation with degenerative change cannot be made with this sequence.

The posterior margin of the disc space is well seen on the sagittal and transaxial projections. The annulus and

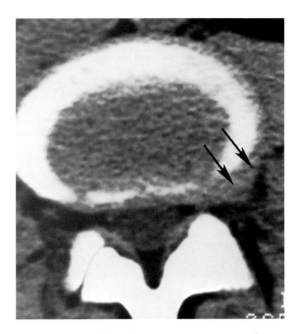

Fig. 13-13 Lateral disc herniation. Herniation of disc material may occur laterally into the intervertebral foramen (arrows). Extreme lateral herniations compress the nerve root exiting at the corresponding level. This type of herniation cannot be detected with myelography but is seen with CT as high density material within the intervertebral canal.

the posterior longitudinal ligament are seen as a single linear structure of very low signal intensity behind the vertebral bodies. The ligaments cannot be separated from the cortical bone.

Herniation of disc material is seen as disc-equivalent intensity tissue in the epidural space. On the T_1-weighted images it is slightly hyperintense to the CSF and hypointense to the epidural fat (Fig. 13-14). On T_2-weighted images, including GRE images, the disc material is nearly isointense with the CSF; and the disc herniation is primarily diagnosed by defining the elevated posterior ligament and annulus. Large herniations are obvious. Tears of the annulus may be seen as interruptions of the annular-ligament line (Fig. 13-15). Small herniations may be difficult to differentiate from annular bulge except by the contour on the transaxial images, as discussed in the section on CT scanning. Lateral herniations into the intervertebral foramen are best seen on the transaxial images.

Degenerative changes of the bone adjacent to disc space produce characteristic signal abnormalities on the T_1-weighted images. In the early stages there is de-

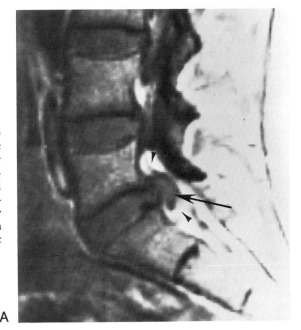

Fig. 13-14 Posterolateral disc herniation, MRI. (A)
Parasagittal T$_1$-weighted image (SE 900/20). A large disc
extrusion is present in the epidural space (arrow) and is clearly
outlined by the high signal intensity epidural fat (arrowheads). **(B)** Para-axial view shows the herniated disc material
in the left epidural space (arrow). The disc material is intermediate density between high intensity epidural fat and low
intensity CSF within the dural tube (wavy arrow). Aside from
intensity factors, the principles for diagnosis of herniated disc
with MRI are the same as with CT scanning.

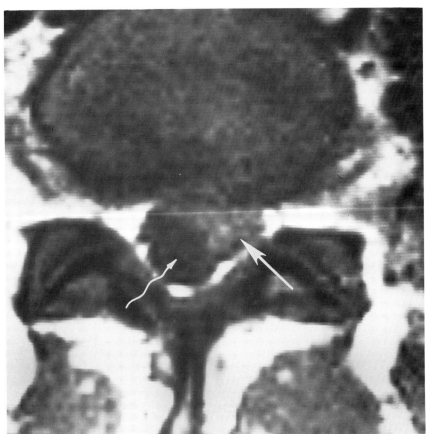

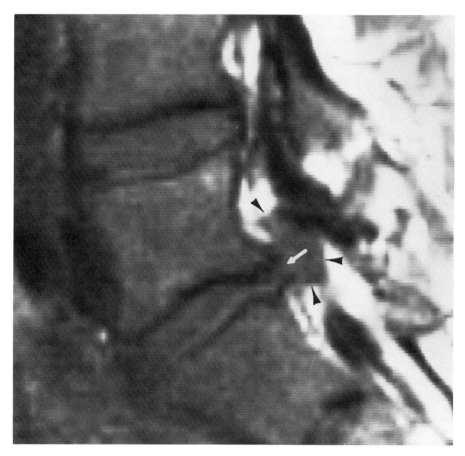

Fig. 13-15 Annular tear. Parasagittal MRI shows disruption of the posterior annular fibers (white arrow) associated with a large disc extrusion (arrowheads). The disc interspace is narrowed (SE 900/20).

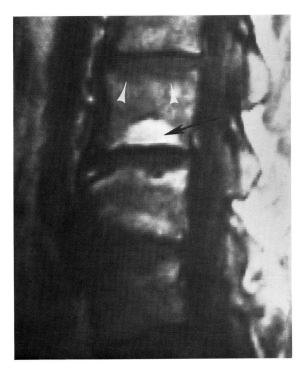

Fig. 13-16 Bone changes of degenerative disc disease. Parasagittal MRI (SE 900/20) shows early stage changes of hypointensity adjacent to the disc space (white arrowheads) and high intensity signal representing the late stage of fatty infiltration (black arrow).

creased signal intensity adjacent to the end-plates, which is thought to represent edema infiltrating the normal marrow. Fibrofatty infiltration occurs in the later stages, producing high signal intensity (Fig. 13-16). The end-plates remain sharply defined, differentiating this process from the early changes of osteomyelitis and discitis. Large regional osteophytes may result in very low signal along the vertebral margins. Discs with normal T_2 signal intensity are almost never associated with disc herniation, except in cases of acute trauma.

Postoperative Lumbar Spine

A significant number of persons who have had prior lumbar surgery develop recurrent symptoms, sometimes termed the "failed-back syndrome." These patients are often referred to the imaging specialist to differentiate between the possible causes.

CAUSES OF THE FAILED-BACK SYNDROME

Inappropriate patient selection for surgery

Lateral stenosis

Postoperative epidural scarring

Recurrent disc herniation or lateral disc

Central spinal stenosis

Infection

Operation at the wrong level

Arachnoiditis

Facet subluxation or fracture

Bone overgrowth and spinal stenosis

Failure of bone graft fusion

Foreign body

Pseudomeningocele

Hemorrhage

The most common causes of the "failed back" are inappropriate patient selection for surgery, a lateral recess or canal stenosis that was not treated, arachnoiditis, and postoperative scarring. Recurrent disc herniation is relatively uncommon. The most difficult diagnostic problem is the differentiation of recurrent disc from scar at the level of the prior surgery. Recurrent disc herniation requires surgical removal, whereas scarring cannot be treated successfully with excision.

The myelogram has little use in the evaluation of the postoperative patient. Most postoperative myelograms are abnormal to some degree, showing failure of contrast filling of the nerve root sleeves at the level of surgery and minor irregularities of the margin of the subarachnoid space. Herniated discs produce rounded defects in the contrast column, but it is difficult to differentiate the defect produced by disc from that of postoperative scar and arachnoiditis.

Computed tomographic scanning is useful for postoperative imaging. The level of the prior surgery can be defined reliably by the partial absence of the ligamentum flavum and lamina at the site of the disc exploration (Fig. 13-17). A partial facetectomy is identified by the absence of the medial part of the superior facet with

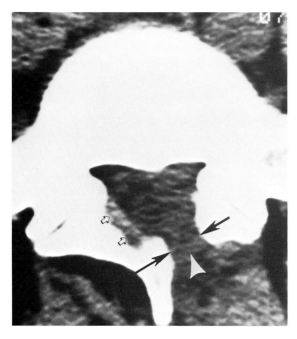

Fig. 13-17 Postoperative hemilaminectomy and epidural scarring. CT scan shows the absence of the left lamina and ligamentum flavum (black arrows). Homogeneous increased density in the left side of the epidural space represents scarring (white arrowhead). The ligamentum flavum is well seen on the right (open arrows).

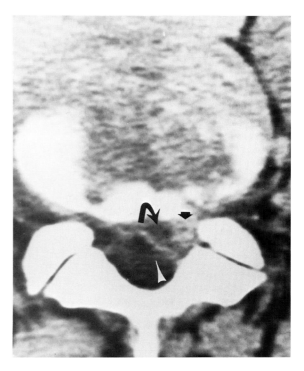

Fig. 13-18 Postoperative recurrent disc herniation. Contrast-enhanced CT scan shows homogeneous enhancement of epidural scar on the left (black arrow). The nonenhancing region more centrally represents recurrent disc herniation (curved arrow). The herniated disc material is causing compression of the dural tube (white arrowhead).

a sharp margin remaining. Facet fractures, spinal stenosis, and infections can all be diagnosed. Bone windows are essential.

The most difficult differential is between postoperative scar and recurrent disc herniation. The diagnosis of recurrent disc herniation is based on the same criteria as in the nonoperated spine. There must be a well circumscribed, rounded density greater than that of the dural sac that is causing a mass effect. Displacement of the theca and nerve roots is critical for making the diagnosis. Displacement away from the disc space is unusual with scarring alone. If present, calcification is diagnostic of herniation. Scar tends to be a relatively homogeneous cuff of tissue density in the epidural space confined to the side of surgery. Most often the theca is retracted toward the scar density. Nerve roots may be surrounded and difficult to identify. High dose intravenous contrast enhancement can sometimes distinguish scar from disc herniation. The scar generally enhances,

whereas the disc material does not (Fig. 13-18). Chronic recurrent herniation may be outlined by an intensely enhancing rim of dense scar.

The MRI technique is useful for recognition of recurrent disc herniation and its differentiation from scar. Both T_1- and T_2-weighted images are obtained. The transaxial plane is most useful. Scar is relatively hyperintense with the CSF of the dural sac on T_1-weighted sequences, isointense on proton density images, and moderately hypointense on T_2-weighted images (Fig. 13-19). Herniated disc material is usually of low signal intensity on heavily T_2-weighted images (Fig. 13-20). Gd-DTPA can be used as with CT scanning, producing enhancement of the epidural scar on the T_1-weighted images. The herniated disc material does not enhance. The imaging characteristics of scar and recurrent disc herniation are summarized in box (p 386).

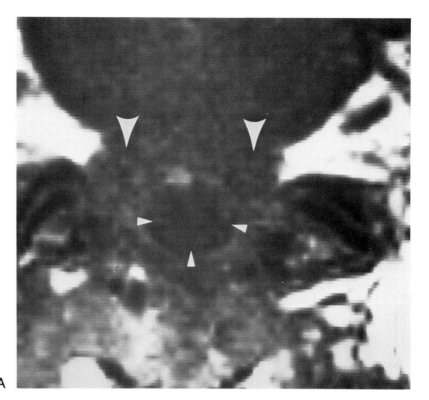

A

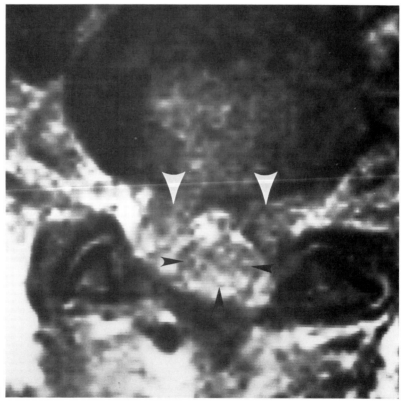

Fig. 13-19 Postoperative epidural scar, bilateral laminectomy, MRI. (A) T$_1$-weighted study shows epidural scar as homogeneous signal intensity (large arrowheads) that is relatively hyperintense to the CSF within the dural tube (small arrowheads). The scar is well outlined by the high intensity epidural fat. (B) Proton density images (SE 2500/40) show the epidural scar (white arrowheads) as nearly isointense with the CSF within the dural tube (black arrowheads). (*Figure continues.*)

B

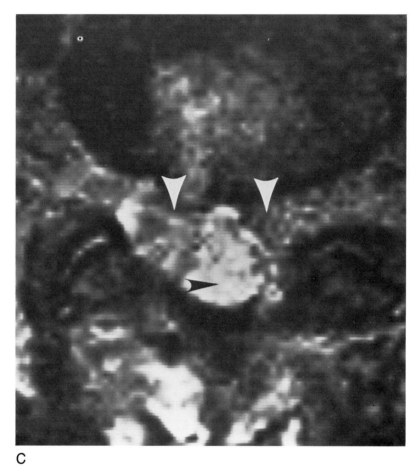

C

Fig. 13-19 (*Continued*) **(C)** T$_2$-weighted image (SE 2500/90) shows the epidural scarring as homogeneous hypointensity (white arrowheads) compared with the high signal intensity of the CSF (black arrowhead). The epidural fat and epidural scar are nearly isointense.

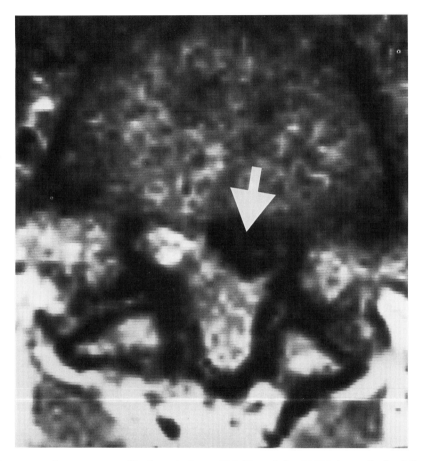

Fig. 13-20 Postoperative recurrent disc herniation, MRI. T_2-weighted MRI shows the focal disc herniation as extreme hypointensity (arrow). (SE 2500/90)

CT AND MRI CHARACTERISTICS OF
EPIDURAL SCAR

Scar

CT density slightly lower than HNP

MRI T_2 intensity slightly higher than HNP

Relatively homogeneous

Occurs only on the side of the surgery

Conforms to the contour of the dural sac

May retract the sac (rarely displaces the sac)

May be away from the disc space

Shows enhancement with intravenous contrast

Disc herniation

CT density greater than scar

MRI T_2 intensity less than scar

Occurs at disc space level

Causes displacement of thecal sac and nerve roots

Does not contrast-enhance

Arachnoiditis

Arachnoiditis is most common after lumbar surgery but may occur after trauma or infection. Previously, Pantopaque myelography was the most common cause. Intra-arachnoid adhesions develop, producing characteristic findings with imaging. There is clumping of nerve roots within the dural tube (Figs. 13-21 and 13-22), and the roots may become adherent to the margins of the dura. If all the nerve roots are adherent laterally, the thecal sac may appear "empty." Bizarre patterns can develop on the myelogram (Fig. 13-23). Focal clumps may produce myelographic defects that suggest disc herniation. If the fibrosis is particularly severe, the dural tube can be "blocked" by adhesions (see Fig. 14-28). This situation is seen as high signal intensity within the sac on T_1-weighted MRI. The pain of arachnoiditis may be severe and unrelenting.

Cervical Spondylosis and Disc Herniation

Cervical spondylosis results from disc degeneration, which creates pathology similar to that described for the lumbar spine except for some variation in the distribution of the lesions. The uncovertebral joints (of Luschka) are affected, creating osteophytes that protrude from the posterolateral uncinate processes into the intervertebral foramina (Fig. 13-24). Posterior osteophyte formation from the disc margins may be large, creating transverse spondylytic bars. Partial fusion of the segments may result from the hypertrophic bridges. The C5-C6 and C6-C7 levels are those most frequently diseased (80 percent). It is less common at the C4-C5 and C3-C4 levels. The osteophytes produce radiculopathy when they compress the nerve root in the lateral part of the spinal canal or intervertebral foramen. The exiting nerve root normally occupies no more than 25 percent of the neural foramen, so severe narrowing is necessary before radicular symptoms are produced. Posterior growth of the osteophytic bars narrows the spinal canal and, if severe, produces a myelopathy from cord compression.

Significant calcification or ossification of the posterior longitudinal ligament may occur and is most frequent in the cervical region. The ossified ligaments may be so thick they severely narrow the spinal canal, causing a myelopathy. The thick calcific density can be seen on plain films as well as CT scans (Fig. 13-25) and MRI.

Herniation of the nucleus occurs spontaneously or with trauma. It may be central or posterolateral and is often referred to as a "soft disc" herniation. "Hard disc" (a misnomer) refers to osteophytosis. Disc herniations and spondylytic bars are both capable of producing radiculopathy or myelopathy.

Plain film radiography is basic to the evaluation of cervical spondylosis. Oblique views are necessary to evaluate the intervertebral foramina. In the early stages, there is loss of the normal lordosis, indicating some restriction of motion. The disc spaces become narrowed. Large osteophytes are seen on both anterior and posterior margins of the vertebral bodies. The parasagittal dimension of the spinal canal can be estimated by measuring from the posterior margin of an osteophyte to the anterior margin of the spinous process. From C4 to C7 this dimension is normally more than 12 mm. A

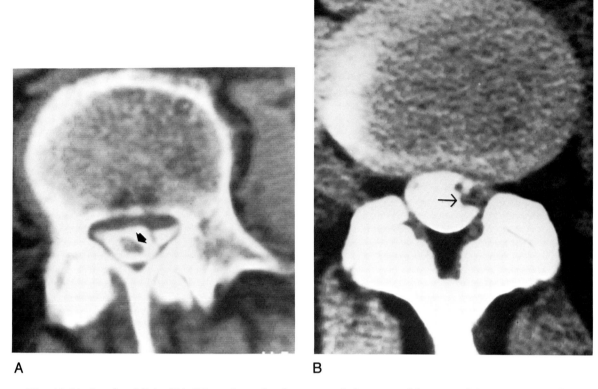

A   B

Fig. 13-21 Arachnoiditis. (A) CT myelography shows central clumping of the roots of the cauda equina from adhesive arachnoiditis (arrow). **(B)** Here the nerve roots are adherent with the lateral margin (arrow). This abnormality may simulate disc herniation on myelography.

Fig. 13-22 Adhesive arachnoiditis, MRI. Parasagittal T_1-weighted image shows adhesion of the roots of the cauda equina into a central cord (white arrows). This patient has had laminectomy and removal of the spinous processes from L3 through L5 (black arrows). Degenerative disc disease with gas disc phenomenon and a slight retrolisthesis is present at L3-L4 (arrowheads).

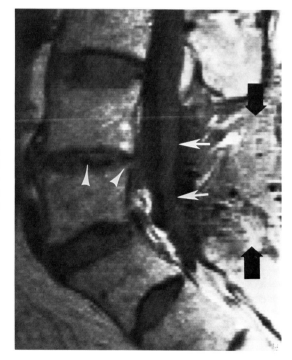

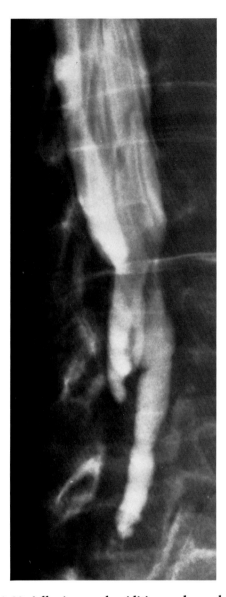

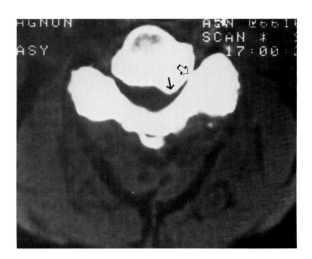

Fig. 13-24 Cervical osteophytes. Transaxial CT scan shows a large osteophyte from the left uncinate process (black arrow). It protrudes into the spinal canal and into the intervertebral foramen (open arrow), where it may cause constriction of the exiting nerve root.

Fig. 13-23 Adhesive arachnoiditis, myelography. The roots of the cauda equina are adherent, and the lower lumbar subarachnoid space is obliterated. The myelographic patterns of arachnoiditis are infinite.

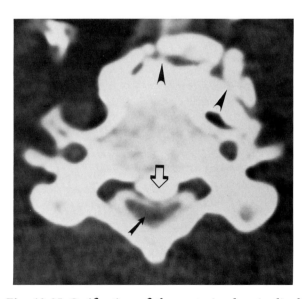

Fig. 13-25 Ossification of the posterior longitudinal ligament. CT myelography shows thickening and ossification of the posterior longitudinal ligament (open arrow), which causes significant compression of the dural tube and spinal cord (black arrow). The cord compression produces myelopathy. Large anterior osteophytes are present (arrowheads).

dimension of less than 10 mm indicates a high probability of spinal cord compression and myelopathy. Myelography, CT myelography, or MRI is necessary for the anatomic diagnosis of cord compression.

Myelography is still an important test for evaluating cervical spondylosis. The contrast should fill the entire cervical dural sac. Osteophytes from uncinate process

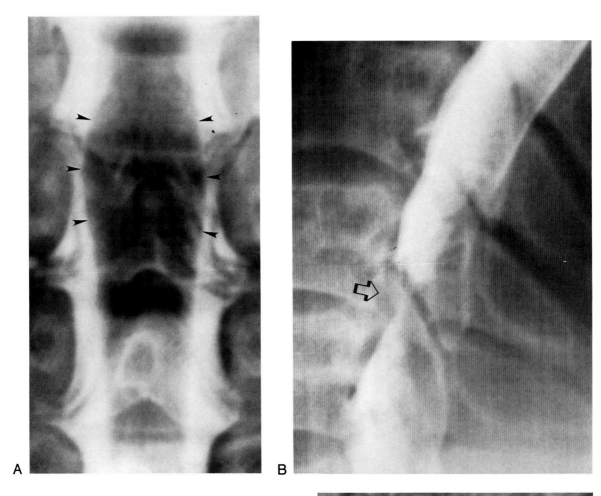

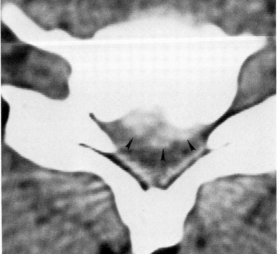

Fig. 13-26 Large cervical disc herniation. (A) AP myelography shows apparent widening (pseudoenlargement) of the cord due to compression by the large disc herniation (arrowheads). **(B)** Lateral view shows the posterior displacement of the contrast-outlined dural tube by the large disc herniation (arrow). Herniated disc material has migrated superiorly behind the vertebral body. **(C)** CT scan shows the high density herniated disc material within the spinal canal (arrowheads).

or a small (2 to 4 mm) posterolateral disc herniation produce a small defect in the contrast-filled nerve root sleeves. These defects occur commonly with aging, and most are asymptomatic. Correlation of myelographic defects with the precise level of the radiculopathy is mandatory. Suspected symptomatic lesions can be confirmed with CT myelography or MRI.

Anterior transverse defects are produced by both osteophytes and central disc herniations. Central herniations are more common in the cervical region than the lumbar region. "Ridges" may be present at many levels, and their significance is determined primarily by correlation with the level of any radiculopathy or myelopathy. If the spinal cord is compressed, the subarachnoid space is attenuated and the cord appears widened on the

frontal projection (Fig. 13-26). It may mimic an intramedullary tumor. The lateral projection shows the hypertrophied bone ridges or disc herniation responsible for cord widening. Lateral disc herniations produce lateral defects on the contrast column at the disc level (Fig. 13-27).

With CT, cervical disc herniation may be seen as a high density epidural lesion on routine examination (Fig. 13-26C), but the lack of much epidural fat makes most herniations difficult to detect. CT myelography has much greater sensitivity, which shows the disc herniation displacing the contrast-filled thecal sac (Fig. 13-28). Thin sections (2 mm) are required. Disc herniations can be differentiated from osteophytes. Bone window images allow evaluation of the intervertebral foramina for encroachment by osteophytes.

The diagnosis of cord compression by disc, osteophyte, or a narrow canal requires CT myelography. To diagnose cord compression, the subarachnoid space must be nearly obliterated and the spinal cord flattened or distorted (Fig. 13-25).

The preferred initial method for evaluating cervical spondylosis disc herniation and myelopathy is MRI. Thin-section parasagittal and transaxial images are obtained (Fig. 13-29). T_1-weighted SE and T_2*-weighted

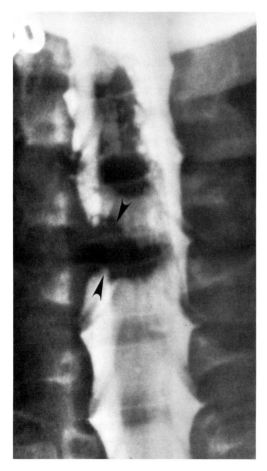

Fig. 13-27 Lateral cervical disc herniation. AP myelography shows a large, lateral, extradural-type defect at the level of the disc space representing the disc herniation (arrowheads).

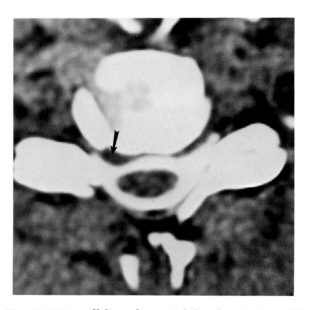

Fig. 13-28 Small lateral cervical disc herniation. CT myelography shows the disc herniation as a slight displacement of the contrast-outlined dural tube and nerve root sleeve (arrow). CT myelography is the most sensitive examination for detecting small cervical disc herniations.

Fig. 13-29 Cervical disc herniation, MRI. (A) Proton density image shows disc herniation with displacement of the dural tube (arrow). **(B)** Transaxial GRE T_2*-weighted image shows the hypointense disc herniation displacing the hyperintense dural tube (arrowheads).

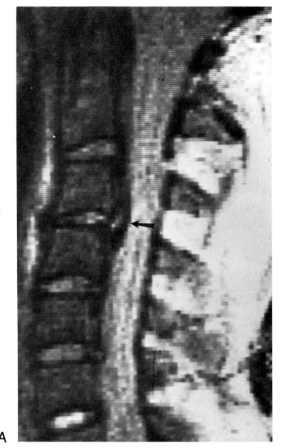

A

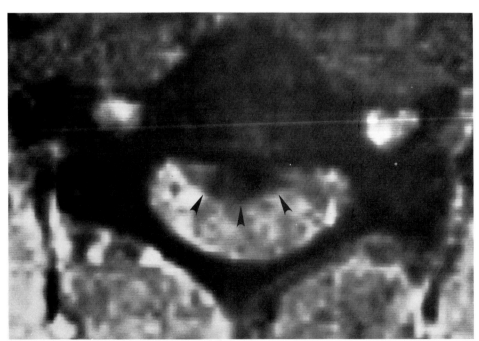

B

GRE sequences are the most useful. The degree of cord compression can be determined. GRE imaging with T_2^* weighting produces a myelographic effect to better define the posterior margin of disc herniation and the degree of spinal stenosis. The transaxial plane is used to detect small herniations that cause radiculopathy. GRE imaging is excellent for defining osteophytes, but very short TE sequences (less than 15 msec) are needed to reduce magnetic susceptibility artifacts, which accentuate the size of osteophytes. In the cervical region, the intensity of the T_2 signal in the disc spaces (on SE images) is a less reliable indicator of degenerative disc disease because of the small size of the cervical nucleus pulposus. Myelography followed by CT myelography remains the most sensitive technique for evaluating cervical radiculopathy caused by small disc herniations that are not seen with MRI.

Thoracic Disc Herniation

Thoracic disc herniation is uncommon. It accounts for about 0.5 percent of all disc herniations; 75 percent of the herniations occur below T3, with most being at T11-T12. Multiple disc herniations may occur. Plain film myelography is reportedly diagnostic in only 56 percent of cases. CT scanning, usually as CT myelography, has improved the diagnostic results. The CT examination is performed similar to the lumbar study. The same criteria are used for the diagnosis of disc herniation, although many disc herniations are calcified and may be confused with meningioma. MRI is generally not as sensitive as CT myelography for the detection of thoracic disc herniation, but it has the advantage of being able to easily examine a greater length of the spine. The clinical diagnosis is also difficult, as there is no distinct symptom complex.

Discography

Discography is the direct injection of a water-soluble contrast material into the disc space and radiographically observing its distribution. The contrast injected into the nucleus pulposus pushes aside the disc matrix, forming pools of contrast. The pattern of the pools depends on the degree of degeneration of the disc nucleus and the surrounding annulus.

The needle is placed under fluoroscopic control, using an oblique extradural approach. The nature of any pain produced is noted and correlated with the patient's symptoms.

In the completely normal disc, the contrast forms a coalescent collection of pools around the uniformly compressed nucleus. It appears as a more or less elliptical dense blob of contrast within the center of the disc space. Only 0.5 ml of contrast is accepted, and there is no pain.

When early degenerative changes have occurred, there are varying degrees of fibrosis of the nucleus and separation of the nucleus from the vertebral end-plates. The separation causes the injected contrast to pool adjacent to the end-plates, which appear bilobular with the central portion free of contrast.

With more severe degrees of degeneration, there is greater irregularity of the increasingly fibrous nucleus. Clefts form in the annulus. The annular clefts are demonstrated by contrast extending peripherally from the nucleus and, in the more degenerated conditions, completely through the annulus to the posterior or anterior longitudinal ligaments. The severely degenerated disc accepts large amounts of contrast, up to 1.2 ml, and the patient's pain may be reproduced by the injection.

With annular rupture, the injected contrast extends through the annulus and escapes the disc space, often deflected upward or downward by a still intact posterior longitudinal ligament. Annular rupture may occur at any stage of disc degeneration. There is correlation of the degree of hydration of the discs as demonstrated by T_2-weighted MRI and the degenerative changes as defined by discography.

The usefulness of discography has not been clearly established and so is controversial. Because degenerative patterns have been seen in studies in asymptomatic persons, many radiologists believe that with the availability of CT scanning and MRI there is no place for discography. However, there are some clinicians and radiologists who believe that discography can give specific information in patients who have persistent, long-term back pain without radiculopathy and no evidence of disc herniation on myelography, CT scans, or MRI. In this situation, some believe that demonstration of a posterior annular tear, associated with reproduction of the patient's pain, is significant, and that anterior interbody fusion at that level can relieve the pain.

Lumbar Facet Arthropathy

Lumbar facet arthropathy is almost always caused by increased stress placed on the joints as a result of degenerative disc disease. The lumbar facets receive sensory innervation from overlapping segments of the posterior rami of the spinal nerves, so the pain produced by the arthropathy is deep and poorly localized. Pain of the "facet syndrome" is difficult to distinguish from the pain produced by degenerated disc disease.

The most frequent CT finding of facet arthropathy is osteophyte formation at the margins of the joint. The superior facet is the one most frequently affected. These osteophytes may narrow the spinal canal, the lateral recesses, and the lateral neural canal (intervertebral foramen). The facet joint space narrows to less than 2 mm, and a gas disc phenomenon may occur. Hypermobility results from the laxity of the periarticular ligaments, producing spondylolisthesis or retrolisthesis. Ossification may extend into the ligamentum flavum. There is subchondral sclerosis and cystic degeneration, and a synovial cyst sometimes containing gas may enlarge into the epidural space. CT scanning is the most accurate technique for defining facet arthropathy and its consequences (Fig. 13-3).

Lumbar Spinal Stenosis

Spinal stenosis is characterized as either lateral or central, developmental or degenerative (acquired). Degenerative lateral stenosis is the most common form of spinal stenosis. With this disorder, osteophytes narrow the lateral recesses or the lateral neural canals, causing radiculopathy. Central stenosis, narrowing of the spinal canal, is less common and when severe causes the cauda equina syndrome. All forms of degenerative spinal stenosis occur during the later phases of the spondylitic process and usually in persons over the age of 50. Other causes of acquired stenosis include the degenerative type of spondylolisthesis (L4-L5), ossification of the posterior longitudinal ligament and ligamentum flavum, Paget's disease, trauma, and spinal fusion.

Developmental narrowing of the spinal canal rarely causes symptoms unless there is superimposed degenerative change. Small lesions become symptomatic in this group. Congenital stenosis may occur as an isolated spinal deformity, with achondroplasia, and with Morquio's disease.

Lateral spinal stenosis refers to narrowing of the lateral recesses or lateral neural canals. Axial CT sections through the level of the pedicles demonstrate the lateral recesses. They are bounded anteriorly by the posterolateral vertebral body, posteriorly by the base of the superior facet, and laterally by the pedicle. The lateral recess contains the segmental nerve root as it exits the

dura but before curving to exit below the pedicle. Osteophytes from the superior facet encroach on the recess, causing nerve root entrapment. Bulging of the annulus can further compromise the recess. The nerve root is flattened, and the epidural fat surrounding the root in the canal is obliterated. This type of stenosis is seen most frequently at the L5-S1 level.

There are no absolute criteria for the diagnosis of lateral recess stenosis. The recess is said to be narrowed if it measures 3 mm or less in height, but the diagnosis is based more on visualization of the compressed nerve root within the recess (Fig. 13-30 and Fig. 13-11).

The lateral neural canal (intervertebral foramen) may also become narrowed by a similar process. Resorption of the disc and the narrowing of the disc space cause upward and forward movement of the superior facet into the foramen resulting in nerve root compression. Bulging of the annulus and osteophyte formation from the posterolateral rim of the adjacent vertebral body may further compromise the canal. Thin section scanning or reformatting of the images in the lateral or oblique planes may be necessary to make a definitive diagnosis. MRI gives excellent views of the foramen

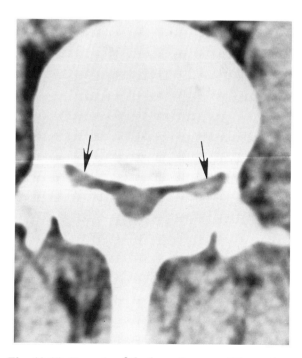

Fig. 13-30 Stenosis of the lateral recess. CT scan shows significant narrowing of both lateral recesses with compression of the exiting nerve roots (arrows). The epidural fat within the recesses is nearly totally obliterated.

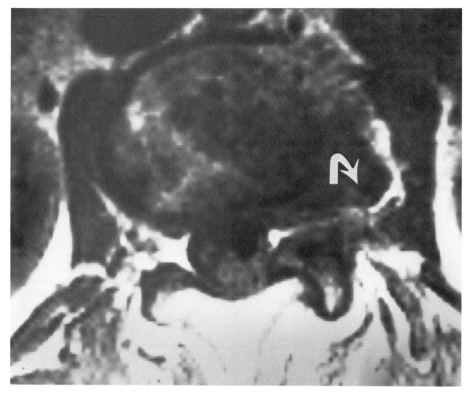

A

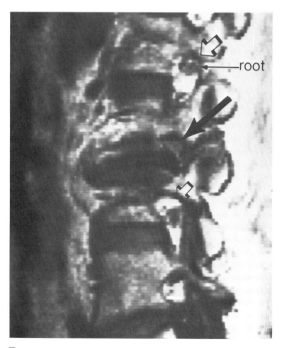

B

Fig. 13-31 Lateral canal stenosis, MRI. (A) T_1-weighted image in the transaxial view shows the low signal intensity of a large osteophyte obliterating the left lateral neural canal (arrow). It may be difficult to differentiate disc herniation from an osteophyte. **(B)** Parasagittal view shows obliteration of the lateral neural canal, with displacement of epidural fat and compression of the nerve root (black arrow). The normal intervertebral foramina are seen above and below (open arrows).

and segmental root (Fig. 13-31). Disc material can also herniate into the lateral canal.

The myelographic findings for recess and canal stenosis are nonspecific. Shortening, widening, and poor opacification of the nerve root sheaths may be seen, but these changes can also be seen with disc herniation, arachnoiditis, and anatomic variation. The CT and MRI scans are far superior for evaluating lateral stenosis.

Central spinal stenosis is narrowing of the spinal canal. Acquired stenosis from degenerative change is the most common cause of central spinal stenosis and occurs most frequently at the L4-L5 level. The canal is narrowed from the posterolateral aspect by the enlarged osteophytic and encrusted inferior facets. Osteophytes and a bulging annulus also narrow the canal from the anterior aspect. Additionally, the lamina and the ligamentum flavum may be thickened (more than 5 mm). Because of the hypertrophy of the inferior facets, the interfacet distance is narrowed. It usually measures more than 16 mm but may become less than 10 mm with severe stenosis. A parasagittal dimension of less

than 12 mm suggests stenosis. This dimension is the least important and may remain normal even with severe stenosis of the canal.

The CT scan, particularly as CT myelography, is the most accurate technique for diagnosing central spinal stenosis (Fig. 13-32). Bone hypertrophy is easily seen.

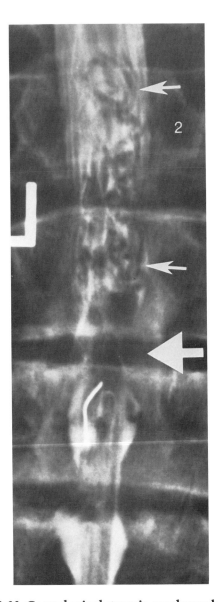

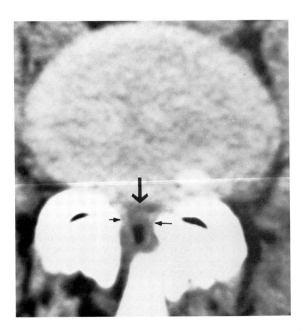

Fig. 13-32 Central spinal stenosis, CT scan. Transaxial view shows extreme narrowing of the central spinal canal (large arrow) due to inferior facet hypertrophy (small arrows). With this degree of narrowing there is a high probability of cauda equina compression. Spinal stenosis may be congenital or acquired.

Fig. 13-33 Central spinal stenosis, myelography. High grade constriction is present at the L3-L4 level (large white arrow). Less severe constriction is present at L4-L5, but it is still causing displacement of the nerve roots to the central portion of the canal. Note the buckling of the nerve roots above the severe constriction (small arrows).

The epidural fat is obliterated as the dural sac is constricted. Contrast within the thecal sac demonstrates the compromise of the subarachnoid space and displacement of the CSF with cauda equina constriction (see Fig. 13-35B).

With myelography, the dural sac usually shows undulating constrictions that are narrowest at the level of the disc spaces. Severe stenosis causes a complete block. The nerve roots are displaced centrally in the canal, and there may be "buckling" of the roots above or below the level of the constriction (Fig. 13-33). Although many of the anterior defects may mimic herniation of the disc, these defects are almost always caused by annular bulging and osteophytes. Herniation of disc material is generally not a part of this late phase of spondylosis.

The MRI scan is also capable of defining spinal stenosis, but the degree of cauda equina constriction is generally more difficult to evaluate than with CT myelography. Transaxial T_2-weighted SE or GRE images to produce a "myelographic" effect help to diagnose nerve root constriction (Fig. 13-34). The sagittal plane may understate the degree of canal narrowing as the canal is most severely narrowed from side to side. On the T_1-weighted images the dural tube is more intense than average at the site of constriction because nerve roots rather than CSF fill the intradural space. Buckling of the nerve roots may be seen (Fig. 13-37A).

Spinal stenosis may be acquired from other disease processes, particularly Paget's disease (Fig. 13-35) fracture (see Fig. 14-22) and degenerative spondylolisthesis (Fig. 13-37).

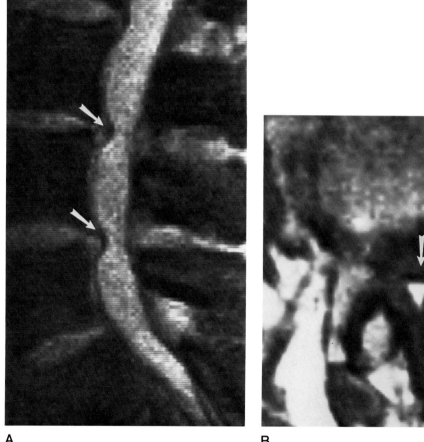

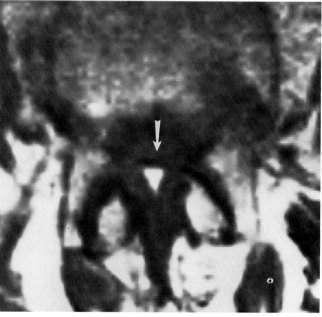

A   B

Fig. 13-34 Central spinal stenosis, MRI. (A) FISP 20 GRE 300/10 image shows good myelographic effect within the dural tube. Two disc herniations are present, causing spinal stenosis (arrows). **(B)** There is hypertrophy of the facets and ligamentum flavum. Only a small amount of high intensity epidural fat remains in the posterior angle. The cauda equina fills the constricted dural sac (arrow).

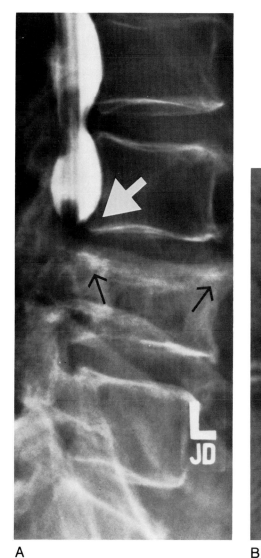

A

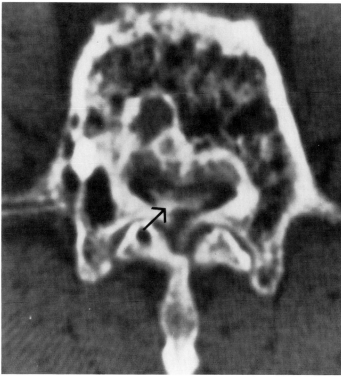

B

Fig. 13-35 Spinal stenosis, Paget's disease. (A) Lateral myelographic study shows a complete block to the inferior flow of contrast at the L3-L4 level (white arrow) secondary to enlargement of L4 by Paget's disease (black arrows). A moderate annular bulge is present at L2-L3. **(B)** Transaxial CT scan shows the typical vertebral changes of Paget's disease with enlargement of the vertebral body, irregular ossification, and thickening of the cortex, which constricts the spinal canal. Minimal contrast is seeen in a constricted dural tube (arrow).

Spondylolisthesis

Spondylolisthesis is the anterior displacement of a superior vertebral body over the body below. It occurs in about 5 percent of the adult population and is most frequent at the L5-S1 level. There are two types, lytic and degenerative.

Lytic spondylolisthesis, by far the most common type, is the result of a fracture or fibrous cleft in the pars interarticularis of L5. This cleft divides the posterior elements into two portions: (1) an anterosuperior portion consisting of the pedicle, superior facet, and transverse process; and (2) a posteroinferior portion consisting of the inferior facet, lamina, and spinous process.

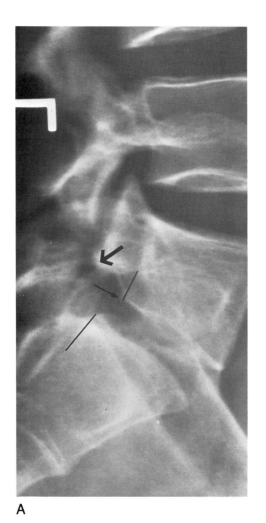

A

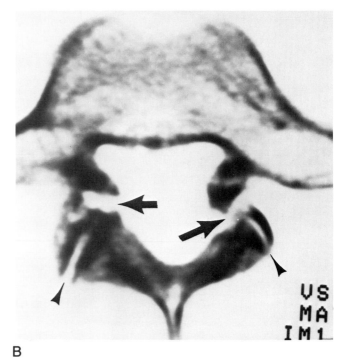

B

C

Fig. 13-36 Spondylolisthesis, lytic type. (A) Grade I spondylolisthesis is present at L5-S1 (thin arrow). Note the cleft in the pars interarticularis (large arrow). (B) Transaxial CT scan shows the bilateral clefts through the pars interarticularis (arrows). These clefts are distinct from the facet joints (arrowheads). Note the enlargement of the spinal canal with a slight figure-of-eight configuration. (C) CT scan through the level of the disc space shows the forward slightly rotated slippage of L5 over S1 (opposed black arrows). The annulus and disc bridge the increased gap (curved black arrow) between the posterior margins of L5 and S1 (arrowheads). This density must not be misinterpreted as disc herniation. Note that the spinal canal is not narrowed with lytic spondylolisthesis.

The disconnection of the support of the inferior facet allows the forward slippage of L5 over S1. The clefts are bilateral 85 percent of the time. The etiology is controversial but is generally considered to be post-traumatic.

Plain films demonstrate the forward displacement of L5 with relation to S1 (Fig. 13-36). It is classified according to the degree of slippage, from grade I (less than 25 percent anterior displacement) by quarters through grade IV (75 percent to total displacement). Generally, the oblique films are best for showing the cleft in the pars interarticularis between the two facets.

The CT scan shows the pars defect as a horizontal cleft, often with surrounding sclerosis, just anterior to the facets at the level of the pedicles (Fig. 13-36B). It must be differentiated from the clefts of the facet joints themselves, which occur at the level of the disc space. The jagged defect can be seen on sagittal reformatted images. L5 slips forward on S1, and the annulus is stretched between the displaced posterior margins of the vertebral bodies. It appears as a broad band of soft tissue density just above the posterior superior rim of S1 and must not be misinterpreted as herniated disc material (Fig. 13-36C). The spinal canal appears enlarged, often with a characteristic "double" appearance somewhat resembling a figure-of-eight. The sagittal reformation images give an accurate estimate of the size of the canal.

Disc herniation at the level of slippage is unusual (less than 25 percent). However, there is about a 30 percent incidence of disc herniation at the level above.

With the forward displacement, there is vertical narrowing of the intervertebral foramina at L5 (lateral canals) as the annulus and osteophytes protrude into the canal. The degree of foraminal narrowing increases with the degree of forward slippage. Significant compromise of the lateral canals may occur in 30 to 40 percent of patients.

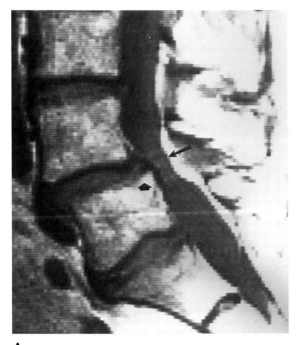

A

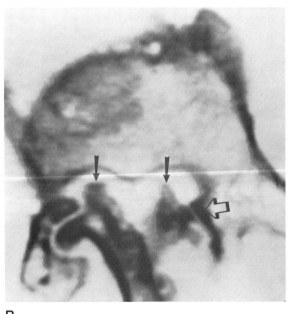

B

Fig. 13-37 Spondylolisthesis, degenerative type. (A) Parasagittal T_1-weighted MRI shows grade I spondylolisthesis at L4-L5 (short arrow). Note the signincant spinal stenosis caused by the anterior slippage of L4 (long arrow). The increased signal intensity within the dural tube at the level of stenosis represents bunched nerve roots. **(B)** Transaxial CT scan shows the hypertrophic change and forward overriding of the superior facets of L4 into the spinal canal and lateral recesses (black arrows). The lamina are also moved forward and cause posterior constriction of the central spinal canal. The left facet is oriented in a near-sagittal plane (open arrow).

Degenerative spondylolisthesis is secondary to destructive degenerative disease of the facet joints. Facets oriented in the sagittal plane augment the process. The key factor is hypermobility of the facet joints almost always at L4-L5. The inferior facet of L4 rides forward on the superior facet of L5, causing compression of the lateral recesses. Still attached to the pedicles, the laminae move forward to cause spinal stenosis and compression of the thecal sac from behind. There is a characteristic S-shaped deformity of the dural tube, when seen from the side by MRI or myelography, that may cause significant cauda equina compression (Fig. 13-37).

Other types of spondylolisthesis are traumatic, iatrogenic (removal of facets), and pathologic (Paget's disease and rarely tumors).

Retrolisthesis

Retrolisthesis commonly occurs in both the cervical and lumbar spine secondary to disc degeneration with disc space narrowing. The upper vertebral body is drawn backward as the superior facets descend the posteriorly inclined inferior facets (Fig. 13-22). Retrolisthesis may cause compromise of the lateral canals

---

MOST COMMON TUMOR TYPES ACCORDING TO AGE

Children
- Astrocytoma
- Ependymoma
- Congenital (teratoma, dermoid, lipoma)
- Ewing's sarcoma
- Eosinophilic granuloma
- Neuroblastoma
- Ganglioneuroma

Adolescents/young adults
- Osteoid osteoma
- Osteoblastoma
- Giant cell tumor
- Aneurysmal bone cyst
- Eosinophilic granuloma
- Ewing's sarcoma
- Osteochondroma
- Syringohydromyelia
- Hemangioma (AVM)
- Hemangioblastoma

Adults
- Metastatic tumors (over 50 years), breast, prostate, kidney, lymphoma, lung
- Neurofibroma (average age 39 years)
- Meningioma (average age 45 years; 85% occur in females)
- Myeloma (50–70 years)
- Astrocytoma
- Ependymoma
- Lymphoma

MOST COMMON TUMORS BY LEVEL

Any level
- Metastasis
- Myeloma

Craniocervical junction
- Meningioma

Cervical level
- Neurofibroma (especially C2)
- Astrocytoma

Thoracic level
- Meningioma
- Neurofibroma

Thoracolumbar level
- Ependymoma of the conus medullaris
- Hemangioma
- Lymphoma

Lumbar level
- Ependymoma of the filum terminale
- Lipoma
- Dermoid
- Lymphoma

Sacral level
- Chordoma
- Giant cell tumor

because of the relative upward displacement of the inferior facets into the foramina.

TUMORS AND TUMOR-LIKE LESIONS OF THE SPINE AND SPINAL CORD

Tumors and tumor-like conditions of the spine can be classified into four topographic categories. Such classification is useful, as the presentation and differential diagnosis are unique to each category. In order of frequency of occurrence, these groups are (1) tumors of the vertebral column, (2) tumors of the epidural space, (3) tumors of the intradural-extramedullary space, and (4) tumors of the spinal cord (intramedullary). Listings of the frequency of tumors according to various categories are given in Table 13-2 (see also boxes p 400).

Clinical Presentation

Extramedullary tumors generally impinge on the cord as they enlarge. First, there is compression of the nerve roots, causing localized pain at the level of the tumor or radicular pain in the distribution of the dermatome involved. Paresthesia may occur and is an important sign. Subsequently, the cord is involved. The fiber tracts and cord neurons that are closest to the expanding lesion are first compressed, resulting in a Brown-Sequard syndrome or some modification of it. This syndrome consists in ipsilateral spastic paralysis below the level of the lesion, ipsilateral loss of position and vibratory sensation, and contralateral loss of pain and temperature sensation. Because of irritation or destruction of both the posterior and anterior horn cells, there is pain, paresthesia, or anesthesia in dermatome distribution as well as flaccid paralysis of muscles innervated by

Table 13-2 Type of Tumor and Tumor-like Lesion by Tissue Space

Mass Location	Adults	Children
Extradural		
Common	Herniated disc	Neuroblastoma
	Metastasis	Ganglioneuroma
	Osseous with epidural spread	Leukemia
	Spread from retroperitoneum	Lymphoma
	Direct to epidural space	Lipoma
Uncommon	Myeloma	
	Lymphoma	
	Hematoma	
	Abscess (epidural empyema)	
Intradural-extramedullary		
Common	Neurofibroma (45%)	"Drop" metastasis
	Meningioma	Medulloblastoma
Rare	"Drop" metastasis	Ependymoma
	Melanoma	Dermoid
	Carcinomatosis	
	Arachnoiditis	
	Subdural empyema	
Intramedullary		
Common	Glioma (95%)	Glioma
	Ependymoma (65%)	Ependymoma
	Astrocytoma (35%)	Astrocytoma
Rare	Hemangioblastoma	Lipoma
	Neuronal tumors	
	Melanoma	
	Neurofibroma	
	Metastasis	
	Granuloma (sarcoid)	
	Myelitis and multiple sclerosis	
	Syringohydromyelia	

the motor neurons of the level. With complete compression, there is paraparesis and total loss of sensory function below the lesion.

The development of any of these symptoms represents an emergency. The potential for reversibility critically depends on early diagnosis and treatment. Once paraparesis develops, the prognosis for recovery is poor. This pattern of neurologic involvement of the spinal cord is most often caused by metastatic tumor or myeloma of the spinal column. Lymphoma, epidural abscess, epidural hematoma, and trauma with disc herniation or bone displacement are the other relatively common entities encountered.

Intramedullary lesions produce a different set of findings. Classically, these lesions first compress the lateral spinal thalamic sensory tracts as they cross ventral to the central canal, producing bilateral loss of pain and temperature sensation from dermatomes at the level of involvement. Because other sensory functions remain intact, the syndrome is referred to as sensory dissociation. As the lesion within the cord expands it compresses the anterior horn cells, causing segmental flaccid paralysis with subsequent muscular atrophy. With compression of the lateral pyramidal tracts, there is spastic paresis of lower segmental muscle groups. This type of presentation occurs most commonly with syringomyelia. Spine cord tumors usually present with motor findings and pain as the prominent features.

TUMORS OF THE VERTEBRAL COLUMN

As a group, tumors of the vertebral column are those most commonly encountered. Most are metastatic. The tumors are listed in the box.

Metastatic Tumors

Metastases account for most of the tumors of the spinal column. They usually result from hematogenous spread, often via Batson's valveless venous plexus. The tumors most commonly involve the vertebral bodies, and there are often multiple lesions at the time of diagnosis. The less common solitary lesion is most likely to be from a carcinoma of the lung, kidney, or thyroid. The thoracic segments are those most commonly involved, followed by the lumbar, sacral, and cervical

---

TUMORS OF THE VERTEBRAL COLUMN

Adults
- Common
- Metastatic tumors
  - Breast
  - Lung
  - Prostate
  - Kidney
  - Gastrointestinal tract
  - Lymphoma
  - Thyroid
- Myeloma

- Uncommon
  - Hemangioma
  - Chordoma
  - Giant cell
  - Osteoid osteoma
  - Osteoblastoma
  - Aneurysmal bone cyst
  - Chondrosarcoma
  - Osteosarcoma

Children/adolescents
- Ewing's sarcoma
- Eosinophilic granuloma

---

segments. Direct metastatic tumor of the spinal cord and epidural space is rare.

Technetium 99m phosphate and diphosphonate radionuclide bone scans and MRI (see below) are the most sensitive diagnostic tests for the presence of metastatic tumor in the spine. The radionuclide accumulates in the region of increased bone formation, produced by most metastatic tumors (Fig. 13-38A). The sensitivity of the test is about 95 percent, which is double the sensitivity of plain film radiography. The specificity (true negative) of the radionuclide scan is also about 95 percent. However, the predictive value of a positive test is not as high, as there are a number of disease processes that can produce nonspecific radionuclide uptake, particularly degenerative change. Lesions diffusely distrib-

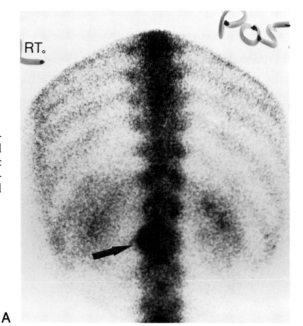

Fig. 13-38 Metastatic tumor to the spine. (A) Radionuclide bone scan shows uptake of label in the right L2 vertebral body, representing bone reaction to a metastatic deposit (arrow). **(B)** Lytic metastasis. The "absent pedicle sign" indicates lytic involvement of the right pedicle and proximal lamina of L1 (arrows).

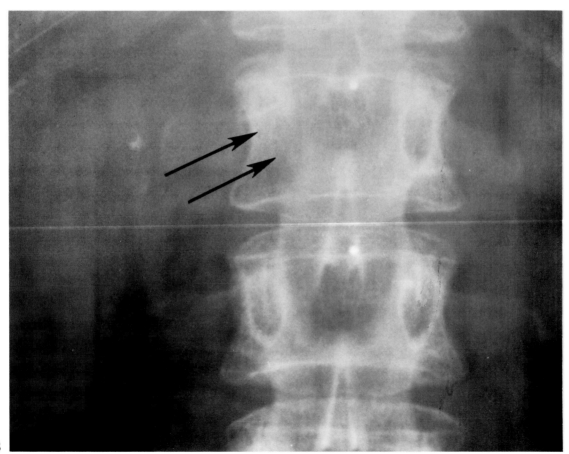

uted throughout the axial skeleton may produce a uniformly dense scan, sometimes referred to as the "super scan." False-negative scans result from lesions that are purely lytic or are growing rapidly.

Plain film radiography is basic to the evaluation of metastatic tumors of the spine. The fundamental changes are alterations in the bone density and architecture. Metastatic tumors may have an osteolytic, osteoblastic, or mixed pattern. Fifty percent of the bone mineral content must be lost for the osteolytic lesions to be detectable with plain film techniques. The metas-

tases have a strong predilection for the vertebral bodies but frequently spread to involve the base of a pedicle, producing the "absent pedicle sign" (Fig. 13-38B). Although the entire vertebral body may be destroyed or demineralized, the end-plates and adjacent disc spaces are usually preserved. Pathologic compression fracture is common. Loss of posterior height of the vertebral body usually occurs, differentiating a pathologic fracture from simple post-traumatic wedging (Fig. 13-39). Osteoblastic metastases are most commonly from metastatic carcinoma of the prostate, mucin-secreting carcinoma of the gastrointestinal tract (colon or pancreas), and breast carcinoma. Mast cell tumors cause sclerosis within bone but are rare. As a rule, the cortex is not thickened, and the bone is not enlarged with blastic metastatic disease, differentiating it from Paget's disease (Fig. 13-35). Mixed osteoblastic and osteolytic metastases represent a combination of the resorptive and reparative functions, and produce a complex inho-

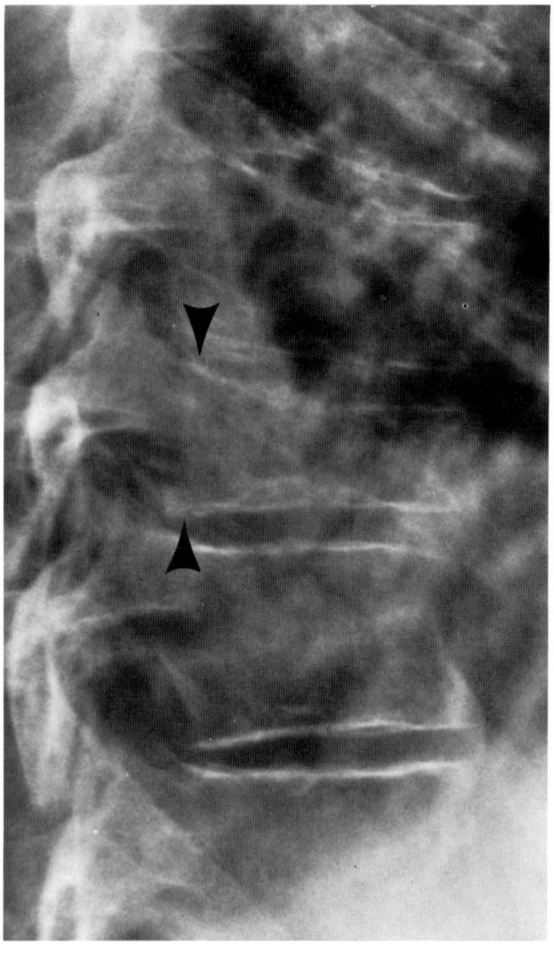

Fig. 13-39 Pathologic compression fracture. Lytic metastasis involves a thoracic vertebral body, resulting in a compression fracture. Note the loss of the height of the posterior portion (arrowheads). This point differentiates the pathologic fracture from a post-traumatic wedge compression fracture (see Fig. 14-19).

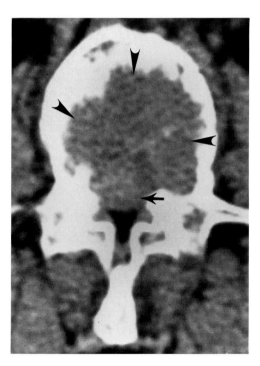

Fig. 13-40 Lytic metastasis, CT scan. Transaxial CT scan shows a large destructive tumor within the vertebral body (arrowheads). It has broken through the cortex posteriorly into the epidural space (arrow). Large, purely lytic lesions are most commonly metastases from lung or kidney, or they are myeloma. The radionuclide scan and plain film radiography could be normal with a tumor such as this one.

mogeneous pattern. These lesions most commonly occur with metastasis from breast carcinoma.

The CT scans with bone windows are far more sensitive for detecting the presence of tumor than plain films and may demonstrate metastatic destruction when the radionuclide bone scan is negative (Fig. 13-40). The principles are the same as for plain film

radiography. Epidural extension of tumor may be seen, especially with myelography or CT myelography (Fig. 13-41). Percutaneous biopsy can be done with CT guidance.

The MRI technique is sensitive to the presence of metastatic tumor and defines epidural growth and cord compression. Metastatic tumor causes prolongation of both T_1 and T_2 relaxation times. Tumor deposits appear relatively hypointense on the T_1-weighted images (Figs. 13-42 and 13-43) and hyperintense on T_2-weighted images. Replacement of high intensity marrow fat also contributes to the visibility of the deposits on the T_1-weighted images, making this sequence the most useful. GRE T_2*-weighted images may show the tumors as high signal intensity (Fig. 13-42C). Gd-DTPA enhancement is generally not useful for defining bone metastasis and may enhance tumor deposits slightly, so they become isointense with the marrow and therefore undetectable. MRI has the advantage of being able to examine the entire spine and epidural space at one time and without manipulation of the patient.

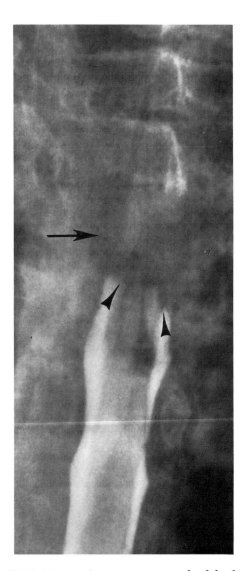

Fig. 13-41 Metastatic tumor to vertebral body with epidural extension. Myelography shows a complete block to the cephalad flow of contrast (arrowheads) by an epidural mass. This appearance is typical of an epidural block seen en face. Note the bone destruction of the vertebral body and posterior neural arch (arrow).

Postirradiation Change in the Spine

Radiation kills marrow cells but not fat. As early as 1 month after radiation therapy, MRI examination of the spine shows hyperintensity of the vertebral bodies due to predominance of remaining fat within the marrow cavities. Recurrent tumor may be seen as foci of low signal intensity. On CT scans irregular bone sclerosis and healing can be seen within regions previously demineralized.

Myeloma

Myeloma, a malignant tumor of marrow plasma cells, usually occurs at multiple sites but sometimes presents as a solitary lesion. It is most common in the 50- to 70-year age range and is almost never seen before age 40. It most frequently begins in the axial skeleton. Because it is a diffuse disease, marrow aspiration is usually positive for myeloma cells, even when bone appears normal. A serum M-component immunoglobulin is present in more than 90 percent of patients.

Myeloma produces purely osteolytic lesions within the vertebral bodies. It is infrequent in the posterior neural arch of the spine, a helpful differential point for

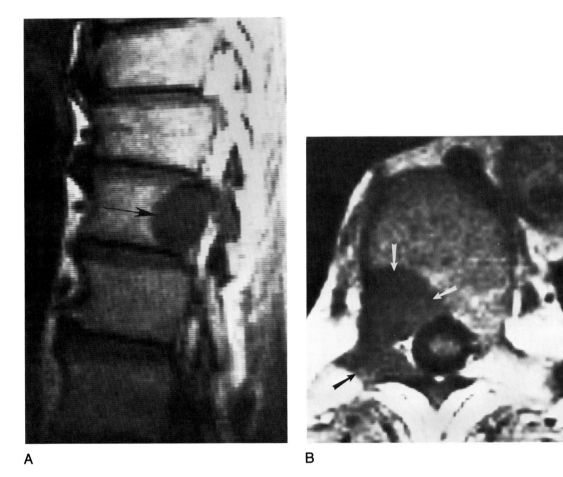

A   B

Fig. 13-42 Metastatic tumor, lung carcinoma, MRI. (A) T_1-weighted parasagittal MRI shows the tumor mass as a relative hypointensity replacing the relatively hyperintense fatty marrow (arrow). **(B)** Transaxial T_1-weighted study shows the tumor in the posterior vertebral body (white arrows) extending into the right pedicle (black arrow). (*Figure continues.*)

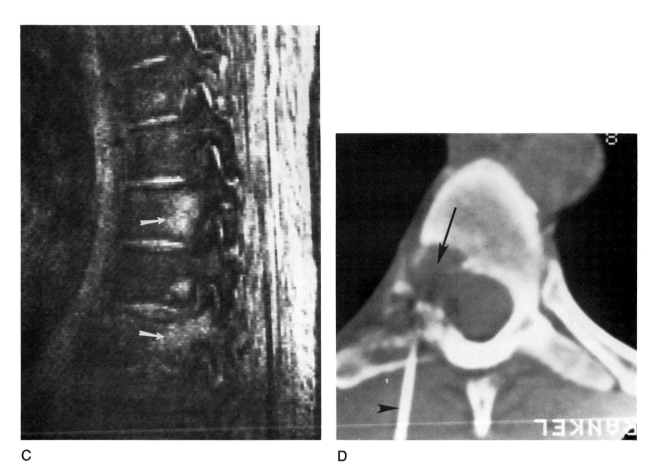

C   D

Fig. 13-42 (*Continued*) (**C**) Parasagittal GRE flash 20 450/10 shows metastatic deposit as high signal intensity (arrows). (**D**) CT scan shows the lytic destruction of the right pedicle and transverse process (arrow). A percutaneous biopsy needle is seen entering posteriorly (arrowhead).

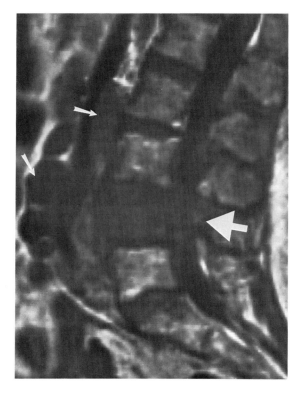

Fig. 13-43 Lymphoma, MRI. There is loss of the usual high signal intensity within the L4 vertebral body, representing involvement with lymphoma. Lymphoma is within the spinal canal as well (large arrow). Note the lymphadenopathy in the prespinal region (small arrows). Patchy loss of signal in other vertebral levels indicates diffuse involvement.

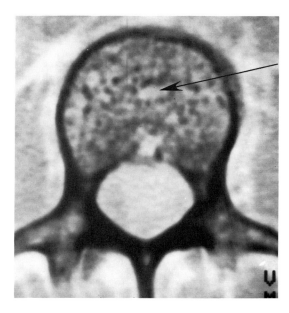

Fig. 13-44 Myeloma. Transaxial CT scan with bone windows show enlargement of the marrow spaces of the vertebral body without focal bone destruction (arrow). This change is typical of early myeloma and is difficult to differentiate from osteoporosis. The pedicles and transverse processes are not involved.

distinguishing myeloma from metastatic osteolytic tumor. The early bone changes mimic osteoporosis or hemangioma (Fig. 13-44). The tumor may break out of the confines of the vertebral body, causing a paraspinal or epidural mass. Because bone destruction is complete, vertebral collapse is common.

Hemangioma

Hemangiomas are common benign tumors of capillaries or other blood vessels. They occur in up to 10 percent of persons, most frequently at the region of the thoracolumbar junction. Almost all are within the vertebral body, where the abnormal vessels replace the cancellous bone. The remaining trabeculae thicken and are seen as thick striations coursing through the lesion. With CT scanning, the trabeculae are seen on end as

multiple, rounded, bone densities within the marrow cavity. This pattern may rarely occur with myeloma or metastasis. Although unusual, vertebral collapse or expansion of the hemangioma into the epidural space may cause cord compression. The hemangioma is hyperintense on both T_1- and T_2-weighted MRI (Fig. 13-45).

Chordoma

Chordoma is a malignant tumor arising from the remnants of the fetal notochord within the vertebral body. It is found most commonly in men 50 to 70 years old. Eighty-five percent are found in the sacrum. The clivus, cervical spine and petrous bone are the other common locations. The tumor may be eccentric.

The tumors are slow-growing and may be large at the time of presentation. They cause lytic destruction with exophytic tumor growth (Fig. 13-46). Sacral neuropathy causes bladder dysfunction and pain. Calcification may be seen within the tumor, particularly in tumors of the clivus; and there may be a thin rim of peripheral calcification. It may not be possible to dif-

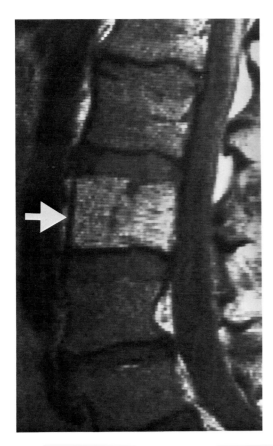

Fig. 13-45 Hemangioma, MRI. Parasagittal T_1-weighted MRI shows a hemangioma of the vertebral body as hyperintense (arrow). Hemangiomas are also hyperintense on T_2-weighted images.

ferentiate the tumor from metastasis or giant cell tumor except by biopsy.

Giant Cell Tumor

Giant cell tumors arise from the stromal elements of the marrow space. Ninety percent of the tumors are benign when first diagnosed, but up to 30 percent of these lesions become malignant, especially if radiation therapy is given for treatment of residual tumor. They occur overwhelmingly within the sacrum and become large. The bone is destroyed and the periosteum expanded, usually into a thin rim with ossification around the periphery of the tumor. The tumor may break through the periosteum into the anterior or posterior

paraspinal spaces. The peak occurrence is in the 20- to 30-year age range, with 2:1 female predominance.

Osteoid Osteoma

Osteoid osteoma is a small benign lesion of bone consisting of a 1- to 5-mm nidus of vascularized osteoid tissue that resembles an osteoblastoma (giant osteoid osteoma). It probably is a reactive lesion, possibly to an infectious agent.

The nidus is surrounded by a dense reaction of bone sclerosis. In the spine it almost always occurs in the cortex of the facets, with the sclerosis spreading into the pars interarticularis, lamina, or pedicles. The peak incidence is between 10 and 25 years of age, with a 2:1 male predominance.

Characteristically, the lesion is painful, although the pain may be relieved to some extent by aspirin. The nidus must be removed if the pain is to be reliably relieved. Plain films, tomography, CT scans, and radionuclide bone scanning can be used to localize and identify the lesion. Radiographic verification of removal of the non-ossified nidus is desirable.

Osteoblastoma

An osteoblastoma resembles the tissue of the nidus of an osteoid osteoma, yet the tumor is much more aggressive and progressively enlarges. It is found almost exclusively in the posterior neural arch in persons 10 to 20 years of age with a 2:1 male predominance. The lesion is expansile and often breaks through the cortical bone to produce a soft tissue mass. A thin rim of bone sclerosis may surround the tumor. Speckled calcification within the osteoid matrix is the rule. The lesion may resemble an osteosarcoma, chondrosarcoma, or aneurysmal bone cyst.

Aneurysmal Bone Cyst

An aneurysmal bone cyst is a benign expansile lesion of the posterior neural arch consisting of blood-filled spaces and osteoclasts. It occurs in children and young adults (5 to 25 years of age). Possibly a reaction to trauma or hemorrhage, it is seen as a rapidly growing radiolucent cyst-like lesion with a thin cortical rim of calcium. Trabeculae may cross the central portion of the cyst. Cord compression can occur.

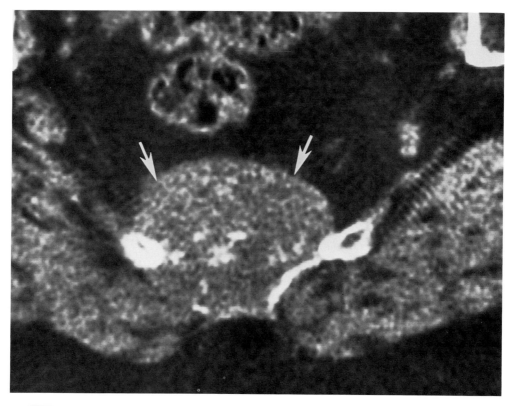

Fig. 13-46 Chordoma, CT scan. A large mass representing chordoma has destroyed the lower sacrum and coccyx and extends anteriorly into the pelvis (arrows).

Chondrosarcoma

Chondrosarcoma is a malignant tumor that produces cartilage. It occurs in the 30- to 50-year age range, growing slowly with the potential to metastasize. The tumors are difficult to treat and stubbornly recur after surgical excision. They are not radiosensitive. They occur within the vertebral body and cause an osteolytic appearance with punctate calcifications within the tumor matrix. They usually do not cross a disc space. It may be impossible to differentiate the lesion from a chordoma when it occurs in the sacrum.

Osteochondroma

An osteochondroma represents local dysplasia of the cartilage at an epiphyseal growth plate usually within a pedicle. It generally becomes symptomatic during ado-lescence. There may be spinal cord compression, deformities of the spine, and, rarely, malignant degeneration. The cortex of the lesion is continuous with the cortex of the neural arch. CT scanning is the best method to identify this rare lesion.

Eosinophilic Granuloma

Eosinophilic granuloma is the most benign form of histiocytosis X, a neoplastic granulomatous proliferation of reticulum cells. It is a lesion of childhood and young adulthood. The lesions are lytic and may be solitary or multiple, sometimes superimposed within the same vertebral body to produce a "bone within a bone" appearance on the radiographs. Calve's vertebra plana, an isolated complete collapse of a vertebral body so that it comes to resemble a dense disc of bone, is almost always the result of eosinophilic granuloma.

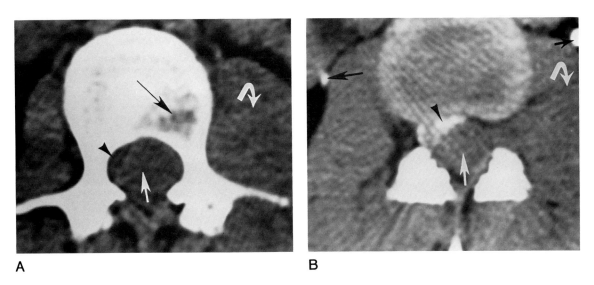

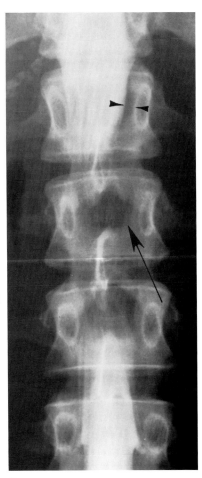

Fig. 13-47 Ewing's sarcoma. (A) Routine transaxial CT scan shows a small destructive lesion in the left side of the vertebral body (black arrow). A large paraspinal mass associated with it (curved arrow) extends into the epidural space (white arrow), compressing the hypodense dural tube (arrowhead). **(B)** CT myelography proves the epidural extension of tumor (white arrow) severely compressing the contrast-filled dural tube (arrowhead). The large left paraspinal mass is seen (curved arrow). Note the excretion of the myelographic contrast within the ureters (black arrows). **(C)** Myelography shows a typical large epidural mass. The dural tube is severely compressed over two segments (arrow). The dural tube is displaced away from the pedicle at the superior end (arrowheads), proving the epidural location of the tumor mass.

Ewing's Sarcoma

Ewing's sarcoma is a highly malignant tumor arising in the bone marrow in children or young adults. It generally produces a lytic lesion with a characteristically large noncalcified paraspinal soft tissue mass (Fig. 13-47).

EXTRADURAL TUMORS AND MASS LESIONS

Extradural tumors are the most common type of tumor found within the spinal canal. The extradural nature of the mass can be defined by the displacement of the dural tube away from the margins of the spinal canal. This characteristic displacement can be seen with myelography (Fig. 13-47C), CT myelography, and MRI. When a lesion is large or there is a complete "block," it may be impossible to accurately categorize its precise origin. Most neoplastic masses in the extradural space are malignant.

Metastasis

Metastasis is by far the most common epidural tumor encountered. It almost always results from exophytic growth of vertebral metastasis into the epidural space. Hematogenous epidural metastasis is rare. This subject was discussed in a preceding section about tumors of the vertebral column.

IMAGING SIGNS OF EXTRADURAL LESIONS

Displacement of dura away from the pedicle or vertebral body (Fig. 13-47C)

Displacement of the cord away from the lesion

Narrowing of the subarachnoid space on the side of the lesion (Fig. 13-51)

Indistinct margin of lesion, often with "feathering" on myelography (Fig. 13-69A)

Often associated with bone lesion (Fig. 13-41)

Lymphoma

Lymphoma is a relatively common extradural tumor that is mostly found in the lumbar region. It may be primary within the epidural space in the spinal canal (Fig. 13-48), or it may spread into the epidural space from a retroperitoneal focus (Figs. 13-43 and 13-49). The adjacent bone is sometimes involved. By the time of recognition, the tumor is usually widespread in the retroperitoneum, intervertebral foramina, and spinal canal; and it may extend over several levels. On CT and MRI the tumor is seen as a homogeneous mass displacing the epidural and paraspinal fat. It is slightly hypointense on T_1-weighted and slightly hyperintense on T_2-weighted MR images.

Neuroblastoma, Ganglioneuroma

Neuroblastoma and ganglioneuroma are tumors of children and young adults, arising from either the adrenal gland or the sympathetic paraspinal neural chain that extends from the base of the skull to the pelvis. Direct intraspinal spread of the tumor, which occurs in about 20 percent of cases, is best recognized with CT myelography or MRI (Fig. 13-50). Widening of the intervertebral foramina is common, and there may be local bone destruction. Calcification within the mass is common (Fig. 13-51). The epidural spread of tumor may extend a few segments away from the primary paravertebral mass. It is important to identify intraspinal spread prior to surgical excision of these tumors. Often it is not possible to reliably differentiate benign from malignant tumors without biopsy or excision.

Infection

Most commonly, an epidural inflammatory mass is secondary to osteomyelitis of the vertebral body, but a spontaneous epidural abscess (empyema) or cellulitis can occur. The inflammatory tissue may mimic tumor, particularly lymphoma. Epidural infection is discussed in a subsequent section on inflammation of the spine.

Hematoma

Spontaneous hematoma can occur in the epidural space, particularly in elderly persons who are taking anticoagulants of any type, including aspirin. Occasionally, an epidural hemorrhage occurs in younger persons with

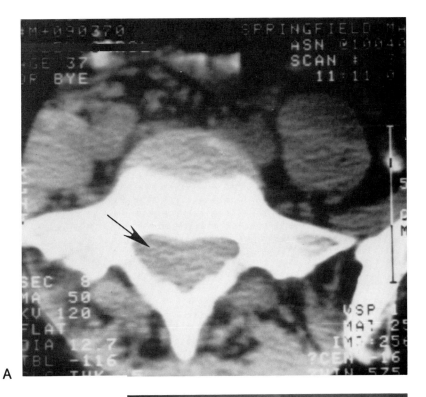

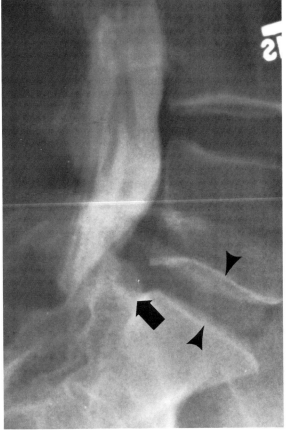

Fig. 13-48 Lymphoma. (A) Transaxial CT scan shows soft tissue density obliterating the epidural fat of the spinal canal (arrow). It represents primary epidural lymphoma. **(B)** Lumbar myelography shows the epidural mass (arrow). It could be misinterpreted as a large disc herniation. However, note the normal disc interspace (arrowheads), which would be unusual in association with such a large herniation.

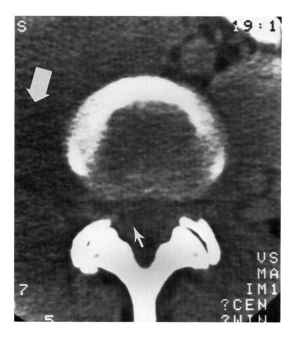

Fig. 13-49 Burkitt's lymphoma, AIDS. Transaxial CT scan shows a large extranodal mass of lymphoma in the paraspinal region on the right (large arrow). It extends through the intervertebral foramen into the epidural space of the spinal canal (small arrow).

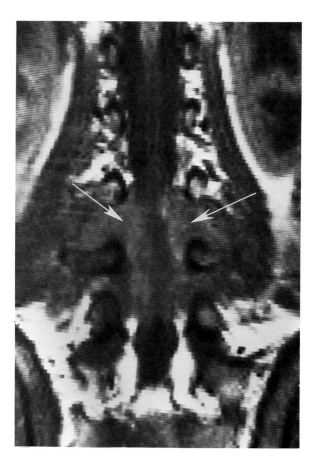

Fig. 13-50 Neuroblastoma. Coronal MRI of the lower lumbar region shows retroperitoneal neuroblastoma extending through the intervertebral foramina into the epidural space bilaterally (arrows). Normal epidural space and fat within the intervertebral foramina are seen at superior levels.

no apparent underlying predisposition. The mass of blood may be large and cause cord compression, but more often it simply causes pain in a dermatome distribution.

The typical findings of an epidural mass are seen with myelography. The CT scan usually demonstrates a nonspecific mass with density slightly greater than that of the dural sac (Fig. 13-52). In the acute phase, MRI shows the signal intensity of a high protein fluid, but high signal intensity blood on T_1- and T_2-weighted images in later subacute and chronic phases.

INTRADURAL EXTRAMEDULLARY LESIONS

Intradural extramedullary lesions are mostly benign and constitute the second most common type of tumor within the spinal canal. In adults the tumor is almost always either a meningioma or a neurofibroma. Intradural metastases are rare. In children, intradural lesions are usually congenital, such as a lipoma or epidermoid inclusion, but intradural "drop metastases" occur with specific intracranial tumors, particularly medulloblastoma, ependymoma, and dysgerminoma.

The intradural extramedullary location of the lesion is determined by seeing, with myelography or MRI, displacement of the spinal cord away from the margins of the dural tube. The lateral margins of the dura remain in close relation with the spinal canal. There is frequently a "capping" type defect seen with myelography, still the most accurate method to diagnose these lesions. Some tumors have an extradural component as well. Gd-DTPA shows enhancement of many of the lesions, increasing their visibility with MRI.

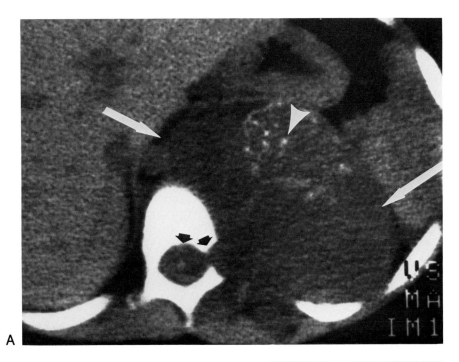

A

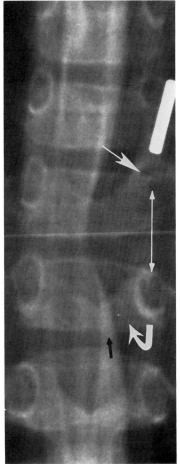

B

Fig. 13-51 Ganglioneuroma. (A) Transaxial CT scan shows a large relatively hypodense mass in a left paraspinal region (white arrows). The mass has enlarged the left intervertebral canal and extends into the epidural space (black arrows). Calcification is present within the tumor (arrowhead). The tumor has locally invaded through the posterior chest wall. **(B)** AP myelography shows characteristic findings of an epidural mass. The dura is displaced away from the pedicle (curved arrow). The subarachnoid space tapers to obliteration at the maximal point of the mass (black arrow). A left intervertebral foramen is widened (opposed arrows), and there is inferior erosion of a pedicle (white arrow).

IMAGING SIGNS OF INTRADURAL EXTRAMEDULLARY LESIONS

"Capping" defect with sharp margin to lesion

Displacement of the cord away from the dural margin

Widening of the subarachnoid space on the side of the lesion (Fig. 13-53)

No bone abnormality (except with "dumbbell" lesions)

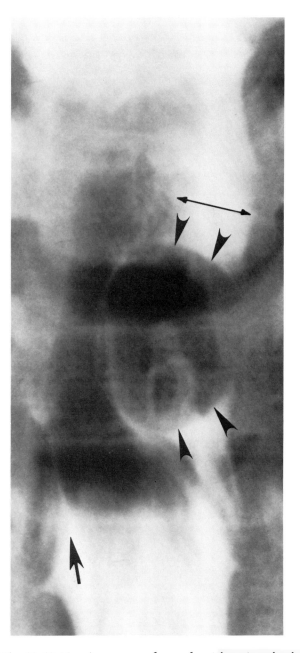

Neurinoma (Schwannoma, "Neurofibroma")

The neurinoma may also be correctly termed a schwannoma, as it arises from the sheath cells of the posterior nerve roots. It is seen most commonly in the 20- to 40-year age group. There is no sex predilection, and the tumor may occur at any site along the neuraxis, except the C1 level. It may be familial. Multiple neurinomas occur with neurofibromatosis.

The lesions produce the characteristic intradural ex-

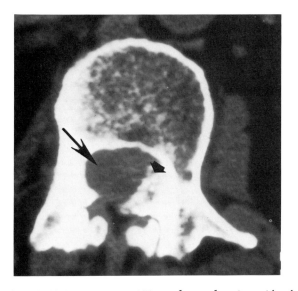

Fig. 13-52 Hematoma, CT myelography. An epidural hematoma occurred spontaneously in this patient. A nonspecific epidural mass is seen (long arrow) compressing the dural tube, which is filled with contrast (short arrow).

Fig. 13-53 Neurinoma, myelography. A large intradural neurinoma is outlined by the myelographic contrast material. A cap defect is seen (arrowheads) The subarachnoid space is widened on the side of the tumor (opposed arrows), and the cord is displaced away from the lesion, narrowing the contralateral subarachnoid space (arrow). These abnormalities are the "classic" findings of an intradural extramedullary lesion.

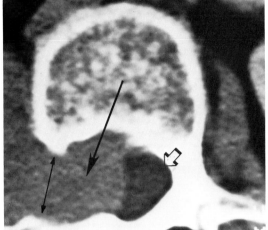

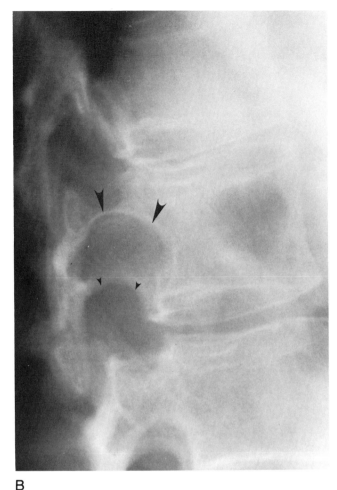

A   B

Fig. 13-54 "Dumbbell" neurinoma. (A) Contrast-enhanced CT scan shows a homogeneously enhancing dumbbell neurinoma extending from the intradural space through the intervertebral foramen into the right paraspinal space (long arrow). The enhanced tumor is hyperdense to the dural tube and spinal cord (open arrow). The intervertebral foramen is widened (opposed arrows). **(B)** Lateral spine radiograph shows enlargement of the intervertebral foramen on the side of the tumor (large arrowheads). A normal intervertebral foramen is seen on the opposite side (small arrowheads).

tramedullary type of appearance on plain film myelography. A "cap" defect is almost always seen within the subarachnoid space, and the cord is usually displaced (Fig. 13-53). The lesions tend to grow out of the dura through the nerve root sleeves and enter the lateral neural foramen, causing it to become enlarged ("dumbbell tumors") (Fig. 13-54). The resulting paraspinal mass can become large. Calcification does not occur. The tumors are vascular and show hypervascular "blushing" with angiography and contrast enhance-

ment with MRI and CT scanning (Fig. 13-54A). MRI easily identifies these tumors and differentiates them from cystic lesions. They are generally isointense or hypointense to the spinal cord on the T_1-weighted images and moderately hyperintense on the T_2-weighted images (Fig. 13-55).

When the tumors are large or multiple within the spinal canal, they may cause scalloping of the posterior margins of the vertebral bodies and separation or thinning of the pedicles. Most commonly, neurinomas

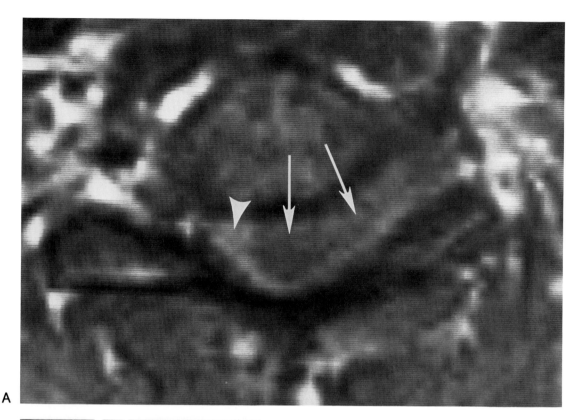

A

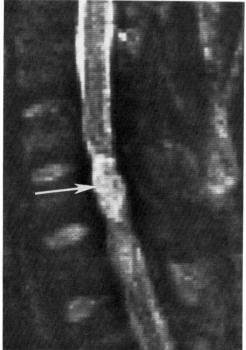

B

Fig. 13-55 Neurinoma, MRI. (A) Transaxial T_1-weighted MRI through the cervical spine shows a slightly hypointense dumbbell neurinoma within the spinal canal and left intervertebral formen (arrows). The more intense appearing spinal cord (arrowhead) is compressed to the right. **(B)** parasagittal T_2-weighted MRI shows the neurinoma as a hyperintense mass (arrow).

cause a radicular syndrome; but if large enough, the spinal cord can become compressed with the production of a Brown-Sequard syndrome.

Meningioma

Meningioma is a benign tumor that arises from the meninges of the dura. It occurs most commonly after the age of 40 in the thoracic region and almost always from the posterior dural surface. Other common sites are the foramen magnum and the cervical region. There is a 4:1 female predominance. The lesion may calcify, which differentiates it from neurofibroma. A rare calcified anterior intraspinal meningioma may be difficult or impossible to differentiate from the much

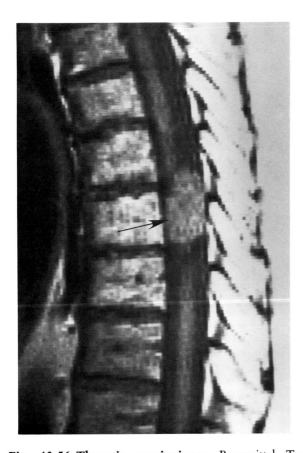

Fig. 13-56 Thoracic meningioma. Parasagittal T_1-weighted MRI shows an intradural extramedullary meningioma (arrow). It is nearly isointense with the spinal cord. The cord is displaced anteriorly and laterally with posterior widening of the subarachnoid space, findings typical of an intradural extramedullary mass.

more common calcified herniated thoracic disc. Meningiomas rarely grow out of the dural sac and do not produce any significant paraspinal mass. Except perhaps at the foramen magnum, associated bone sclerosis does not occur with spinal meningioma.

The lesions are easily seen by MRI, which is the preferred method of diagnosis. The tumor is isointense to the cord on T_1-weighted images (Fig. 13-56) and slightly hyperintense on T_2-weighted images. It is seen as a "negative" defect within the CSF on the T_2-weighted images. Meningioma is hyperintense after Gd-DTPA enhancement.

With myelography, the typical intradural extramedullary type of defect is seen. The characteristic location, age, and sex of the patient suggests the correct tissue diagnosis. A meningioma is difficult to demonstrate with plain CT scanning but can easily be seen with CT myelography. The lesion enhances with intravenous contrast, differentiating it from a fluid-filled cyst or meningocele.

Metastasis

Metastasis may occur within the subarachnoid space. It is most likely to result from lymphoma, leukemia, breast carcinoma, or melanoma. Drop metastasis from primary intracranial tumors are more common in children, especially from a medulloblastoma, ependymoma, neuroblastoma, or atypical teratoma of the pineal region. On myelography and CT myelography, the tumor deposits appear as rounded filling defects within the contrast column (Fig. 13-57) and may be "matted," mimicking the changes of arachnoiditis. Complete block to the flow of intrathecal contrast is possible. MRI has high sensitivity and shows these lesions (Fig. 13-58), particularly on the T_1-weighted Gd-DTPA images, as hyperintense masses within the CSF. The intradural metastasis cannot be seen on plain CT scans. (See also Fig. 5-24.)

INTRAMEDULLARY TUMORS AND MASS LESIONS

The hallmark of intramedullary tumor is enlargement of the spinal cord, usually over several vertebral levels. With small lesions, the widening may be subtle or undetectable. Myelography and CT myelography can outline the dimensions and configuration of the cord but cannot identify the inner anatomy.

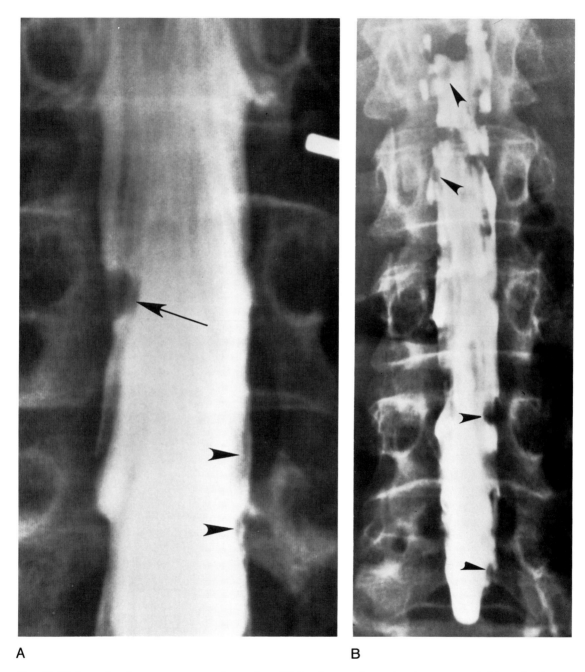

A   B

Fig. 13-57 Intradural metastases, myelography. (A) Lumbar myelography shows a rounded intradural mass (arrow) and irregular, flat masses along the lateral dural surface (arrowheads). They represent metastatic tumor deposits. **(B)** Multiple round masses are seen in the lumbar region, representing metastases (arrowheads).

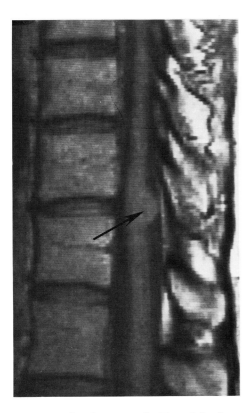

Fig. 13-58 Intradural metastasis. T_1-weighted parasagittal MRI shows an intradural thoracic mass representing metastatic deposit from breast carcinoma. When seen as a single lesion, it cannot reliably be differentiated from a meningioma.

The MRI method has significant advantage over other techniques for defining intramedullary pathology. Not only can the outline of the cord be seen, but signal abnormalities within the cord can identify focal lesions, differentiating between cyst and solid tumor. Gd-DTPA can further define focal lesions and increases

---

IMAGING SIGNS OF INTRAMEDULLARY LESIONS

Cord enlargement, usually over several segments

Circumferential narrowing of the subarachnoid space at the site of cord enlargement

Tapering of margins with normal cord

No displacement of the dura (Figs. 13-59 – 13-63)

---

the sensitivity of the examination, although the enhancement of cord tumors is not as consistent as with intracranial tumors. The specific tumor type cannot be diagnosed reliably by MRI signal characteristics.

Glioma

Ependymoma of the spinal cord and filum terminale accounts for about 60 percent of all intramedullary neoplasms. This tumor almost always presents in the lumbar or sacral region and rarely extends as high as the thoracic cord (see Fig. 13-60). As with all intramedullary tumors, the cord is widened and fills the subarachnoid space at the level of the tumor mass. On plain film myelography, the cord must be seen to be widened in two projections. This criterion excludes the spurious apparent enlargement seen when the cord is compressed by an extradural lesion such as a herniated disc or spondylytic ridge (pseudoenlargement) (Fig. 13-26). In the absence of dysraphism, a mass within the filum terminale is almost always an ependymoma.

Astrocytoma is the next most common type of intramedullary tumor, accounting for about 33 percent of tumors of the spinal cord. It occurs predominantly in the cervical cord. It is the most frequently encountered cord tumor in children. The tumor may become large, extending through the entire cord (Fig. 13-59). Cystic change is common. The imaging findings are identical to those of ependymoma. Oligodendroglioma and glioblastoma multiforme are rare.

The tumors may become large, extending over many segments; rarely, nearly the whole spinal cord is involved (Fig. 13-59). The spinal canal may become enlarged to accommodate the tumor with the pedicles separated and thinned along their medial margins. This situation occurs most commonly at the L1-L3 level (Fig. 13-60). Because the discs are resistant to remodeling from tumor, the posterior margins of the vertebral bodies may become scalloped and can be pronounced.

The tumor within the cord, as well as any cystic component, is clearly demonstrated by MRI. The solid tumor is seen as high intensity on heavily T_2-weighted images (Fig. 13-61). Compared with syringomyelia, tumor cysts show relatively high signal intensity on both T_1- and T_2-weighted images because of contained protein and lack of fluid motion (Fig. 13-62). Gd-DTPA enhancement occurs in the solid components (Fig. 13-63) and clearly differentiates solid tumor from cysts and syringomyelia. The full extent of the tumor is most easily evaluated with MRI.

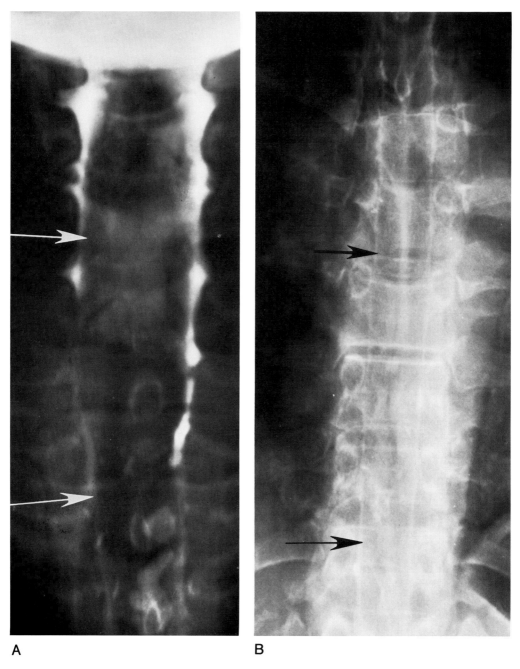

A   B

Fig. 13-59 Astrocytoma of spinal cord. (A) Cervical myelography shows gross enlargement of the cervical spinal cord over many segments (arrows). The subarachnoid space is circumferentially narrowed. **(B)** The tumor extends througout the entire cord (arrows). The compressed subarachnoid space is represented by a thin line of contrast.

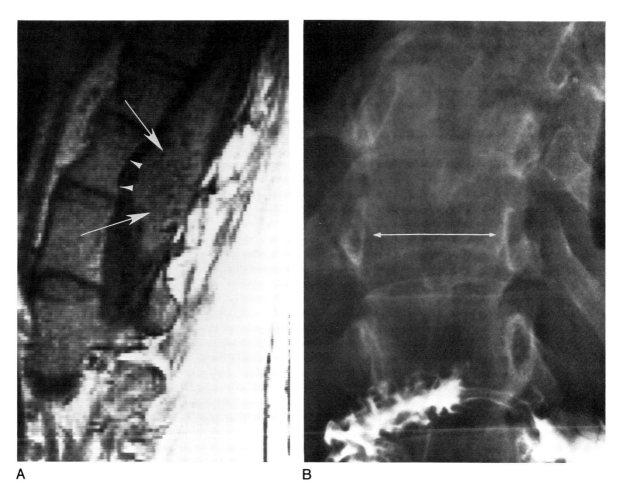

A

B

Fig. 13-60 Ependymoma of the conus medullaris. (A) Parasagittal T$_1$-weighted MRI shows isointense enlargement of the conus medullaris (arrows). Note the scalloping of the posterior margins of the vertebral bodies (arrowheads). **(B)** AP spine view shows scoliosis, widening of the spinal canal (opposed arrows), and flattening of the medial margins of the pedicles.

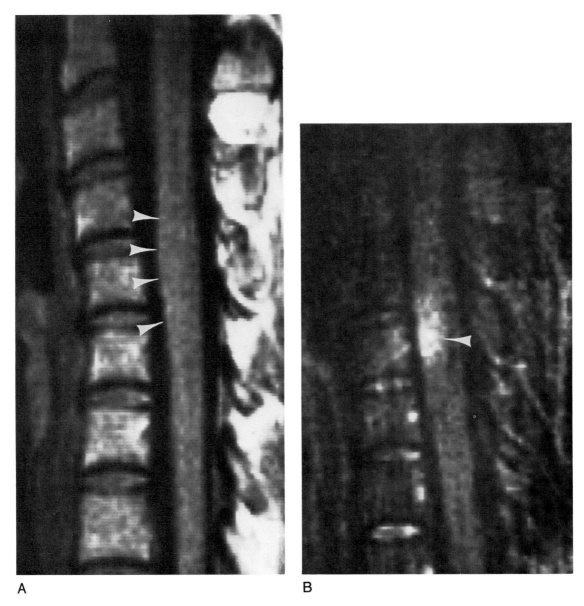

A   B

Fig. 13-61 Astrocytoma. (A) Parasagittal T_1-weighted image shows subtle enlargement of the mid-cervical cord (arrowheads). **(B)** T_2-weighted study shows high signal intensity representing the tumor mass (arrowheads). This appearance is nonspecific, and multiple sclerosis, cord metastasis, and inflammatory lesions such as sarcoid could produce these findings.

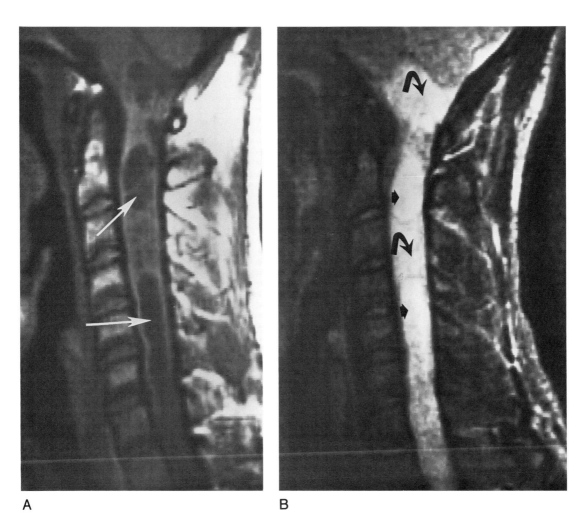

A   B

Fig. 13-62 Cystic astrocytoma. (A) Transaxial T_1-weighted MRI shows diffuse enlargement of the medulla and cervical cord. Multiple cysts are seen containing fluid slightly hyperintense to CSF (white arrows). **(B)** T_2-weighted study (SE 2500/80) shows that the cyst contains very hyperintense fluid (small arrows). The intervening solid tumor shows high T_2 signal intensity (curved arrows) but slightly less intense than the cysts.

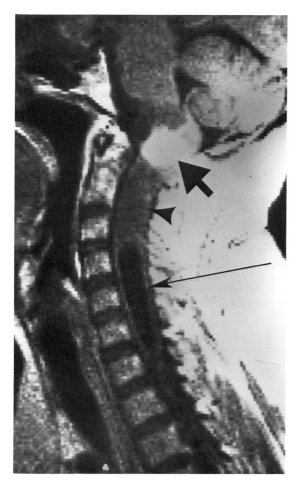

Fig. 13-63 Astrocytoma, Gd-DTPA enhancement. Parasagittal T_1-weighted MRI shows intense enhancement of the medullary portion of the tumor (fat arrow). The upper cervical solid tumor does not enhance (arrowhead). A cyst is present at the inferior portion of the tumor (long arrow).

Hemangioblastoma

Hemangioblastoma is a malignant vascular tumor that may present within the cord as a single mass or as multiple tumors. It occurs as an isolated tumor or in association with the Von Hippel-Lindau syndrome. The lesion enlarges the cord and may be associated with enlarged vascular channels on the cord surface, which can be demonstrated with plain film myelography, CT myelography, and as flow-void with MRI. Selective spinal cord angiography shows a highly vascular lesion with small intrinsic vessels, creating an intense "blush." Arteriovenous shunting may be present to some extent but not nearly so predominantly as with an

arteriovenous malformation (AVM). The blush lasts into the venous phase, reminiscent of the blush seen with meningioma. Cysts may be present. The solid tumor shows contrast enhancement and high T_2 signal on MRI.

Lipoma

Lipoma is a rare tumor that occurs in adults, even without associated spinal dysraphism. The lesion may be in any intradural space, although it tends to arise in the posterior part of the thecal sac or cord, most commonly in the lumbosacral region (Fig. 13-64). It is frequently related to the filum terminale. Widening of the spinal canal can occur with large lesions. CT scans and MRI can specifically identify these lesions from their characteristic signal signatures. Occasionally, these tumors extend outside the dura and may reach the skin.

Dermoid

Although usually associated with the dysraphic syndrome, the epithelial cystic lesions known as dermoids may occur as an isolated lesion. They have no specific CT characteristics and may be of high or low density depending on the nature of the debris within the cyst. On MRI they tend to be inhomogeneous with variable

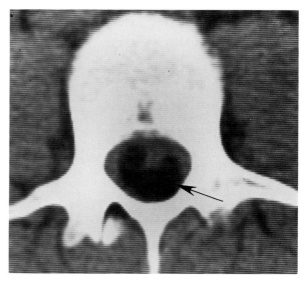

Fig. 13-64 Intraspinal lipoma. Transaxial CT scan shows hypodense tissue within the spinal canal, representing a lipoma (arrow). Most lipomas are related to the filum terminale.

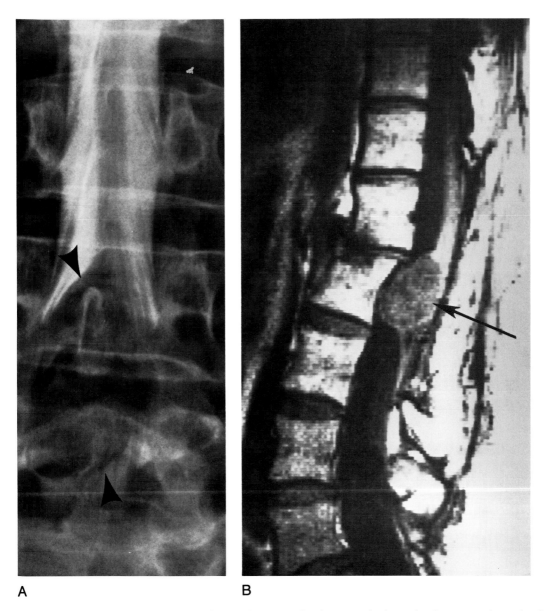

A   B

Fig. 13-65 Dermoid. (A) Myelography shows a large intradural mass in the lower lumbar region (arrowheads). The differential diagnosis includes lipoma and ependymoma. **(B)** Parasagittal T$_1$ MRI in another patient shows an intradural slightly hypointense mass attached to the conus medullaris (arrow). This dermoid was thought to result from prior trauma and surgery.

signal intensities. They are usually intradural-extrame-dullary in location but may be within the cord (Fig. 13-65). They are known to occur following lumbar puncture or surgery, probably as a result of introducing viable epithelial cells deep into the spinal canal.

INFLAMMATION

Pyogenic Infections

Pyogenic infections of the spine are becoming increasingly common. The process may be difficult to diagnose, and frequently patients suffer for months without appropriate diagnosis or treatment.

Pain is the most common symptom, and it is often relentless. Fever is inconsistent and low grade. The process is relatively slow, and the problem may go on for months or even years. The erythrocyte sedimentation rate (ESR) is almost always elevated. Most commonly patients have had superficial skin infections or have undergone a recent urologic or gynecologic procedure. Intravenous drug abusers are at risk. Sometimes no risk factor is present.

The infections may occur at any age but are more common in persons over age 60. Batson's plexus undoubtedly plays an important role in the spread of infection to the spine, and because of its proximity to the pelvic organs the lumbar spine is the area most frequently involved. Rarely, the infectious process is multicentric. *Staphylococcus aureus* is by far the most common pyogenic infectious agent affecting the spine, but any organism may cause the infection.

The hallmark radiographic findings are vertebral end-plate erosion and disc space narrowing (Fig. 13-66). Pyogenic infection of the spine is actually an osteomyelitis of the vertebral body with secondary involvement of the disc space (discitis) and the opposite vertebral body. It may take 2 to 3 months from the onset of pain before the spine changes become detectable. The end-plate erosion may be subtle, and plain film tomography may help in better definition.

Characteristically, the anterior two-thirds of the vertebral bodies are involved, and the posterior spinal arch is not affected. Eventually there is symmetric erosion of the two adjacent vertebral bodies with associated obliteration of the disc space (Fig. 13-67A&B). Only late in the untreated process is there vertebral

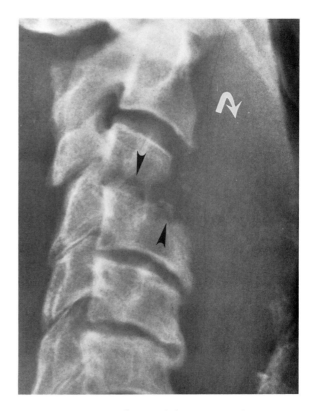

Fig. 13-66 Osteomyelitis and disc space infection. Lateral cervical spine in a patient with extensive laminectomy shows vertebral end-plate erosion on both sides of a narrow disc interspace (arrowheads). Considerable destruction has occurred anteriorly at C3. A large prevertebral abscess is present (curved arrow).

body collapse. These changes are distinct from tumor of the spine. Tumor causes destruction or sclerosis of the vertebral body and may involve multiple levels, but as a rule there is preservation of the end-plates and the disc space.

After 2 to 3 months, hypertrophic bone change occurs, causing osteophytes and sclerosis about the vertebral body. Eventual fusion between the adjacent vertebral bodies may result. A small paravertebral abscess mass is common, but it is not seen on the plain films unless the mass is unusually large and displaces or obliterates the psoas muscle. The abscess within the disc space may bulge into the anterior portion of the spinal canal, but cord or nerve root compression and empyema are unusual.

Sometime prior to the plain film changes, the radionuclide technetium bone scan becomes positive, the

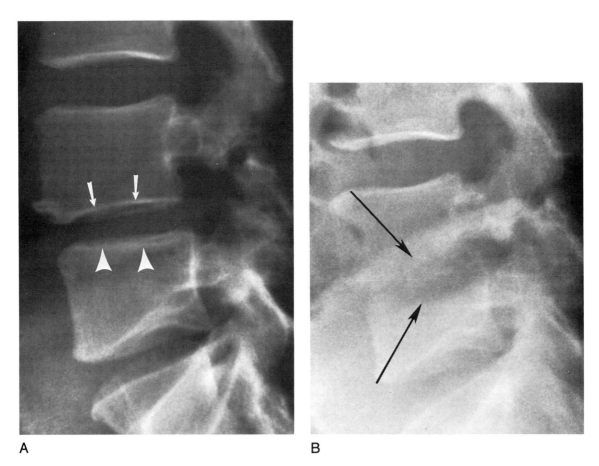

A   B

Fig. 13-67 Osteomyelitis and disc space infection. (A) Initial radiograph of the lower lumbar spine shows disc interspace narrowing at the L4-L5 level. The superior end-plate of L5 is indistinct (arrowheads), whereas the inferior end-plate of L4 is nearly normal (arrows). These plain film changes are typical of early vertebral ostemyelitis and discitis. **(B)** Radiograph obtained 6 weeks later shows marked progression of the findings with severe erosion of both end-plates (arrows) surrounding the obliterated disc space. There is partial collapse of the L5 vertebral body with spondylolisthesis. (*Figure continues.*)

process being represented as a "hot" spot in the vertebral body or two adjacent vertebral bodies. The finding is nonspecific, and the diagnosis can be surmised only because of the elevated ESR and any suggestive history. The gallium- or indium-tagged leukocyte scan is usually not positive in the early stages of the disease but later becomes positive in more than 50 percent of cases (Fig. 13-67D&E).

The most sensitive imaging examination for the detection of vertebral osteomyelitis is MRI. The findings are characteristic. Loss of height of the disc space and blurring of the end-plates are seen. On the T_1-weighted images, decreased signal intensity occurs within the portions of the vertebral bodies adjacent to the disc space and usually within the disc space itself. High signal intensity is seen in these regions on the T_2-weighted images. These disc space changes are almost never seen with tumor. There is resolution with effective antibiotic therapy (Fig. 13-67F&G).

Also useful for diagnosing and managing spinal infections is CT scanning. Regions of bone destruction adjacent to the end-plates can be seen with appropriate windows. There is a small paravertebral swelling or mass visible in virtually all cases. If the infection is chronic, reactive bone formation is detected surrounding the disc space, usually anteriorly (Fig. 13-67C).

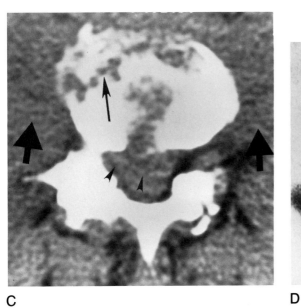

C

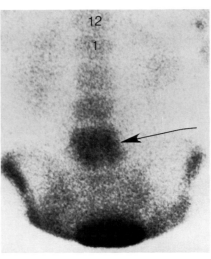

D

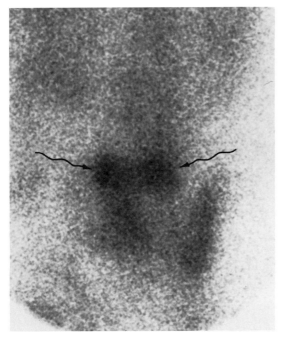

E

Fig. 13-67 (*Continued*) **(C)** CT scan through the inferior L4 level shows the combination of lytic destruction with reactive new bone formation (thin arrow). A large paraspinal inflammatory mass is present (large arrows). The inflammation has extended posteriorly, causing obliteration of the epidural fat on the right and compression of the dural tube (arrowheads). **(D)** Technetium radionuclide bone scan shows increased uptake at both L4 and L5 vertebral bodies with no visible intervening disc interspace (arrow). **(E)** Gallium scan shows increased uptake at the L4-L5 level. Note that the uptake extends beyond the margins of the vertebral body, representing the paraspinal spread of infection (arrows). (*Figure continues*)

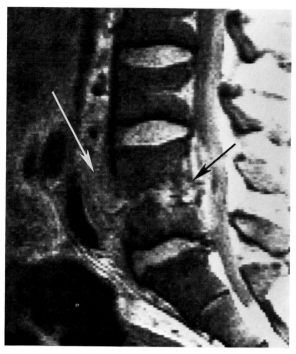

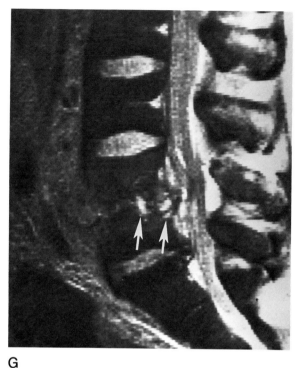

F

G

Fig. 13-67 (*Continued*) **(F)** SE 1000/22 MRI shows erosion of the disc interspace at L4-L5 (black arrow). The inflammatory reaction extends into the prevertebral space (white arrow). **(G)** Proton density MRI (SE 2500/40) shows some high signal within the posterior portion of the disc interspace and epidural extension of the infection (arrows).

There are no specific findings to differentiate between the various pyogenic organisms. The etiology of infection of the spine can be determined only by tissue biopsy and culture. The CT scan is especially useful for selecting the region of the largest inflammatory mass and greatest bone destruction to guide placement of a percutaneous biopsy needle.

Nonpyogenic Infections

Coccidioides immitis, Cryptococcus neoformans, Aspergillus fumigatus, Brucella, and *Echinococcus* may cause spinal infection especially in endemic regions. The lesions are generally osteolytic with no surrounding sclerosis. There may be disc space narrowing and a small paravertebral mass, but these findings are not as constant as with nonpyogenic infections. *Actinomyces israelii,* found in the mouth and often associated with mandibular infection, may cause infection of the spine, especially

the cervical segments. This infection spreads to involve adjacent structures. The process is mixed lytic and sclerotic, and there is a large paravertebral abscess with sinus tracts. Biopsy and serologic findings may make the specific diagnosis.

Tuberculosis

Spinal tuberculosis results from hematogenous spread from pulmonary tuberculosis. Some evidence of the lung infection is almost always present. The infection is an osteomyelitis usually at the thoracolumbar junction. It begins adjacent to the vertebral end-plate, spreading quickly into the adjacent disc space. The bone lesion is purely osteolytic with poor margination and regional osteoporosis. Cartilage is destroyed, resulting in a narrowed or obliterated disc space. The infection spreads to the opposite vertebral body. Vertebral collapse is common, resulting in a gibbus deformity. Uncommonly, the posterior arch becomes involved; such involvement almost never occurs with pyogenic infections.

Characteristically, there is a large paravertebral abscess, often large enough to be seen on plain films. The size of the mass may be disproportionately larger than the degree of vertebral body destruction. Multiple contiguous vertebral bodies may become involved with the infection as the infection spreads superiorly and inferiorly underneath the poorly attached anterior longitudinal ligament. The infection erodes the anterior borders of the more distant vertebral bodies, causing a "gouge" defect. In the chronic phase, extensive mottled calcification is deposited within the paravertebral abscess.

Epidural Abscess (Empyema)

An epidural abscess usually occurs as a metastatic infection from a distant site. Less commonly, it may occur secondary to an adjacent osteomyelitis of the spinal column (Fig. 13-66) or with iatrogenic infection from surgery or lumbar puncture. *Staphylococcus* is the most common organism. It is a serious infection, and the abscess may spread rapidly throughout the loose fatty tissue of the spinal canal. Patients are acutely ill with fever, progressing motor and sensory neurologic deficits, and spine tenderness. Cord compression and death may result. The abscess must be drained, which often requires extensive laminectomy. The infection occurs with equal frequency at all levels of the spine.

The best initial examination is MRI. The inflammatory change is seen on T_1-weighted images as obliteration of the normal epidural fat density and displacement of the dural tube. On the T_2-weighted images the infection is seen as high signal intensity epidural tissue (Fig. 13-68). Paraspinal inflammatory reaction may also be present. CT myelography can be used to make the diagnosis (Fig. 13-69). The spinal puncture is made at an asymptomatic level to avoid contamination of the subarachnoid space.

Subdural Empyema

The spinal subdural space is a rare location for infection within the spinal canal. Such infection usually results from the spread of adjacent epidural infection through the dura into the subdural extra-arachnoid space, although it may occur in isolation. When seen in isola-

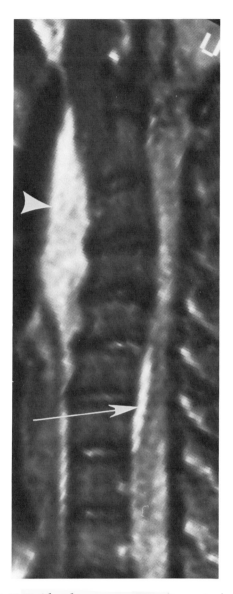

Fig. 13-68 Epidural empyema, MRI. Parasagittal proton density (SE 2500/40) image shows high signal intensity in the anterior epidural space causing dural compression (arrow). Also note the prevertebral retropharyngeal abscess (arrowhead).

tion, the presentation is similar to epidural infection, except that there is no associated localized pain or tenderness in the back. The myelographic findings are the same as with epidural infection, although the MRI or CT scan may not show obliteration of the epidural fat. MRI may show increased intensity within the dural tube on T_1-weighted images.

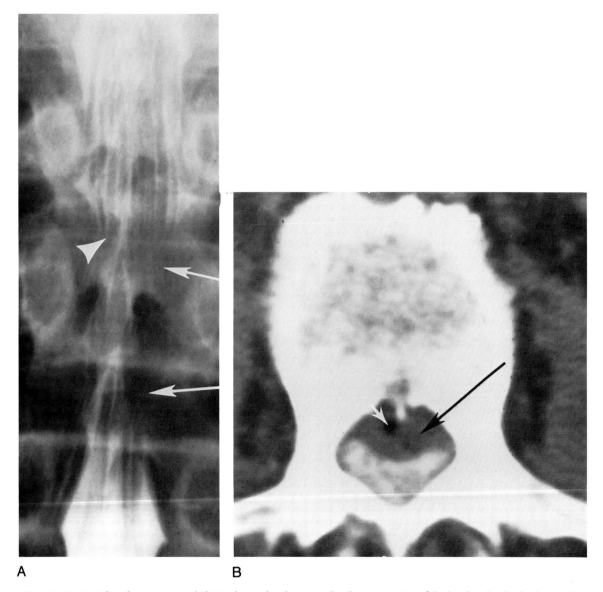

A

B

Fig. 13-69 Epidural empyema. (A) Myelography shows epidural compression of the lumbar dural tube (arrows). Note the "feathering" at the superior margin of the block produced by the nerve roots (arrowhead). This myelographic finding is nonspecific and can be produced by any epidural mass, particularly lymphoma. Acute fever suggests the diagnosis of epidural infection. **(B)** CT scan in the same patient shows the anterior epidural inflammatory mass (black arrow). The gas bubble (white arrow) makes the diagnosis of infection likely. Note that there are no bone or paravertebral abnormalities. Contrast fills the compressed dural sac.

Hypertrophic Pachymeningitis

Hypertrophic pachymeningitis may occur as an isolated finding or in association with the mucopolysaccharidoses. The meninges and dura are markedly thickened, causing compression of nerve roots and in severe cases the spinal cord. Plain films are normal or show the bone changes associated with Morquio's disease.

Acute Transverse Myelitis

Acute transverse myelitis occurs in young adults, producing rapid onset of symptoms mimicking cord compression. Although the etiology is elusive, the syndrome is associated with viral infections and radiation therapy. Some investigators believe that the process is a form of multiple sclerosis.

The myelographic findings during the acute phases are usually normal, and the diagnosis is one of the exclusion of other disease processes. However, the cord may show intrinsic enlargement that is indistinguishable from a small cord tumor. On MRI, the signal on T_2-weighted images is generally not increased (Fig. 13-70). The CSF shows a low grade pleocytosis. The cord disease causes both motor and sensory loss with local radicular changes. Long tract signs appear later.

Guillain-Barré Syndrome

The Guillain-Barré syndrome is another form of myelitis and radiculitis that is strictly limited to the anterior horn cells or peripheral nerves, causing a flaccid, usually ascending paralysis. Sensory changes do not occur. Myelography is normal, and the cord shows no enlargement.

Infections of the Spinal Cord

Infections of the spinal cord are rare. Pyogenic infection, especially with *Staphylococcus,* is the most common and usually occurs in association with known infection elsewhere. Granulomas, particularly of fungal and sarcoid origin, may also occur. The cord shows nonspecific enlargement and high T_2 signal with MRI. The differentiation from tumor may be possible only at surgical exploration.

CRANIOVERTEBRAL JUNCTION

The craniovertebral junction is considered separately, as there are unique features of pathology that affect this region. Lesions at this level of the spine are notoriously difficult to diagnose clinically. Symptoms of ataxia, weakness of the lower extremities, and tingling of the fingers are nonspecific and often suggest disease at other levels.

The superior imaging technique for evaluating this region is MRI. If MRI is not available, plain film radiography and CT myelography/cisternography may be used. Developmental abnormalities are common, producing symptoms of compression of the upper spinal

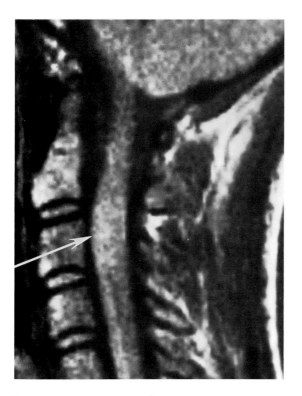

Fig. 13-70 Transverse myelitis. T_1-weighted MRI shows slight expansion of the upper cervical cord (arrow), a nonspecific finding. (The T_2-weighted image showed no high signal intensity.) It was thought to represent transverse myelitis. The same change might be found with a small tumor, multiple sclerosis, or focal cord infection, although the latter processes usually show high signal intensity on the T_2-weighted images. (Courtesy of Dr. Paul Markarian, Mercy Hospital, Springfield, MA.)

cord and medulla that do not become a clinical problem until adulthood. The average age for the onset of symptoms is 28 years.

Basilar Impression (Invagination)

Basilar impression can be a developmental abnormality or occur as a result of softening of the bone at the base of the skull, as in Paget's disease or osteogenesis imperfecta. The abnormality consists in superior displacement of the upper cervical spine into the base of the skull secondary to upward curving of the margins of the foramen magnum. The diagnosis is generally made by plain skull film analysis using any one of a number of reference lines drawn at the base (Fig. 13-71). Using the lateral projection, Chamberlain's line is drawn from the posterior margin of the hard palate back to the anterosuperior margin of the posterior rim of the foramen magnum. If more than 8 mm of the odontoid process projects above this line, basilar impression is a strong possibility.

The abnormality may cause direct compression of the lower brain stem because of the small size of the foramen magnum. Importantly, basilar impression is frequently associated with other abnormalities, particularly the Chiari type I malformation and syringohydromyelia. MRI of the region is done in persons with congenital basilar invagination.

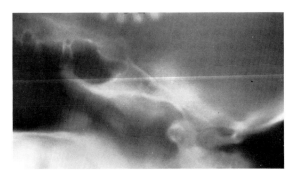

Fig. 13-71 Basilar impression and platybasia. Lateral tomography demonstrates upward invagination of the cervical spine, with 50 percent of the ondontoid projecting above Chamberlain's line. This finding represents basilar impression. Note the flattening of the basal angle formed between the planum sphenoidale and the posterior margin of the clivus, called platybasia. (From Heinz, 1984, with permission.)

Platybasia

Although often misunderstood, the term platybasia refers only to a relatively obtuse angle formed by the planum sphenoidale and the dorsal margin of the plane of the clivus (Fig. 13-71). If this angle is more than 143 degrees, the skull has a flattened appearance and platybasia is determined to exist. It has no significance except as an alert to the presence of other possible anomalies, particularly at the craniovertebral junction.

Occipitalization of the Atlas

Occipitalization of the atlas results from failure of separation of the anterior arch of C1 from the inferior tip of the clivus. There may also be fusion of the transverse processes and the posterior arch into the occipital bone. The atlanto-occipital joints may be normal or fused. The odontoid process is often deformed and is high in the anterior portion of the foramen magnum (Fig. 13-74).

The major importance of this malformation is its association with compressive syndromes of the medulla, especially if the AP dimension of the foramen magnum is reduced to less than 2 cm. Thickening of the adjacent ligaments, dural bands, and the Chiari type I malformation (in 15 percent) are the usual causes of the neural compression. Weakness and ataxia in the lower extremities are the most frequent symptoms followed by upper extremity findings and neck pain.

Other segmental fusions (Klippel-Feil) of the cervical spine are frequently present, especially at the C2-C3 level (Fig. 13-72). The observation of fusion anomalies at any level of the cervical spine calls for a careful search for occipitalization of the atlas. CT myelography and cisternography as well as MRI scanning can demonstrate the associated anomalies (Chiari I, syrinx), cord compression, or angulation that may be present.

Odontoid Dysplasia and Atlantoaxial Hypermobility

Odontoid dysplasia, including aplasia and hypoplasia, is most commonly seen in association with dwarf syndromes but may occur in normal children or adults. The odontoid may not completely fuse with the axis, leaving a persistent synchondrosis (fibrous union). At best, nonfusion is difficult to differentiate from a fracture. The absence of prior neck trauma is important for

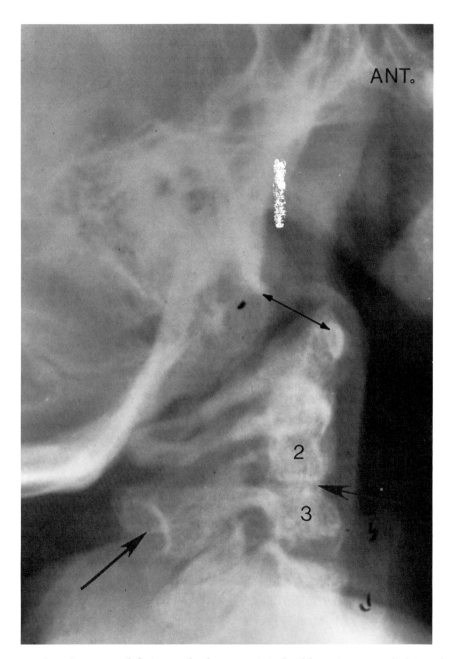

Fig. 13-72 Kippel-Feil segmental fusion and atlanto-occipital subluxation. Lateral plain radiograph of a child shows congenital fusion of the C2-C3 level involving the vertebral bodies and the posterior arches (arrows). In addition, this patient has atlanto-occipital luxation (opposed arrows), which may be due to laxity of ligaments in patients with Down and Ehlers-Danlos syndromes. (Courtesy of Dr. Leon Kruger, The Shriner's Hospital for Crippled Children, Springfield, MA.)

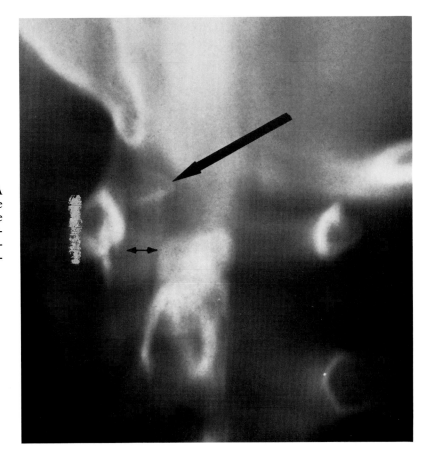

Fig. 13-73 Os odontoideum. A small malformed odontoid (large arrow) is widely separated from the axis. There is instability of the atlantoaxial articulation with anterior displacement of the atlas (opposed arrows).

making the diagnosis as well as the performance of both flexion and extension views in the lateral projection to determine if instability is present.

Os odontoideum (ossiculum terminale) refers to complete separation from the axis of a malformed small odontoid (Fig. 13-73). This situation allows hypermobility at the C1-C2 level, which can be seen with flexion and extension lateral plain films. The odontoid remnant may be fused with the clivus.

Hypoplasia of the dens may be associated with instability (Fig. 13-74). The odontoid may be absent (aplasia) and this is always associated with instability.

Atlantoaxial subluxation may occur in the absence of bone anomalies at the craniovertebral junction. Most commonly, it results from abnormality of the transverse ligament, usually from erosive change produced by rheumatoid disease (Fig. 13-75). It also occurs in persons with ligamentous laxity such as in Down or Ehlers-Danlos syndrome. Rarely, it occurs in isolation.

The diagnosis is made when in the lateral flexion

view there is more than 5 mm of separation of the odontoid from the anterior arch of C1 in children under 12 years of age or more than 3 mm separation in adults. Chronic instability is almost always associated with cord compression syndromes. Ligamentous instability may also result in hypermobility at the craniovertebral junction, especially in Down syndrome (Fig. 13-72).

Chiari I Malformation

Chiari I malformation is probably an acquired abnormality that is distinct from the Chiari II type malformation. It consists in a downward position of the cerebellar tonsils, usually to the level of C1. The tonsils are deformed into a pyramidal shape and are closely applied to the posterolateral portion of the medulla. Ligamentous thickening at the foramen magnum may also be present. The anomaly occurs with or without other craniovertebral bone abnormalities and is frequently

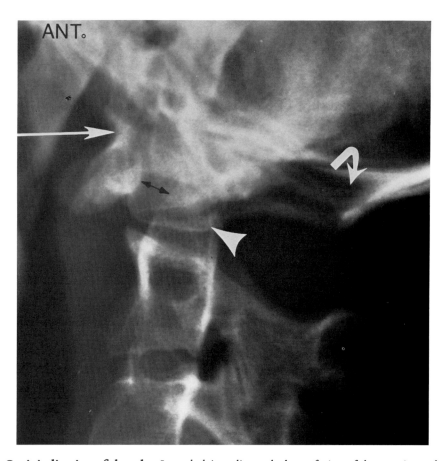

Fig. 13-74 Occipitalization of the atlas. Lateral plain radiograph shows fusion of the anterior arch of C1 with the base of the clivus (arrow). The posterior arch is also fused to the occipital bone (curved arrow). The odontoid is hypoplastic (arrowhead), and there is widening of the dentoatlantal interval (opposed arrows).

associated with syringomyelia. The abnormality most often becomes symptomatic during early adolescence or young adulthood, causing pain in the posterior neck with a cord compressive syndrome or ataxia.

The diagnosis is best made with MRI (Fig. 13-76) or CT myelography. Plain CT scans of the upper cervical region cannot reliably define the position of the tonsils. Relief of the compression usually results in disappearance of the symptoms.

Tumors

Meningioma is by far the most common tumor encountered at the craniovertebral junction. Patients most often present in the 35- to 55-year range with local pain, corticospinal tract symptoms, or high cervical radicular pain. The tumors almost always occur an-

teriorly or anterolaterally in the intradural extramedullary space.

With MRI the mass is shown to be anterior to the cord with the typical signal characteristics of meningioma. With CT scanning the tumor is seen as a homogeneously enhancing lesion. Bone sclerosis is rare. Vertebral or ipsilateral external carotid angiography shows the typical hypervascular tumor with a prolonged homogeneous blush. Myelography demonstrates the mass in the upper subarachnoid space.

Neurinoma occurs rarely at the craniovertebral level. It may involve the lower cranial nerves and usually enlarges the neuroforamina. Neurinoma is almost never found on the C1 root. Because the tumors involve the nerve roots, they are laterally positioned in the spinal canal.

Metastatic tumor can be found in the craniovertebral

Fig. 13-75 Rheumatoid arthritis, atlantoaxial hyper-mobility. (A) Increased space is present between the anterior arch of the atlas and the odontoid (long arrow). The odontoid is eroded by the inflammatory process (small arrow). Rheumatoid changes are also present in the facets (arrowhead), which allows anterior listhesis at multiple levels. **(B)** Transaxial view shows severe odontoid erosion (arrow) as well as erosion of the anterior arch of C1 (arrowheads). The atlantoaxial displacement is reduced when the patient is supine.

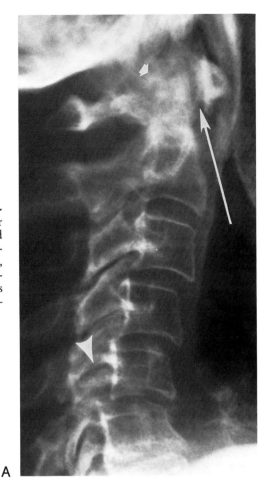

A

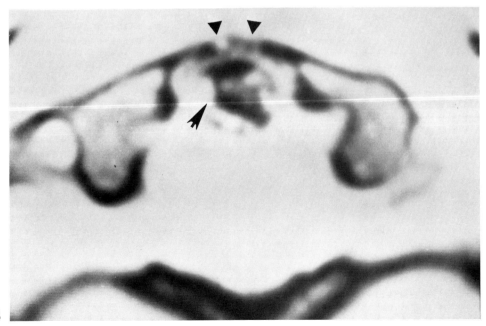

B

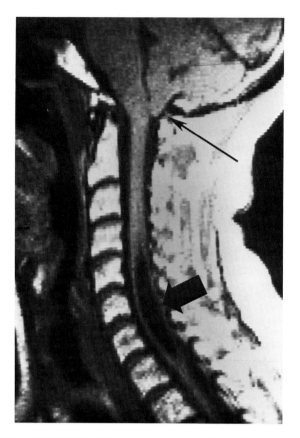

Fig. 13-76 Chiari I, syringomyelia. T_1-weighted MRI shows the downward displacement of pointed cerebellar tonsils into the upper cervical spinal canal (thin arrow). Syringomyelia is present in the lower cervical spinal cord (fat arrow).

region. Destructive or blastic lesions occur in the atlas, odontoid, and skull base. Large carcinomas of the posterior nasopharynx and hypopharynx may directly invade the anterior margin of the foramen magnum or upper cervical spine.

CONGENITAL ANOMALIES

At birth there are usually one or two ossification centers in the vertebral bodies. If two are present, they are divided by either a sagittal or a coronal cleft. The neural arch (pedicles, lamina, transverse processes, spinous process) has a single ossification center on each side. The odontoid process contains two ossification centers divided by a sagittal cleft, and the tip has one or two separate centers. The odontoid forms from the same somite as the distal clivus.

The neural arches fuse posteriorly beginning in the first year. The lumbar segments fuse first, followed by the thoracic segments and sacral segments. The cervical arches fuse last at the end of the third year. The neurocentral synchondrosis, the junction between the posterior neural arch (pedicles) and the vertebral bodies, begins fusion at age 2 in the cervical region and completes the process in the lumbar region by age 5. The sacrum does not become fully ossified until about age 5.

The dural sac and spinal cord have a rounded configuration during the first year of life but become somewhat more oval thereafter with the long dimension in the transverse plane. The spinal canal is originally larger than the vertebral bodies but becomes equal to the bodies at about 6 to 8 years. Thereafter the canals are smaller than the transverse dimension of the adjacent vertebral body. The cord normally enlarges at the C3-C6 level and again at the T10-T11 level. Because of the normal thoracic kyphosis the thoracic cord is anterior in the spinal canal, whereas at other levels it lies posteriorly. The conus medullaris comes to lie at T12-L1, its usual adult level, by age 2 months. There is some variation in the level, but a conus below the middle of L2 is considered abnormally low. The filum terminale, normally measuring 1.0 to 1.5 mm in diameter, extends from the lower point of the tapered conus medullaris and courses inferiorly to attach to the sacrum in the posterior aspect of the canal. The descending nerve roots form the cauda equina and are usually oriented in a V configuration within the sac as viewed on transaxial CT myelography or MRI.

Dysraphism

The term spinal dysraphism encompasses a large group of disorders that originate from defects in the formation of the neural tube. These fusion abnormalities may involve any part of the spinal axis and include hemivertebrae, cleft vertebrae, segmental fusions of vertebral bodies or lamina, spinal bifida occulta, or widely spread neural arches. Neural tissue involvement with the dysraphic abnormality may be manifested by a thickened filum terminale with tethering of the cord, dural ectasia, meningocele, myelomeningocele, diastematomyelia, diplomyelia, neurenteric cyst, or the Chiari type II malformation. Overgrowth of sequestered tissue may lead to abnormal tissue collections such as lipoma, epidermoid, dermoid, and teratoma. In 50 percent the dysraphic abnormalities are associated with an overlying cutaneous lesion, such as a hairy patch, pigmentation, vascular malformation, dermal sinus, subcutaneous lipoma, or obvious meningocele sac (spinal bifida cystica). Combinations of these lesions are the rule. Almost always, the dysraphic syndromes present during infancy or childhood. It is important to realize

that the degree of neural derangement does not always correlate with the degree of the vertebral segmental abnormality.

Spina Bifida Occulta

Spina bifida occulta is a posterior defect in the fusion of the lamina but without cutaneous abnormality or meningeal protrusion through the defect. It occurs most commonly at the L5 or S1 level. With spinal bifida

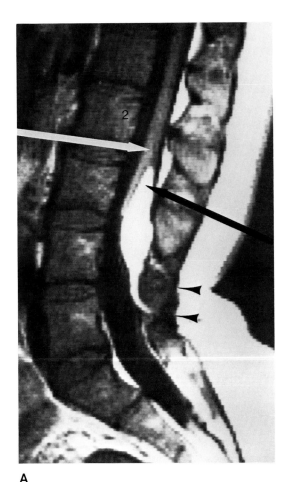

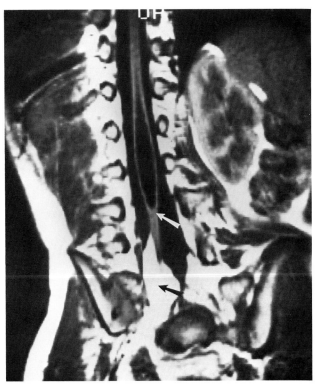

A B

Fig. 13-77 Spinal dysraphism: tethered cord, lipoma. (A) Parasagittal T_1-weighted MRI shows a low conus medullaris due to tethering (white arrow). A lipoma is present and extends into the conus medullaris (black arrow). Dysraphism is present is the lower lumbar region (arrowheads), and the lipoma tracks posteriorly through the defect. The spinal canal is widened. **(B)** Coronal MRI in another patient shows the low conus medullaris and tethering with syringomyelia of the lower spinal cord (white arrow). A large lipoma fills the lower sacral canal (black arrow). The pedicles are widely separated from the dysraphism.

occulta the posterior arches are closely approximated with cortical margins on the adjacent lamina. There may be overlap and peculiar configurations. Spina bifida occulta is usually of no clinical significance.

Tethered Cord

Tethering of the conus medullaris is the most common of the dysraphic syndromes. It is almost always associated with some form of spinal dysraphism. The spinal cord does not disjoin from the surrounding tissue and becomes relatively fixed and stretched, resulting in functional derangements within the conus and neuronal damage, which may become irreversible.

With tethering, the conus is almost always below the middle of L2. The causes of tethering include spinal lipoma (Fig. 13-77A), thickened filum terminale (more than 2 mm), diastematomyelia, and myelomeningocele. Syringomyelia may be present (Fig. 13-77B). These abnormalities can all be readily recognized with MRI or CT myelography.

The symptoms usually begin during infancy or early childhood but occasionally as late as adulthood. Foot deformities (especially pes cavus), scoliosis, leg weakness or numbness, muscular atrophy, and bladder dysfunction are the common problems. Surgery is directed at relieving the tethering and often prevents further progression, although rarely do the neurologic deficits improve.

Meningocele

Meningocele is herniation of the meninges outside the spinal canal through a dysraphic cleft (Fig. 13-78). If neural elements are incorporated in the herniation, it is termed *myelomeningocele*. A *lipomyelomeningocele* contains a lipoma in addition to the other elements. If the herniation is outside the dura but within the spinal canal, it is called an *intraspinal meningocele* (Fig. 13-79). Meningocele and myelomeningocele are almost always associated with the Chiari II malformation, but lipomeningocele and intraspinal meningocele are not. Meningoceles of all types are associated with diastematomyelia, hydromyelia, and scoliosis.

The various types of meningocele can be differentiated with CT myelography and MRI. With myelomeningocele, neural elements can be seen coursing from the sac. The flattened tethered cord forms a pla-

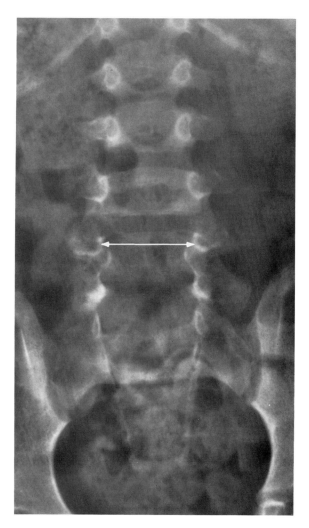

Fig. 13-78 Dysraphism. AP view of the lumbar spine shows gross enlargement of the lower lumbar spinal canal with separation of the pedicles (opposed arrows). The lamina and spinous processes are absent at the L4 and L5 levels. This abnormality was associated with a myelomeningocele.

code underneath the skin with the nerve roots exiting forward through the sac. These lesions are most common at the thoracolumbar level but may occur at a lower level.

Lipomeningoceles are rare. The lipomatous tissue, easily recognized with CT scans and MRI, is located underneath the skin sometimes separated from the placode of the myelomeningocele sac. It often infiltrates the neural elements and the intradural space. When it does, it is virtually impossible to remove.

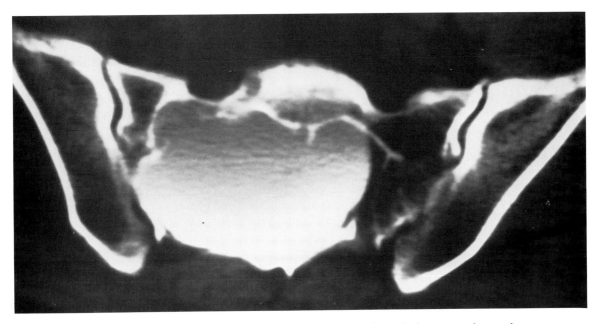

Fig. 13-79 Intraspinal meningocele. Transaxial CT myelography through the sacrum shows a large contrast-filled sac within a grossly dysraphic and expanded sacral spinal canal. The meningocele is confined to the region of the canal. There are no nerve roots within this sac.

Diastematomyelia

Diastematomyelia is a congenital splitting of the spinal cord into halves. Each half contains its corresponding anterior and posterior horn cells and the ipsilateral nerve roots. Most commonly, the separated cord is contained within one dural sac; but the sac may be split by a bone or cartilaginous spicule dividing the dura and the cord (Fig. 13-80). If a spicule is present, it almost always arises from the posterior portion of the vertebral body and crosses through the canal to a lamina. True dipolmyelia, duplication of the cord into two complete but separate structures, is rare.

The plain radiographs almost always show a spinal bifida occulta at the level. The bone of the spicule may be seen (Fig. 13-80A). The vertebral body and the local disc space are narrowed or fused and often deformed (Fig. 13-81B). The pedicles are separated but retain their normal shape. Most lesions occur at the upper lumbar level, but rarely they have been reported as high as C3 and in the sacrum. Scoliosis and other spinal deformities are usually present. Some report that the incidence of diastematomyelia in persons with congenital scoliosis may be as high as 5 percent.

The diagnosis is best made with MRI (Fig. 13-81) or CT myelography (Fig. 13-80B). The spur and the division of the cord and dural sac are easily identified. The ipsilateral nerve roots can be seen exiting from the cord. The split in the cord usually extends superiorly from the level of the spur. Without the spur, the split may extend inferiorly completely through to the conus. There may be tethering of the bifida conus (Fig. 13-81B). Rarely, multiple spurs are present.

Clinically, the lesion may have any of the cutaneous markers associated with the dysraphic syndromes. Pes cavus and other orthopedic deformities are common. The clinical symptoms are less severe in those without the spur. Surgery is directed at relieving the mechanical tension on the cord including the tethering.

Syringohydromyelia

Practically, it is impossible to distinguish syringomyelia (cystic formation within the cord not lined by ependyma and separate from the central canal) from hydromyelia (cystic enlargement of the central canal, which is lined by ependyma). Gardner proposed the term syr-

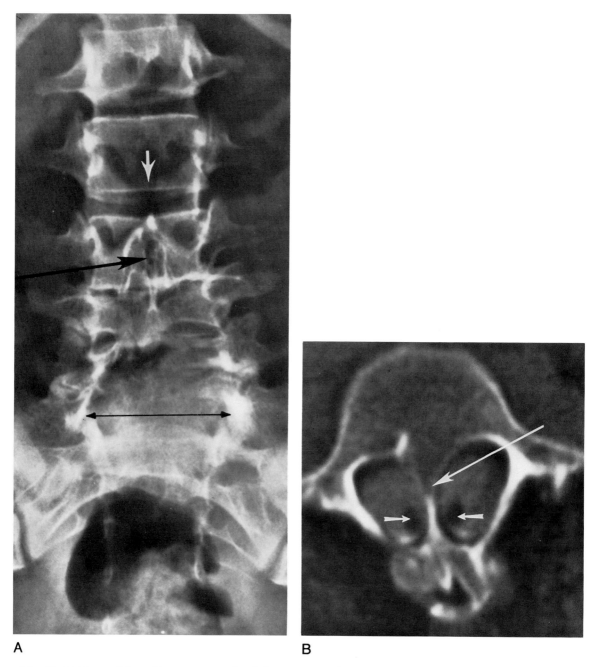

A   B

Fig. 13-80 Dysraphism, diastematomyelia. (A) A meningocele is present with a grossly widened lower lumbar and sacral canal (opposed arrows). Above it, at L3, a diastem (bone spicule) is seen coursing between the lamina and the vertebral body (black arrow). Spina bifida is present at L2 (white arrow). **(B)** Transaxial CT myelography shows the diastem dividing the spinal canal (long arrow), a tethered and divided spinal cord (small arrows), and a divided dural tube.

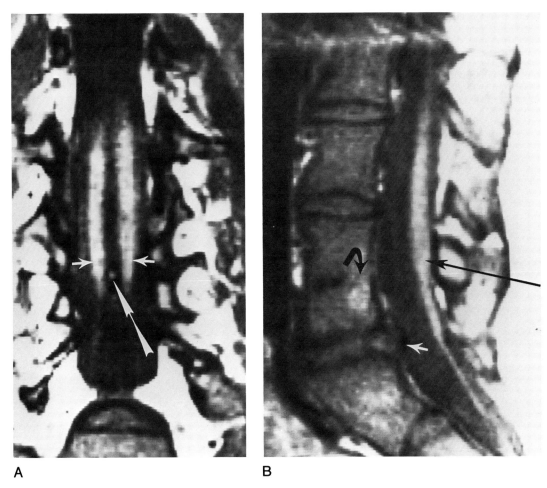

Fig. 13-81 Dysraphism, diastematomyelia. (A) Coronal MRI shows a dysraphic lower spinal canal. The tethered cord is divided in half (small arrows) by a diastem, which is difficult to recognize (long arrow). Note the small amount of marrow fat within the center of the bone spicule. **(B)** Parasagittal MRI just off the midline shows one-half of the tethered cord (long arrow). Vertebral body fusion is present at the level of the diastem (curved arrow). A moderate-size disc herniation is seen at L5-S1 (white arrow). The filum is thickened. (SE 600/15)

A   B

ingohydromyelia, which combines the two processes into one category. Post-traumatic cysts and cysts associated with tumors are still commonly termed syringomyelia in the literature.

The cystic change within the cord is most common in the cervical region but often extends inferiorly into the thoracic and rarely the lumbar region. It is unusual for the cyst to extend above C2, although syringobulbia (involvement of the pons and upper medulla) is found infrequently. In children the cyst almost always causes cord enlargement, which may be associated with widening of the spinal canal. Syringohydromyelia is most often associated with one of the dysraphic anomalies, the Chiari I malformation, craniovertebral anomalies, and congenital scoliosis. It may be seen as an isolated finding.

The superior method for diagnosis is MRI (Fig. 13-82A). The cystic cavity is seen as CSF-equivalent signal intensity within the spinal cord. The cord may be widened or collapsed (Fig. 13-82B&C), depending on patient position. Atrophy is common; and when collapsed, the cord may appear small.

With CT myelography the outline of the cord is obvious. The cyst may be seen on the initial postcon-

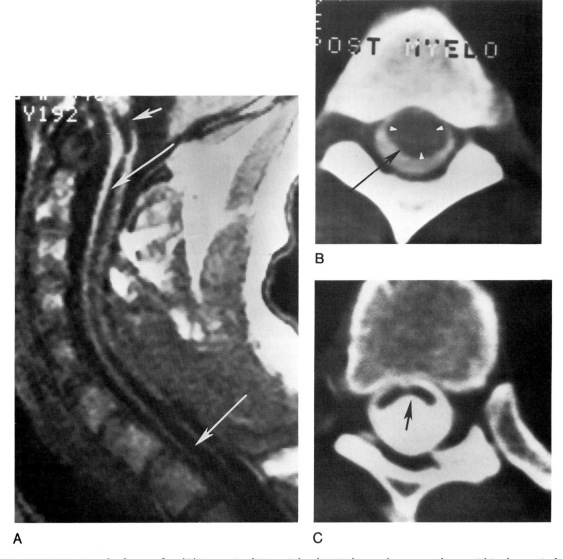

Fig. 13-82 Syringohydromyelia. (A) Parasagittal T_1-weighted MRI shows a long central cyst within the cervical spinal cord (long arrows). There appears to be an open obex (small arrow). **(B)** Transaxial CT myelography shows an enlarged cord (arrow). Faint contrast filling of the large central cyst is barely seen (arrowheads). **(C)** At a lower level, the atrophic cord is collapsed when the patient is supine (arrow).

trast examination as a low density abnormality within the cord. More likely, it is found with a 6-hour delayed examination. At this time some of the contrast agent enters the cyst cavity, either through an open obex at the inferior floor of the fourth ventricle or by diffusion through the cord parenchyma (Fig. 13-82B). The region of the foramen magnum is studied to detect a Chiari malformation.

Chiari II Malformation

The Chiari II malformation is discussed in Chapter 12 as a congenital anomaly of the brain.

Neurenteric Cyst

The neurenteric cyst is a rare lesion that results from persistence of the embryonic canal (of Kovalevsky) between the yolk sac and the notochordal canal. Usually it is found in the thoracic region. It is always associated with some form of anterior dysraphism of the vertebral body, and the sclerotic margins of the persistent canal can be seen in the frontal projection on plain films and on CT examination. There are associated duplications of the bowel. The cyst of the lesion may be anterior to the spine or within the spinal canal (Fig. 13-83) or cord. The cyst may fill with contrast from the subarachnoid space.

Arachnoidal Cyst

Arachnoidal cysts occur rarely with the dysraphic syndrome, with neurofibromatosis, or from prior meningitis. They may also occur as isolated idiopathic lesions. They are usually intradural but may extend outside the dura within the spinal canal or paravertebral tissues. They may be either communicating or noncommunicating with the subarachnoid spaces. Arachnoid cysts characteristically occur in the posterior portion of the spinal canal, often causing a complete block at myelog-

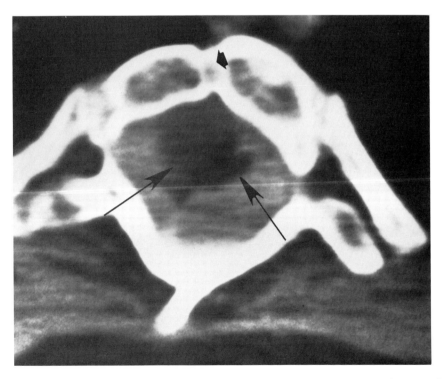

Fig. 13-83 Neurenteric cyst. Transaxial CT myelography shows a neurenteric cyst extending into the dural tube and spinal cord (arrows). The anterior canal of Kovalevsky can be seen coursing through the deformed vertebral body (small arrow).

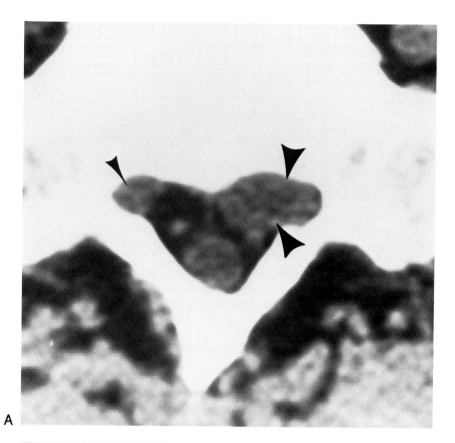

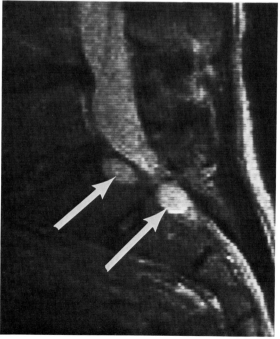

Fig. 13-84 Perineural cyst. (A) Transaxial CT scan shows a CSF-equivalent-density lesion in the left lateral recess of S1 (large arrowheads). The lateral recess is enlarged, and the left S2 nerve root is displaced posteriorly. A small cyst is present on the right (small arrowhead). **(B)** T$_2$-weighted MRI shows the high CSF-intensity signal of perineural cyst at S1 and S2 (arrows).

raphy. The lesion may be large, extending over many segments and producing widening of the canal and posterior scalloping of the vertebral bodies. Both CT scanning and MRI can usually diagnose the cystic nature of the lesion. At the caudal end of the dural sac it may be impossible to differentiate an arachnoid cyst from an intraspinal meningocele.

Perineural enlargements of the arachnoid occur frequently but are usually asymptomatic. The main problem is to differentiate a cyst from disc herniation on CT scans (Fig. 13-84). Myelography and MRI easily identify the cysts.

DEVELOPMENTAL MASS LESIONS

Almost always midline, developmental mass lesions are the result of sequestration or overgrowth of normal tissues. They are most often encountered in association with the dysraphic syndrome, although isolated tumor masses do occur.

Lipoma

Lipoma is the most prevalent form of the midline developmental mass and usually is associated with a spinal defect or myelomeningocele. It is most commonly located in the subcutaneous tissue over the spinal defect but often is seen anteriorly within the dural tube and filum terminale. However, the caudal nerves are usually simply displaced and not incorporated within the fatty mass. Occasionally, it extends superiorly within the filum into the conus medullaris (Fig. 13-77). The extent of the mass can be evaluated easily with either CT scanning or MRI.

Dermal Sinus and Dermoid

Congenital sinus tracts occur frequently at the lower end of the spine. Those that occur above the gluteal crease have a potential for entrance into the dural sac. Most true dermal sinus tracts enter the dura. They may connect with intradural dermoid cysts or extend into the conus. Those that extend inward are usually associated with demonstrable spinal dysraphism, although the defect may be subtle. The tracts need to be removed as they have the potential to cause bacterial meningitis.

Teratoma

The teratoma is a rare lesion that may occur within the dura or spinal cord. It is usually associated with regional dysraphism. The lesion may be large, extending over many levels and widening the canal. It most commonly occurs in the thoracic region. A sacrococcygeal teratoma presents as a pelvic mass and usually is not associated with the dysraphic syndrome.

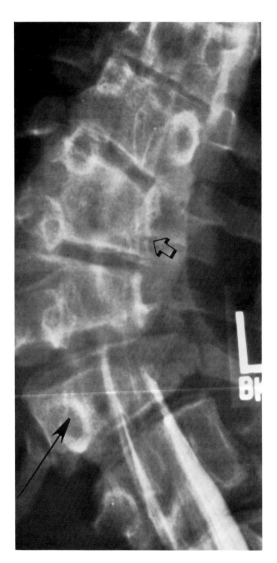

Fig. 13-85 Congenital scoliosis. Congenital scoliosis is often caused by vertebral anomalies such as hemivertebrae (black arrow) and segmental fusion (open arrow). Congenital scoliosis is often associated with other spinal anomalies affecting the cord.

SCOLIOSIS

Seventy percent of scoliosis is idiopathic, occurring primarily in adolescent girls. Most frequently, the primary thoracic curve is convex to the right extending from T4 to L1 with a secondary curve convex to the left from L1 to L5. Usually only plain film radiographs are required for evaluation, and they are obtained with the person in the erect position. The angle of the scoliosis is determined by drawing lines parallel to the end-plates of the most superior and inferior vertebral bodies of the primary curve, constructing perpendicular lines from them, and then measuring the angle at the point of intersection. Bending films may be requested to deter-

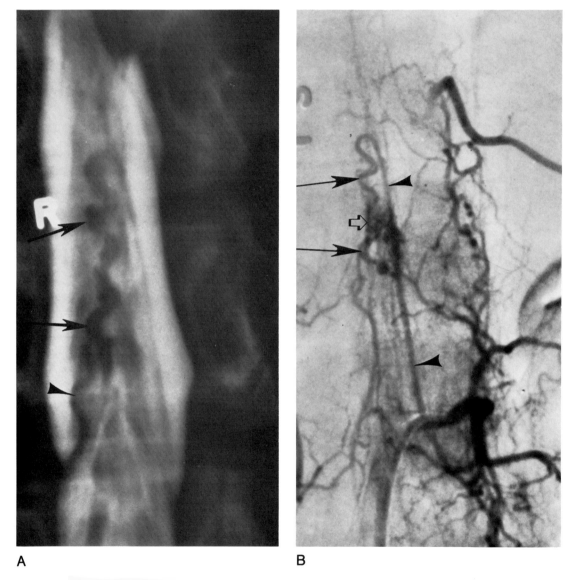

A   B

Fig. 13-86 Spinal cord AVM. (A) Myelography shows a serpiginous filling defect on the anterior surface of the conus medullaris, representing the enlarged feeding artery (arrows). A radicular feeder is seen entering from below (arrowhead). **(B)** Spinal angiography with the catheter in a left lumbar artery opacifies the large artery of Adamkiewicz (arrowheads), which fills the enlarged, serpiginous anterior spinal artery (arrows). A small tangle of abnormal vessels represents the malformation (open arrow). A smaller segmental artery enters from the right inferiorly as seen on myelography. This malformation is type 2.

mine the flexibility of the spine prior to surgical intervention.

Scoliosis can occur because of tumor, infection, hemivertebrae (Fig. 13-85), dysraphism, muscular imbalance, and postirradiation damage to the spine. Congenital spine anomalies and the early onset of scoliosis is often associated with syringohydromyelia, diastematomyelia and chiari I malformation. Scoliosis may also occur in association with neurofibromatosis. Myelography, CT myelography, or MRI scanning may be indicated for congenital scoliosis patients to detect associated lesions prior to corrective surgical manipulation.

ATROPHY

Spinal cord atrophy occurs after trauma (see Fig. 14-29), with syringomyelia (Fig. 13-82), or as a consequence of progressive spondylosis. The cord is decreased in size, and the visualized subarachnoid space is necessarily enlarged except in those with spinal stenosis. The cord tends to be smaller in the AP dimension than in the transverse dimension, as the cord is tethered bilaterally by the nonelastic dentate ligaments. The anterior median fissure is widened. The atrophy may be focal or extend over many segments, particularly when associated with syringomyelia.

ARTERIOVENOUS MALFORMATIONS OF THE SPINAL CORD

Arteriovenous malformations (AVMs) of the spinal cord are rare lesions and are most commonly encountered as unexpected findings on myelography. Rarely, they cause spinal subarachnoid hemorrhage or cord hematoma. A cutaneous hemangioma is present in 25 percent of these cases. Most occur in the thoracolumbar region.

There are three types of malformation encountered: (1) "adult type," consisting of a small, compact, serpiginous malformation often on the posterior surface of the cord and supplied by a single feeding artery; (2) a tangle of small vessels often fed by a single artery; and (3) the "juvenile type," with a large malformation fed by many arteries and found mostly in children.

The diagnosis is made with selective spinal angiography (Figs. 13-86 and 13-87). A compulsive selective study of all of the radicular arteries must be done to

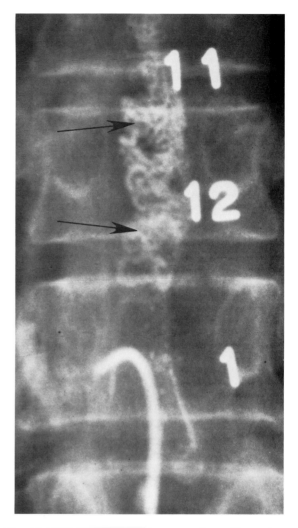

Fig. 13-87 Spinal AVM. A large vascular malformation is opacified in the lower spinal cord (arrows).

define all of the feeders of the malformation. It is important to define the AP position of the AVM within the cord. An AVM must be differentiated from a hemangioblastoma of the cord, which appears similar but tends to have tightly packed, small vessels and produces a more homogeneous tumor "blush."

SUGGESTED READINGS

Bassett LW, Gold RH, Webber MM: Radionuclide bone imaging. Radiol Clin North Am 19:675, 1981

Beres J, Pech P, Berns TF, et al: Spinal epidural lymphomas: CT features in seven patients. AJNR 7:327, 1986

Breger RK, Williams AL, Daniels DL, et al: Contrast enhancement in spinal MR imaging. AJNR 10:633, 1989

Brown BM, Schwartz RH, Frank E, Blank NK: Preoperative evaluation of cervical radiculopathy and myelopathy by surface-coil MR imaging. AJNR 9:859, 1988

Bundschuk CV, Modic MT, Ross JS, et al: Epidural fibrosis and recurrent disk herniation in the lumbar spine. AJNR 9:169, 1988

Christenson PC: The radiologic study of the normal spine: cervical, thoracic, lumbar and sacral. Radiol Clin North Am 15:133, 1977

Czervionke LF, Daniels DL, Ho PSP, et al: Cervical neural foramina: correlative anatomic and MR imaging study. Radiology 169:753, 1988

Daniels DL, Hyde JS, Kneeland JB, et al: The cervical nerves and foramina: local-coil MR imaging. AJNR 7:129, 1986

Donovan-Post MJ (ed): Computed Tomography of the Spine. Williams & Wilkins, Baltimore, 1984

Dorwart RH, Genant HK: Anatomy of the lumbar spine. Radiol Clin North Am 21:201, 1983

Dorwart RH, Vogler JB III, Helms CA: Spinal stenosis. Radiol Clin North Am 21:301, 1983

Epstein BS, Epstein JA, Jones MD: Lumbar spinal stenosis. Radiol Clin North Am 15:227, 1977: Cervical spinal stenosis. Radiol Clin North Am 15:215, 1977

Flannigan BD, Lufkin RB, McGlade, et al: MR imaging of the cervical spine: neurovascular anatomy. AJNR 8:27, 1987

Gardner WJ, Abdullah AF, McCormack LJ: The varying expressions of embryonal atresia of the fourth ventricle in adults. J. Neurosurg 14:591, 1957

Haughton VM: Disc disease, degenerative spine disease, and tight spinal canal. p. 865. In Heinz ER (ed): Neuroradiology. Churchill Livingstone, New York, 1984

Haughton VM, Williams AL: Computed Tomography of the Spine. CV Mosby, St. Louis, 1982

Heinz ER: Craniovertebral abnormalities. p. 849. In Heinz ER (ed): Neuroradiology. Churchill Livingstone, New York, 1984

Hinks RS, Quencer RM: Motion artifacts in brain and spine MR. Radiol Clin North Am 26:737, 1988

Horton JA, Latchaw RE, Gold LHA, Pang D: Embolization of intramedullary arteriovenous malformations of the spinal cord. AJNR 7:113, 1986

Hyman RA, Gorey MT: Imaging strategies for MR of the spine. Radiol Clin North Am 26:505, 1988

Jackson DE Jr, Atlas SW, Mani JR, et al: Intraspinal synovial cysts: MR imaging. Radiology 170:527, 1989

Karnaze MG, Gado MH, Sartor KJ, Hodges FJ: Comparison of MR and CT myelography in imaging the cervical and thoracic spine. AJNR 8:983, 1987

Lee SH, Coleman PE, Hahn FJ: Magnetic resonance imaging of degenerative disk disease of the spine. Radiol Clin North Am 26:949, 1988

Minami S, Sagoh T, Nishimura K, et al: Spinal arteriovenous malformation: MR imaging. Radiology 169:109, 1988

Modic MT, Masaryk T, Boumphrey F, et al: Lumbar herniated disk disease and canal stenosis: propsective evaluation by surface coil MR, CT and myelography. AJNR 7:709, 1986

Newton TH, Potts DG (eds): Computed Tomography of the Spine and Spinal Cord. Spinal Dysraphism. Vol. 1. Clavadel, San Anselmo, CA, 1983

Orrison WW, Eldevik OP, Sackett JF: Lateral C1-2 puncture for cervical myelography. III. Historical, anatomic and technical considerations. Radiology 146:401, 1983

Pagani JJ, Libshitz HI: Imaging bone metastasis. Radiol Clin North Am 20:545, 1982

Parizel PM, Balériaux D, Rodesch G, et al: Gd-DTPA-enhanced MR imaging of spinal tumors. AJNR 10:249, 1989

Penning L, Wilmink JT, van Woerden HH, Knol E: CT myelographic findings in degenerative disorders of the cervical spine: clinical significance. AJNR 7:119, 1986

Pettersson H, Harwood-Nash DCF: CT and Myelography of the Spine and Cord. Techniques, Anatomy and Pathology in Children. Springer-Verlag, Berlin, 1982

Porter BA, Shields AF, Olson DO: Magnetic resonance imaging of bone marrow disorders. Radiol Clin North Am 24:269, 1986

Raghavan N, Barkovich AJ, Edwards M, Norman D: MR imaging in the tethered spinal cord syndrome. AJNR 10:27, 1989

Robertson HJ, Smith RD. Cervical myelography: survey of modes of practice and major complications. Radiology 174:79, 1990

Ross JS, Delamarter R, Huestle MG, et al: Gadolinium-DTPA-enhanced MR imaging of the postoperative lumbar spine: time course and mechanism of enhancement. AJNR 10:37, 1989

Ross JS, Masaryk TJ, Modic MT: MR imaging of lumbar arachnoiditis. AJNR 8:885, 1987

Sage MR: Techniques in imaging of the spine. Part I. Plain-film radiology. p. 777. In Heinz ER (ed): Neuroradiology. Churchill Livingstone, New York, 1984

Smoker WRK, Godersky JC, Knutzon RK, et al: The role of MR imaging in evaluating metastatic spinal disease. AJNR 8:901, 1987

Teplick JG, Lassey PA, Berman A, Haskin ME: Diagnosis and evaluation of spondylolisthesis and/or spondylolysis on axial CT. AJNR 7:479, 1986

Williams AL: CT diagnosis of degenerative disc disease. Radiol Clin North Am 21:289, 1983

Yang PJ, Seeger JF, Dzioba RB, et al: High-dose IV contrast in CT scanning of the postoperative lumbar spine. AJNR 7:703, 1986

Zimmerman RA, Bilaniuk LT: Imaging of tumors of the spinal canal and cord. Radiol Clin North Am 26:965, 1988

14

Spinal Trauma

The diagnosis of spinal injury is one of the most significant tasks of the radiologist. An understanding of both the forces of injury and the structural and functional components of the spine make it possible to analyze spinal derangements. Almost all fractures and dislocations occur in specific patterns.

MECHANISM OF INJURY

According to the two-column theory of the spine of Holdsworth and colleagues, there are two gross segments of the spine: the anterior and the posterior. These segments can be thought of as two parallel supporting columns. The anterior component consists of the vertebral body, intervertebral disc, annulus fibrosis, and anterior and posterior longitudinal ligaments. The posterior component consists of the pedicles, articular masses (pillars), lamina, spinous process, and posterior ligaments (ligamentum flavum, interspinous ligament, joint capsules). The three-column theory of Denis categorizes the posterior vertebral body, annulus, and posterior longitudinal ligament as being a third significant component.

There are basic principles relating vector force to the type of injury produced. The fundamental two-column theory indicates that a flexion injury causes compression of the anterior column (vertebral body) and distraction of the posterior column (spinous process, facets). An extension injury causes distraction of the anterior column and compression of the posterior column. Axial compression causes fractures of the anterior and the posterior columns. Shear causes craniovertebral separation or fracture-dislocations at the disc space, par-

ticularly at the thoracolumbar junction. Lateral flexion causes fracture of the articular masses, and rotation results in unilateral facet joint dislocation. Because of anatomic variations, certain injuries are common to specific levels. The details of specific injuries are discussed below and are organized according to the spinal level and mechanism of the injury.

The motion of the spine occurs at the intervertebral disc and the synovial diarthrodial (free motion) facet joints. At all levels, the major stability of the spine is provided by the ligaments, particularly the ligamentum flavum and the posterior longitudinal ligament. When these ligaments are disrupted, the spine becomes unstable.

Spinal Stability

The goal of treatment for spinal injuries is to provide complete healing with preservation of normal, painless function of the spine and protection from future neurologic damage. When planning treatment, the concept of spinal stability is employed. Injuries that are unstable need fixation with prolonged traction, casting, or surgical fusion.

Stability has a complex definition that implies (1) maintenance of normal physiologic motion and limits of motion under normal conditions and during conditions of minor trauma; (2) stability of structure, so there is no further deformation or displacement of the spine; and (3) no progressive compression of neural tissue. There is no completely satisfactory system for classification of acute injuries as stable or unstable, although White has offered a useful measurement. From cadaver studies he found that the spine becomes unstable if there is more than a 3.5-mm anterior displacement of a vertebral body or an intervertebral angulation of more than 11 degrees. When this amount of displacement occurred, there was always disruption of the major posterior ligaments. In general, if only the anterior column (vertebral body) or the posterior column (facet, lamina, and spinous process) is fractured and there is no displacement, the spine is stable. If both are fractured and there is displacement, the spine is unstable. For many injuries, however, it is difficult or impossible to determine stability.

IMAGING

Cervical Spine

Plain film radiography demonstrates most injuries and so remains the primary and essential imaging study. CT scanning is of use for certain fractures and can be used to image levels that are not well examined with plain films. It is especially good for defining retropulsion of fragments into the spinal canal and for detecting fractures of the posterior arch. MRI is sometimes useful for examining the acute injury with incomplete spinal cord injury and for detecting late complications. With CT scanning available, plain tomography has little advantage except for horizontally oriented fractures, particularly of the odontoid process.

The lateral projection plain film radiograph is the most important in the evaluation of cervical spine injury. About 70 percent of fractures are recognized on this view; and except for the Jefferson fracture of the atlas, it demonstrates all of the important unstable fractures. When severe trauma has occurred to the cervical spine, this initial lateral view is obtained with a horizontal beam and the patient supine. Most significant injuries show some displacement on this view. However, it is a "relocating" position for cervical displacements, and the alignment of the spine may appear normal even in the presence of significant unstable spinal injury. If the supine study is normal, additional lateral radiographs are obtained with controlled flexion-extension views to detect previously occult displacements.

Because a large number of injuries occur at the C7 level, it is essential that this level be examined. An oblique, "swimmer's" projection or CT scans of this level can be obtained if the lateral film is inadequate.

In the neutral position, the anterior and posterior borders of the vertebral bodies, as well as the anterior margin of the posterior vertebral arch, form a gentle C curve, with slight lordosis (Fig. 14-1). Except at the C1-C2 level, there is equal space between the posterior spinous processes. The margins of the facet joints are aligned (Fig. 14-2). Any sudden change in angulation, displacement, or apposition suggests an injury. An exception is at the C7 level, where the superior facet is long and the posterior margin of the inferior facet of C6 does not align with the posterior margin of the superior facet of C7. A groove is frequently present on the superior facet of C7 (Fig. 14-1A).

There are predictable normal displacements (less than complete dislocations) with motion of the cervical spine. With flexion, the spinous processes separate nearly equally, with somewhat larger separation of the C1-C2 interspinous space. The posterior borders of the vertebral bodies define a smooth anterior curve, about uniform in children but maximal in the lower regions in adults. As a consequence of the forward sliding of the vertebral bodies, small steps are formed at each level (Fig. 14-1C).

Pseudosubluxation is the term generally applied to the hypermobility of the C2-C3 level and, to a somewhat lesser extent, to the C3-C4 level in infants and children. The anterior displacement is attributed to laxity of the ligaments. The physiologic displacement may be difficult to differentiate from pathologic displacement associated with flexion sprain. The posterior cervical line is helpful. This line is drawn from the anterior margin of the posterior arch of C1 to the anterior margin of the posterior arch of C3. The anterior margin of the posterior arch of C2 does not normally extend more than 2 mm in front of this line. If the posterior arch moves forward more than this, flexion sprain may be diagnosed.

With extension, reverse motion occurs. The spinous processes are closely apposed, and there is an accentuation of the cervical lordosis. Slight posterior steps result, again defining a gentle curve (Fig. 14-1A).

Cervical spondylosis affects the alignment of the spine. With degenerative narrowing of the disc space, a slight retrolisthesis may result. With arthrosis of the intervertebral facets, a slight anterolisthesis may result from laxity of the articular ligaments.

The relation of the anterior arch of C1 and the dens (the atlantodental interval) is evaluated on the lateral projection. In the neutral and extension positions, the

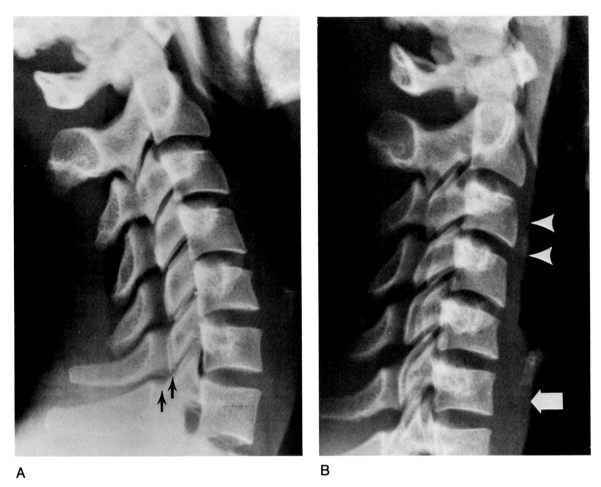

Fig. 14-1 Normal flexion-extension of the cervical spine. (A) Extension view. There is slight posterior overlap of the facet joints with extension. Note the normal anterior offset of the C6 facet with relation to C7 (black arrows). **(B)** Normal neutral position. There is slight anterior displacement of the middle vertebral bodies secondary to the effects of gravity. Note the normal retropharyngeal space (white arrowheads) and retrotracheal space (white arrow). *(Figure continues.)*

interval is small, on the order of 1 mm. With flexion the interval may widen, but it should not exceed 3 mm in the adult or 5 mm in young children. If these dimensions are exceeded, C1-C2 instability may be diagnosed.

The lateral projection also provides a good view of the anterior cervical soft tissues (Fig. 14-1B). With many types of cervical injury there is an associated prevertebral hematoma. It causes a mass effect that can be seen as increased thickness to the prevertebral retropharyngeal or retrotracheal spaces. There may be anterior displacement of the prevertebral "fat stripe." The

hematoma may be large or small. It may be the only finding with occult fractures of the upper cervical spine, especially hyperextension injuries, but significant cervical spine injury frequently occurs without soft tissue hematoma or edema. The normal prevertebral soft tissue measurements are given in Table 14-1.

On the AP projection the posterior spinous processes are normally midline. Rotational injury results in displacement of the spinous processes away from the direction of the rotation. Other findings may include widening of a vertebral body, which indicates burst fracture, displacements from shear, and fractures of the

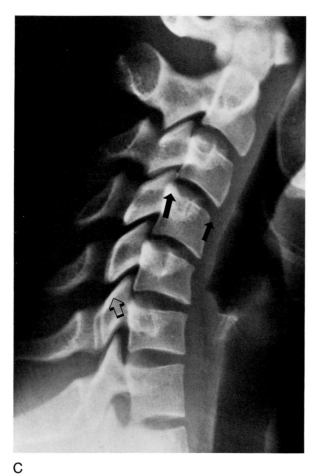

C

Fig. 14-1 *(Continued)* **(C)** Normal flexion view. There is stepwise anterior displacement of the vertebral bodies (black arrows). Separation may also occur at the posterior facet joints (open arrow).

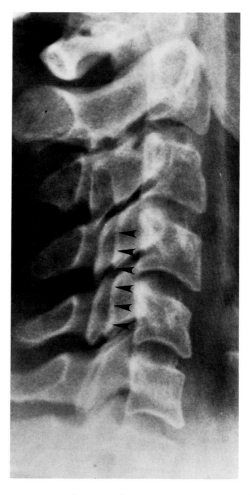

Fig. 14-2 Normal cervical spine. Note alignment of the posterior margins of both columns of pillars (arrowheads), which is best seen on this slightly oblique view.

pillars. The space of the uncovertebral joints are normally small and uniform throughout. With rotational injuries, there may be separation of the joints.

The pillar projection better defines the articular pillars. The central ray is angled about 45 degrees caudad

Table 14-1 Cervical Prevertebral Soft Tissue Measurements

Site	Average (mm)	Range (mm)
Retropharyngeal space	3.5	2–7
Retrotracheal space		
Children	7.9	5–14
Adults	14	5–22

(Modified from Gehweiler et al., 1980, with permission.)

with the head turned away from the side of interest. This view demonstrates compression fractures of the pillar, which are most common at the C6 level.

The AP "open mouth" view of the C1 level is part of the complete cervical spine examination and shows the axis and atlas to advantage. It is used to detect fractures of the atlas (Jefferson type) and dens. The evaluation of this view is often difficult, mainly because of the numerous variations in the relation of the atlas and axis with head position. Fracture of the ring of the atlas results in lateral offset of the lateral masses of the atlas on both sides. Whenever there is doubt about a fracture of the atlas, a CT scan is performed.

There are normally two ossification centers for the

odontoid and occasionally an accessory ossification center at the tip. Fusion of the dens at the subdental synchondrosis occurs at about 5 to 7 years of age. This fused synchondrosis may be visualized for many years as a condensation of bone along the fusion line at the base of the dens. It must not be confused with a compression fracture. Frequently the dens does not completely fuse with the axis, leaving an open horizontal synchondrosis at the base. This lucent line has slightly sclerotic borders. The dens may have a split in its superior portion from nonfused ossification centers. A vertical nonfused synchondrosis may also occur in the anterior arch of the atlas.

The right and left oblique views are performed with the body turned 45 degrees, which visualizes the intervertebral foramina on the side opposite to the direction of turning and is best for visualizing rotational injuries. If there is rotational injury, the superior pillar at the level of the injury is anteriorly displaced into the upper portion of the intervertebral foramen and the facets do not align. The offset of the uncovertebral joints can also be seen in this projection. A list of the significant signs of cervical spinal trauma is given in the box.

Thoracic and Lumbar Spine

Injuries in the thoracic and lumbar spine are less common, and there are fewer injury patterns. Lateral and AP views suffice for detection in most cases. The same principles discussed above apply to these regions. CT scanning is useful for defining the full extent of the injury and the presence of fragments within the spinal canal.

HYPERFLEXION INJURIES

Complete Bilateral Facet Joint Dislocation

Complete bilateral facet joint dislocation is the most common type of hyperflexion injury and accounts for about 13 percent of all cervical spine injuries. It occurs most often at the C5-C6 and C6-C7 levels and results from severe hyperflexion. The injury is due to falls (particularly down stairs), automobile accidents, and contact sports.

The force is directed from below at the occipital region of the skull. From this strong upward and forward force, there is complete disruption of all of the posterior ligaments, the annulus of the disc space, and usually the anterior longitudinal ligament. Such injury allows the facet joints to dislocate completely, with the pillars above becoming locked anteriorly to the pillars below. Occasionally, the dislocation of the facet joints is partial, with the posterior tip of the superior pillar just in contact with the anterosuperior aspect of the inferior pillar.

The dislocation is best seen on the lateral radiograph (Fig. 14-3). There is anterior displacement of the vertebral body by 50 percent or more, overriding and locking of the pillars into the intervertebral foramina, and widening of the interspinous distance. Other minor fractures may occur of the vertebral body or pillars.

SIGNIFICANT SIGNS OF CERVICAL TRAUMA

Retropharyngeal and retrotracheal hematoma
Abnormal vertebral alignment
    Acute kyphotic angulation
    Widened interspinous space
    Rotation of a segment
    Displacement of a vertebral body
Abnormal joints
    Widened atlanto-dental interval
    Widened or narrowed intervertebral disc
    Widened facet joint
    Widened uncovertebral joint
    Widened or displaced atlantoaxial joint
Fractures
    Vertebral body
        Avulsions from anterior vertebra body
        Compression of the vertebral body
        Linear fracture, vertical or horizontal
    Vertebral arch
        Pillar
        Spinous process
        Lamina, horizontal or vertical
        Pedicle
        Transverse process

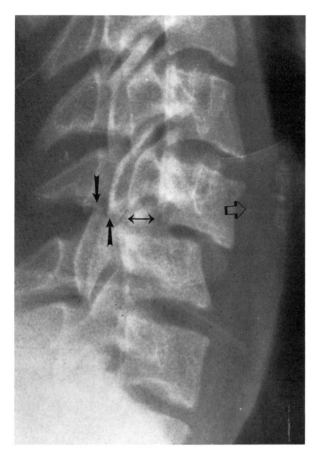

Fig. 14-3 Hyperflexion dislocation (bilateral "locked facets"). There is 50 percent anterior displacement of C4 on C5 (horizontal connected arrows). The articulating pillars are totaly displaced and locked (opposing black arrows). Note the prevertebral hematoma (open arrow).

Significant neurologic injury is common. The injury is unstable and requires reduction and fixation.

Hyperflexion Sprain (Subluxation)

Hyperflexion sprain is a much less severe form of the hyperflexion dislocation described above. The force of injury is much less, resulting in partial injury to the posterior ligament complex. The anterior displacement stops short of complete dislocation, and the spine reduces to nearly its normal alignment.

The horizontal beam lateral radiograph may be normal, and the injury may become apparent only on the flexion or upright lateral view. Extension realigns the spine. Usually, there is only slight separation of the posterior facet joints, the posterior intervertebral disc, and the interspinous distance at the level of injury. An associated avulsion fracture of the posterior arch or compression of a vertebral body sometimes occurs (Fig. 14-4). Neurologic damage is rare.

The posterior ligament complex is always weakened or disrupted with this injury. However, the severity of the injury can be estimated only by the displacement with flexion. The posterior ligaments heal poorly, and up to 50 percent show delayed evidence of instability with increased anterior displacement at the level of injury. Follow-up radiographs are performed 3 months after the injury.

It may be difficult, if not impossible, to distinguish "hypermobility" from slight sprain. Subtle compression of a vertebral body or avulsion of the posterior arch is sought, as it may be the only firm indication of injury. Clinical correlation and follow-up films are necessary in this situation.

Spinous Process Fracture

About 15 percent of persons with cervical spine injury have a fracture of the spinous process (Fig. 14-4). Most of these injuries occur as part of a fracture complex. Only 2 percent have an isolated spinous process fracture (clay-shoveler's fracture).

It occurs predominantly at C6-T1 near the base of the spinous process and results from hyperflexion and the pull of the trapezius and rhomboid muscles and the nonelastic interspinous ligament. Small avulsion fractures may occur at the posterior tip of the process, resulting from the attachment of the ligamentum nuchae being torn out. There is a high association with occult hyperflexion sprain. An isolated spinous process fracture is stable.

Hyperflexion-Rotation Injury (Unilateral Facet Dislocation)

Unilateral dislocation of a facet joint is the characteristic injury of simultaneously occurring hyperflexion and rotation forces. It often results in the unilateral "locked facet." This injury accounts for about 4 percent of all cervical spine injuries and is most common at the C4-C7 levels (Fig. 14-5).

The superior vertebral body at the level of injury rotates around a pillar, causing the opposite superior

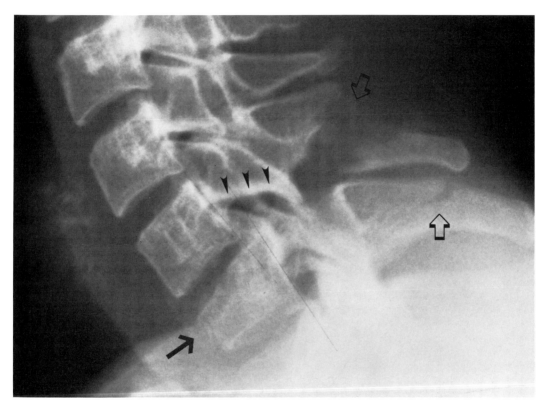

Fig. 14-4 Hyperflexion sprain and spinous process fracture. There is anterior displacement of C6 on C7 with separation of the facet joints (arrowheads) indicating sprain. Fractures are seen through the spinous processes (open arrows). There is also compression of the C7 vertebral body (black arrow).

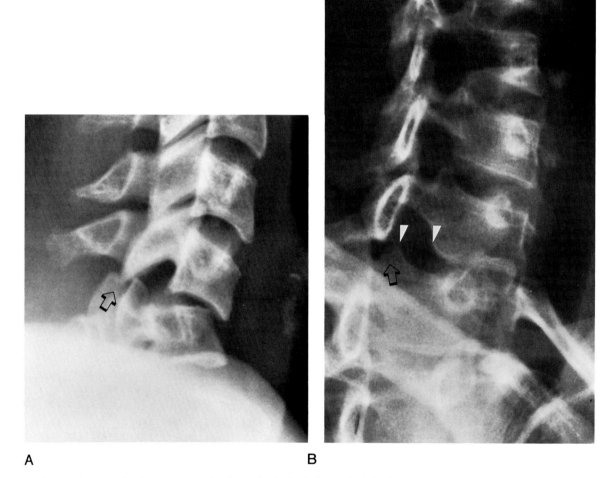

A　　　　　　　　　　　　　　　B

Fig. 14-5 Hyperflexion rotation (unilateral "locked facets"). (A) The lateral projection shows the unilateral facet locking (arrow) with less than 50 percent anterior offset of the displaced segment. There is widening of the interspinous space posteriorly. **(B)** Oblique view shows rotational displacement of the superior articular pillar into the intervertebral foramen (open arrow). Note the wide separation of the uncovertebral joint (arrowheads).

HYPERFLEXION-ROTATION, UNILATERAL "LOCKED FACETS"

Anterior displacement of superior vertebral body, <50% width

Rotation of vertebral body

Articular pillar rotated to move into intervertebral foramen

Unilateral widening of uncovertebral joint

Displacement of spinous process toward side of facet joint dislocation.

pillar to dislocate forward over the inferior pillar, finally coming to lie in the intervertebral foramen. Usually the pillar becomes locked in this forward position. The superior tip of the inferior pillar may be fractured. The capsules of the facet joints on both sides are torn, and the interspinous ligament is always ruptured. However, the posterior longitudinal ligament and the annulus of the disc space are variably injured and may remain intact. Laminar fracture is rare.

Multiple radiographic views are necessary to define the injury. The oblique projection is the best for showing the dislocated facet, and the AP projection is the best for showing the rotational component of the injury.

When the dislocated pillar is in the "locked" position, the injury is stable, and there may be difficulty reducing the spine to its normal alignment. Once the dislocation has been reduced, the spine is usually unstable and needs fixation for proper healing. Dislocations that are more than 4 months old are considered to be stable. No attempt at reduction is made at this point, as it might result in new neurologic injury. Almost all of the neurologic injuries involve a nerve root or the brachial plexus.

On the lateral radiograph the hyperflexion unilateral "locked facet" injury often cannot be differentiated from the hyperextension-compression fracture-dislocation. The two injuries can be differentiated by demonstration of more severe pillar and posterior arch fractures that occur with the hyperextension compression injury. CT scanning is useful for identifying these fractures.

HYPERFLEXION-COMPRESSION INJURIES

"Teardrop" Hyperflexion Fracture-Dislocation

The teardrop hyperflexion fracture dislocation injury occurs less often than hyperflexion dislocation, accounting for about 5 percent of cervical injuries. Almost all of the fractures occur at the C5 level. The injury is the worst result of a severe compressive hyperflexion force. Lesser force results in only wedge compression of the vertebral body or wedge fracture with hyperflexion sprain (Fig. 14-4).

The combination of hyperflexion and compressive forces results in the compressive vector being moved in an arc. The compression force begins with a straight downward vector but converts to a backward directed

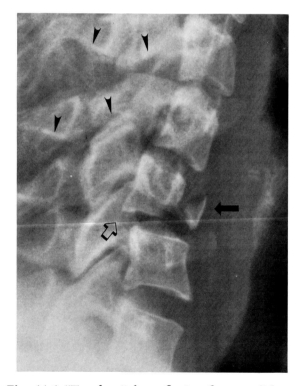

Fig. 14-6 "Teardrop" hyperflexion fracture-dislocation. The anterior avulsed fracture can be seen with its typical rotation (black arrow). There is retropulsion of the vertebral segment into the spinal canal (open arrow). Injuries have also occurred at more superior levels with widened interspinous spaces and facet joint displacement (arrowheads).

vector, which causes the fractured vertebral body to be rotated downward and backward. The resistance of the vertebral body below produces the avulsion "teardrop" fracture.

The avulsed fragment is displaced and rotated anteriorly (Fig. 14-6). The fractured vertebral body is shoved backward into the spinal canal, producing a kyphotic angulation. The interspinous distance is widened because of the disruptive forces applied to the posterior column. The disc space, the posterior longitudinal ligament, and the posterior ligament complex are disrupted, rendering the spine unstable. Frequently there are fractures of the pedicles or lamina. Additional posterior injuries may occur at other levels.

This fracture complex is particularly common after a diving injury but also results from falls and automobile accidents. The injury is best demonstrated on the lateral radiograph. Neurologic damage is frequent and correlates with the degree of retropulsion of the vertebral body into the spinal canal. This hyperflexion compression injury is distinguished from the hyperextension fracture-dislocation and the compression "burst" fractures discussed below.

Simple Wedge Compression Fracture

The isolated simple wedge compression fracture is the simplest type of hyperflexion-compression injury. It results from the effect of a relatively mild compressive force acting along the anterior aspect of the vertebral column. The fracture almost always occurs at the C5 or C6 level and may be seen at both levels simultaneously. Although there is a hyperflexion component to the forces applied, usually the force is slight so the posterior ligament complex stretches but does not rupture. However, with stronger force, the fracture may be associated with hyperflexion sprain. Occasionally, there is an associated arch fracture (lamina, spinous process, pedicle, or transverse process) from the pull of the intact ligaments. When it occurs as an isolated injury, it is stable and is almost never associated with significant neurologic damage.

The injury is best demonstrated on the lateral radiograph and is identified as a loss of the height of the anterior portion of the vertebral body. Care must be taken to differentiate the injury from the normally occurring slight decrease in vertical height of the anterior portions of C5 and C6. Such differentiation may be impossible in the case of minor fractures, and the clinical setting determines the likelihood of fracture.

The compression wedge fracture is most frequently associated with other injuries of the cervical spine, particularly hyperflexion sprain and unilateral or bilateral locking facet (Fig. 14-4). Therefore whenever a wedge fracture is identified, a flexion view and a CT scan are obtained to determine the presence of occult posterior injury. Follow-up radiographs are repeated in 3 months to detect delayed instability from further collapse or associated sprain.

Avulsion Fracture of the Vertebral Body

With slightly greater compressive force, an avulsion of the anterosuperior aspect of a vertebral body may occur (Fig. 14-7). It must be differentiated from the avulsion from the anteroinferior aspect of the vertebral body that generally occurs with hyperextension and may indicate severe occult disruption (see next section).

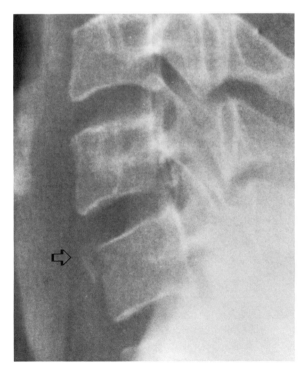

Fig. 14-7 Avulsion fracture of the vertebral body. This fracture of the anterosuperior aspect of the vertebral body is due to hyperflexion with mild compression (arrow).

HYPEREXTENSION-DISRUPTION INJURY

Accounting for about 2 percent of all spine injuries, the hyperextension sprain is infamous for its lack of radiologic findings in association with severe spinal cord injury. The injury, which may occur at any level, is the result of a hyperextension-disruptive force applied to the forehead, face, jaw, or throat. The upward and backward force compresses the spinous processes and the articular pillars so they act as a fulcrum around which the anterior portion of the vertebral bodies rotate. This condition causes rupture of the anterior longitudinal ligament and the intervertebral disc, which is either bisected or torn from the inferior end-plate of the vertebral body above. From the anteroinferior aspect of this vertebral body, a small bone fragment may be avulsed by the annulus. Importantly, aside from prevertebral soft tissue swelling, this fragment may provide the only clue of the significant occult injury.

The high incidence of severe neurologic damage results from the nature of the spinal disruption. The vertebral bodies above the level of the disruption dislocate posteriorly, pinching the spinal cord on the fixed upper margin of the lamina below. Minor injuries cause posterior cord syndromes, with loss of position sense and motor weakness, but complete cord injury is more common. This injury is a momentary dislocation, and the cervical spine reduces to its normal anatomic position, which accounts for the normal radiographic findings in the presence of severe neurologic dysfunction. The injury is unstable to extension motion.

HYPEREXTENSION-DISRUPTION INJURY

Severe cord injury with little radiographic abnormality

Prominent prevertebral swelling

Small avulsion "chips" from the anteroinferior margin of vertebral body

Gas phenomenon of a disc space

Widening of the injured disc space (may be subtle)

The diagnosis may have to be made by assumption, in the characteristic clinical setting. The injury almost always occurs in persons over 50 years old. It is considered to be a result of the greater susceptibility of degenerated discs to the forces of disruption.

Presented with a person who has spinal cord injury and a normal spine radiograph, it is imperative that there be no extension of the neck. Because of the "pincer effect," small posterior movements of the neck may cause significant neurologic damage. It is especially true if the person is somnolent or if tracheal intubation is attempted. Never attempt a deliberate extension or "hanging" head radiography in an attempt to prove the diagnosis. MRI may diagnose this condition by demonstration of cord injury, prevertebral hematoma and disruption of the anterior longitudinal ligament.

HYPEREXTENSION-COMPRESSION INJURY

Hyperextension-Compression Fracture-Dislocation

Hyperextension-compression fracture-dislocation is a common injury complex in the cervical spine, accounting for about 10 percent of cervical spine injuries. It occurs at the C4 through C7 level. The injury is thought to be a result of both hyperextension and compression forces moving the head in a posterior arc. At first, the downward compression force is applied to the posterior arch, causing variable fractures of the pillars, lamina, spinous process, and pedicles. Once they have fractured, the vertebral body is free to move anteriorly because of the combined forces acting through the arc, causing rupture of the disc space below.

Usually, only one articular pillar is fractured owing to a rotational component to the force. The pillar is comminuted and is characteristically rotated into the horizontal plane (Figs. 14-8 and 14-9), allowing the facet joint to be visualized on the AP projection. The horizontal position can also be recognized on the lateral and oblique projections. Varying degrees of comminution of the arch occurs. Bone fragments may be displaced into an intervertebral foramen. The injuries may occur at two contiguous levels (Fig. 14-10). Multiple projections are needed for accurate diagnosis. Most of the injuries occur as a result of automobile accidents.

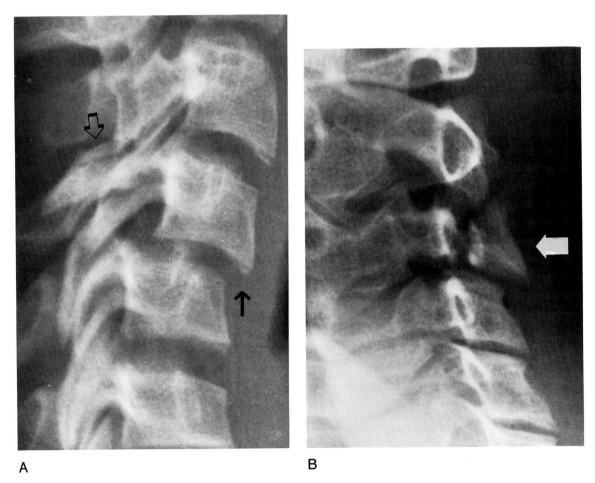

Fig. 14-8 Hyperextension compression fracture-dislocation. (A) Lateral radiograph shows anterior displacement of a vertebral segment (black arrow), with a fractured and horizontally rotated pillar (open arrow) **(B)** Oblique view shows fractured pillar, which is horizontally rotated and laterally displaced (arrow).

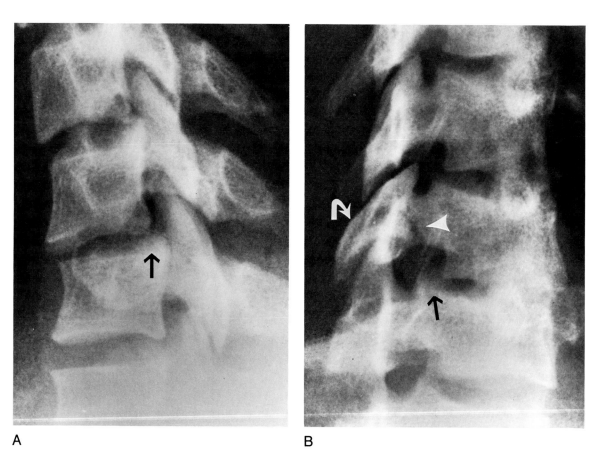

A

B

Fig. 14-9 Hyperextension compression fracture-dislocation. (A) Lateral radiograph shows subtle anterior offset of a vertebral segment (arrow). **(B)** Oblique view shows fracture through the pedicle (white arrowhead), horizontal rotation of the pillar (curved arrow), and widening of the uncovertebral joint (black arrow).

HYPEREXTENSION-COMPRESSION INJURY

Anterior Displacement of the vertebral body with rotation

Horizontal rotation of the fractured articular pillar

Anterior displacement of a pillar into the intervertebral foramen

Posterior arch fractures

Separation of uncovertebral joint

The CT scan shows the injury to good advantage (Fig. 14-11). The rotation of the vertebral body is well demonstrated with separation of the uncovertebral joints. The fractures of the pillar and posterior arch are easily seen, and any displaced bone fragments can be identified.

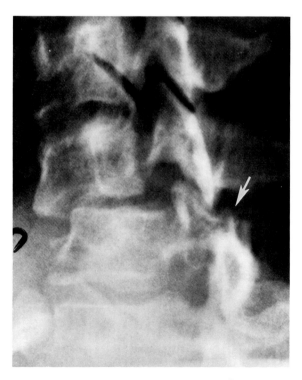

Fig. 14-10 Hyperextension compression fracture-dislocation. Sometimes it is the pillar from the nondisplaced segment that is fractured (arrow).

This fracture-dislocation is generally considered unstable because of the posterior arch fractures and the disconnection of the arch from the vertebral body. There is usually little or no neurologic injury. Treatment consists in restoration of anatomic alignment and stabilization by prolonged immobilization. Early posterior fusion is not satisfactory because of the disconnection of the vertebral body from the posterior arch.

The anterior displacement of the vertebral body suggests a flexion-rotation type of injury, with unilateral locking facets. The two injuries may appear identical on the lateral radiograph. The differentiation of the two injuries is based primarily on the presence of a pillar fracture other than simple avulsion. Hyperflexion injuries do not produce compression fractures of the pillars.

Pillar Fracture

The isolated pillar fracture results from a lesser force with more rotational component than the hyperextension fracture-dislocation discussed in the preceding section. A vertical fracture of the pillar causes retropulsion and sometimes lateral displacement of a fracture fragment, which is seen on the lateral, oblique, and pillar views. The CT scan shows the fracture well. The injury may result in radiculopathy.

VERTICAL COMPRESSION INJURY

The "burst" fracture of the vertebral body results from a pure compressive force that is applied at precisely the instant the spine is held straight. It is found exclusively in the cervical and lumbar spinal segments. The normal kyphosis of the thoracic spine converts an axially directed force into a forward rotational-compressive force, causing a wedge-type fracture. Vertical compression may cause fracture of the C1 ring (Jefferson fracture), which is discussed in a following section.

The bursting-type injury is the result of the nucleus pulposus breaking through the thin inferior end-plate of a vertebral body. This upward herniation of the nucleus into the centrum of the vertebral body causes the comminuted fracture and outward displacement ("bursting") of the fracture fragments. There is always a vertical fracture of the vertebral body (Fig. 14-12), which differentiates the burst fracture from the simple wedge fracture. The "burst" fracture may occur alone

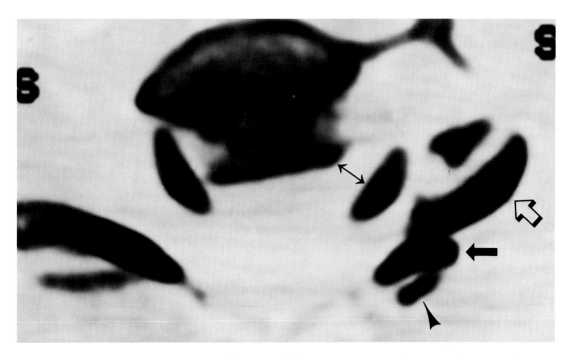

Fig. 14-11 Hyperextension compression fracture-dislocation, CT scan. The transaxial CT scan shows rotation of a vertebral body segment with widening of the uncovertebral joint (opposed arrows). The left superior pillar is fractured and rotated horizontally and anteriorly into the intervertebral foramen (open arrow). It is displaced anterior to the intact inferior pillar (solid black arrow). A fragment of the superior pillar remains posteriorly (arrowhead).

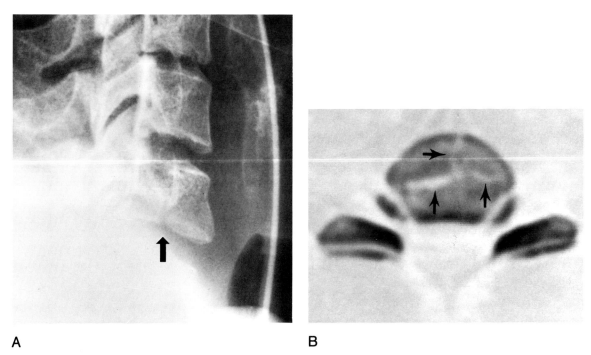

A   B

Fig. 14-12 Burst fracture. (A) Lateral cervical spine view shows vertically oriented fracture through the mid-vertebral body with subtle anterior displacement of the fracture fragment (arrow). **(B)** Transaxial CT scan shows the vertically oriented fracture lines of the burst injury (arrows).

BURST FRACTURE

Vertical fracture through the vertebral body

Widening of the margins of the vertebral body

Loss of height of vertebral body

Retropulsion of a fracture fragment

Fractures of the posterior arch

---

or as part of the hyperflexion-compression teardrop fracture dislocation. Major neurologic injury often results from retropulsion of a fracture fragment into the spinal canal. The CT scan is useful for defining all the components of the injury.

The burst compression fracture may be severe and associated with considerable disruption of the posterior arch, pillars, pedicles, and disc space. In this situation the spine is unstable and requires internal fixation. Sometimes axial traction relocates retropulsed fragments, but often surgical removal of the fragment is necessary.

CRANIOVERTEBRAL JUNCTION

The occiput, atlas, and axis together constitute the region of the craniovertebral junction. The anatomy of this region differs from the remainder of the spine. The same forces that affect the lower cervical spine cause the injury to the craniovertebral junction, but unique fractures occur as a result of the impact of the base of the skull on C1 and C2. Neurologic injury is uncommon, probably because of the wide spinal canal at this level.

Fractures and dislocations of the craniovertebral region account for 35 percent of all cervical injuries. The injuries may result from hyperextension, hyperflexion and vertical compression. Axis (C2) injuries occur about four times as frequently as atlas (C1) injuries. The two most common injuries of the axis are fracture of the dens, accounting for about 13 percent of all cervical injures, and bilateral pedicle fracture with dislocation, the hangman's fracture, accounting for about 7 percent of all cervical injuries. Because of the often subtle findings on radiographs and the infrequent association of neurologic injury, fractures and dislocation may be difficult to diagnose. Controlled flexion-extension lateral

---

FRACTURES AND DISLOCATIONS OF THE CRANIOVERTEBRAL JUNCTION

Odontoid (dens)
 Superior type I (rare)
 Transverse, type II (most common)
 Body of axis, type III
Pure atlantoaxial dislocation
 Transverse ligament rupture
Atlantoaxial rotatory dislocation
Vertebral arch fractures
 Bilateral pedicles (hangman's)
 Unilateral pedicle (unusual)
 Spinous process and lamina
Vertebral Body Avulsion
Fractures of the atlas
 Jefferson fracture
 Posterior arch fracture
 Avulsion, anteroinferior margin
 Horizontal fracture of the arch
Atlanto-occipital junction
 Craniovertebral separation
Associated injuries at lower levels

---

filming, plain film tomography, and CT scanning may be necessary. There is a high association of injuries at lower levels of the cervical spine.

Fracture of the Dens (Atlantoaxial Fracture-Dislocation)

The most common injury at the atlantoaxial level is fracture of the dens. The mechanism of the injury determines the direction of the displacement of the dens. The most common anterior displacement results from hyperflexion, with the strong transverse component of the cruciate ligament holding fast and shearing off the dens. With posterior dislocation, hyperextension causes the anterior arch of the atlas to move posteriorly, shearing the dens. Lateral displacement is rare. The displacements may be subtle, and there may simply be slight angulation with respect to the posterior margin of the body of the axis.

The fracture may be at any level in the dens. The rare type I fracture occurs near the superior tip of the dens. Type II is a transverse fracture near the base of the dens but not within the body of the axis; it heals poorly. Type III is a fracture of the foundation of the dens in the anterosuperior portion of the body of the axis (Fig. 14-13); it is more stable than the type II fracture and heals much more readily.

In the absence of any displacement, radiographic diagnosis of a fracture of the dens is often difficult. Subtle changes in alignment or minute breaks in the cortical margin of the dens or anterior axis may be all that is apparent on the plain radiographs. Tomography may be necessary to demonstrate the fracture, particularly if it is oriented in an oblique plane. Delayed to-

mography may demonstrate a fracture not seen initially. A fracture must be differentiated from (1) failure of fusion of the dens with the body of the axis at the subdental synchondrosis, and (2) Mach bands that result from the overlap of the margins of the anterior and posterior arches of C1 and the teeth. With persistent synchondrosis there are sclerotic margins to the linear defect and no instability. CT may demonstrate a type III fracture that is occult on plain films. Controlled flexion-extension views may be necessary to make the diagnosis but are avoided if possible.

Neurologic injury occurs in only a few of the patients with odontoid fracture-dislocation. Many persons with the fracture complain only of neck stiffness or pain, sometimes with an associated torticollis. Persons with odontoid fracture often seek medical attention weeks after the injury.

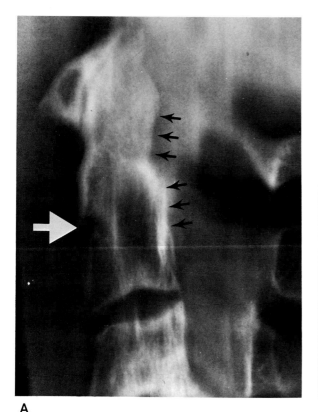

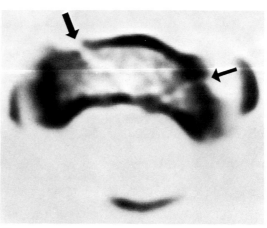

A **B**

Fig. 14-13 Odontoid fracture, type III. (A) Lateral tomography shows a cortical fracture of the anterior axis (white arrow). There is a subtle change in the alignment of the odontoid with the inferior body of the axis (black arrows). **(B)** Transaxial CT scan shows a fracture through the body of the axis (arrows).

Pure Atlantoaxial Dislocation

Pure atlantoaxial dislocation occurs infrequently. It results from a severe hyperflexion injury that causes disruption of the transverse ligament of the atlas, which normally holds the odontoid close against the anterior arch of the atlas. The factors that determine whether the ligament ruptures or the dens fractures are not known, except in the obvious cases of rheumatoid arthritis, ankylosing spondylitis, Down syndrome, infection, metastatic tumor, or other processes that weaken the ligaments.

The diagnosis is made with the lateral projection. The predental space is widened to more than 3 mm in adults and 5 mm in children under age 12. Controlled flexion views may be necessary to make the diagnosis.

The injury is unstable and requires fixation. Patients present with either upper neck pain or cord dysfunction. Cord injury is more common with this injury than with the fracture-dislocation of the dens.

Atlantoaxial Rotatory Dislocation (Fixation)

Atlantoaxial rotatory dislocation is uncommon. It results from excessive rotation of the atlas, although the degree of rotation necessary to cause fixed dislocation is variable. It is usually at least 45 degrees with respect to the transverse plane of the axis. The mechanism of the injury is not well understood.

The dislocation may occur spontaneously, after trauma, after respiratory infection, or after surgical procedures, particularly those of the head and neck region. The fixed rotation causes torticollis. However, most persons with torticollis do not have demonstrable rotatory dislocation of the atlas.

The diagnosis depends on the demonstration of abnormal motion of the atlantoaxial junction with attempted rotation, which is best seen with fluoroscopy or cineradiography. Normally, the atlas moves at least the first 20 degrees without motion of the axis or the lower cervical spine. With rotatory fixation, the abnormal relation of the atlas and the axis persists in all positions. When the transverse ligament is also disrupted, the atlas may displace forward as well as rotate, and the predental space is abnormally wide. The spinal canal may become narrowed, causing cord compression. A CT scan can also demonstrate the fixed rotatory dislocation (Fig. 14-14).

Hangman's Fracture

Sometimes referred to as traumatic spondylolisthesis of C2, the fracture-dislocation known as hangman's fracture is complex. It may result from variable forces, but hyperextension is the most common cause. The pedi-

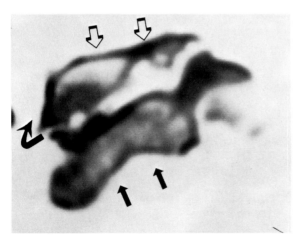

A

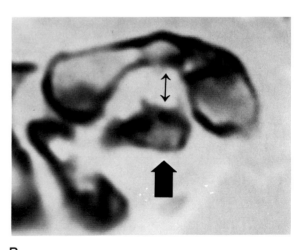

B

Fig. 14-14 Atlantoaxial rotatory dislocation, CT scans. (A) The rotated atlas (open arrows) is locked in front of the axis (black arrows). **(B)** The atlas is also displaced anteriorly with widening of the predental space (opposed arrows). The large black arrow points to the dens.

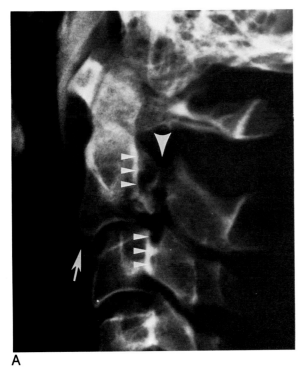

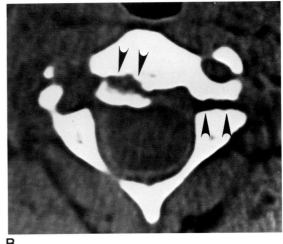

A   B

Fig. 14-15 Hangman's fracture. (A) Lateral radiograph shows fractures through the pedicles (large white arrowhead) and anterior displacement of the C2 vertebral body (small arrowheads). A small avulsion fracture is also present (arrow). **(B)** Transaxial CT scan shows fracture through the left pedicle and the base of the right pedicle within the vertebral body (arrowheads).

cles are fractured bilaterally, and there is variable anterior displacement of the vertebral body depending on the degree of disruption of the anterior ligaments and disc space. There may be dislocation of one or both of the facet joints, in which case the posterior ligaments are also disrupted and the posterior arch moves forward as well. There is usually a prevertebral hematoma. Simultaneous hyperflexion injuries are frequent in the lower cervical spine. The injury is best diagnosed with the lateral plain radiograph (Fig. 14-15).

The bilateral pedicle fracture disconnects the posterior arch from the vertebral body of the axis, making the spine unstable at this level. Neurologic injury is uncommon except with facet dislocation. Most hangman's fractures can be reduced with traction, and they heal after immobilization in a cast or brace. With facet dislocation, anterior fusion may be necessary because of the insbility of the posterior arch.

HANGMAN'S FRACTURE (C2)

Bilateral fractures of the pedicles
Anterior dislocation of the body of the axis
Anterior rotation of C2
Wedge compression of C3 (occasional)
Injuries at lower levels

Vertebral Body Fractures

An avulsion fracture from the anteroinferior margin is the most common fracture of the body of the axis (Fig. 14-15). It is thought to be the result of a hyperextension. Its main importance is its high association with other injuries of the cervical spine.

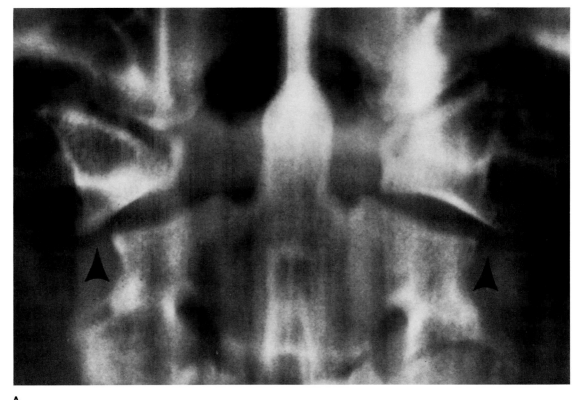

A

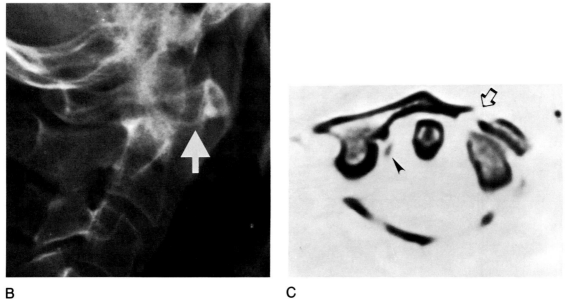

B   **C**

Fig. 14-16 Jefferson fracture of C1. (A) AP view through the mouth shows bilateral lateral offset of the lateral masses of C1 (arrowheads). **(B)** Lateral view shows widening of the predental space, indicating rupture of the transverse ligament (arrow). **(C)** Transaxial CT scan shows fracture through the left anterior ring (arrow). It is a unilateral Jefferson fracture. Note avulsion of the transverse ligament (arrowhead).

Jefferson Fracture

The classic Jefferson fracture complex consists of four fractures: two fractures on each side involving the anterior and posterior arches of C1. It is a burst fracture of the atlas that results from an axial compressive force transmitted through the occipital condyles to the lateral masses. A uniformly distributed compressive force produces symmetric fractures of the ring, allowing the ring to expand equally in all directions. Both lateral masses are displaced laterally about the same distance. It the force is strong enough, the transverse ligament is ruptured. A compressive force distributed more to one side fractures the anterior and posterior ring on that side only, producing more displacement of one lateral mass. This injury is a common variation of the Jefferson-type fracture, which is sometimes referred to as a lateral mass fracture.

The through-the-mouth AP projection is the most useful plain film examination. With the true Jefferson fracture the lateral margins of both lateral masses overhang the lateral margins of both superior articular surfaces of the axis (Fig. 14-16). When the total lateral displacement (the sum of the overhang of each lateral mass) is 9 mm or more, the transverse ligament is also ruptured. A controlled flexion view in the lateral projection may be necessary to define ligament stability. Unilateral displacement from unilateral fracture of a lateral mass may be difficult to diagnose by plain film. CT scans are diagnostic of fractures of the atlas (Fig. 14-16) and are obtained in most cases, particularly when the plain film diagnosis is uncertain.

When associated with disruption of the transverse ligament, the Jefferson fracture is unstable; otherwise it is a stable injury. Neurologic injury is infrequent. Vertebral artery damage may result from the lateral displacement. Traction may reduce the separation of the fragments. Immobilization usually results in healing.

Posterior Arch Fracture

Isolated posterior arch fracture of C1 usually occurs just posterior to the transverse process. These fractures result from hyperextension, which crushes the thin pos-

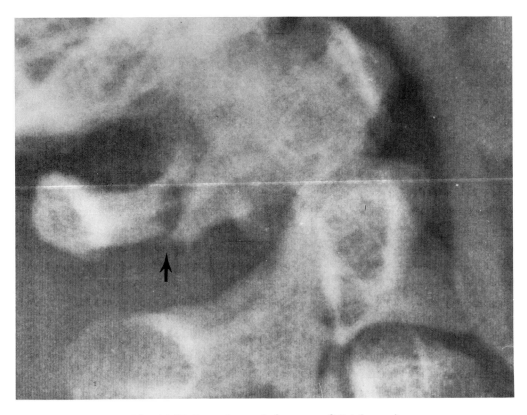

Fig. 14-17 Posterior arch fracture of C-1 (arrow).

terior ring between the occiput and the large spinous process of the axis. The fracture may be unilateral or bilateral. The diagnosis can be made with the lateral radiograph or CT scanning (Fig. 14-17).

The fracture is stable and heals well with collar immobilization. There is a frequent association with hyperextension fractures at lower levels, particularly type II fracture of the dens.

Horizontal Fracture of the Atlas

The horizontal fracture of the atlas is also produced by hyperextension and can be considered a variant of an avulsion-type fracture. The avulsion probably results from the pull of the anterior longitudinal ligament and the longus colli muscles. The fracture itself has little importance but is highly associated with other hyperextension injuries of the axis or lower cervical spine.

Atlanto-Occipital Dislocation

Separation of the cranium from the spine is a result of severe shear and is almost always immediately fatal. The medulla is usually transected. All surviving persons have neurologic damage. Almost all cases are of the anterior-type dislocation, i.e., the skull is anteriorly displaced off the spine (Fig. 14-18).

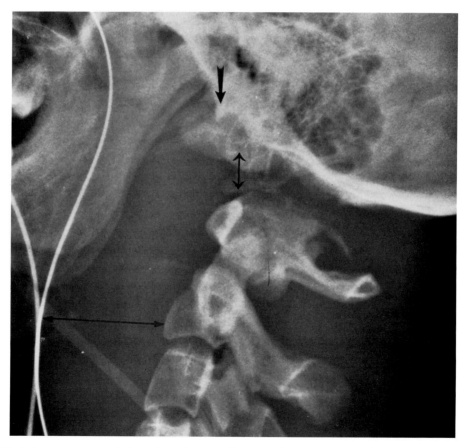

Fig. 14-18 Atlanto-occipital dislocation. Lateral radiograph shows anterior displacement of the skull with relation to the cervical spine. There is wide separation between the base of the clivus (black arrow) and the anterior arch of C1 (vertical opposed arrows). A large prevertebral hematoma is a constant finding with this injury (horizontal opposed arrows).

THORACIC AND LUMBAR SPINE INJURIES

Compression Fractures

Anterior compression fracture is the most common fracture of the thoracic and lumbar spine in all age ranges. As with all injuries of the lower spine, it occurs most frequently at the thoracolumbar junction.

The injury results from a compressive force applied with the spine held in flexion. Because the flexion motion pivots about a fulcrum that is centered at the nucleus pulposus, it is the anterior portion of the vertebral body and intervertebral disc that suffers the greatest force. The anterosuperior portion of the vertebral body is the first to fracture, usually seen as a buckling of the cortex. With increasing force, there is increasing compression of the vertebral body into a wedge shape. With severe injury, there is near-total flattening of the anterior body and anterior angulation of the spine. Any herniation of the nucleus is almost always anterior. In the lumbar spine, the large disc space allows the upper vertebral segment to slide forward, producing a shearing force on the vertebral disc. This sequence may cause avulsion of the superior end-plate of the vertebral body below (Fig. 14-19).

It may be difficult to determine the age of a vertebral compression fracture. It is generally not possible to be more specific than classifying the fracture as either "recent" or "remote." Healing takes about 3 months and results in the loss of the zone of bone condensation and smoothing of the margins of avulsions or cortical breaks.

Uncomplicated compression fractures are stable. However, hyperflexion with a disruptive force applied posteriorly may rupture the ligamentous complex, which is recognized by widening of the interspinous distance. Occasionally, there is delayed collapse of a fractured vertebral body, resulting in a significant kyphotic gibbus. Therefore follow-up radiographs are necessary 3 months after the injury.

A vertebral compression fracture must be differentiated from a pathologic fracture (see section on metastatic disease to the spine in Chapter 13). A compression fracture in persons less than 50 years old without a clear history of appropriate trauma is likely to be a pathologic fracture, and tumor may be found in as many as 50 percent of these cases. In older persons with

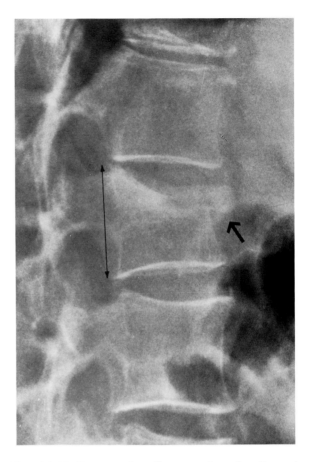

Fig. 14-19 Compression fracture. Lateral radiograph showing preservation of the posterior height of the vertebral body (opposed arrows) and anterior avulsion (arrow). The anterior vertebral body is compressed from above.

osteoporosis, compression fractures are much more commonly the result of minor trauma, and the incidence of pathologic fracture here decreases to about 20 percent.

Fracture-Dislocation

Almost all fracture-dislocations of the thoracic and lumbar spine are produced by hyperflexion force alone or with rotation, compression or shear. Because of the inherent strength of the thoracic and lumbar regions of the spine, dislocations are the result of severe forces. The fractures tend to involve multiple levels and have a high association with severe neurologic damage (Fig. 14-20).

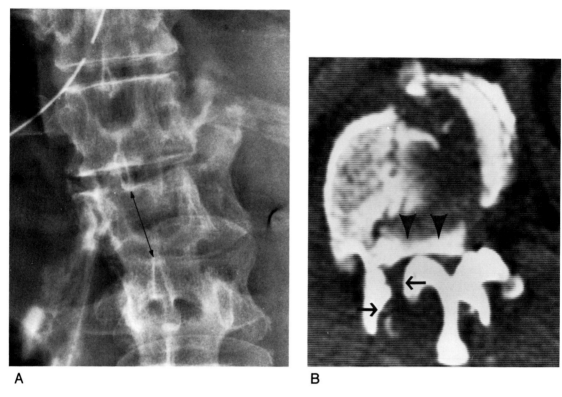

A   B

Fig. 14-20 Fracture-dislocation of T12-L1. (A) AP radiograph showing displacement with compression. There is wide separation between the spinous processes posteriorly (opposed arrows). **(B)** Transaxial CT scan shows dislocation of the facets (arrows), avulsion of the left anterolateral vertebral body, burst fracture, and retropulsion into the spinal canal (black arrowheads).

The same principles of hyperflexion injury discussed for injuries of the cervical spine apply to injuries of the lumbar spine. There is anterior compression and posterior distraction. Stability of the spine is determined by the integrity of the posterior ligament complex and the posterior longitudinal ligament (the third column of Denis). This complex is disrupted when there is widening of the interspinous distance, displacement of the vertebral body, or widening of the posterior disc space. If a rotational force is involved, there may be unilateral offset of the facets and a characteristic "slice"-type avulsion fracture of the superior end-plate of the subjacent vertebral body. A shearing force may result in fracture of the pars interarticularis.

The injury may be difficult to detect radiographically, as a supine position of the patient tends to relocate the spine into a nearly normal alignment. Subtle displacements may be the only plain film clue to the presence of a severe fracture. CT scanning defines the injuries.

"Seatbelt"-Type Injury

The seatbelt-type injury is similar to the hyperflexion injury, although the fulcrum of the flexion motion is more anteriorly positioned in the body. This situation produces more of a distractive force posteriorly and little compression of the vertebral bodies. The injury occurs not only with lap-type seatbelts but with any restraint that allows the upper body to be thrown into acute hyperflexion over the restraint. For example, the injury occurs when a person riding a snowmobile or trail bike encounters a waist-high fence wire or rail.

The spine is ripped apart by the bending disruptive force. The nature of the fracture depends on the outcome of the tension between ligaments and bone.

There may be only ligamentous rupture with intact bone, or there may be varied horizontal fractures through the posterior arch and vertebral body. Two types of fracture are common.

1. *Smith fracture.* This horizontal fracture goes through the transverse process, extends into the pedicle and pars interarticularis, and goes forward into the posterosuperior vertebral body, where a small fragment is avulsed from the posterosuperior end-plate.
2. *Slice ("Chance") fracture.* There is complete horizontal splitting of the posterior arch, extending into the superior portion of the vertebral body and often curving upward to reach the end-plate. The fracture goes posteriorly through the spinous process (Fig. 14-21).

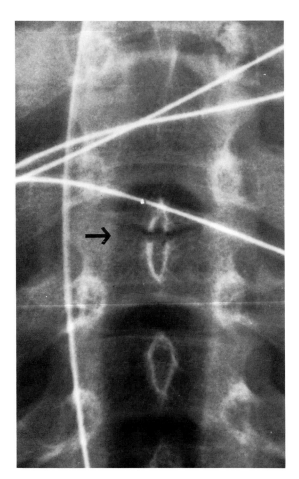

Fig. 14-21 Slice fracture. A horizontal fracture extends through the posterior arch into the spinous process (arrow).

Burst Fracture

The burst fracture is a result of axial compression. The mechanism is the same as that described for fracture of the cervical spine. There is upward forcing of disc material into the vertebral body, causing it to split. Retropulsion of the posterior fragment of the vertebral body is common and causes neurologic compression (Figs. 14-22 and 14-23). More than 25 percent compromise of the spinal canal is considered significant. Frequently, there is fracture of the posterior arch. Once thought to be a stable injury, the fracture is now considered unstable. Treatment is directed at removing fragments within the spinal canal and stabilizing the spine to avoid later collapse.

HYPEREXTENSION FRACTURE-DISLOCATION

Hyperextension fracture-dislocation is a rare injury that consists of fracture of the pars interarticularis or lamina. It causes spondylolisthesis.

INJURIES WITHOUT FRACTURE OR DISLOCATION

Injury of the spinal cord may occur without disruption of the spine. These injuries cannot be diagnosed with plain film radiography or routine CT scanning but require MRI, myelography, or CT myelography.

Nerve Root Avulsion

With injuries of the upper extremities or pelvis, avulsion of nerve roots from the cervical or sacral region may occur because of distraction of the nerve roots. The roots are pulled from their origins in the cord in the cervical region or are torn from the cauda equina in the lumbosacral region. Usually there is tearing of the nerve root sleeve from the dural sac so a pseudomeningocele is formed.

Myelography or CT myelography is the best means of making the diagnosis (Fig. 14-24). The myelographic contrast outlines the disruption of the nerve root sleeve. Sometimes the avulsion of the nerve root from the cord can be demonstrated.

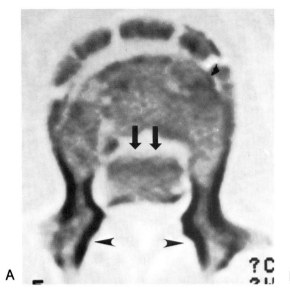

A

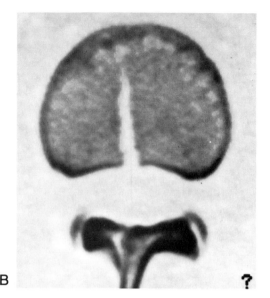

B

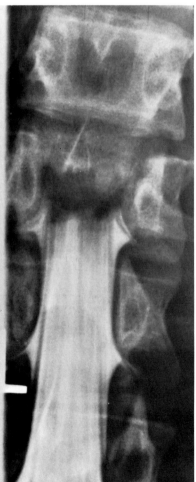

C

Fig. 14-22 Burst fracture, lumbar spine. (A) Transaxial CT scan shows typical retropulsion of a fragment into the spinal canal (arrows). Note the nonvisualization of the inferior facets from the level above, indicating facet joint dislocation (arrowheads). **(B)** Lower view of vertebral body shows the vertical burst fracture. **(C)** Myelography showing total extradural type block by the retropulsed fragment.

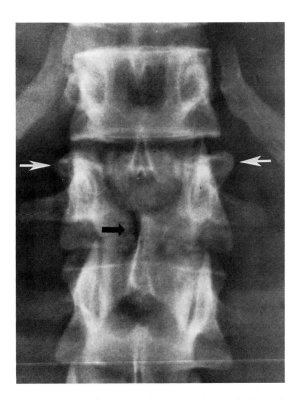

Fig. 14-23 Burst fracture of L1. AP radiograph shows loss of height and widening of the L1 vertebral body (white arrows). Fracture can be seen extending through the lamina posteriorly on the right (black arrow). These subtle changes must be recognized, as frequently this view is the only one available on the acutely traumatized patient.

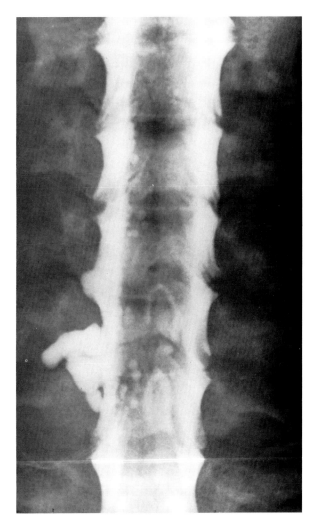

Fig. 14-24 Torn dural sac. This study followed an avulsion injury of the cervical nerve roots. A pseudomeningocele is demonstrated with a Pantopaque myelogram. (From Osborne, 1984, with permission.)

Spinal Cord Contusion

Contusion or hemorrhage may occur within the spinal cord causing a central cord syndrome (Fig. 14-25). It may occur without fracture or dislocation of the spine and is seen primarily in those with spondylosis. The hypermobility of the spine and osteophytes compress the cord, resulting in the hemorrhage or contusion. This problem is best demonstrated with MRI, which shows the signal intensity of edema or hemorrhage within a swollen cord. Myelography or CT myelography shows only the cord swelling. If spinal stenosis is present, decompression sometimes produces improvement.

MAJOR DELAYED POST-TRAUMATIC COMPLICATIONS

Delayed malalignment of an injury thought to be stable

Failure of healing with malalignment

Unrecognized displaced fracture fragment that later results in neurologic dysfunction (Fig. 14-26)

Post-traumatic syringomyelia (Fig. 14-27)

Post-traumatic arachnoiditis (Fig. 14-28)

Occlusion or pseudoaneurysm of the vertebral artery

Post-traumatic atrophy of the spinal cord (Fig. (14-29)

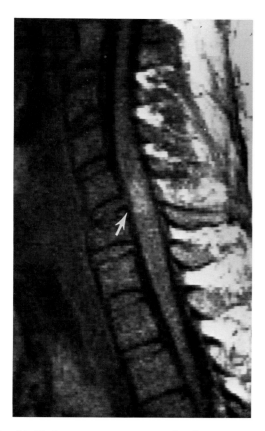

Fig. 14-25 Acute post-traumatic disc herniation with cord hemorrhage. MRI 1 week after injury shows disc herniation with increased intensity within the cord (arrow) on T_1-weighted image. The cord is swollen. (SE600/20)

Acute Post-Traumatic Disc Herniation

Acute disc herniation may result from trauma. It causes pain or neurologic dysfunction with little or no radiographic change seen. MRI is the best means of demonstrating the herniation (Fig. 14-25).

Delayed Complications of Fracture and Dislocations

Most delayed problems due to injury present with persistent or new symptoms following the injury. Focal radiculopathy suggests a change in position or a displaced bone fragment (Fig. 14-26); progressive myelopathy suggests syringomyelia (Fig. 14-27); and arachnoiditis causes pain (Fig. 14-28). Plain film radiography, CT scanning, and MRI can be used appropriately to make the diagnosis. Angiography of the vertebral artery may be necessary if vascular injury is suspected, although MRI may determine vessel occlusion or dissection.

MRI and Myelography in Acute Spinal Injury

A complete spinal cord injury is present when the patient has no neurologic function below the level of injury. There is little that can be done to help this

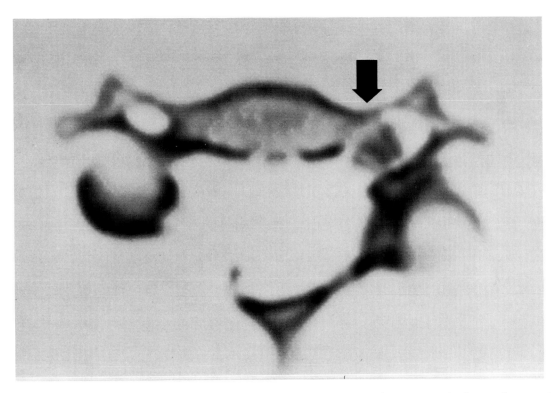

Fig. 14-26 Fragment displaced into intervertebral foramen. Transaxial CT scan easily shows a fragment in the foramen, causing radiculopathy (arrow). Such fragments can also cause vertebral artery injury.

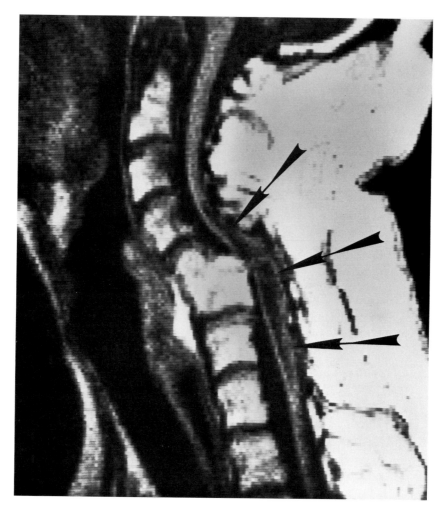

Fig. 14-27 Post-traumatic syrinx. T_1-weighted MRI shows post-traumatic syringomyelia as a region of low signal within the cord (arrows). Expansion of the cyst can lead to progressive neurologic dysfunction.

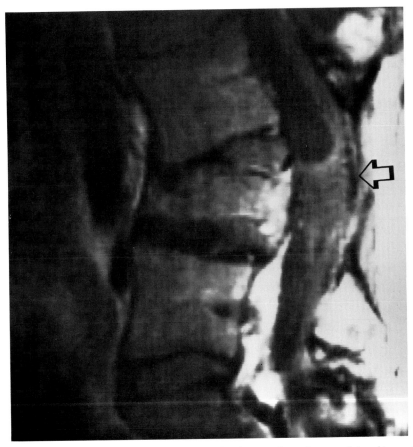

Fig. 14-28 Post-traumatic arachnoiditis. MRI T_1-weighted image shows increased signal intensity in the region normally occupied by the CSF within the dura (arrow).

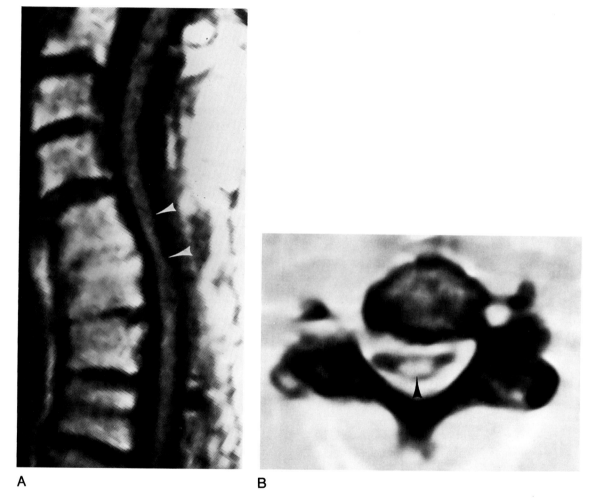

A

B

Fig. 14-29 Post-traumatic cord atrophy. (A) MRI examination shows a small cord through the region of the fracture site (arrowheads). **(B)** Transaxial CT myelography shows the small size of the cervical cord (arrowhead).

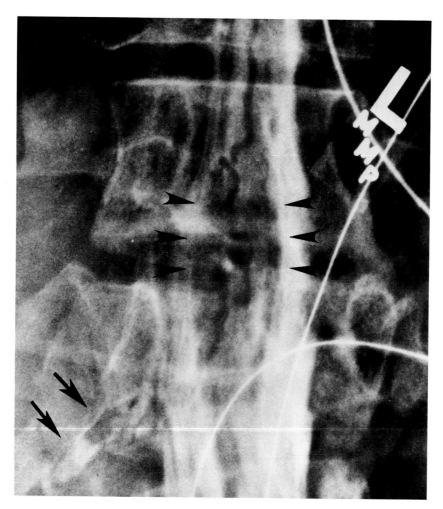

Fig. 14-30 Hematomyelia and dural tear. Myelography shows widening of the conus medullaris (arrowheads). In addition, there is extravasation of contrast from the dural tear (arrows).

situation except to prevent ascending neurologic decline by stabilizing the bone injury and providing good physiologic supportive measures. MRI and myelography are unnecessary.

With incomplete spinal cord injury, decompression and stabilization can result in neurologic improvement. MRI and myelography may be of some benefit in this group (Fig. 14-29). The primary aim is to identify mechanical cord compression caused by spinal stenosis, displaced fragments of bone, disc herniation, or epidural hematoma, i.e., extramedullary compressive lesions. Relief of the cord compression may lead to partial recovery of function and prevention of additional neurologic decline. If an intramedullary hematoma is found, there is no benefit accrued by its decompression (Fig. 14-30).

The MRI scans may provide some prognostic information after injury, as the finding of cord edema rather than hemorrhage implies a greater chance for neurologic recovery. During the acute phase (less than 7 days) MRI shows both cord edema and hemorrhage as low intensity on the T_1-weighted images, but only edema produces high signal on the T_2-weighted images. Gradient echo images also show acute hemorrhage as low signal. After 1 week, hemorrhage shows as high signal intensity on both the T_1- and T_2-weighted images (Fig. 14-25).

SUGGESTED READINGS

Atlas SW, Regenbogen V, Rogers LF, Kim KS: The radiographic characterization of burst fractures of the spine. AJNR 7:675, 1986

Cervical Spine Research Society: The Cervical Spine. 2nd Ed. JB Lippincott, Philadelphia, 1989

Denis F: Updated classification of thoracolumbar fractures. Orthop Trans 6:8, 1982.

Donovan-Post MJ: Computed tomography of spinal trauma. In Donovan-Post MJ (ed): Computed Tomography of the Spine. Williams & Wilkins, Baltimore, 1984

Donovan-Post MJ, Green BA: The use of computed tomography in spinal trauma. Radiol Clin North Am 21:327, 1983

Edeiken-Monroe B, Wagner LK, Harris JH Jr: Hyperextension dislocation as the cervical spine. AJNR 7:135, 1986

Gehweiler JA Jr, Osborne RL, Becker RF: The radiology of vertebral trauma. WB Saunders, Philadelphia, 1980

Harris JH Jr, Edeiken-Monroe B: Radiology of Acute Cervical Spine Trauma. 2nd Ed. Williams & Wilkins, Baltimore, 1987

Holdsworth FW: Fractures, dislocations and fracture-dislocations of the spine. J Bone Joint Surg [Br] 45:6, 1963

Holdsworth FW: Fractures, dislocations and fracture-dislocations of the spine. J Bone Joint Surg [AM] 52[A]:1534, 1970

Kim KS, Chen HH, Russell EJ, Rogers LF: Flexion teardrop fracture of the cervical spine: radiographic characteristics. AJNR 9:1221, 1988

Kowalski HM, Cohen WA, Cooper P, Wisoff JH: Pitfalls in the CT diagnosis of atlantoaxial rotatory subluxation. AJNR 8:697, 1987

Kulkarni MV, Bondurant FJ, Rose SL, et al: 1.5 Tesla magnetic resonance imaging of acute spinal trauma. Radiographics 8:1059, 1988

Osborne D: Spinal trauma. p. 887. In Heinz ER (ed): Neuroradiology. Churchill Livingstone, New York, 1984

Quencer RM: The injured spinal cord. Radiol Clin North Am 26:1025, 1988

White AA, Panjabi MM: Clinical biomechanics of the spine. Lippincott, Philadelphia, 1978

Index

Page numbers followed by an f indicate figures; those followed by a t indicate tables.

487